THE ENCYCLOPEDIA OF

DRUG ABUSE

Esther Gwinnell, M.D.
and
Christine Adamec

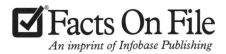

An imprint of Infobase Publishing

The Encyclopedia of Drug Abuse

Facts On File, Inc.
An imprint of Infobase Publishing
132 West 31st Street
New York NY 10001

Library of Congress Cataloging-in-Publication Data

Gwinnell, Esther.
The encyclopedia of drug abuse / by Esther Gwinnell and Christine Adamec.—1st ed.
p. ; cm.
Includes bibliographical references and index.
ISBN-13: 978-0-8160-6330-7 (alk. paper)
ISBN-10: 0-8160-6330-3 (alk. paper)
1. Substance abuse—Encyclopedias. 2. Drug abuse—Encyclopedias. I. Adamec, Christine A., 1949- II. Title.
[DNLM: 1. Substance-Related Disorders—Encyclopedias—English. 2. Pharmaceutical Preparations—Encyclopedias—English. WM 13 G994e 2008]
RC563.4.G97 2008
616.86'003—dc22   2007021439

Facts On File books are available at special discounts when purchased in bulk quantities for businesses, associations, institutions, or sales promotions. Please call our Special Sales Department in New York at (212) 967-8800 or (800) 322-8755.

You can find Facts On File on the World Wide Web at http://www.factsonfile.com

Text and cover design by Cathy Rincon
Illustrations by Sholto Ainslie

Printed in the United States of America

VB Hermitage 10 9 8 7 6 5 4 3 2

This book is printed on acid-free paper and contains 30% post-consumer recycled content.

Christine Adamec and Dr. Gwinnell wish to thank Marie Mercer, reference librarian at the DeGroodt Public Library in Palm Bay, Florida, for her expert assistance in locating hard-to-find reference materials.

CONTENTS

FOREWORD

"Every junkie is a setting sun."

—Neil Young

During the past decade, it seemed that every day brought new information about the physiology of the human brain. New brain imaging techniques, chemical markers for neurotransmitters, new medications, and new understanding of the working of those medications have expanded our knowledge exponentially.

At the same time, methamphetamine and opiate addictions have also expanded. The crisis of home-made or readily available and dangerous addictive drugs has led to workplace drug testing and attempts to maintain drug-free zones near schools or businesses. The new understanding of ways in which these addictive drugs actually change the brain has not yet produced the kind of effective treatments that are available for other diseases.

The combination of 12-step programs is still only partially effective in treating those who are addicted to street drugs and prescription drugs. The numbers are much smaller than we would hope, and every day, new addicts are created. Nonetheless, physicians, patients, and families strive to cure, to overcome, to prevent, and to resist drug addition.

New medications are becoming available to treat opiate addiction and alcoholism. Trials of medications to help with amphetamine addictions are under way, and new uses for other drugs are being explored. There is synergy between trying to find new medications and learning about the true effect on the brain of the various addictive substances. Now we have proof that opiates and other drugs actu-ally change receptor sites in the brain. The physical change in the brain promotes continued addiction in ways that were never understood before.

We are still losing people to the needle and the pipe. Generations are destroyed by drugs, as parents who are drug addicts raise their children in profoundly destructive ways, producing new generations susceptible to drug addiction who then raise their own children in homes of squalor and violence.

If knowledge has any power, I want this book to have that power to inform and instruct. Lives can be saved and addicts can recover and heal, and that can also be carried down the generations, with healthier, happier families. Workplaces are safer when workers are not under the influence of intoxicants. Patients are safer when doctors are not abusing drugs, and all of us are safer when drivers are clean and sober.

Some years ago, one of my patients died from an accidental overdose of street drugs. There were very few options for treatment at that time, and he was just not successful in overcoming a terrible addiction combined with a psychiatric illness. Now we have a half-dozen possible treatments that were not available then, and it makes me glad for the future and sad for the past. I look forward to a new edition of this book in a decade. Who knows what wonders will be yet ahead and what challenges will develop?

"As the circle of light increases, so does the circumference of darkness around it."

—Albert Einstein

—Esther Gwinnell, M.D.

PREFACE

Many people depend on prescribed medications such as benzodiazepines to cope with serious anxiety disorders, while others rely on narcotic pain medications to enable them to live relatively normal lives rather than being disabled by suffering from the severe pain that is caused by, for example, cancer, chronic back pain, or other debilitating conditions. In addition, others use stimulants to treat such problems as attention deficit hyperactivity disorder, narcolepsy, and other illnesses. Most people agree that these medications are essential in our modern-day society.

Yet there are also many people who abuse or are dependent on (addicted to) some of the same drugs that help so many others. In addition, some people abuse illicit substances, such as marijuana and heroin, as well as legal substances, such as alcohol and many prescribed medications. Sometimes abusers resort to criminal acts, including committing felonies, in order to obtain drugs. They cause great hardship to themselves and their families as well as to society at large.

Substance abuse has been a problem for thousands of years, although the particular drugs of abuse change periodically. In ancient times, people may have abused hallucinogens such as mescaline or similar drugs used as part of ceremonies in order to induce a dreamlike state. The ancient Incan royalty, nobility, and athletes, chewed coca leaves (from which cocaine is derived) for stimulation. In contrast, in the 21st century, the most popular legal drug used and abused by millions of Americans is alcohol, while the most popular illegal drug abused (and also used by millions) is marijuana.

Addiction and the abuse of drugs and/or alcohol are difficult and complex problems for which simple answers do not exist, and for which a multifaceted and forward-thinking approach often may be more effective.

For example, when a drug is accepted in society but is suddenly banned outright, as when the Eighteenth Amendment (commonly referred to as Prohibition) abruptly banned the use of alcohol, such action does not eliminate the desire for the substance. Instead, organized criminals, seizing an opportunity, manufactured and supplied many different types of alcohol to willing consumers for a considerable profit, until Prohibition was repealed and alcohol became once again a drug that was lawful for adults to consume.

Because of the failure of Prohibition, some people believe that all drugs should be "legalized," assuming that this action would drive down the prices of drugs and reduce jail and prison sentences. There is a valid argument for legalization. Yet, at the same time, the public expects from its government a certain degree of protection, and were the use of drugs such as methamphetamine or heroin suddenly legalized (as is unlikely), if and when harm was caused by individuals using these drugs, there would be a public outcry. As a result, a balance must be maintained between what rights individuals should enjoy and what controls society imposes on them. This book does not purport to resolve such key issues but rather seeks to provide information to clarify the issues.

In this volume, issues related to this complex balancing act, such as the use of narcotics (such as

OXYCONTIN, OXYCODONE, HYDROCODONE, and other drugs and drug combinations) for pain control versus the abuse of these same narcotics by others seeking to obtain a state of euphoria or oblivion, are discussed.

Another conundrum is how individuals who are dependent on alcohol or drugs should be treated. Laws in the United States allow individuals to refuse treatment, no matter how ill they appear to physicians and others; however, at the same time, they may be punished with incarceration if they commit crimes while under the influence of drugs or alcohol, such as leaving the scene of a car crash in which someone was injured, stealing items to pay for drugs, prostituting themselves to obtain drugs, and committing many other criminal acts that are often inextricably linked to drug use. A variety of entries in this volume discuss aspects of this issue, including crime and criminals, gangs, jail inmates, and law enforcement.

There are many myths and misconceptions about drug abuse, and the key myths are explored in the entries in this volume. For example, one prominent myth is that minorities are the primary abusers of drugs and alcohol; however, with the exception of a high rate of alcohol abuse among American Indians and Alaska Natives, the highest proportion of substance abusers are whites. This is true across the board, no matter which drug is considered, whether it is cocaine, methamphetamine, anabolic steroids, or any other of the entire gamut of illicit drugs.

Whites are also more likely to abuse prescription drugs than individuals of other races. This does not mean that minorities do not have drug problems—many do—however, it does mean that the problem of drug abuse is not primarily confined to individuals of particular minority ethnicities and races. This issue is discussed in the separate entries on various drugs, as well as in the specific entry on racial/ethnic differences and drug and alcohol abuse.

Another common myth is that adolescents are the primary drug abusers and that drug abuse is simply a transient "stage" in the lives of many teenagers. Although some adolescents do abuse drugs and alcohol, studies such as the National Survey on Drug Use and Health have demonstrated, however, that in nearly all cases (with the exception of the abuse of inhalants), the largest proportion of drug and alcohol abusers are young adults, ages 18–25. In addition, college students, usually in their late teens and early twenties, are also heavy abusers of both alcohol and drugs, although often their noncollege peers are heavier abusers of substances. As a result, this volume offers separate entries on adolescents, college students, and young adults and their particular issues with substance abuse.

A third common myth is that alcohol is a "safe" drug compared to marijuana, cocaine, and other drugs that are often used illicitly. Instead, although alcohol can be purchased legally by those individuals ages 21 and older (and is often also consumed by those who are underage), it is a very dangerous drug that can lead to fatalities caused by car crashes and personal violence.

Thousands of people die of causes related to health issues caused by the chronic consumption of alcohol, such as cancer, cirrhosis of the liver, heart attack, and stroke, to name the most serious illnesses. Children born to alcohol abusers may suffer from severe and lifelong developmental disabilities, such as fetal alcohol syndrome. These issues are discussed in the entries on injuries caused by alcohol and/or illicit drugs, alcohol abuse and dependence and health problems, and fetal alcohol syndrome.

Another common myth is that chronic marijuana abuse is harmless. Although occasional use usually will not cause serious problems, studies have shown that frequent use is associated with increased risks for criminal acts and violence, despite the image of marijuana as a "mellow" drug. This myth is discussed at length in the entry on marijuana.

Last, a common myth is that most people take illegal drugs or abuse prescription drugs simply in order to get "high." Although that goal is certainly an element of abuse, many abusers and addicts have or develop serious psychiatric problems, such as antisocial personality disorder, anxiety disorders, attention deficit hyperactivity disorder (often untreated), bipolar disorder, depression, or schizophrenia and all are related to their substance abuse and dependence. Each of these psychiatric disorders is discussed as a separate entry in this encyclopedia.

Drug and alcohol abuse are likely to continue to be major problems in our society, but with increased knowledge, better solutions can be sought and identified. Knowledge is power.

My coauthor and I hope that readers will find this book informative, interesting, and thought-provoking.

—Christine Adamec

INTRODUCTION

THE HISTORY OF DRUG ABUSE

Narcotics and other addictive drugs as well as alcohol (also a drug) are substances that have been used since ancient times to treat illness, accompany religious rituals or family celebrations, stimulate the mind, or sedate and soothe the emotions. They have also been abused for millennia. In many cases, drugs that were once considered acceptable by society later became unacceptable or even illegal. For example, opiates and cocaine were generally considered acceptable substances in the 19th century and were commonly used by many people for medical and nonmedical (recreational) reasons; however, the nonmedical use of these drugs became illegal in the 20th century and medical uses were sharply curtailed.

In addition, the use of marijuana was not perceived as a problem in past centuries, although it is an illegal drug in the United States today. As well, alcohol was lawfully manufactured and consumed in most states in past centuries until its manufacture was banned by the Eighteenth Amendment (Prohibition) in 1917, because attitudes toward alcohol use were extremely negative at that time. Prohibition was eventually repealed and the manufacture of alcohol became legal and acceptable once again.

This historical overview describes drug and alcohol abuse through time, starting with drug abuse, then moving on to alcohol abuse, past to present. Note that societal attitudes toward those who abuse or are dependent on (addicted to) drugs and/or alcohol have periodically changed in a cyclical manner. In some periods, substance abuse has been tolerated, whereas in other ages, the abuser is demonized as an immoral and even an evil person. In addition, drugs and alcohol themselves, as substances, have alternately been ignored, tolerated, or viewed as inherently wicked and corrupting influences.

Considering Drug Abuse Through History

The use and abuse of drugs are not modern phenomena and probably predate written language. The icon of the opium poppy was depicted in the ancient language of Sumeria in southern Iraq, dating back to 3100 BCE. The Ebers Papyrus, which dates to 1500 BCE, includes about 800 prescriptions, including those that use the berry of the poppy; thus, the value of the opium poppy was clearly known to the ancients thousands of years ago.

Many well-respected people in the past either used or were addicted to drugs such as opium, laudanum, morphine, and cocaine, including the poet Elizabeth Barrett Browning, the authors Guy de Maupassant and Louisa May Alcott, and many other luminaries. The famous nurse Florence Nightingale was a user of opium, and she wrote to her friend in 1866 that nothing helped her illness but "a curious new-fangled little operation of putting opium under the skin," clearly referring to injection by a hypodermic needle. The inventor Thomas Edison was a cocaine user, as was Sigmund Freud, the creator of psychoanalysis. King George III of England (1738–1820) took opium for his rheumatism.

Looking back earlier in time, the epic poems written by the great Greek poet Homer referred to the use of opium, and in the *Odyssey*, opium is described as the drug that quiets all pains and quarrels. The famous Greek physician Galen created lists of individuals in his era who were authorities on the use of opium. In the time of Pliny the Elder, an excess of opium was often used as a means of suicide, as described in Pliny's account of the suicide of the father of Publius Licinius Caecina, a Roman senator.

In the 11th and 12th centuries, returning crusaders took opium back to Europe from Arab lands. At first the use of the drug was very limited, but eventually opium was perceived and used as a powerful analgesic.

In the Middle Ages, according to Charles F. Levinthal in *Drugs, Society and Criminal Justice*, Viking warriors who consumed hallucinogenic mushrooms were known as "Berserkers." In later years, violent and irrational behavior became known as *berserk* behavior. Also in medieval times, women who believed themselves to be witches created a variety of concoctions and brews. Some self-proclaimed witches relied upon the sweat glands of toads (which had hallucinogenic qualities) for their purportedly magical concoctions.

Marijuana has been used for many years, and according to Levinthal, the first reference to cannabis was in writings in 2737 BCE, when the drug was used to treat gout, malaria, rheumatism, and other maladies. However, there were periods when marijuana was negatively perceived; for example, in 1484, Pope Innocent VII condemned the use of hemp (marijuana) in the Black Mass, a proscription that presumably indicates that some people used the drug.

Drug Abuse in the Eighteenth Century

Prior to the Revolutionary War in what is now the United States, many colonists relied on so-called patent medicines imported from Britain for a variety of ailments. Many of these drugs contained opium. After the Revolutionary War, sales of drugs from American medicine makers were boosted

because it seemed far more patriotic to buy from within the country than to purchase from a recent enemy. Drug sales from Britain never regained their former popularity.

According to David F. Musto in *The American Disease: Origins of Narcotic Control*, opium was commonly available in America before 1800, in multidrug prescriptions. Says Musto, "Valued for its calming and soporific effects, opium was also a specific against symptoms of gastrointestinal illnesses such as cholera, food poisoning, and parasites."

The High Prevalence of Drug Abuse in the Nineteenth Century

The use of drugs in the 19th century was, in retrospect, almost shockingly common. According to Levinthal, an estimated 25 percent of the population in the United States in the 19th century relied upon either morphine or opium, and these and other drugs were widely available to the general public. They were often included in popular nostrums purchased at the local apothecary (pharmacy) with no prescription. Yet to individuals in the 21st century, the idea that opium and its products (as well as cocaine) were freely available to men, women, and children and even administered to infants in the past is difficult to understand or grasp.

Barbara Hodgson offers some perspective in her book *In the Arms of Morpheus: The Tragic History of Laudanum, Morphine, and Patent Medicines:*

> Before the twentieth century, those who were ill had little choice but to turn to a substance such as opium. At least three conditions paved the way for this situation. First, opium was a vital means of coping with cholera, dysentery and tuberculosis, diseases borne of horrific living conditions such as those of the Industrial Revolution, because it reduced the physical manifestations of the disease—for example, diarrhea and coughing. Second, many diseases were incurable; opium eased the pain brought on by these ailments. And last, because opium was effective, available and cheap, those who distrusted or couldn't afford medical help diagnosed and treated their ailments themselves.

Opium was used by physicians to treat severe pain, menstrual problems, dysentery, arthritis, diabetes, pneumonia, sexually transmitted diseases, and many other ailments. It was actually effective in treating dysentery because opiates tend to cause constipation. Opiates were and still are effective at treating pain; however, they have no antibiotic or antiviral action, nor do they treat diabetes, and thus they were and are not efficacious in treating bacterial or viral diseases. However, the drug did make many sick people feel better.

Opium was available in powdered and gum forms, although most people consumed opium in some type of solution. Many people drank their opium in laudanum (a mixture of opium and other ingredients), and many of these solutions included up to 90 proof alcohol.

Patent Medications Were Very Popular

After the Civil War, sales of patent drugs escalated. Most of the drugs were not actually patented, but some were trademarked. However, these remedies together were referred to as patent medications. There were no controls over these medications; they were freely obtainable and obtained. Most consumers had no idea of what was included in their favorite remedies.

Says the author John Parascandola in his article on patent medications in *Caduceus,* "After the Civil War, patent medicine quackery really entered its golden age. Thousands of products flooded the market. As the cost of getting into business was relatively small and no great knowledge was required, many would-be entrepreneurs entered the field." In many cases, these drugs were worthless to trusting consumers, and in some cases, individuals became addicted to narcotic-laced remedies.

Medicine makers advertised their concoctions in calendars, almanacs, coloring books, and cookbooks, and in many other ways. Some sellers offered medicine shows, where they marketed their drugs in public and combined the sales pitch with a puppet show, magic show, or animal act.

Mail order drugs were also readily available to the population. According to Stephen R. Kandall, the author of *Substance and Shadow: Women and Addiction in the United States,* many Americans relied on patent medicines purchased through Sears Roebuck and similar mail-order catalogues. Some concoctions had names that may amuse the public today, such as Pink Pills for Pale People and Mrs. Winslow's Soothing Syrup.

Some of the popular patent medications that were sold by mail or in apothecaries and were specifically targeted to infants and children contained narcotics; for example, Mrs. Winslow's Soothing Syrup contained morphine (as well as sugar syrup, anise, caraway, fennel, and alcohol) and was given to infants for teething pain or other common problems of infancy.

Cough syrups commonly included narcotics; for example, according to Parascandola in his article in *Caduceus,* Dr. Bull's Cough Syrup comprised morphine sulfate dissolved in syrup.

Women and Opiates in the Nineteenth Century

In the 19th century, experts estimate that women used opium at a rate at least three times greater than that of men. In part, this was because the drug was commonly recommended or administered to them by physicians as a cure-all solution for numerous complaints. In addition, alcohol use among women was greatly frowned upon, while the use of opium and laudanum was widely accepted. Women were also heavy consumers of popular nostrums laced with opium and morphine. Most addicted women had no trouble obtaining their "medicine" whenever they needed it.

Opium and morphine were prescribed for menstrual difficulties, headaches, and many other common ailments suffered by females. As a result, some women became addicted to drugs. Says Kandall in *Substance and Shadow: Women and Addiction in the United States,* "Addiction to opiates touched all social levels—society women identifying with the artistic or intellectual set, rural and working-class women coping with long hours and loneliness, and prostitutes in city streets and opium dens. It is hardly surprising that such a large proportion of America's opiate addicts were women."

The Introduction of Morphine in the Nineteenth Century

Morphine was isolated from opium in 1803 by Frederick Wilhelm Adam Sertürner in Germany, who called his creation "morphium," which was later shortened to *morphine.* Morphine was only about one-tenth the weight of raw opium but it was ten times stronger.

Morphine first became available in the United States in the 1830s but its popularity surged several decades later. The drug was frequently used to treat wounded soldiers in the Civil War and some developed a lifelong addiction to the drug. In addition, widows and family members of soldiers who died in the war often took morphine or other opiates to deal with their grief.

Morphine was commonly used in the second half of the 19th century, particularly after the development of the hypodermic needle, which was introduced in the United States in 1856. At that time, doctors believed that since injected morphine did not travel through the digestive system, then there would be no craving for the drug, and thus, morphine would not be addicting. Of course, they were wrong in this assumption.

People in the 19th century also took morphine as a treatment for sexually transmitted diseases, such as syphilis, as well as for a broad host of other diseases and medical conditions, such as sciatica, cholera, hernia, and even sunstroke.

Americans could purchase syringes by mail from catalogues, and some fashionable women carried their morphine syringes in special pouches attached to their belts or sashes. Many individuals, including physicians, had no idea of the dangers that were associated with reusing needles. Because of this lack of knowledge, unsterile needles caused severe skin abscesses in many users.

Says Morgan in *Drugs in America: A Social History 1800–1980*, "Even before warnings about addiction began in the 1870s, many commentators thought hypodermic medication overused. One doctor reported in 1877 that a colleague showed him an old syringe 'with as much pleasure as an old veteran would show his trusty blade, and claiming that he had used it more than one thousand times.'"

Cocaine Becomes a Popular Nineteenth-Century Drug

Another drug commonly used in the latter part of the 19th century was cocaine. Cocaine was originally isolated from the coca plant in the 1850s and given its name by the German chemist Alfred Niemann. But the use of the coca plant preceded the development of cocaine for many centuries and the ancient Inca chewed coca for energy and stamina.

In the 1860s and into the early 20th century, the patent medicine industry used cocaine in many nostrums, although most people had no idea they were ingesting a potentially addicting drug, since there were no labeling requirements and few people, including physicians, knew that cocaine was addictive.

In 1884, the ophthalmologist Karl Koller wrote about the anesthetic properties of cocaine, and many surgeons worldwide were intrigued. At that time, doctors actively sought an anesthetic alternative to the highly unreliable ether, and cocaine seemed ideal.

Cocaine became popular among physicians when a young neurologist, Sigmund Freud, wrote a monograph about the beneficial effects of cocaine in 1884. Cocaine was subsequently used to ease the pain of labor for mothers in delivery and many physicians nationwide (and worldwide) perceived cocaine as an effective analgesic for a variety of ailments. One common use of cocaine was as a treatment for hay fever and sinus congestion. Cocaine was also used to treat cholera, yellow fever, and sexually transmitted diseases, such as syphilis. As with opiates, cocaine has no antibiotic or antiviral qualities, although it provides pain relief.

Cocaine was sometimes used as a treatment for those addicted to opiates, and Freud allegedly recommended cocaine to a friend who was a morphine addict; however, this individual subsequently became addicted to cocaine. In fact, cocaine was recommended by many physicians of the time as a treatment for opiate addiction, and according to some accounts, this treatment worked without inducing a new addiction to cocaine. However, in other cases, as with Dr. Freud's friend, the patient simply exchanged one addiction for another.

Cocaine was also used as a physical stimulant (particularly for the heart), a mental stimulant (there were no available antidepressants at that time), a drug for gastric distress, a treatment for kidney disease, and, as mentioned, a medication for colds, hay fever, and sinus troubles. The Civil War general Ulysses S. Grant experienced severe pain from terminal throat cancer and used cocaine to help him finish writing his memoirs before his death.

In addition to being included in tonics, wines, and soft drinks, cocaine was offered in a smokable form of the drug: cocaine cigarettes and a cocaine cigar. Smoking several of these cigars was marketed as a good way for men to get rid of the "blues."

However, when cocaine was used nonmedically, often by young urban males, this abuse was widely disparaged, and the term *cocaine fiend* was frequently used to describe and deride such young men.

Cocaine and Coca-Cola

John Styth Pemberton, a druggist from Atlanta, Georgia, initially used cocaine in his "French Wine of Coca, the Ideal Tonic" in 1866, modeling it on Vin Mariani. Vin Mariani was an extremely popular beverage in Europe, created by Angelo Mariani, a Corsican chemist, and it was also consumed in the United States. Because of a temperance attitude in Atlanta, Pemberton removed the alcohol from his product, using kola nuts (which contain natural caffeine) and cocaine to make the drink he named Coca-Cola. The first Coca-Cola was sold at Jacob's Pharmacy in Atlanta on May 8, 1886, according to the Library of Congress. (Cocaine was removed from the soft drink in 1903 according to the *Southern Medical Journal.*)

The new drink was a major success and was marketed as an "ideal brain tonic" that could treat migraines, depression, and neuralgia. Coca-Cola was marketed as a "temperance drink" (for those opposed to the use of alcohol) as well as an "intellectual beverage."

The cola syrup was originally mixed with tap water, but when mixed with carbonated water to provide quick relief to a headache sufferer, the new drink was a success and carbonated water was added as a new ingredient to the product. Pemberton sold his formula to the drink before his death. Coca-Cola was actively promoted and continues to be a major success story.

Cocaine as a Means to Spur Laborers

In the late 19th and early 20th centuries, some employers who hired workers (often minority members) for difficult physical labor encouraged the use of cocaine and even supplied the drug to them in some cases, according to Joseph F. Spillane in *Cocaine: From Medical Marvel to Modern Menace in the United States, 1884–1920.*

According to Spillane, "Many saw the drug as a means of increasing production and manipulating their workforce. Levee construction camps operating along the Mississippi River reportedly supplied cocaine to workers, as did many southern road construction camps."

In addition, says Spillane, "Textile mills were particularly likely to have cocaine introduced by workers, supervisors or employers. In Manchester, Connecticut, the home of many silk mills, one employer attempted to ease problems caused by irritating dust from the production process by supplying workers with a menthol and cocaine spray, to be taken on the job. In Maine, operatives from the textiles mills in Lewiston purchased cocaine for their workers."

The fact that many such workers were blacks may partly explain why cocaine was a problem drug among some blacks of the time.

Marijuana in the Nineteenth Century

Cannabis sativa (marijuana) first became of interest in the United States in the mid-19th century, as did hashish. Some doctors prescribed a tincture of cannabis for oral use or injection. Most users mixed marijuana with food or smoked it. According to Morgan, cannabis was available in candy, food, and some drinks, all ready for purchase and with no controls on its use or consumption. Says Morgan: "Between 1840 and 1900, dozens of articles in the medical journals suggested cannabis for innumerable ailments, and it entered the pharmacopoeia in 1870. It seemed useful as an anticonvulsant and relaxant, even in cases of tetanus and hydrophobia [rabies]. Doctors experimented with it widely, often to alleviate disorders for which they had no other remedies."

Marijuana was used to treat insomnia and migraine, especially the migraines of women. In addition, it was used to treat labor pains, postpartum psychosis, and sexually transmitted diseases, such as gonorrhea. Some physicians used marijuana to treat opium addiction.

By the end of the century, the use of marijuana by the general public declined, and it did not again become a popular drug for several generations, from the 1960s to the present.

The Introduction of Heroin

Although heroin was first synthesized from morphine in 1874, it was introduced by the Bayer Company in 1898. Heroin was three times stronger than morphine and believed to be nonaddictive. The drug was recommended to tuberculosis patients for chronic cough, but many other applications developed quickly, and heroin was an ingredient in many patent medications. Considered a wonder drug that could relieve virtually any complaint, heroin was even included in remedies for colicky and teething infants. Often heroin was combined with a high dose of alcohol in home remedies.

Experts initially believed heroin was much less addicting than morphine, because lower dosages of heroin were needed for effect; however, the reality was that heroin was much more potent than morphine, and therefore more addictive.

Drug Abuse in the Twentieth Century

In the early 20th century, many individuals believed that drug addiction was treatable or at least tolerable. However, since most addicts were middle- and upper-class women, often addiction was simply ignored. For those who sought treatment in the early part of the century (mostly men), facilities for individuals afflicted with drug abuse dotted the nation and primarily served those who could afford to pay their fees. The treatments of that time (hot baths, purgatives, and so forth) did not work, but the point is that attitudes toward the addict were not negative. This situation changed.

By about 1920, physicians were deeply split between those who felt it acceptable and humane to treat drug addicts with maintenance doses of the drug to which individuals were addicted and those doctors who considered it immoral to sell "dope" to so-called dope fiends. Many physicians believed that there was no organic basis for addiction, and consequently, anyone addicted to drugs should be compelled to stop taking drugs altogether. Some key figures, such as Dr. Lawrence Kolb, Sr., of the United States Public Health Service, believed normal people could not become addicted to drugs and only psychopathic individuals would develop an addiction. He believed a normal person would experience no euphoria from a morphine injection, whereas a psychopath would experience such a high.

Many modern studies have shown that some individuals have a genetic predisposition toward substance abuse; however, their physiological reaction to an initial injection of opiates is, as far as is known, the same as or similar to the experience of those who have no familial predispositions toward addiction.

Reform of Patent Medications

Reformers became distressed by opium-laced remedies in the early part of the 20th century, and in 1905, Samuel Hopkins Adams ran his "Great American Fraud" series in *Collier's* magazine, attacking suppliers of these nostrums. This series was influential in affecting public attitudes. In addition, after the passage in 1906 of the federal Pure Food and Drug Act, which required labeling of narcotics and alcohol on the bottle, the narcotic content of most patent medications diminished.

According to Musto, the morphine content of Mrs. Winslow's Soothing Syrup declined from 0.4 grain per ounce in 1908 to 0.16 grain in 1911, and morphine was totally removed from the product by 1915.

Early Twentieth-Century Theories on Addiction and Pathology

According to Spillane in *Federal Drug Control*, prior to World War I, many physicians believed in the antibody theory of addiction: that drug use somehow created antibodies in the blood of addicts, who, as a result, were helpless to end their drug addiction.

Says Spillane, "These physiological changes were [believed to be] beyond the control of the addict, and many doctors accepted that these changes required maintenance doses to be given indefinitely. Many of the leading supporters of the narcotic clinics had been schooled in versions of the antibody theory." Researchers now know that chronic drug use can result in brain changes, although these are not caused by antibodies or reactions to viruses, as far as is known.

By 1919, the theory that antibodies caused addiction was no longer in favor, and instead, addicts were believed to be mentally defective or psycho-pathic, with no willpower to resist addictive drugs. Law enforcement was seen as the answer to keep addicts away from the drugs they craved. Because of this punitive attitude and change in policy, most narcotic maintenance clinics were closed by 1921.

Drugs in Wartime:
World War II and the Vietnam War

In World War II, amphetamines in the form of Benzedrine and other drugs were freely given to Axis soldiers and sailors who needed to stay awake in battle conditions. These drugs were also used by the Allies (the United States, Britain, etc.) to keep *their* soldiers awake.

During the Vietnam War, service members were not given drugs by the government as in World War II; however, many drugs were freely available to military men and women stationed in Southeast Asia. Interestingly, most service members who used drugs in Vietnam readily gave them up when they returned home to the United States, even though some developed long-term addictions to heroin and other drugs.

According to Levinthal, an estimated 11 percent of the troops who returned from Vietnam were regular abusers of heroin and 22 percent had tried the drug at least one time, and there were great concerns about what was believed to be large numbers of these addicts returning to the United States. The heroin in Vietnam was very pure—90 to 98 percent pure, versus the heroin in the United States then, which was 2–10 percent pure. However, only 1–2 percent of the returned Vietnam War veterans continued to abuse heroin when they came home, whether it was because the drug was too costly in the United States or too difficult to obtain, or they were relieved to be back home (or the result of other factors or a combination of factors).

Tranquilizers, Barbiturates, and Diet Drugs

In the 1950s to the 1970s, many people (mostly women) were prescribed tranquilizers for a broad array of complaints. Physicians prescribed Methe-drine, an amphetamine, for overweight patients. Calming drugs such as diazepam (Valium) became extremely popular. Says Kandall, "Like their nine-teenth-century counterparts, who had recom-mended opiate-laden 'soothing syrups' and related compounds for patients suffering from psychic stress, overzealous physicians began to prescribe these medications with little sense of control, once again reaching for the prescription pad to treat women's neuroses and maladjustments."

In 1974, an estimated two-thirds of the new prescriptions written by doctors for Valium were for women, as were 71 percent of the new prescrip-tions for Librium, another tranquilizing drug.

Drugs and the General Public
in the 1960s and 1970s

The abuse of illegal drugs in the United States skyrocketed in the late 1960s and early 1970s, and experts are still sorting out the reasons for this high rate of drug abuse. Dr. Timothy Leary, one of the few tenured professors to be fired from Harvard University, openly advocated the use of LYSERGIC ACID DIETHYLAMIDE (LSD), with his catch phrase "Tune in, turn on and drop out." D-lyser-gic acid diethylamide was first noted by Dr. Albert Hofmann of Sandoz Laboratories in Basel, Switzer-land, in 1943. He accidentally took a small amount of LDS-25, the shortened name for the drug, and noted its hallucinogenic effects.

Dr. Leary also experimented with other hallu-cinogenic drugs, such as psilocybin. Some college students and young adults followed Leary's advice, abusing LSD, as well as other hallucinogenic drugs. However, these drugs were never as popular as mar-ijuana, which was commonly found on college cam-puses in the late 1960s and the 1970s. Such drug use continues today although at much lower levels than in the sixties and seventies of the 20th century.

President Richard Nixon declared a "total war on drugs" after his election in 1968, and as a result of his efforts the Comprehensive Drug Abuse Pre-vention and Control Act was passed in 1970. The Nixon administration also funded treatment pro-grams for heroin addicts, including detoxification programs and methadone maintenance clinics.

Under the administration of President Ron-ald Reagan, a tougher stance against drugs was adopted. Congress enacted the Comprehensive Crime Control Act, increasing penalties for the abuse of drugs and the scope of asset forfeitures that could be made against drug violators.

Cocaine became popular again in the 1970s and early 1980s, glamorized by Hollywood. According to the Drug Enforcement Agency, the amount of illicit cocaine that entered the United States increased from 19 metric tons in 1977 to 51 metric tons in 1980. Cocaine was the drug of movie stars, college students, and young professionals. It was also used as an appetite suppressant by some.

Drugs in the Mid- to Late Twentieth Century

In the middle part of the 20th century, tranquilizers in the benzodiazepine class were introduced. Chlordiazepoxide (Librium) was introduced to the market in 1960 and diazepam (Valium) was introduced in 1963. These drugs were popular drugs of abuse for about the next 10–15 years but have since largely fallen out of favor. They are still used as medications to treat individuals who have anxiety disorders. For example, in 1972, Valium was the first most popularly prescribed drug of any type of drug, and Librium was the third most popular drug. In 1975, when the popularity of these drugs peaked, it is estimated that 85 million prescriptions were written in the United States.

The primary users were women and some experts say that doctors were too ready with their prescription pads, just as they were generous providers of laudanum and morphine to females in the late 19th century.

Nancy Reagan, wife of President Ronald Reagan, launched an antidrug campaign in 1985, with the slogan "Just say no." Although it was much ridiculed, the campaign did draw attention to the problems associated with drug abuse and addiction. Some experts believe it was the emergence of crack cocaine that led to the escalation of a drug war by the federal government, as exemplified by the Anti–Drug Abuse Act of 1986. This law increased the role of the military in controlling drugs at the federal level and created mandatory prison sentences for drug offenders.

In 1986, President Reagan sought to get drugs out of the workplace and schools, making them "drug-free," and initiated the drug testing of some government workers in sensitive occupations. This decision was attacked by the American Civil Liberties Union and other groups, but drug testing has remained firmly entrenched in the United States to this day for many workers, students, and prospective employees.

Crack cocaine was of particular concern to law enforcement officials in the 1980s, and the penalties for the use or sale of this drug were severe, prompting some experts to wonder aloud why the sale or possession of crack cocaine was punished far more assiduously than was that of powdered cocaine, also an addicting drug. Some experts speculated racial issues were present, because most abusers of crack at that time were African Americans, while the majority of abusers of powdered cocaine were white.

In the latter part of the 20th century, it became increasingly popular for adolescents and young adults to attend all-night dance parties, also called *raves*, at which drugs were freely available. Marijuana, methamphetamine, and many other drugs were routinely bought and sold at these events, as were hallucinogenic drugs: METHYLENEDIOXYMETHAMPHETAMINE (MDMA/ECSTASY), PHENCYCLIDINE (PCP), LSD, and others. Eventually, law enforcement authorities cracked down on these functions, which became less common. However, it is still possible for adolescents and young adults to obtain illicit drugs from each other as well as from drug dealers.

Laws on Addictive Drugs

Prior to the passage of the first federal laws on drugs, many states and some cities had restrictions; for example, in 1875, San Francisco created an opium ordinance, and in 1877, Nevada enacted the first state opium law. Tennessee passed a law banning the sale of cocaine in 1901. By 1914, before the passage of the Harrison Narcotic Law, nearly every state had banned the sale of cocaine.

Says Spillane, "Because the earliest laws dealt with sales, not possession, sellers caught with drugs would often be charged with disorderly conduct or some other offense. In this way, an arresting officer could take a seller into custody without having to prove that a sale had taken place."

In 1914, the Harrison Narcotic Act was passed by Congress. This law was created largely because of the Hague Opium Convention of 1912, an international treaty the United States had signed that required the United States to develop restrictions on cocaine and opiates. The law took effect on March 1, 1915. The law allowed the federal government to tax those who managed drugs, such as pharmacists and physicians, and it also required them to register with the federal government and pay a federal tax of one dollar per year. Patent medications with only a small amount of heroin, opium, cocaine, or morphine were exempt from the law. The law went into effect in 1915.

After the implementation of the Harrison Narcotics Act, pharmacists could only fill prescriptions for narcotics that were written by physicians or dentists (with some exceptions), and the law did not allow for refills of prescriptions.

Shortly after the passage of the Harrison Act, the government created a requirement that taxed drugs also had to be stamped, and anyone who had unstamped drugs was breaking the law. Several U.S. Supreme Court decisions that followed the Harrison Act led to the interpretation that physicians could not prescribe any narcotics for "nonmedical" use. As a result, addicted individuals could not receive maintenance doses of the drugs to which they were addicted.

In part because some physicians believed addiction was largely physician-driven in the late 19th century, many physicians did not fight the increasingly rigid rulings by the Treasury Department, which oversaw the laws enacted as a result of the Harrison Act. In *Webb v. United States* in 1919, the U.S. Supreme Court ruled it was illegal to prescribe morphine to an addict to keep him or her comfortable. In 1922, in *U.S. v. Behrman,* an even more restrictive ruling, the Supreme Court ruled that it was illegal for a doctor to prescribe drugs to an addict.

Dr. Charles Linder of Seattle was prosecuted for giving a prescription of four tablets to a person he thought was an addict but who was actually an informant for the Treasury Department. Dr. Linder fought his prosecution and in 1925, in *Linder v. U.S.,* the Supreme Court overturned his conviction. However, according to author White, despite this ruling, the Treasury Department continued to intimidate physicians about treating addicts, and more than 25,000 doctors were indicted between 1914 and 1938, and 3,000 of them went to jail.

Desperate addicts went from physician to physician seeking narcotics, and some injured themselves or faked infections in order to obtain their drugs.

In 1922, the Jones-Miller Act, which increased narcotics violation fines to $5,000 and prison terms to up to 10 years, was passed. According to White, "In less than a decade, the status of the addict had shifted from that of legitimate patient to that of willful criminal."

Some addicts were incarcerated, and according to Winger and colleagues in *A Handbook on Drug and Alcohol Abuse: The Biomedical Aspects,* prison overcrowding resulted. Incarceration did not help addicts or change their behavior, so a new concept, that of *narcotic farms,* was developed and enacted by Congress in 1928. It was believed that hard work and clean living at one of the farms in Lexington, Kentucky, or Fort Worth, Texas, would rehabilitate drug addicts.

Say the authors, "By involving addicts in the hard but productive labor required by agriculture, in the context of clean healthy rural life, these combined prisons and farms were intended to develop moral character, the lack of which had caused these unfortunate people to become addicted." However, the narcotic farms were largely unsuccessful, possibly because many addicts eventually returned to the environment in which their addiction developed.

In 1970, the Comprehensive Drug Abuse and Control Act was passed; this law created the initial concept that drugs could be scheduled in terms of their addictive potential. Title II of this law was the Controlled Substances Act (CSA), which placed addictive drugs into five separate categories based on their addictive potential. (The entire act is often referred to as the Controlled Substances Act.)

In the CSA, drugs in Schedule I were illegal drugs such as marijuana and heroin, while drugs in the other schedules were drugs with medical use but an abuse potential; for example, Schedule II drugs included opiates also used legitimately to treat pain but which were sometimes abused. Cocaine was included in Schedule II because it was (and sometimes still is) used by ophthalmologists in treating eye disease.

The Drug Enforcement Administration (DEA) was created as a result of the Comprehensive Drug Abuse Prevention and Control Act. The DEA was given all federal law enforcement powers over narcotics, with the exception of those crossing the borders of the United States and its ports of entry, for which responsibility was assigned to the U.S. Customs Service. Today the DEA has agents in the United States and in many countries abroad, where they collect information on drug trafficking and coordinate seizures with foreign governments.

President Bill Clinton appointed a "drug czar" and convinced Congress to increase the budget for drug interdiction. Clinton signed the Comprehensive Methamphetamine Control Act in 1996, to increase penalties for manufacturing and/or selling methamphetamine.

Under the administration of President George W. Bush, the Combat Methamphetamine Epidemic Act of 2005 was passed; the law requires retailers to keep chemicals that can be used as precursors behind store counters or in a locked cabinet inaccessible to customers. The war against drug abuse continues actively today.

Class, Gender, and Race: Societal Attitudes toward Addiction Often Depend on Who Is Addicted

Some historians have pointed out that societal attitudes toward addiction are largely driven by views toward the groups who are perceived as addicted. For example, in the 19th century, most addicts were middle- and upper-class white women, and addiction was generally tolerated. However, in the 20th century, when addiction became more of a problem among young adult males using drugs recreationally (and sometimes becoming addicted to them), drug addicts were often demonized as evil. This issue may be considered in the light of the 21st century, when prescription drug abuse and addiction are often regarded as almost a white-collar type of crime, whereas the abuse of crack cocaine and heroin is seen as very bad or wicked.

Simply put, most middle-class and upper-class individuals in the 21st century do not abuse crack or heroin, although they may abuse prescription drugs or even powdered cocaine. According to Caroline Jean Acker in *Creating the American Junkie: Addiction Research in the Classic Era of Narcotic Control*, "We now have in the United States a two-tier system of response to drug dependence: treatment for the middle and upper classes and incarceration for most others, including the poor, the uninsured, ethnic minorities, and immigrants. Employment status, race, gender, and class all influence which response an individual encounters."

According to Charles F. Levinthal in *Drugs, Society, and Criminal Justice* and according to other authors, racist fears have played a significant role in the way drugs have been regarded in the United States; for example, some individuals in the early 20th century mistakenly believed cocaine would spur African Americans to rape white women in the South, while opium use would result in unwanted sexual contact between Chinese individuals and white Americans. Marijuana was believed to make Latinos violent.

In addition, some individuals feared that cocaine abuse among blacks would cause them to attack whites. Says the author David Musto, "The fear of the cocainized black coincided with the peak of lynchings, legal segregation, and voting laws all designed to remove political and social power from him. Fear of cocaine might have contributed to the dread the black would rise above 'his place,' as well as reflecting the extent to which cocaine may have released defiance and retribution. So far, evidence does not suggest that cocaine caused a crime wave but rather that anticipation of black rebellion inspired white alarm."

The fear was so intense that bizarre myths developed, such as the myth that blacks using cocaine would be impervious to .32 caliber bullets, as a result of which some police departments switched to .38 caliber revolvers.

Musto says by 1914, politicians, physicians, pharmacists, and the news media were convinced opiates and cocaine caused regular users to become criminals and/or to lose their mind, and these drugs were associated with outcast subgroups or foreigners. Says Musto, "Cocaine raised the specter of the wild Negro, opium the devious Chinese, morphine the tramps in the slums; it was feared that use of all these drugs was spreading into the 'higher classes.'"

In the late 1980s (and arguably in the present) many experts believed that there were distinctive differences in the way addicted individuals were treated, depending on their race, socioeconomic status, and employment status. According to Acker in *Creating the American Junkie:*

> For the poor, the unemployed, the uneducated, the uninsured, and people of color, drug use was more likely to occur in a setting of concentrated social problems, and users were typically subject to arrest and incarceration. For the middle and upper classes, for those with jobs, education, and health coverage, legal sanctions were less common, and numerous resources were available to support individuals seeking to end destructive drug use. These might include an employer willing to hold a job while the individual completed treatment and health insurance or personal assets to cover the cost of treatment.

Drug and Alcohol Abuse and Dependence in the Twenty-first Century

Concern over drugs has become institutionalized and is an everyday issue that many people do not even consider. For example, many employers require drug testing (and a clean result) before they will hire an individual, regardless of the type of job and even when there has been no past history of drug abuse. If an individual *has* been a drug user who was arrested for a drug offense, he or she may be subjected to random drug checks by a probation or parole department. Drug tests are sold in pharmacies so that parents can check for possible drug use, usually by their adolescent children. If an individual behaves in an aberrant or unusual manner, many people think or even state aloud that the person must be on drugs.

Popular Drugs in the Twenty-first Century

The most popular drug of abuse in the 21st century is alcohol, followed by marijuana. Among those in treatment, the third most commonly abused drug after alcohol and marijuana is cocaine. In general young adults and high school students are the most likely to abuse illicit drugs as well as to misuse prescription drugs. For example, among young adults 19–28 years old in 2004, 57.4 percent had ever used marijuana.

Some states have attempted to legalize marijuana use for those who are ill with cancer or chronic painful diseases and have passed laws allowing such use; however, the federal government actively opposes such laws. However, there is one marijuana drug supported by the federal government: dronabinol (Marinol), an oral medication developed with the assistance of the Drug Enforcement Administration. Experts who favor smoking marijuana are dismissive of this drug and it is unknown how commonly it is used.

Some drugs are of particular concern. For example, although most people do not abuse methamphetamine, the abuse of this drug is slightly up or remains the same among some high school students. According to information from the Monitoring the Future reports for 2004 and 2005, 3.1 percent of 8th graders had ever used methamphetamine in 2005, compared to 2.5 percent in 2004. In addition, 1.8 percent of the 8th graders had used the drug in the past year in 2005, compared to 1.5 percent in 2004.

The rate of methamphetamine abuse among young adults ages 19–28 and college students in particular is significantly higher than that of high school students. In 2004, 9 percent of young adults had ever used methamphetamine, compared to 5.2 percent of college students.

Methamphetamine is a dangerous drug, and the number of emergency department admissions increased from 13 per 100,000 admissions in 1993 to 56 per 100,000 in 2003, the most recent information as of this writing.

Another area of concern is the misuse of prescription drugs, which is particularly high among college students and young adults ages 19–28 years old. For example, in 2004, 14.9 percent of young adults had ever abused tranquilizers, compared to 10.6 percent of college students. Barbiturates were also abused; 9.7 percent of young adults had ever abused barbiturates, as had 7.2 percent of college students.

In considering the abuse of narcotic painkillers in 2004, individuals ages 18–25 years were most likely to have abused this type of drug: 11.9 percent had misused narcotics in the past year, and 3.8 percent had abused them in the past month, according to a report on prescription drug abuse from the Executive Office of the President. Among those ages 12–17, 7.4 percent had abused prescription narcotics in the past year and

1.9 percent had abused them in the past month. Clearly, prescription drug abuse is a serious problem in the United States.

Drug Abuse: A Global Problem in Modern Times

Today modern societies are actively interconnected by the Internet and cell phones. Transactions can be made rapidly in response to information available through current modern communications. Unfortunately, drug dealers also frequently use this enhanced communication system to communicate with their suppliers as well as drug customers. In addition, some drug dealers set up sophisticated systems to manage drug smuggling and sales, although there are still street corner drug dealers who sell drugs in public and take the risks associated with open sales.

In addition, international trade is vital to the economy of the United States, Canada, and other Western countries. At the same time, increased trade with other countries sometimes involves criminal elements of these societies, who seek to purvey illegal and dangerous drugs.

It is also important to note that drug abuse is not limited to the United States and Canada but is a worldwide problem. According to the *World Drug Report 2006*, published by the World Health Organization, 200 million people, or 5 percent of the people in the world, have used illegal drugs in the past 12 months. There are an estimated 25 million people who are addicted to drugs in the world, about 0.6 percent of the global population ages 15–64 years.

As in the United States, the most popular drug worldwide in 2004 was cannabis (marijuana), used by 162 million people. The next most abused type were amphetamines (including amphetamines and methamphetamine and excluding Ecstasy), abused by 35 million people globally, followed by abusers of opiates (16 million people), and of this number 11 million were heroin abusers. Cocaine was abused by 13 million individuals worldwide.

In considering drug seizures worldwide in 2004, cannabis represented 53 percent of all seizures. (The World Health Organization includes marijuana, hashish, and hashish oil within their definition of cannabis.) Opiates represented 15 percent of all drug seizures around the globe. Amphetamine-like stimulants (such as amphetamines, methamphetamine, and Ecstasy) represented 10 percent of all seizures, and cocaine represented 9 percent of global drug seizures. Together, these categories of drugs represented 87 percent of all world drug seizures in 2004.

The majority of the global opium production in 2005 occurred in Afghanistan (89 percent). An estimated 16 million people, less than 1 percent of the global population (0.4 percent), abuse opiates. According to the World Health Organization, 54 percent of the world's abusers of opiates live in Asia, followed by 25 percent in Europe, 14 percent in the Americas (North America and South America), 6 percent in Africa, and 1 percent in Oceania (Pacific Ocean countries, including Australia).

The greatest uses of opiates occur along the drug trafficking routes from Afghanistan. Some countries have a very high rate of abuse; for example, according to a World Health Organization estimate, there are 1.2 million opiate abusers in Iran, or 2.8 percent of the country's population, ages 15–64 years. Rates are also high in Kyrgyzstan (2.3 percent of the 15- to 64-year-old population) and Kazakhstan (1.3 percent).

In considering worldwide cocaine abuse, according to the World Health Organization, about 13.4 million people, less than 1 percent of the global population (0.3 percent), abuse cocaine. The highest abuse in 2005 was seen in North America, which had nearly half of all the worldwide cocaine abusers. The largest cocaine market (40 percent of all cocaine users in the world) was the United States, followed by western and central Europe. An estimated 2.8 percent of the population in the United States ages 15–64 abused cocaine in 2004, followed by 1.1 percent in western and central Europe.

Treatment for Drug Abuse through the Ages

In past years, drug addicts have been treated with other drugs of abuse (although it was unknown at the time that these drugs were subject to abuse), such as cocaine, morphine, marijuana, and heroin. As mentioned, addicts have also been placed on narcotic farms, where it was believed that clean living and hard work would rehabilitate them.

However, studies indicated that as many as 96 percent of those treated resumed addiction, usually within about six months of their discharge.

At some points in history, addicts were believed to be incorrigible, and they were often jailed. There was a movement at one point to require commitment of addicts to institutions, since it was believed that they could not be cured. According to White, many addicts were civilly committed in California, Illinois, and New York in the 1960s into state psychiatric hospitals for one to three years. Addicts in the past have also been placed in workhouses or poorhouses, along with the insane, the elderly, and orphaned children.

Frequently, treatment for addiction was confined to compelling the individual to go through withdrawal, although sometimes tapering off drugs was allowed. Often whether tapering was used depended on the status of the addict, and a genteel lady of the early 20th century was far more likely to receive drug tapering than a young man labeled as a cocaine fiend or a black male who may have become addicted to the drug by an employer who was seeking to get more work out of him.

Treatment of Addicted Women

Kandall says that although there was some concern about addiction in the late 19th century, it was not until the early 1970s that women addicts were directly acknowledged and helped. Says Kandall, "While it is true that some women were passive beneficiaries of such drug treatment efforts as sanitariums, drug clinics, and methadone maintenance programs, not until the 1970s, following the emergence of the Women's Movement and various self-help initiatives, did addicted women finally begin to receive attention in their own right. Even then, drug-using women, especially those belonging to racial and ethnic minorities, faced hostility, prejudicial reporting to legal and child protection authorities, and criminal prosecution for drug-related conduct during pregnancy."

Kandall also said confrontational treatment programs that sought to attack the ego of addicted men usually failed or were harmful to addicted women, who already had very fragile egos and experienced intense guilt and shame about their addiction.

Unusual Treatments

Unusual treatments for drug addiction abounded in the first half of the 20th century; for example, in the 1930s, some doctors used insulin to induce a mild coma, which they believed would then reduce the craving for opiates. Addicts at the Colorado State Penitentiary received a particularly unusual treatment, described by White: "The procedure used at the Penitentiary involved raising blisters on the abdomen of the addict, withdrawing serum from the blisters with a hypodermic syringe, and then injecting the serum into the patient's arm. This procedure was repeated four to five times a day for a week to ten days in order to effect the 'cure.'"

Methadone Maintenance

In 1964, Drs. Vincent Dole and Marie Nyswander began their pioneering research with transitioning heroin and morphine addicts to methadone. Their work indicated to them that methadone was an effective alternative to heroin or morphine because it did not cause wild mood swings or euphoria yet would satisfy the craving for narcotics. They proposed a methadone maintenance program as a treatment. They believed that addiction was a disease at a time when most addicts were perceived as immoral and criminal people. In some cities, addicts accounted for about half of inmates of jails. As a result of their groundbreaking work, their first methadone clinic opened in New York City in 1965 and was later followed by others nationwide.

There was opposition to methadone maintenance from many groups. Some black militants believed methadone was a vehicle to enslave them, and one group threatened to burn down a methadone clinic in New Haven, Connecticut. Other opposition arose from neighborhoods that did not want a methadone clinic in their areas. However, the greatest opposition was that of the federal government. Federal narcotics agents worried about drug diversion of the methadone to those outside the clinic who could abuse it (a valid concern), and had difficulty accepting the concept of maintenance on a narcotic. As a result of these concerns, the 1974 Narcotic Addict Treatment Act, which gave control to the Justice Department over who could dispense methadone as a maintenance drug, was passed; that system continues into the 21st century.

There continue to be major arguments for and against methadone maintenance; for example, addicts in this program avoid unsterile needles from drug sharing and hence they avoid this particular risk for the transmission of sexually transmitted diseases. They also receive a drug that is approved by the Food and Drug Administration (FDA), rather than drugs on the street, which are often adulterated with other substances and whose purity varies widely.

Many addicts on the program can lead normal lives and hold jobs. On the negative side, methadone is a narcotic and individuals in methadone maintenance programs are still addicts. In addition, some methadone patients receive an extra amount of methadone to get them through a long weekend or for other reasons and they sell the drug. Some methadone users continue to abuse other drugs. As a result, methadone maintenance programs continue to be regarded as controversial by some experts.

Modern Treatments

Today, medications such as buprenorphine and naltrexone are used to treat individuals addicted to narcotics, although some heroin addicts remain on methadone maintenance programs. Benzodiazepines may be used to treat individuals who experience difficult detoxification from drugs.

Most drug addicts who are treated receive outpatient therapy, although some receive treatment in a hospital or a rehabilitative setting. Often the wealthy are more likely to receive treatment, since they can pay the fees and do not have to go on a waiting list to receive treatment. Another reason why many addicts do not receive treatment is that they refuse treatment or fail to acknowledge that they have a problem.

In the 21st century, there are increasing numbers of facilities that deal with the diverse needs of addicts, including those who are mentally ill in addition to being addicted to drugs, women who are pregnant addicts, gay and lesbian addicts, adolescent addicts, and so forth, although arguably there are still insufficient facilities to deal with the needs of most addicted individuals.

As in centuries past, most addicts who undergo residential treatment eventually return to their home environment and face the same stressors and inducements to use drugs they had in the past. Membership in twelve-step organizations such as Narcotics Anonymous or Cocaine Anonymous can be helpful, as well as regular counseling sessions.

Considering the Historical Use of Alcohol

Alcohol has been a "social lubricant" as well as a drug of abuse for thousands of years. Fermented honey was probably the first form of alcohol, used in about 8000 B.C.E. The ancient Egyptians made their own beer in 3700 B.C.E. Wine was referred to in the ancient Code of Hammurabi in about 1700 B.C.E.

The ancient Egyptians provided home treatment for people who were dependent on wine or beer, and the Greeks and Romans supported the idea of public institutions for alcoholics.

In the 1700s, gin was very cheap and also very much abused by much of the population in Europe. According to Levinthal, gin consumption in England had increased by 22 times over the consumption in 1685.

In the United States, and in the early days of the Pilgrims, alcohol was considered an acceptable part of life in everyday rituals, although public drunkenness was frowned upon.

In later years, as in the late 19th century and the early 20th century, excessive alcohol consumption was increasingly considered socially unacceptable, and some individuals turned to drugs laced with morphine or cocaine, regarding themselves as on a higher plane than those who relied upon alcohol. In addition, others used patent medicines that included both drugs and alcohol—although often they were unaware of the contents of the drugs they used.

Alcoholic Nostrums

A survey in the *Ladies' Home Journal* revealed that 75 percent of the women in the Women's Christian Temperance Union (WCTU) who were polled were regular consumers of alcohol-laced products, such as Lydia Pinkham's Vegetable Compound. The WCTU was an anti-alcohol organization popular in the 1890s. This was not necessarily a hypocritical act, as in those days, the producers of patent medicines were not compelled to include the ingredients of their products on the labels of the drugs. So the WCTU women probably did not know that they were consuming the item that they so actively lobbied against. However, some of them apparently *did* realize that alcohol was included in these remedies, and they justified their use as medicinal and therefore acceptable.

It is interesting to note that Lydia Pinkham's Vegetable Compound, used to treat illnesses among women, was a concoction that was 20 percent alcohol (40 proof). Ironically, the Pinkhams had refused to sell alcohol in their grocery store in Lynn, Massachusetts, in the 1870s, in contrast to other grocery stores, and this refusal had seriously affected their sales because competitor stores were willing to sell alcohol. In a battle to survive, Lydia Pinkham began selling her vegetable compound, replete with alcohol, which was a rousing and nationwide success.

Alcohol in Early America and the Eighteenth Century

In early America, as in Europe, alcohol was often drunk instead of the often contaminated water or soured milk, and many of the colonists relied heavily on beer, ale, and hard cider. Alcohol was also used to treat headaches, infection, fever, and depression. According to Catherine Gilbert Murdock, "Colonists considered alcohol essential to manual labor; indeed to day-to-day survival. They drank upon waking, with breakfast, lunch, and dinner; during 'grog time' pauses in shop and field work; and at every social event. Employers often paid laborers in drink or drinking binges."

Alcohol was also commonly used during the Revolutionary War and the doctor Benjamin Rush was very concerned about this abuse. He was physician general of the Continental Army and signed the Declaration of Independence.

According to William L. White, "Rush's first professional recognition of the problem of alcohol involved the level of drunkenness among soldiers of the Continental Army—an issue of concern to George Washington as well. In 1777, Rush issued a strong condemnation of the use of distilled spirits;

his condemnation was published and distributed to all soldiers." It was also Dr. Rush who first expressed the idea that a chronic state of intoxication by alcohol was a progressive medical condition and a form of slow suicide. He was also the first doctor to express his belief that the only way to deal with the inebriate was total abstinence from alcohol.

Rush's treatments for alcoholics were painful and dangerous, based on the lack of medical knowledge at the time; for example, he frequently used bloodletting for patients and induced sweating and vomiting.

According to White, the term *alcoholism* was first coined in 1849 by the Swedish doctor Magnus Huss, who described it as a condition of chronic intoxication, physical problems, and the disruption of the individual's normal life. However, Huss's term was not adopted for nearly a century more with the founding of Alcoholics Anonymous in the 1930s. Before then, in most cases, individuals who were dependent on alcohol were referred to as drunkards, inebriates, sots, tipplers, and by other negatively charged labels.

Attitudes toward Alcohol in Victorian America of the Nineteenth Century

Contrary to the situation with opiate abuse and addiction in the 19th century, when most drug addicts were middle- and upper-class females, alcoholism was overwhelmingly a male problem in the 1800s. It was also a very prevalent problem. According to author Levinthal, in 1830, the average per capita consumption of alcohol in the United States was five drinks per day, which is about four times the average level of alcohol consumption in the 21st century. Many people at that time took whiskey breaks at 11 A.M. and 4 P.M. every day except Sunday.

Today it is a basic axiom that Prohibition in the 20th century was a failure, yet historians state that there were valid reasons for a strong desire to eliminate the use of alcohol at that time. According to author Catherine Gilbert Murdock in *Domesticating Drink: Women, Men, and Alcohol in America 1870–1940*, alcohol abuse in the 19th and early 20th centuries was at a massive scale unknown to most Americans in the 21st century.

Says Gilbert Murdock, "Public drunkards were a pathetic, everyday spectacle in villages and cities throughout America. Drink really did kill men and ruin families, and millions of citizens felt that the best way to meet the crisis would be to eliminate alcoholic beverages."

Although many men consumed alcohol, women were actively discouraged from drinking. Gilbert Murdock indicates that one reason was that scientists of the late 19th century believed that even moderate consumption of alcohol would harm each generation that followed, to a successively greater extent, such that their children would be at risk for becoming drinkers and their grandchildren would be at an even greater risk. Clearly, these scientists did not understand that behavior does not affect basic genetic structure or genetic predispositions—at least as far as is known today.

In the latter part of the 19th century, the saloon, a bastion of male drinking, became a popular location for many men. Says Gilbert Murdock, "In a world lacking cheap restaurants, public rest rooms, libraries, meeting halls, even check-cashing facilities, the saloon served as an oasis." Of course, this oasis was not open to females, unless they were barmaids or prostitutes. Gilbert Murdock indicates that the saloon was ubiquitous and in some working-class neighborhoods, there was one saloon for every 400 residents.

The Temperance Movement

Although most people think of women's groups when they think of the passage of the Eighteenth Amendment, which banned the manufacture or sale of alcohol, there were several major predecessors to this law. For example, there were temperance groups in many states, and in 1836, there were 229,000 temperance group members in New York (also known as "drys" versus those opposed to temperance, or "wets"); however, this number declined to 131,000 by 1839. However, temperance was an important cause nationwide and according to Gilbert Murdock, about 10 percent of the population in the United States in the late 1830s were members of temperance societies.

One briefly very successful group were the Washingtonians. This group was formed by 20 men who met every night at a drinking club in Baltimore, Maryland; however, one night, an argument arose over whether proponents of tem-

perance were hypocrites or true believers. Four club members went to a lecture by a minister on the virtues of temperance. They returned and discussed the matter with the others and six of the members decided to form their own temperance club, which they called the Washingtonian Total Abstinence Society. They charged 25 cents to join, and dues of 12 cents per month, meeting weekly.

According to White in *Slaying the Dragon: The History of Addiction Treatment and Recovery in America,*

> Instead of the debates, formal speeches, and abstract principles that had been on the standard temperance meeting agenda, the main bill of fare at a Washingtonian meeting was *experience sharing*—confessions of alcoholic debauchery followed by glorious accounts of personal reformation. Following these opening presentations by established members, newly arrived alcoholics with bloated faces and trembling hands were offered the opportunity to join. As each newcomer came forward, he was asked to tell a little of his own story, then sign the abstinence pledge amid the cheers of onlookers. This ritual of public confession and public signing of the pledge carried great emotional power for those participating.

The Washingtonian movement was extremely popular. It spread throughout the country, and at its height, an estimated 600,000 pledges of abstinence from alcohol were signed. However, by 1845, the organization started to decline and most chapters were no longer active after 1847. Picking up the slack, many fraternal organizations nationwide adopted a temperance philosophy and loomed large between 1842 and 1850. Says White, "The fraternal temperance orders used group cohesion, mutual surveillance, and elaborate cultural trappings—secret handshakes, secret passwords, symbols, elaborate uniforms, and ceremonies—to bolster their resolve to keep the pledge [of sobriety]."

One such group, the Sons of Temperance, was founded in 1842 by 16 men and in the next 10 years grew to more than 250,000 members and chapters in every state. This group's popularity later declined, but by 1882, it still had 73,000 members. This group helped destitute alcoholics and the newly sober, offering many activities, such as plays and organized sports.

Even larger was the Independent Order of Good Templars, founded in 1851 and with 2.9 million members by 1876. This group was dedicated to total abstinence and supported the prohibition of the manufacture and sale of alcohol.

The Women's Christian Temperance Union (WCTU) was a major factor in the temperance movement, and in the early 1890s, the WCTU had nearly 150,000 members nationwide. A key aspect of the WCTU was the underlying belief that women were beings who were somehow above the evils of drink (or should be). Nearly all treatment facilities for alcoholics were for men.

As indicated by Gilbert Murdock in *Domestic Drink: Women, Men, and Alcohol in America 1870–1940*, "Women alcoholics, barred from treatment or sympathy by their own denial and others' prejudices, are one of the great tragedies of the period. Yet one must point out that the association of alcohol and alcoholism with men was essential to the creation of such groups as the WCTU—the development of women's social and political consciousness based on their inherently moral image. In this emphatic gender solidarity, however, women drinkers remained marginalized."

Treatment during the Nineteenth Century

In the latter part of the 19th century, there was a rapid growth of treatment centers for alcoholics. In 1870, there were six such facilities in the United States, which grew to more than 100 facilities by the turn of the century. The first state-funded institution for alcoholics in the country was the Massachusetts State Hospital for Dipsomaniacs and Inebriates, in Foxboro, which opened its doors in 1893.

Treatment for alcoholics in past years ranged from the compassionate to the barbaric, such as forced sterilization of institutionalized alcoholic women in the early 20th century, because it was believed they would have defective children and that they were promiscuous. Some alcoholics received electric shock therapy while others received frontal lobotomies, which Doctors Walter Freeman and James Watts first performed in 1936, believing the procedure would cure alcoholism by eliminating the craving for alcohol.

It did not; one account in William L. White's *Slaying the Dragon: The History of Addiction Treatment and Recovery in America* discusses the case of a patient who was treated for his alcoholism with a lobotomy: "Following the procedure, the patient dressed and, pulling a hat down over his bandaged head, slipped out of the hospital in search of a drink. Freeman and Watts spent Christmas Eve, 1936, searching the bars for this patient, whom they eventually found and returned to the hospital in a state of extreme intoxication."

In the 19th century, aversion therapy was a common method of treatment. According to White, the Swedish Treatment comprised using whiskey to induce aversion: Said White, "In fact, that is all they could drink—whiskey, whiskey-saturated coffee, whiskey-saturated tea, and whiskey-saturated milk. All meals and all snacks, regardless of fare, were saturated with whiskey. Patients wore whiskey-sprayed clothes and slept in whiskey-saturated sheets. The goal was to satiate and sicken the appetite for alcohol and leave one begging for pure water." It is not known whether this treatment was effective.

Counseling was rarely used, unless it was the use of psychoanalysis, which was ineffective at treating alcoholism.

Most treatment institutions that opened in the 19th century were closed by about 1925, with the exception of private facilities and state psychiatric hospitals. By that time, wealthy alcoholics paid for private treatment and those without wealth were institutionalized with the mentally ill under extremely poor circumstances.

Most alcoholics treated in the 19th century were males, and most treatment was ineffectual or even harmful; for example, at the Franklin Reformatory Home for Inebriates, which opened its gates in Philadelphia in 1872, treatment was composed of bed rest as well as the administration of arsenic, strychnine, and electrical shock. In the few treatment centers for female alcoholics, treatment often consisted of abstinence and kindness—which alone were not effective albeit better than poisoning or shocking patients.

The treatments used in the 19th century varied from healthy diets to hydrotherapy, electric shock therapy, and drugs. According to White, some of the drugs used to treat alcoholics between 1860 and 1930 were whiskey, beer, cannabis, belladonna, cocaine, and many others that not only were not effective in treating alcoholism but were also harmful.

Many "miraculous cures," which were inefficacious, were sold to desperate yet hopeful consumers in the 19th century. In some cases, wives and family members were encouraged to treat the alcoholic without his knowledge. The directions were to sprinkle 15–20 drops of Formula A in the alcoholic's first drink, and if that failed to cause vomiting, sprinkle another 15–20 drops in the next drink that was consumed. Formula A contained ipecac, a drug that induces vomiting. Clearly, this was an unethical and dangerous treatment.

Special diets for alcoholics were popular in the 19th century and into the 20th century, especially diets that promoted vegetables or vegetarianism. Some believed that eating red meat could induce a craving for alcohol and thus should be avoided altogether. Many water cures were also popular, such as cold showers or Turkish baths.

Bizarre and Promising Treatments in the Early Twentieth Century

Some treatments for alcoholism in the early part of the 20th century were extremely strange while others were promising. The equine antialcohol antibody was one of the strange treatments. This was an alleged vaccine developed in about 1903 by researchers. They created alcohol dependence in horses and then injected their blood into nonalcoholic horses, who were reportedly revulsed by alcohol. They then made what they believed was an antialcohol antibody from the horse blood and applied it to the skin of human alcoholics. It did not work.

One drug that did prove effective was developed accidentally in 1947, according to White. Danish researchers were testing disulfiram, a drug for the treatment of worms. They each tested the drug on themselves to see whether it was toxic and did not notice any effect. However, later in the day they both had a few drinks, and each had an extremely severe reaction of nausea and vomiting. The researchers, Erik Jacobsen and Jens Hald, then speculated that this drug might be effective in treating alcoholism. Disulfiram (Antabuse) was found to be effective as an aversive treatment and

it is still in use in treatment facilities in the United States and the world.

A popular treatment in the early part of the 20th century was the Lambert-Towns Treatment, which used a regimen during withdrawal from alcohol of such drugs as belladonna, strychnine, digitalis, and hyoscyamus.

Some facilities offered convulsive therapies and induced seizures with drugs. This procedure was largely supplanted by electroconvulsive therapy.

Prohibition: The Eighteenth Amendment

The Eighteenth Amendment, also informally known as Prohibition, passed in 1917 and was ratified in January 1919, after years of extremely active lobbying by temperance groups. This law banned the manufacture and sale of alcoholic beverages, with the hope that problems of alcohol abuse and alcoholism would end. Interestingly, the law did not ban the purchase or consumption of alcohol, and thus individuals who drank were not arrested. Specifically, the law banned "the manufacture, sale, or transportation of intoxicating liquors within, the importation thereof into, or the exportation thereof from the Untied States and all territory subject to the jurisdiction thereof for beverage purposes."

However, many individuals in the United States were actively "wet" (as opposed to the "drys") and continued to obtain alcohol. In fact, fortunes were made among those engaged in running rum and other alcoholic beverages from Canada and other countries to the United States. Prohibition was considered such a failure that President Franklin Roosevelt signed the legislation that became the Twenty-first Amendment, overturning the Eighteenth Amendment, in 1933, and ratification quickly followed by the end of 1933.

Alcoholics Anonymous

No discussion of alcoholism would be complete without at least a mention of Alcoholics Anonymous, a stunningly successful self-help group that began in the United States and has chapters worldwide. Founded in 1935 by Bill W. (William Griffith Wilson) and Dr. Bob (Dr. Robert Smith), the group is a fellowship of fellow alcoholics who assist each other in attaining and maintaining sobriety. Complete abstinence from alcohol is considered necessary and the group's philosophy is included in their Twelve Steps. For example, the first step is to acknowledge powerlessness over alcohol and to admit that one's life is not manageable.

Some critics have argued that it is possible for alcoholics to learn to drink in moderation, rather than avoiding all alcohol for life, but this view appears to be in the minority among many experts.

Twenty-first-Century Treatment for Alcoholism

Today, both inpatient and outpatient treatment is available for alcoholics. Many programs also support membership in Alcoholics Anonymous for recovering alcoholics. Therapy is also useful. Sometimes medications are used to treat alcoholism, such as disulfarm, a drug used for aversion therapy, which causes copious vomiting if the individual consumes even a tiny amount of alcohol. Other drugs that are commonly used to reduce the craving for alcohol are acamprosate (Campral) and naltrexone (ReVia).

Psychotherapy is a common component of treatment, and often a combination of medications and therapy is the most effective treatment for alcoholism. Therapists teach alcoholics how to avoid alcohol and how to deal with others who may encourage or even pressure them to drink. They also help patients cope with stress, because often severe stress can lead to relapse.

Global Alcohol Consumption

According to the Department of Mental Health and Substance Abuse of the World Health Organization (WHO), in 2004, there are an estimated 2 billion people in the world who consume alcoholic beverages and of these, 76.3 have alcohol use disorders (alcohol abuse and alcoholism). Of individuals ages 15 and older in countries that have total recorded alcohol per capita consumption, in terms of liters of pure alcohol, the countries with the average greatest consumption in 2004 were Uganda (19.47 liters per year), Luxembourg (17.54), the Czech Republic (16.21), Ireland (14.46), the Republic of Moldova (13.88), and France (13.54). Consumption in the United States was 8.51.

The countries with the least alcohol consumption, or zero, were Iran, Kuwait, the Libyan Arab Jamahirya, Saudi Arabia, Somalia, and Bangladesh.

In considering beverage-specific consumption, the top consumers of beer were the Czech Republic and Ireland. The top consumers of wine were Luxembourg and France, and the top consumer of spirits was the Republic of Moldova. The United States did not make the top 20 list of consumption in any of these categories.

In terms of alcoholism (alcohol dependence), the WHO report used information from the years 1999–2002 on individuals in 34 countries. The countries with the highest percentage of individuals with alcoholism were Poland (12.2 percent), Brazil (11.2 percent), and Peru (10.6 percent). The rate for the United States was 7.7 percent.

In considering only males who were alcohol dependent, according to the WHO report, the greatest percentages were found in South Africa (27.6 percent), Poland (23.3 percent), and Peru (17.8 percent). The rate in the United States for males was 10.8 percent.

In considering only females who were alcohol dependent, the WHO researchers found the greatest percentages among women in South Africa (9.9 percent), Brazil (5.7 percent), and the United States (4.8 percent).

The WHO report also looked at heavy episodic drinking (between five and seven drinks on any one occasion) among youths in different countries, which varied by country. Very high rates were seen among males in Denmark (62 percent), Poland (41 percent), and the United Kingdom (33 percent). The rate for males in the United States was 11.4 percent.

Among females, high rates of heavy episodic drinking were found in Denmark (54 percent), Ireland (32 percent), and the United Kingdom (27 percent). The rate for females in the United States was 9.9 percent.

Conclusion

Substance abuse has been a problem for millennia and will probably continue to be a problem for many people into the future. This does not mean, however, that the problems generated by drug and alcohol dependence, such as illness, injuries, and deaths, as well as ruined relationships and lost jobs, should be ignored or written off as impossible to solve. Rather, it may mean that individuals today and in the future should take a look at what has been done in the past, considering the mistakes that have been made and seeking to avoid them, and seeking promising alternatives.

It is our hope that it may be possible for society to achieve a balance, recognizing that drug and alcohol abuse are major problems, but not demonizing those who are caught up in addiction. Whenever possible, treatment should be urged upon those who are afflicted with addiction, as well as follow-ups to help them avoid relapse. At the same time, individuals need to learn to take responsibility for the consequences of their actions. It is a difficult balancing act but one that, if it can be achieved, would be well worth it.

Acker, Caroline Jean. "From All Purpose Anodyne to Marker of Deviance: Physicians' Attitudes towards Opiates in the US from 1890 to 1940." In *Drugs and Narcotics in History,* edited by Roy Porter and Mikulas Teich, 114–132. Cambridge: Cambridge University Press, 1995.

———. *Creating the American Junkie: Addiction Research in the Classic Era of Narcotic Control.* Baltimore, Md.: Johns Hopkins University Press, 2002.

Ashenberg Straussner, Shulamith, and Patricia Rose Attia. "Women's Addiction and Treatment through a Historical Lens." In *The Handbook of Addiction Treatment for Women,* edited by Sulamith Ashenbrugh Straussner, New York: Jossey-Bass, 2002.

Berridge, Virginia, and Sarah Mars. "History of Addictions." *Journal of Epidemiology Community Health* 58 (2004): 747–750.

Committee on Addictions of the Group for the Advancement of Psychiatry. "Responsibility and Choice in Addiction." *Psychiatric Services* 53, no. 6 (June 2002): 707–713.

Corley, T. A. B. "Interactions between the British and American Patent Medicine Industries 1708–1914." *Business and Economic History* 16 (1987): 111–129.

Courtwright, David T. *Dark Paradise: A History of Opiate Addiction in America.* Cambridge, Mass.: Harvard University Press, 2001.

Dally, Ann. "Anomalies and Mysteries in the 'War on Drugs.'" In *Drugs and Narcotics in History,* edited by Roy Porter and Mikulas Teich, 199–215. Cambridge: Cambridge University Press, 1995.

Das, G. "Cocaine Abuse in North America: A Milestone in History." *Journal of Clinical Pharmacology* 33 (1993): 296–310.

Department of Mental Health and Substance Abuse. *Global Status Report on Alcohol 2004.* Geneva: Switzerland: World Health Organization, 2004. Available online. URL: http://www.who.int/substance_abuse/publications/global_status_report_2004_overview.pdf. Downloaded July 31, 2006.

De Quincey, Thomas. *Confessions of an English Opium-Eater.* Mineola, N.Y.: Dover, 1995.

Erlen, Jonathon, and Joseph F. Spillane, eds. *Federal Drug Control: The Evolution of Policy and Practice.* Binghamton, N.Y.: Pharmaceutical Products Press, 2004.

Executive Office of the President. *Synthetic Drug Control Strategy: A Focus on Methamphetamine and Prescription Drug Abuse.* Washington, D.C.: Office of National Drug Control Policy.

Hodgson, Barbara. *In the Arms of Morpheus: The Tragic History of Laudanum, Morphine, and Patent Medicines.* Buffalo, N.Y.: Firefly Books, 2001.

Johnston, Lloyd D., et al. *Monitoring the Future: National Survey Results on Drug Use, 1975–2004.* Vol. 2, *College Students and Adults Ages 19–45.* Bethesda, Md.: National Institute on Drug Abuse, National Institutes of Health, 2005.

Kandall, Stephen R. *Substance and Shadow: Women and Addiction in the United States,* Cambridge, Mass.: Harvard University Press, 1996.

Karch, Steven B., M.D. "Cocaine: History, Use, Abuse." *Journal of the Royal Society of Medicine* 92 (August 1999): 393–397.

Levinthal, Charles F. "The History of Drug Use and Drug Legislation." In *Drugs, Society, and Criminal Justice.* Boston: Allyn & Bacon, 2006.

Library of Congress. "Today in History: May 8, "Coca Cola." Available online. URL: http://memory.loc.gov/ammem/today/may08.html. Downloaded July 3, 2006.

Loeb, Lori. "George Fulford and Victorian Patent Medicine Men: Quack Mercenaries or Smilesian Entrepreneurs?" *CBMH/BCHM* 16 (1999): 125–145.

Markel, Howard, M.D. "The Accidental Addict." *New England Journal of Medicine* 352, no. 10 (March 10, 2005): 966–968.

MacCoun, Robert H., and Peter Reuter. *Drug War Heresies: Learning from Other Vices, Times, and Places.* Cambridge: Cambridge University Press, 2001.

Maehle, Andreas-Holder. "Pharmacological Experimentation with Opium in the Eighteenth Century." In *Drugs and Narcotics in History,* edited by Roy Porter and Mikulas Teich, 52–76. Cambridge: Cambridge University Press, 1995.

Meldrum, Marcia L. "A Capsule History of Pain Management." *Journal of the American Medical Association* 290, no. 18 (November 12, 2003): 2,470–2,475.

Morgan, H. Wayne. *Drugs in America. A Social History 1800–1980.* Syracuse, N.Y.: Syracuse University Press, 1981.

Murdock, Catherine Gilbert. *Domesticating Drink: Women, Men, and Alcohol in America, 1870–1940.* Baltimore, Md.: Johns Hopkins University Press, 1998.

Musto, David F. *The American Disease: Origins of Narcotic Control.* 3d ed. New York: Oxford University Press, 1999.

Parascandola, John. "Patent Medicines in Nineteenth-Century America," *Caduceus: A Museum Quarterly for the Health Sciences* 1, no. 1 (Spring 1985): 1–41.

Sandmaier, Marian. *The Invisible Alcoholics: Women and Alcohol.* 2d ed. Blue Ridge Summit, Pa.: TAB Books, 1992.

Scarborough, John. "The Opium Poppy in Hellenistic and Roman Medicine." In *Drugs and Narcotics in History,* edited by Roy Porter and Mikulas Teich, 4–23. Cambridge: Cambridge University Press, 1995.

Schoenberg, Bruce S., M.D. "Coke's the One: The Centennial of the 'Ideal Brain Tonic' That Became a Symbol of America." *Southern Medical Journal* 81, no. 1 (1988): 69–74.

Shanti, Christine M., M.D., and Charles E. Lucas, M.D. "Cocaine and the Critical Care Challenge." *Critical Care Medicine* 31 (2003) 1,851–1,859.

Speaker, Susan L. "Creating a Monster: Newspapers, Magazines, and the Framing of America's Drug Problem," *Molecular Interventions* 2, no. 4 (July 2002): 201–204. Available online. URL: http://molinterv.aspetjournals.org/cgi/reprint.2/4/201.pdf. Downloaded July 15, 2006.

Spillane, Joseph F. "Building a Drug Control Regime, 1919–1930." In *Federal Drug Control: The Evolution of Policy and Practice,* edited by Jonathon Erlen and Joseph F. Spillane, 25–59. Binghamton, N.Y.: Pharmaceutical Products Press, 2004.

———. *Cocaine: From Medical Marvel to Modern Menace in the United States, 1884–1920.* Baltimore, Md.: Johns Hopkins University Press, 2000.

Tracy, Sarah W., and Caroline Jean Acker, eds. *Altering American Consciousness: The History of Alcohol and Drug Use in the United States, 1800–2000.* Amherst, Mass.: University of Massachusetts Press, 2004.

United Nations Office on Drugs and Crime, *World Drug Report 2006.* Vol. 1, *Analysis.* United Nations, June 2006. Available online. URL: http://www.unodc.org/pdf/WDR_2006/wdr2006_volume1.pdf. Downloaded on July 28, 2006.

White, William L. *Slaying the Dragon: The History of Addiction Treatment and Recovery in America.* Bloomington, Ill.: Chestnut Health Systems/Lighthouse Institute, 1998.

Winger, Gail, James H. Woods, and Frederick G. Hofmann. *A Handbook on Drug and Alcohol Abuse: The Biomedical Aspects.* New York: Oxford University Press, 2004.

ENTRIES A to Z

abstinence Refraining from the use of alcohol and/or illicit drugs or misused prescription drugs. Many support groups, such as Alcoholics Anonymous and its spin-off organizations, believe that the individual must forgo all use of the substance to which he or she is addicted and this abstinence must continue for life. They do not believe, for example, that a person who was once an alcoholic can ever have one drink, because they believe that one drink will lead to readdiction.

Because abstinence is very difficult, particularly in the beginning (although some individuals say it continues to be difficult throughout life), support groups can help individuals when they feel a strong craving for ALCOHOL or another substance to refrain from its use.

There are several drugs that promote abstinence from alcohol: DISULFIRAM (Antabuse), ACAMPROSATE (Campral), and NALTREXONE (ReVia). When disulfiram is taken, any amount of alcohol, even a tiny amount that is consumed in food, will lead to extreme nausea and vomiting. The drug is meant to be an aversive way to avoid alcohol and continues to be used in treatment centers nationwide. Other medications that are used to treat alcoholism, such as acamprosate and naltrexone, are intended to decrease alcohol craving rather than react with alcohol intake.

See also ALCOHOLISM.

abuse, alcohol The excessive use of alcohol, which affects an individual's behavior but yet does not rise to the higher level of ALCOHOLISM. However, alcohol abuse can worsen to a dependence (addiction) on alcohol. Many individuals who abuse alcohol also abuse other substances, such as one or more illegal drugs. ALCOHOL is the most commonly abused drug in the United States, followed by MARIJUANA.

Alcohol Abusers
According to the National Institute on Alcohol Abuse and Alcoholism (NIAAA) in the United States, alcohol abusers fit at least *one* of the following criteria that are directly caused by their excessive drinking:

- They fail to fulfill their responsibilities at work, school, or home.
- They drive or operate dangerous equipment while under the influence of alcohol.
- They have been arrested for an alcohol-related problem, such as driving while intoxicated or assaulting another person when drunk.
- They drink despite family or personal relationship problems that are either created or worsened by the excessive drinking.

According to the NIAAA, 4.7 percent of the population of the United States, or 9.7 million people, were alcohol abusers in 2002.

The American Psychiatric Association (APA) has its own definition of substance abuse (including alcohol and other substances) in the *Diagnostic and Statistical Manual of Mental Disorders, Fourth Edition, Text Revision (DSM-IV-TR)*. The APA includes such criteria as recurrent substance use that causes the failure of the individual to fulfill important obligations at work, school, or home, as well as the recurrent substance use in physically hazardous situations and recurrent substance-related legal problems.

See also ADDICTION/DEPENDENCE; ALCOHOL ABUSE AND DEPENDENCE AND HEALTH PROBLEMS; ALCOHOL ABUSE/DEPENDENCE; ALCOHOLISM; DELIRIUM TREMENS; DRUG ABUSE AND DEPENDENCE AND HEALTH PROBLEMS; GENETIC PREDISPOSITIONS AND ENVIRONMENTAL EFFECTS IN SUBSTANCE ABUSE.

American Psychiatric Association. *Diagnostic and Statistical Manual of Mental Disorders*, 4th ed. Washington, D.C.: American Psychiatric Association, 2000.

Grant, Bridget F., et al. "The 12-Month Prevalence and Trends in DSM-IV Alcohol Abuse and Dependence: United States, 1991–1992 and 2001–2002." *Drug and Alcohol Dependence* 74 (2004): 223–234.

abuse, drugs   Drug abuse refers to the excessive use of drugs, whether they are legally prescribed medications (such as NARCOTICS that are prescribed for moderate to severe pain) or illegal drugs; however, this abuse does not rise to the level of drug dependence/ADDICTION. Despite this, a drug abuser may subsequently develop an addiction to drugs.

In general, the drug abuser has a CRAVING for the drug and sometimes may also have developed a TOLERANCE to it, thus needing greater amounts of the drug in order to achieve the same effects desired by the abuser (such as euphoria, intoxication, oblivion, or other effects). However, he or she usually does not experience serious effects from WITHDRAWAL from the drug. In addition, the drug abuser does not center his or her life on acquiring and using the drug.

See also ADDICTION/DEPENDENCE; ADOLESCENTS AND SUBSTANCE ABUSE; ALCOHOL ABUSE AND DEPENDENCE AND HEALTH PROBLEMS; ALPRAZOLAM/ALPRAZOLAM XR (XANAX/XANAX XR) AMPHETAMINE; ANABOLIC STEROIDS; COCAINE; COUGH SYRUP; CRIME AND CRIMINALS; DATE RAPE DRUGS; DEXTROMETHORPHAN; DIAZEPAM; DIVERSION, DRUG; GENETIC PREDISPOSITIONS AND ENVIRONMENTAL EFFECTS IN SUBSTANCE ABUSE; HEROIN; HYDROCODONE; METHADONE; METHAMPHETAMINE; NARCOTICS; OPIATES; OXYCODONE; OXYCONTIN; PROPOXYPHENE; YOUNG ADULTS.

acamprosate (Campral)   A medication that is used to treat alcohol dependence (ALCOHOLISM) that was approved by the Food and Drug Administration for this purpose in 2004 and was first used in the United States in 2005. It is unknown exactly how the drug works, but it may reduce the symptoms that accompany ABSTINENCE from alcohol, such as anxiety and insomnia. In most cases, patients are withdrawn from alcohol for several days or weeks prior to starting acamprosate.

Some studies indicate that a combination of acamprosate and NALTREXONE (ReVia) (another medication used to treat alcoholism), along with behavioral therapy, is the best treatment for alcoholism. This view was discussed in *Alcohol and Alcoholism* in 2006 in relation to a study of 236 patients in Australia. However, another study in a 2006 issue of the *Journal of the American Medical Association*, with 2,383 subjects, indicated that naltrexone and/or behavioral therapy worked significantly better than acamprosate. However, although studies that looked at abstinence showed poor performance for acamprosate, other studies that looked at the absolute decrease in alcohol consumption showed acamprosate to be effective.

See Appendix XV for information on contraindications, serious adverse reactions, and other information, not only for acamprosate but also for DISULFIRAM (Antabuse) and naltrexone, all medications that are used to treat alcoholism.

Acamprosate should not be used by individuals who have severe kidney impairment. Common side effects that may occur with this medication are diarrhea, nausea, abdominal pain, headache, back pain, and chills.

See also DETOXIFICATION; WITHDRAWAL.

Anton, Raymond F., M.D. "Combined Pharmacotherapies and Behavioral Interventions for Alcohol Dependence: The COMBINE Study: A Randomized Controlled Trial." *Journal of the American Medical Association* 295, no. 17 (May 3, 2006): 2,003–2,017.

Feeney, Gerald F. X., et al. "Combined Acamprosate and Naltrexone, with Cognitive Behavioural Therapy Is Superior to Either Medication Alone for Alcohol Abstinence: A Single Centres' Experience with Pharmacotherapy." *Alcohol and Alcoholism* 41, no. 3 (2006): 321–327.

accidental overdose deaths   Deaths that result from an excessive intake of drugs and/or alcohol. Such deaths exclude SUICIDE. Some studies indicate that accidental overdose deaths may be on the increase in the United States. For example, a study in the *American Journal of Preventive Medicine* in 2006 analyzed 1,906 unintentional accidental deaths from medical examiner statistics over the period 1994 to 2003 in New Mexico, the state with the highest rate of drug-induced deaths since 1990.

The researchers found that the rate of unintentional prescription drug overdose death increased from 1.9 people per 100,000 in 1994 to 5.3 per 100,000 in 2003, a 179 percent increase. They also found that the highest rates of unintentional drug overdose involved illegal drugs. In considering *all* the drug overdose deaths, the researchers found that about 77 percent of the people who died were male and about 55 percent were Hispanic, 40 percent were white non-Hispanic, and 2 percent were American Indians. The median age of the decedent was 40 years old. About a third of the drug abuse deaths were caused by both alcohol and drugs in combination.

In limiting the consideration of deaths solely to those caused by prescription drugs alone, the researchers found that 56 percent of the decedents were male, and most were white non-Hispanics (63 percent) or Hispanics (34 percent). The median age at death was 44 years. Most of those who died had lived in metropolitan areas (70 percent).

Opioid painkillers were involved in 77 percent of the deaths caused by prescription drugs, followed by tranquilizers (34 percent), antidepressants (26 percent), and cointoxication with over-the-counter drugs (10 percent). Note that the decedent may have used more than one category of drug that led to death.

The researchers also noted that the proximity to the Mexican border enabled many people to obtain prescription drugs that they could not obtain legally in the United States. They said, "It is probable that drug users chose to use the drugs that are most easily obtained; for instance, in parts of New Mexico near the Mexican border, prescription drugs may be more widely available than illicit drugs."

The researchers also advised physicians prescribing narcotic painkillers, "When prescribing opioid painkillers and other prescription drugs, a healthcare provider's patient encounter should include a discussion of the risks for addiction, the dangers associated with not taking the drug as directed, and the potential interactions that can occur when taking the drug in combination with other prescribed drugs."

See also DEATH; MALICIOUS POISONING.

Mueller, Mark R., et al. "Unintentional Prescription Drug Overdose Deaths in New Mexico, 1994–2003." *American Journal of Preventive Medicine* 30, no. 5 (2006): 423–429.

acquired immune deficiency syndrome (AIDS)/ human immunodeficiency virus (HIV)   Acquired immune deficiency syndrome (AIDS) is the long-term and very serious (and eventually fatal) disease that is caused by the HUMAN IMMUNODEFICIENCY VIRUS (HIV).

An estimated one million people in the United States had HIV/AIDS in 2004. The incidence of AIDS peaked in the United States in 1993 at 80,000 new cases, and the number of annual new cases declined steadily thereafter. In 2004, about 42,500 new cases of AIDS were reported. According to the Centers for Disease Control and Prevention (CDC), 157,252 people were diagnosed with HIV in 33 states in the years 2001–2004. Most people who have HIV or AIDS are male; of 38,553 people who were diagnosed with HIV/AIDS in 2004, 73 percent were male.

In considering the annual rate of reported AIDS cases by areas in the United States in 2004, the rate per 100,000 was the highest in the District of Colombia, or 179.2 people with AIDS per 100,000, followed by 39.7 people per 100,000 in New York and 33.5 per 100,000 in Florida.

An estimated 65 percent of males diagnosed with HIV/AIDS in 2004 contracted the virus through male-to-male sexual contact, according to the CDC. Sixteen percent of males who had HIV/AIDS contracted the virus through heterosexual contact, and 14 percent were infected through injection drug use. A combination of both male-to-male sexual contact and injection drug use led to infection in 5 percent of the male cases. In 1 percent of the cases of the 28,143 males who were diagnosed in 2004, the method of transmission was unknown.

Among the 10,410 females who were diagnosed with HIV/AIDS in 2004, in contrast to infected males, most infected females (78 percent) con-

TABLE I: NUMBER OF CASES AND MEANS OF TRANSMISSION OF AIDS
CASES THROUGH 2004, BY GENDER

Exposure Category	Estimated Number of AIDS Cases through 2004[1]		
	Male	Female	Cumulative Total
Male-to-male sexual contact	441,380	—	441,380
Injection drug use	176,162	72,651	248,813
Male-to-male sexual contact and injection drug use	64,833	—	64,833
Heterosexual contact	59,939	99,175	159,114
Other	14,085	6,636	20,721

[1] Includes persons with a diagnosis of AIDS from the beginning of the epidemic through 2004.
Source: Adapted from Centers for Disease Control and Prevention. "Basic Statistics." Available online. URL: from http://www.cdc.gov/hiv/topics/surveillance/basic.htm. Downloaded On May 11, 2006.

tracted the virus through heterosexual contact, while 20 percent were infected as a result of injection drug use. It is unknown how females obtained the virus in 2 percent of the cases. See Table I for more information.

It should not be assumed that only a few people die of AIDS because of greatly improved medical treatments. In 2004, 15,798 people died of AIDS, including 15,737 adults and adolescents and 61 children under age 13. (See Table II.) It should also be noted that both the numbers of people diagnosed with AIDS and the number of persons living with AIDS has begun to rise from 2002, although the death rate has fallen.

The AIDS infection first attracted the attention of medical experts in medical literature in 1981, when physicians discussed their discovery that young homosexual adults in Los Angeles, New York, and San Francisco were diagnosed with diseases that were not commonly seen in healthy individuals, such as *Pneumocystis carinii* and Kaposi's sarcoma. It was discovered that a virus caused an impairment in immune system resistance, which led to uncom-

mon diseases as well as to death. HIV was isolated as a virus in France in 1983, but it was not known for certain that HIV led to AIDS until 1984.

According to Dennis H. Osmond, the name *human immunodeficiency virus* was chosen in 1986 by the International Committee on the Taxonomy of Viruses. HIV-1 is the designation for the virus that causes AIDS and the broad majority of patients who had AIDS were infected with HIV-1, although in very rare isolated cases, the patient was infected with HIV-2.

When AIDS was first discovered by the general public, there was great concern among many people that the disease could be the end of Western civilization, and it was feared that the disease could be contracted by being in the presence of those infected with HIV. However, the general public eventually accepted that HIV was a blood-borne virus that could be contracted through infected blood or sexual contact with an infected person. In the early days of the awareness of the illness, some few people contracted HIV through contaminated blood obtained from blood transfu-

TABLE II: ESTIMATED NUMBERS OF AIDS DIAGNOSES, DEATHS, AND PERSONS LIVING WITH AIDS, 2001–2005

	2001	2002	2003	2004	2005	Cumulative (1981–2005)
AIDS diagnoses	38,079	38,408	39,666	39,524	40,608	952,629
AIDS deaths	16,980	16,641	17,404	17,453	16,316	530,756
Persons living with AIDS	331,482	353,249	375,511	397,582	421,873	n/a

Source: Centers for Disease Control and Prevention, "A Glance at the HIV/AIDS Epidemic." Department of Health and Human Services, June 2007. Available online. URL: http://www.cdc.gov/hiv/resources/factsheets/At-A-Glance.htm. Downloaded August 27, 2007.

sions; however, this route has long ceased to be a risk because of more extensive testing of blood used for transfusions.

Because of concern about possible discrimination against gays, many states did not report statistics on HIV or AIDS until the 1990s. As of this writing, all states provide statistical data on HIV and AIDS, although the federal government concentrates on data provided from 33 states, which data are used for analysis. (Sometimes statistics are reported in a combined manner, as with HIV/AIDS.)

In the 20th century, many people who had HIV and whose disease had progressed to AIDS died within a short period, such as months. Since that time, however, the situation has vastly improved. Although no cure for HIV or AIDS exists as of this writing, medical breakthroughs have provided effective treatments for many patients who are HIV-positive, so that their lives may be extended for years. As a result, the progression from HIV to AIDS has markedly slowed.

Some babies are born to HIV-infected mothers, and if they are treated as newborns, then they have a much better prognosis. If the mothers were also drug addicted, such as users of injecting drugs such as heroin, the infants must undergo WITHDRAWAL from drugs as well.

The number of new pediatric AIDS cases has markedly decreased since 1994, when the U.S. Public Health Service (PHS) recommended that pregnant women be tested for HIV, and if the test result is positive, be treated. The PHS also recommended that newborn babies be tested as well. In 2003, an estimated 59 cases of pediatric AIDS occurred among children below age 13, compared to 187 cases in 1999. Note that children may also contract HIV as a result of sexual abuse by adults or through sharing of intravenous drugs, as well as by engaging in sex with other children or adolescents who are infected with HIV.

Symptoms and Diagnostic Path

Routine HIV screening is the best way to screen people for HIV/AIDS, and individuals who may be at risk (because of recent sexual contacts with individuals who are infected or those who are considered likely to be infected with the virus for other reasons) should be tested. In addition, intravenous

users of illicit drugs are also at high risk and they should be tested.

Patients may have no symptoms of HIV for years; however, over time, they become ill more frequently and recover much more slowly than others do from common infections and viruses. If the patient who has HIV is untreated, multiple illnesses can cause the condition to deteriorate to the level of AIDS. For example, individuals who have HIV are also prone to development of hepatitis C as well as other forms of liver disease that debilitate the body and can become life-threatening.

HIV is diagnosed with testing, such as with the enzyme immune assay (EIA) test or sometimes with the enzyme-linked immunosorbent assay (ELISA). The test results are usually available within one or two weeks. If the initial test result is positive, it is confirmed with a second test, usually the Western blot test.

There are also rapid HIV tests approved by the Food and Drug Administration (FDA) that can provide results in 20 minutes. If the rapid HIV test result is positive, a further confirming test is given. As of this writing in 2006, the rapid HIV tests approved by the FDA include the OraQuick Advance Rapid HIV1/2 Antibody Test, the Reveal G2 Rapid HIV-1 Antibody Test, the Uni-Gold Recombigen HIV Test, and the Multisport HIV-1/HIV-2 Rapid Test.

Home self-tests for HIV are available for purchase from pharmacies. A home test requires a finger prick of blood that is placed on a special card, which is then sent to a laboratory.

Treatment Options and Outlook

It is extremely important for all HIV patients to receive medical treatment, which can extend their lives for years or indefinitely. In past years, physicians told patients who were HIV-positive that at most, they could expect to live 10 years; however, with the advent of new medications, it is impossible to predict the number of years of survival for most patients. With the introduction in 1996 of highly active antiretroviral therapy (HAART), which is a customized combination of different medications, the outlook for HIV and AIDS greatly improved, although there is still no cure.

Physicians prescribing HAART take into account such factors as the patient's individual level of the virus, the CD4 lymphocyte count, and any clinical symptoms that are present. CD4 lymphocytes are white blood cells that are specifically targeted for infection and destruction by HIV.

Some medications that are used to treat drug addiction may interact with HAART; for example, HAART significantly decreases the level of METHADONE in the bloodstream. This can complicate the treatment of the HEROIN addict who has AIDS or HIV and who is receiving treatment with methadone. All patients who know that they have HIV or AIDS should inform their physician before starting methadone treatment. In addition, methadone clinics may wish to screen patients for HIV.

Researchers are studying whether the same interaction problems are associated with other medications used to treat drug dependence, such as BUPRENORPHINE.

There are also other risks with HAART, for example, an increased risk for neurological problems such as peripheral nerve damage. In addition, HAART has been reported to be linked to increased cholesterol levels as well as to an abnormal blood sugar (glucose) metabolism. Another major problem is medication compliance among patients: Because HAART reduces the viral load, some users mistakenly believe that they are cured and that they do not need to take the medication any longer. They may also believe that they can return to engaging in unsafe sex and/or injecting illegal drugs.

Risk Factors and Preventive Measures

Males who have sex with other males are at an increased risk for contracting HIV, as are those who engage in intravenous drug use involving shared needles. Adults who engage in unprotected heterosexual sex with others at risk for HIV are themselves also at risk for contracting the virus. Members of some races, such as African Americans, have an increased risk for death of AIDS compared to other races or ethnicities.

Sex workers (prostitutes) and individuals who engage in unprotected sex with multiple partners have an increased risk for contracting HIV. Young people have an increased risk for contracting HIV because they are more likely to engage in unsafe sex than older individuals.

Homosexual sex   Men who have sex with other men have a high risk for contracting HIV if they engage in unsafe sex, and as mentioned earlier, the majority of men who have HIV contracted the disease through homosexual sex.

Drug abuse   Drug abuse is strongly related to HIV/AIDS. Many drug abusers inject their drugs intravenously, using needles shared with others who are infected with HIV (as well as with other infections, such as HEPATITIS). They may also share cotton swabs and rinse water, also risky behavior.

In addition, because of the intoxicating and/or addictive effects of many illegal drugs, the risk for sexual contact with infected partners is increased. Since inhibitions are often decreased, the individual may act impulsively and, for example, fail to use condoms or choose to engage in unsafe sex acts, such as anal sex without condoms. In addition, some drug abusers engage in sex in exchange for drugs or for money to purchase the drugs to which they are addicted. One CDC study indicated that smokers of CRACK COCAINE had three times the risk of contracting HIV compared to others.

According to the National Institute on Drug Abuse, some animal studies have shown that some drugs, such as METHAMPHETAMINE, increase HIV viral replication, and thus they should be particularly avoided by individuals diagnosed with HIV or AIDS.

Some particular types of addicts, such as those who abuse multiple drugs, such as COCAINE and HEROIN, have an increased risk for contracting HIV, as do abusers of methamphetamine. At least in part, this risk is likely to be due to the fact that these drugs are often injected.

African Americans have a high risk   Some populations have a greater risk of HIV infection than others; for example, African Americans (including both males and females) accounted for about 13 percent of the population in the United States in 2004, but they represented about half of all diagnosed AIDS cases, or 178,000 people. They were followed by whites (30 percent) and Hispanics (18 percent).

The situation is more dramatic among African-American females, who accounted for 69 percent of the female HIV/AIDS diagnosed in 2003, or 19 times the rate found among white females and five times the rate among Hispanic females. Young African Americans ages 13–19 years represented about 15 percent of all the teenagers in the United States

TABLE III: ESTIMATED NUMBERS OF DIAGNOSES OF AIDS, BY RACE OR ETHNICITY

Race or Ethnicity	Estimated Number of AIDS Cases in 2004	Cumulative Estimated Number of AIDS Cases through 2004[1]
White, not Hispanic	12,013	375,155
Black, not Hispanic	20,965	389,278
Hispanic	8,672	177,164
Asian/Pacific Islander	488	7,317
American Indian/Alaska Native	193	3,084

[1] Includes persons with a diagnosis of AIDS from the beginning of the epidemic through 2004.
Source: Adapted from Centers for Disease Control and Prevention. "Cases of HIV/AIDS by Area of Residence, Diagnosed in 2004—33 States with Confidential Name-Based HIV Infection Reporting." *HIV/AIDS Surveillance Report* Department of Health and Human Services, Atlanta, 2005. Available online URL: http://www.cdc.gov/hiv/topics/surveilance/resources/report/pdf/2004SurveillanceReport.pdf. p. 12. Downloaded May 11, 2006.

in 2004, but they accounted for 66 percent of new AIDS cases. Among African Americans, HIV/AIDS is the leading cause of death among those ages 25–44 years, surpassing heart disease, accidents, cancer, and homicide.

This fact that HIV/AIDS is a serious problem among African Americans does not, however, mean that African Americans have a higher rate of drug addiction than other racial or ethnic minorities. In fact, research indicates that there is a higher rate of drug addiction among whites than African Americans: 8.3 percent for African Americans versus 9.6 percent for whites.

The cause of the markedly higher rate of HIV/AIDS among African Americans may have some explanations beyond drug abuse and addiction. These problems are not markedly greater among blacks compared to whites and other races and ethnicities; nor are African-American men more likely to be homosexual than men of other races.

According to the National Institute on Drug Abuse in their 2006 report, "The noted disparities may in part reflect data showing that African-Americans are predominant among those who become aware of their infection at later stages in the disease process, and who therefore represent lost opportunities for treatment." If this is a valid explanation, this means that individuals of other races who are infected with HIV may obtain treatment earlier in the illness, slowing the rate of progression of HIV to AIDS.

Those with multiple sex partners and/or sex workers As mentioned, individuals who have many sexual partners have a greater risk of con-

tracting HIV/AIDS than those who have sex with one or two partners or who are altogether abstinent. As a result, sex workers such as prostitutes are at risk for contracting HIV, particularly those who fail to take preventive measures, such as requiring males to use condoms. In addition, all individuals who engage in unprotected sex (without a condom) have an increased risk for contracting HIV, as do those who engage in unprotected anal sex.

Young people Young people ages 13 to 24 are at risk for HIV/AIDS, particularly those who are members of minorities. Teenagers and young adults are more likely to engage in unprotected sex than older individuals.

There is also a "generational forgetting" among younger people, who have grown up with the presence of treatments for HIV/AIDS. Because there are known treatments and because many young people are more prone to take risks than older individuals, often "magically" believing that nothing bad could happen to them, the risk for engaging in unsafe behavior leading to infection is greater among adolescents and young adults than in other groups. Some studies have shown that post-HAART-youth are more likely to engage in unsafe behavior than youths prior to the development of HAART.

See also CRIME AND CRIMINALS; DRUG ABUSE AND DEPENDENCE AND HEALTH PROBLEMS; HEROIN; PROSTITUTION; YOUNG ADULTS.

Centers for Disease Control and Prevention. "Basic Statistics." Available online. URL: http://www.cdc.gov/hiv/topics/surveillance/basic.htm. Downloaded May 11, 2006.

Centers for Disease Control and Prevention. "Cases of HIV/AIDS, by Area of Residence, Diagnosed in 2004—33 States with Confidential Name-Based HIV Infection Reporting." *HIV/AIDS Surveillance Report* 16, Public Health Service, 2006.

Centers for Disease Control and Prevention, "Cases of HIV/AIDS by Area of Residence, Diagnosed in 2004—33 States with Confidential Name-Based HIV Infection Reporting." *HIV/AIDS Surveillance Report,* Department of Health and Human Services, Atlanta, 2005. Available online. URL: http://www.cdc.gov/hiv/topics/surveillance/resources/report/pdf/2004Surveillance Report.pdf. Downloaded May 11, 2006.

Centers for Disease Control and Prevention, "A Glance at the HIV/AIDS Epidemic." April 2006. Available online. URL: http://www.cdc.gov/hiv/resources/factsheets/At-A-Glance.htm. Downloaded May 11, 2006

National Institute on Drug Abuse, *HIV/AIDS,* Research Report Series. Available online. URL: http://www.drugabuse.gov/PDF/RRhiv.pdf. Downloaded March 17, 2006.

Osmond, Dennis H., "Epidemiology of HIV/AIDS in the United States." March 2003. Available online. URL: http://hivinsite.ucsf.edu/InSite?page=kb-01-03. Downloaded May 11, 2006.

addiction/dependence Includes both a physical and a psychological need for alcohol and/or prescribed or illegal drugs, as well as accompanying behavior that is harmful to the individual at work and at home. Addicted individuals center their lives around the substance to which they are addicted and are primarily concerned with obtaining the substance and using the substance—other concerns have a far lower priority.

Addicted individuals usually develop a PHYSICAL TOLERANCE to the substance, such that they need a higher dosage of the substance to achieve the same level of effects. They will also suffer the physical reaction of WITHDRAWAL if they cannot or choose not to use the substance to which they are addicted. The difficulty of the withdrawal experience depends on the substance and the degree of dependence and may be as mild as a headache and nausea or as severe as seizures, coma, and risk of death.

It should also be noted that many people who are addicted to one substance also have an addic-tion to other substances as well; for example, the COCAINE addict may also be dependent on alcohol. Many people who are dependent on illegal drugs are also abusers of MARIJUANA. Individuals addicted to METHAMPHETAMINE often abuse alcohol and marijuana.

Some individuals use some drugs in an attempt to reverse the effects of other drugs; for example, they may use STIMULANTS such as cocaine to create euphoria and then later use DEPRESSANTS, such as BENZODIAZEPINES, to enable them to sleep. However, only a physician can appropriately determine what drugs and what dosages of drugs are the safest and best to achieve medical goals. Since people who use illegal drugs or who abuse prescription drugs usually do not consult a physician, they have an increased risk for ACCIDENTAL OVERDOSE DEATHS.

Note that a physical tolerance to a drug alone, however, does not constitute an addiction. The psychological dependence is also an essential element of dependence on drugs and/or alcohol.

Elements of Addiction

There are several key elements that are present in both alcohol and drug dependence, such as an apparent inability to resist the overpowering impulse to abuse the substance or extreme difficulty in doing so. This driving impulse often affects the individual's work performance and may lead to loss of job after job. It often affects marital, romantic, family, and work relationships in a very negative manner.

In addition to the physical tolerance that is present with addiction, individuals who are addicted to alcohol or drugs have a PSYCHOLOGICAL DEPENDENCE on the substance, feeling that they need the drug in order to feel normal. (Indeed, this feeling may be valid, as the symptoms of withdrawal can be very uncomfortable.)

Individuals who are dependent on substances may engage in illegal activities in order to obtain them; for example, the individual who is addicted to prescription drugs may be willing to forge a doctor's prescription, see many doctors in attempts to receive multiple prescriptions from different pharmacies that they can abuse, or take other illegal actions in order to obtain the drug. These actions are committed to receive the concomitant physical and psychological relief that they know that using the drug will generate.

Another element of addiction is the CRAVING to continue to use the substance, which is an integral part of an addiction. This deep-seated compulsion must be recognized and managed by those seeking to help the addict, as well as by addicts themselves, in order for the addict to avoid RELAPSES that can occur after treatment. Even after an individual has undergone treatment or DETOXIFICATION for a substance and the physical addiction is altogether gone, the psychological craving often still lingers, and it can lead the individual back to abuse and then to readdiction to the substance.

Another problem that is associated with addiction and makes recovery difficult is that often individuals who are dependent on drugs or alcohol associate with peers who are themselves dependent on the same substances. As a result, if individuals are treated for their drug or alcohol dependence, but then they return to associating with their peers who continue to abuse or are dependent on substances, it is difficult for these individuals to refrain from resuming first abuse, and then readdiction. Part of the therapeutic process is teaching individuals to value themselves and encouraging them to seek out new friendships among those who are not substance abusers.

In one circumstance, however, former addicts may be helpful to the individual trying to stay off drugs or alcohol, such as twelve-step groups. Often groups of former abusers dedicated to remaining substance-free may help the individual to continue to avoid the substance. National self-help groups such as Alcoholics Anonymous or Narcotics Anonymous may be highly useful to this end.

Symptoms and Diagnostic Path

The symptoms of an addiction depend upon the substance to which the individual is addicted; for example, if the substance is alcohol, the drunken person may be able to drink more than others and seemingly show less response to alcohol, because of a physical tolerance. However, he or she may have a spotty work record and unexplained absences. There may also be relationship and marital difficulties.

If the patient is withdrawing from alcohol, he or she may experience DELIRIUM TREMENS, a syndrome that may include nausea and vomiting, seizures, mental confusion, and other signs and symptoms.

If the addictive substance is a stimulant, the addicted individual may speak more rapidly and behave in an agitated manner. Some drugs, such as methamphetamine, can lead to apparent rapid aging and extreme and undesirable weight loss. Some illegal drugs may cause DELUSIONS and HALLUCINATIONS, such as cocaine, methamphetamine, and HALLUCINOGENIC DRUGS.

Treatment Options and Outlook

The treatment for an addiction depends upon the substance to which the person is addicted. Some people require inpatient treatment, whether they are addicted to alcohol, or illegal drugs such as cocaine, ANABOLIC STEROIDS, or others. Others can recover from their addiction with an effective outpatient treatment program, and most treatment facilities offer outpatient programs.

Medications may be helpful in treatment; for example, BENZODIAZEPINES may ease the symptoms of WITHDRAWAL from alcohol. Some drugs are directly used in treatment, as are NALTREXONE (ReVia) and BUPRENOPHINE, which are used to treat individuals addicted to opiates. METHADONE is used as a treatment (and a substitute drug) for individuals who are addicted to heroin.

Whether the person is in an inpatient or an outpatient treatment program, however, after the release from treatment, follow-up is necessary because many patients experience relapses.

Risk Factors and Preventive Measures

In general, young adult males have the greatest risk for developing an alcohol or drug dependence, although some females also become addicted. Females who were sexually abused as children have an elevated risk of suffering from drug dependence in adulthood.

There is also an apparent genetic risk for alcohol and drug abuse, and thus experts seeking to help the addict should take a family history as well as obtain individual information about the patient.

The best way to prevent addiction altogether is for individuals to refrain from the use or abuse of alcohol and illegal drugs. If prescription drugs are used, the physician's instructions should be followed carefully, and if there are any questions, the pharmacist should be consulted for further information.

All prescription drugs should be kept in a secure place, away from other family members, particularly from adolescents, who may be tempted to experiment with drugs or to share drugs with their friends. This is particularly true of SCHEDULED DRUGS such as NARCOTICS or sedating drugs such as ALPRAZOLAM (XANAX) or DIAZEPAM (VALIUM).

Individuals who legally take stimulant medications for ATTENTION DEFICIT HYPERACTIVITY DISORDER (ADHD), such as various forms of METHYLPHENIDATE, should be advised that they should not openly discuss their use of this drug with others, particularly with adolescents. Although methylphenidate can be very effective in treating individuals who have ADHD, it is also a dangerous drug when it is abused by others for whom it was not prescribed.

See also ABUSE, DRUG; ALCOHOL ABUSE/DEPENDENCE; GENDER DIFFERENCES, ABUSE OF DRUGS AND ALCOHOL; GENETIC PREDISPOSITIONS AND ENVIRONMENTAL EFFECTS IN SUBSTANCE USE DISORDERS.

Courtwright, David T. *Dark Paradise: A History of Opiate Addiction in America.* Cambridge, Mass.: Harvard University Press, 2001.

adolescents and substance abuse Individuals ages 12–17 years old who have substance abuse problems. Adolescents may abuse substances for the following reasons:

- PEER PRESSURE
- curiosity
- failure to consider both the possible short- and long-term consequences of their actions
- magical thinking, assuming that they can handle all problems, including those caused by substance abuse
- emotional disorders, such as DEPRESSION, for which they seek to self-medicate with alcohol and/or illegal drugs
- ATTENTION DEFICIT HYPERACTIVITY DISORDER (ADHD), for which adolescents may self-medicate with

alcohol and/or drugs. (Studies indicate that adolescents who are treated for their ADHD are less likely to become substance abusers than teenagers whose ADHD is untreated.)

- unawareness or disbelief that there are risks and dangers associated with substance abuse (such as addiction, severe side effects, and a lack of control, making the substance abuser more vulnerable to victimization)
- a false feeling of security/immortality

All of these mind-sets are common to adolescents, who may lack the maturity to make reasoned decisions. As a result, teenagers may turn to substance abuse, and they may suffer as a result.

According to the *National Survey on Drug Use and Health,* in 2004, many adolescents did not receive the treatment that they needed for substance abuse. An estimated 2.3 million youths ages 12–17 years (about 9 percent of all youths in this age group) needed treatment for an illicit drug or alcohol problem; however, only about 185,000 youths actually received treatment in a specialized treatment facility. As a result, about 92 percent did not receive treatment in a facility.

Percentages of Youths with Substance Abuse Issues

In the United States, according to the *National Survey on Drug Use and Health,* among all youths who were ages 12 to 17 years in 2004, about 11 percent were current illicit drug users. Some adolescents abused more than one substance, such as both ALCOHOL and MARIJUANA or other combinations of substances. About 7 percent used MARIJUANA, and 4 percent were nonmedical users of prescription drugs (see PRESCRIPTION DRUG ABUSE), 1 percent abused INHALANTS, and less than 1 percent of the adolescents used either HALLUCINOGENIC DRUGS or COCAINE.

It is noteworthy that adolescent drug and alcohol use slightly declined in 2004 from that in preceding years. For example, 15.8 percent of youths had used marijuana in the past year in 2002. By 2004, that percentage had declined to 14.5 percent. The past *month* usage of marijuana also slightly declined, from 8.2 percent in 2002 to 7.6 percent in 2004. (See Table I.)

TABLE I: PREVALENCE RATES OF DRUGS AND ALCOHOL AMONG YOUTHS AGES 12–17: 2002–2004

	2002	2003	2004
Marijuana			
Lifetime	20.6	19.6	19.0
Past Year	15.8	15.0	14.5
Past Month	8.2	7.9	7.6
Cocaine			
Lifetime	2.7	2.6	2.4
Past Year	2.1	1.8	1.6
Past Month	0.6	0.6	0.5
Ecstasy			
Lifetime	3.3	2.4	2.1
Past Year	2.2	1.3	1.2
Past Month	0.5	0.4	0.3
LSD			
Lifetime	2.7	1.6	1.2
Past Year	1.3	0.6	0.6
Past Month	0.2	0.2	0.2
Inhalants			
Lifetime	10.5	10.7	11.0
Past Year	4.4	4.5	4.6
Past Month	1.2	1.3	1.2
Alcohol			
Lifetime	43.4	42.9	42.0
Past Year	34.6	34.3	33.9
Past Month	17.6	17.7	17.6

Source: Adapted from Office of Applied Studies, Substance Abuse and Mental Health Services Administration. *Overview of Findings from the 2004 National Survey on Drug Use and Health.* Publication no. SMA 05-4061. Rockville, Md.: Department of Health and Human Services, September 2005, p. 39.

TABLE II: SUBSTANCE DEPENDENCE OR ABUSE FOR SPECIFIC SUBSTANCES IN THE PAST YEAR, AGES 12–17 YEARS, BY PERCENTAGE, 2002–2004

Past Year Dependence or Abuse	2002	2003	2004
Illicit drug	5.6	5.1	5.3
Marijuana and Hashish	4.3	3.8	3.9
Cocaine	0.4	0.3	0.4
Heroin	0.1	0.0	0.1
Hallucinogens	0.6	0.4	0.5
Inhalants	0.4	0.4	0.5
Nonmedical Use of Psychotherapeutics[1]	1.3	1.4	1.5
Pain Relievers	1.0	1.1	1.2
Tranquilizers	0.4	0.4	0.3
Stimulants	0.4	0.4	0.3
Sedatives	0.1	0.2	0.1
Alcohol	5.9	5.9	6.0
Illicit drug or alcohol	8.9	8.9	8.8
Both illicit drug and alcohol	2.5	2.2	2.5

[1] Nonmedical use of prescription-type pain relievers, tranquilizers, stimulants, or sedatives; does not include over-the-counter drugs.
Source: Adapted from Office of Applied Studies, Substance Abuse and Mental Health Services Administration. *Overview of Findings from the 2004 National Survey on Drug Use and Health.* Publication no. SMA 05-4061. Rockville, Md.: Department of Health and Human Services, September 2005.

With regard to substance abuse or dependence (addiction), the percentages of youths abusing drugs were significantly lower in 2004. (See Table II.) As can be seen from the table, from 2002 to 2004, the largest percentages of youths either abused alcohol or were dependent on an illegal drug or alcohol. The second largest category of youths were those who abused alcohol or who were alcoholics. For example, 6 percent of youths abused alcohol in 2004 and 8.8 percent abused either illicit drugs or alcohol. It should also be noted that the percentages of youths who were abusing prescription drugs was slightly up, from 1.3 percent in 2002 to 1.5 percent in 2004.

Considering Some Specific Drugs

According to the *National Survey on Drug Use and Health,* in considering the rates of first-time drug use for specific drugs, among youths ages 12–17 years, 5.0 percent used marijuana for the first time in 2004. With regard to inhalants, most individuals who used inhalants were below age 18 years, and 75 percent were younger than age 18 when they first used an inhalant, with the average age of first use of 16 years in 2004. The largest users of inhalants were 14–15 years old, although their percentage of use was small (1.6 percent).

Most users of cocaine and HEROIN are older than adolescents (ages 12–17). For example, the average age of first use of cocaine was 20 years old in 2004, and the average age of the first use of heroin was 24.4 years. In addition, the average age of users of METHYLENEDIOXYMETHAMPHETAMINE (MDMA/ECSTASY) was 19.5 years in 2004.

The average age of those using prescription drugs nonmedically for the first time was as follows: 29.3

years for sedatives, 25.2 years for tranquilizers, and 24.1 years for stimulants. Among new users of METHAMPHETAMINE, the average age was 22.1 years. Thus, drugs that were the greatest risks for adolescents were marijuana and inhalants (as well as alcohol, for which the average age of first use was 17.5 years in 2004).

Patterns among Youths and Drug Abuse

Researchers for the *National Survey on Drug Use and Health* found distinct patterns among those youths who were more likely to abuse alcohol and drugs, including differences in gender, age, race, and ethnicity; perceived parental attitudes toward illegal drugs; attitudes toward school; the belief that religious beliefs were important; and fighting and delinquent behavior.

Gender Among youths ages 12–17 years in 2004 in the United States, the rate of overall substance abuse was nearly identical for girls and boys: 9.0 percent for females and 8.7 percent for males. However, with regard to the abuse of MARIJUANA, significantly more girls abused the drug. In fact, since 2002, more girls than boys started using marijuana for each year, and in 2004, 675,000 girls started using marijuana, compared to 577,000 boys who had an onset of marijuana use.

It is also true that teenage girls are more likely than adolescent boys to engage in PRESCRIPTION DRUG ABUSE. In 2004, 14.4 percent of adolescent girls had misused prescription drugs in their lives, compared to 12.5 percent of teenage boys. In considering prescription drug abuse in the past month, 4.1 percent of teenage girls had abused prescription drugs, compared to 3.2 percent of teenage boys.

These abuses may be at least in part due to a rate of DEPRESSION among adolescent girls that is more than double that among teenage boys; for example, 2.40 million teenage girls had ever suffered a major depressive episode in 2004, compared to 1.07 million of adolescent males.

Drug abuse and age The *National Survey on Drug Use and Health* further broke down the risk of drug use within the age group of 12–17 years. For example, among youths ages 12–13 years old, the dominant form of drug abuse (excluding alcohol) was the abuse of prescription drugs (1.7 percent). In contrast, among 14- to 15-year-olds,

TABLE III: ABUSE OF SPECIFIC DRUGS BY YOUTHS AGES 12–17, BY DRUG AND BY AGE GROUPING, PERCENTAGES, 2004

Drugs Abused	Ages 12–13	Ages 14–15	Ages 16–17
Marijuana	1.1	7.3	14.5
Prescription Drugs Used Nonmedically	1.7	4.1	5.1
Inhalants	1.2	1.6	0.9

Source: Adapted from Substance Abuse and Mental Health Services Administration. *Overview of Findings for the 2004 National Survey on Drug Use and Health.* Rockville, Md.: Department of Health and Human Services, September 2005, p. 14.

the dominant drug of abuse was marijuana, and 7.3 percent in this age group had used this drug. Among youths ages 16–17, marijuana was also the dominant drug of abuse, and 14.5 percent used this drug. Less than 1 percent of this group abused inhalants. (See Table III.)

Race/ethnicity Some racial groups of adolescents had a higher rate of illegal drug use than others. For example, the rate of current illegal drug use among American Indians or Alaska Natives (together considered as one group) was 26.0 percent, which is greater than twice the rate among all youths, or 10.6 percent. (See Table IV.) The highest percentage of current illegal drug use was among individuals of two or more races, or 12.2 percent, followed by whites (11.1 percent).

Parental approval and substance use Parental attitudes toward drugs often have an impact on the drug use of their children. According to the *National Survey on Drug Use and Health* in 2004, among youths who perceived strong parental disapproval of the idea of their adolescent children's trying marijuana or hashish once or twice, their use was about a sixth (5.1 percent) compared to the rate among those who did *not* perceive their parents would strongly disapprove (30.0 percent). Note: This does not mean that if children use drugs, their parents approve of this use.

Attitudes toward school Findings from the *National Survey on Drug Use and Health* revealed a significant difference in drug use when comparing students who reported that they liked or "kind of liked" school compared to those who disliked or hated school. For example, in considering mari-

TABLE IV: RATE OF CURRENT ILLICIT DRUG USE AMONG
YOUTHS AGES 12–17, BY RACE AND PERCENTAGE, 2004

American Indians or Alaska Natives	26.0
Two or more races	12.2
Whites	11.1
Hispanics	10.2
African Americans	9.3
Asians	6.0
All youths	10.6

Source: Adapted from Substance Abuse and Mental Health Services
Administration. Overview of Findings for the 2004 National Survey
on Drug Use and Health. Rockville, Md.: Department of Health and
Human Services, September 2005, p. 18.

juana use, students who said that they either liked
or kind of liked school had a past month marijuana
use of 6.0 percent. In contrast, students who said
that they "didn't like very much" or "hated" school
had a rate of 14.6 percent of marijuana use in the
past month, more than twice the rate of the more
satisfied students.

Religious beliefs   Youths who professed religious
beliefs had a lower rate of illicit drug use, according to the *National Survey on Drug Use and Health.*
Among those who said that they believed religious
beliefs were very important, 8.1 percent had used
an illegal drug in the past month, compared to 18.5
percent who disagreed that religious beliefs were
important. Thus, the impact of religious beliefs
decreased the use of illegal drugs by more than half
among adolescents.

Fighting and delinquent behavior   Serious
fights among adolescents age 12–17 are also linked
to drug use. In 2004, the *National Survey on Drug Use
and Health* reported that 18.9 percent of youths who
were in serious fights at school or at work used illegal drugs, compared to 8.1 percent of youths who
not been involved in fighting. Also, among youths
who had stolen or attempted to steal something,
40.9 percent engaged in illicit drug use, compared
to 9.1 percent who did not steal but did use illegal
drugs, about one-fourth the rate of the would-be or
actual young thieves.

*Alcohol abuse and patterns among adoles-
cents*   Alcohol is a major drug of abuse for adolescents ages 12–17 years old. According to the
National Survey on Drug Use and Health, 17.6 percent
of youths were current drinkers in 2004. About 11

percent were binge drinkers (individuals having five
or more drinks on at least one occasion in the past
two weeks) and 2.7 percent were heavy drinkers.

Among youths ages 12–17 years, males and
females have about the same rate of alcohol use,
with adolescent girls having a slightly *greater* percentage, or 17.2 percent of males and 18.0 percent
of females. However, among an older population
of young adults, males had a much higher rate of
past month alcohol use than females; for example,
56.0 percent of females age 18–25 years reported
past month alcohol use, compared to 64.9 percent
of males within this same age group.

Race and ethnicity and alcohol   In considering
current alcohol use (not binge drinking or heavy
drinking), according to the *National Survey on Drug
Abuse and Health,* the rates were highest (at or above
18 percent) for whites, American Indians/Alaska
Natives, and Hispanics. They were lowest for blacks
(9.8 percent) and Asians (9.4 percent).

BINGE DRINKING among youths was highest
among American Indians/Alaska Natives (25.8 percent) in 2004, followed by Hispanics (24.0 percent),
whites (23.8 percent), blacks (18.3 percent), and
Asians (12.4 percent).

Driving under the influence of alcohol   According to the *National Survey on Drug Abuse and Health,*
approximately 10.2 percent of youths ages 16–17
years old drove under the influence of alcohol in
2004. This percentage doubled to 20.2 percent
among young adults, ages 18–20 years old, and it
further increased to 28.2 percent for those individuals ages 21–25 years old.

Adolescents and drug diversion   Adolescents
ages 12–17 have an increased risk of engaging in
drug diversion, which refers to giving as well as
either selling or buying legally prescribed drugs
for the purpose of abuse. Often prescribed drugs
are purchased from other students, who may sell
their stimulant medications that are prescribed to
treat attention deficit hyperactivity disorder, such
as METHYLPHENIDATE (RITALIN/CONCERTA/FOCADIN,
ETC.). Others find and steal medications from home,
such as narcotic painkillers that belong to their parents or other family members.

In a study of students in grades 7, 9, 10, and 12
in CANADA, reported in 2001 in the *Canadian Medical Association Journal,* of the 5 percent of students

who were medically prescribed stimulants, 15 percent said that they had given away some of their medication and 7 percent said they had sold their medication. Males were more likely to sell their medicine than females. In addition, 4 percent of these students said their medicine had been stolen from them and 3 percent said their medicine was taken by force. Giving away drugs is just as illegal as selling them to others.

Another study of students who were treated with psychostimulant drugs for ADHD based its results on 1,723 students in the Detroit, Michigan, area, ranging in age from grades 6 through 11 in the United States. Reported in *Substance Use & Misuse* in 2004, the study found that 23 percent of students who were taking legally prescribed stimulants said that they were approached by others who wanted them to give, sell, or trade their stimulant medications.

See also ATTENTION DEFICIT HYPERACTIVITY DISORDER; DIVERSION, DRUG; DRUG COURTS; GENETIC PREDISPOSITIONS AND ENVIRONMENTAL EFFECTS IN SUBSTANCE USE DISORDERS; METHYLPHENIDATE; PEER PRESSURE; RUNAWAY/THROWAWAY YOUTHS; YOUNG ADULTS; ZERO TOLERANCE LAWS.

McCabe, S. E., C. J. Teter, and C. J. Boyd. "The Use, Misuse and Diversion of Prescription Stimulants among Middle and High School Students." *Substance Use & Misuse* 39, no. 7 (2004): 1,095–1,116.
Poulin, Christiane. "Medical and Nonmedical Stimulant Use among Adolescents: From Sanctioned to Unsanctioned Use." *Canadian Medical Association Journal* 165, no. 8 (2001): 1,039–1,044.
Substance Abuse and Mental Health Services Administration, *Overview of Findings for the 2004 National Survey on Drug Use and Health*. Rockville, Md.: Department of Health and Human Services, September 2005.

adverse reaction Unexpected medical result of the use of a legal or illegal medication, including prescription medications or over-the-counter drugs. For example, the abuse of METHAMPHETAMINE may cause seizures, hyperthermia, or other serious and even life-threatening reactions in many individuals. It should be noted that even herbal remedies may cause adverse reactions.

An adverse reaction may range from a relatively minor one to a far more serious reaction. In some cases, an adverse reaction may be life-threatening and require EMERGENCY TREATMENT. Some individuals experience adverse reactions as a result of combining one or more drugs with alcohol.

In some cases, a combination of substances, such as a prescription drug and/or alcohol and an illegal drug, may cause harmful effects.

Alcohol, even in small amounts, may cause an adverse reaction to medications used for many different types of common medical problems. (See Table I.)

See also ACCIDENTAL OVERDOSE DEATHS; DATE RAPE DRUGS; DRUG INTERACTIONS; MALICIOUS POISONING.

TABLE I: INTERACTIONS BETWEEN ALCOHOL AND COMMON MEDICATIONS (BOTH PRESCRIPTION AND OVER-THE-COUNTER DRUGS)		
Symptoms/Disorders	Common Medications and Selected Brand Names (Generic Names in Parentheses)	Some Possible Reactions with Alcohol
Allergies/Colds/Flu	Alavert (loratadine) Allegra, Allegra-D Benadryl (diphenhydramine) Clarinex (desloratadine) Claritin, Claritin-D (loratadine) Dimetapp Cold & Allergy (brompheniramine) Sudafed Sinus & Allergy (chlorpheniramine) Triaminic Cold & Allergy (chlorpheniramine) Tylenol Allergy Sinus (chlorpheniramine and acetaminophen) Tylenol Cold & Flu (chlorpheniramine and acetaminophen) Zyrtec (cetirizine)	Drowsiness, dizziness; increased risk for overdose

Symptoms/Disorders	Common Medications and Selected Brand Names (Generic Names in Parentheses)	Some Possible Reactions with Alcohol
Angina (chest pain), coronary heart disease	Isordil (isosorbide) Nitroglycerin	Rapid heartbeat, sudden changes in blood pressure, dizziness, fainting
Anxiety and epilepsy	Ativan (lorazepam) Klonopin (clonazepam) Librium (chlordiazepoxide) Paxil (paroxetine) Valium (diazepam) Xanax (alprazolam)	Drowsiness, dizziness; increased risk for overdose; slowed or difficult breathing; impaired motor control; unusual behavior; and memory problems
	Herbal preparations (kava kava)	Liver damage, drowsiness
Arthritis	Celebrex (celecoxib) Naprosyn (naproxen) Voltaren (diclofenac)	Ulcers, stomach bleeding, liver problems
Blood clots	Coumadin (warfarin)	Occasional drinking may lead to internal bleeding; heavier drinking also may cause bleeding or may have the opposite effect, resulting in possible blood clots, strokes, or heart attacks
Cough	Delsym, Robitussin Cough (dextromethorphan) Robitussin A-C (guaifenesin and codeine)	Drowsiness, dizziness; increased risk for overdose
Depression	Anafranil (clomipramine) Celexa (citalopram) Desyrel (trazodone) Effexor (venlafaxine) Elavil (amitriptyline) Lexapro (escitalopram) Luvox (fluvoxamine) Norpramin (desipramine) Paxil (paroxetine) Prozac (fluoxetine) Serzone (nefazodone) Wellbutrin (bupropion) Zoloft (sertraline)	Drowsiness, dizziness; increased risk for overdose; increased feelings of depression or hopelessness in adolescents (suicide)
Diabetes	Glucophage (metformin) Micronase (glyburide) Orinase (tolbutamide)	Abnormally low blood sugar levels, flushing reaction (nausea, vomiting, headache, rapid heartbeat, sudden changes in blood pressure)
Enlarged prostate	Cardura (doxazosin) Flomax (tamsulosin) Hytrin (terazosin) Minipress (prazosin)	Dizziness, light headedness, fainting

(table continues)

TABLE I *(continued)*

Symptoms/Disorders	Common Medications and Selected Brand Names (Generic Names in Parentheses)	Some Possible Reactions with Alcohol
Heartburn, indigestion, sour stomach	Axid (nizatidine) Reglan (metoclopramide) Tagamet (cimetidine) Zantac (ranitidine)	Rapid heartbeat, sudden changes in blood pressure (metoclopramide); increased alcohol effect
High blood pressure	Accupril (quinapril) Capozide (hydrochlorothiazide) Cardura (doxazosin) Catapres (clonidine) Cozaar (losartan) Hytrin (terazosin) Lopressor HCT (hydrochlorothiazide) Lotensin (benzapril) Minipress (prazosin) Vaseretic (enalapril)	Dizziness, fainting, drowsiness; heart problems such as changes in the heart's regular heartbeat (arrhythmia)
High cholesterol	Advicor (lovastain and niacin) Altocor (lovastatin) Crestor (rosuvastatin) Lipitor (atorvastatin) Mevacor (lovastatin) Niaspan (niacin) Pravachol (pravastatin) Pravigard (pravastatin and aspirin) Vytorin (ezetimbe and simvastatin) Zocor (simvastatin)	Liver damage (all medications); increased flushing and itching (niacin); increased stomach bleeding (pravastatin and aspirin)
Infections	Macrodantin (nitrofurantoin) Flagyl (metronidazole) Grisactin (griseofulvin) Nizoral (ketoconazole) Nydrazid (isoniazid) Seromycin (cycloserine) Tindamax (tinidazole)	Fast heartbeat, sudden changes in blood pressure; stomach pain, upset stomach, vomiting, headache, or flushing or redness of the face; liver damage (isoniazid, ketokonazole)
Muscle pain	Flexeril (cyclobenzaprine) Soma (carisoprodol)	Drowsiness, dizziness; increased risk of seizures; increased risk for overdose; slowed or difficult breathing; impaired motor control; unusual behavior; memory problems
Nausea, motion sickness	Antivert (meclizine) Atarax (hydroxyzine) Dramamine (dimenhydrinate) Phenergan (promethazine)	Drowsiness, dizziness; increased risk for overdose
Pain (such as headache, muscle ache, minor arthritis pain), fever, inflammation	Advil (ibuprofen) Aleve (naproxen) Excedrin (aspirin, acetaminophen) Motrin (ibuprofen) Tylenol (acetaminophen)	Stomach upset, bleeding and ulcers; liver damage (acetaminophen); rapid heartbeat

Symptoms/Disorders	Common Medications and Selected Brand Names (Generic Names in Parentheses)	Some Possible Reactions with Alcohol
Seizures	Dilantin (phenytoin) Klonopin (clonazepam phenobarbital)	Drowsiness, dizziness; increased risk for seizures
Severe pain from injury, postsurgical care, oral surgery, migraines	Darvocet-N (propoxyphene) Demerol (meperidine) Fiornal with codeine (butalbital and codeine) Percocet (oxycodone) Vicodin (hydrocodone)	Drowsiness, dizziness; increased risk for overdose; slowed or difficult breathing; impaired motor control; unusual behavior; memory problems
Sleep problems	Ambien (zolpidem) Lunesta (eszopiclone) Prosom (estazolam) Restoril (temazepam) Sominex (diphenhydramine) Unisom (doxylamine)	Drowsiness, sleepiness, dizziness; slowed or difficult breathing; impaired motor control; unusual behavior; memory problems
	Herbal preparations (chamomile, valerian, lavender)	Increased drowsiness

Note: This list does not include all medications that may interact with alcohol and offers only a sampling of such drugs. In addition, the list does not include all ingredients found in every medication. A pharmacist should be consulted for more information on harmful interactions with alcohol.
Source: Adapted from National Institute on Alcohol Abuse and Alcoholism. "Harmful Interactions: Mixing Alcohol with Medicines." Rockville, Md.: National Institute on Alcohol Abuse and Alcoholism, August 2005. Available online. URL: http://pubs.niaaa.nih.gov/publications/Medicine/Harmful_Interactions.pdf. Downloaded August 22, 2007.

Afghanistan   An Asian country that is bounded by Iran, Pakistan, Tajikistan, Turkmenistan, and Uzbekistan and that relies heavily on the revenues received from the illicit sale of HEROIN. Afghanistan produces the majority (about 87 percent) of all the opium that is grown in the entire world, according to the World Health Organization report in 2006. Every province in Afghanistan reportedly engages in cultivating opium poppies, almost solely for the production of heroin for the world market.

Most of the heroin that is used by addicts in the United States is produced in South America; however, some heroin from Afghanistan is smuggled into the United States through traffickers in Europe and Central Asia. Europe and Asia are the primary markets for heroin produced in Afghanistan. About 95 percent of the heroin that is abused in the United Kingdom is from Afghanistan, and other European and Asian countries are also heavy consumers of the heroin that is produced there. ORGANIZED CRIME groups in Russia and other countries are heavily involved in heroin trafficking from Afghanistan.

According to a cover story in the *Wall Street Journal* in 2006, CLANDESTINE LABORATORIES in Afghani-

stan have been so active and effective at producing the heroin that is derived from opium poppies that they have significantly driven the price of the drug down in Europe, from an estimated $251 per gram in 1990 to $75 a gram in 2006. In 2006, an estimated 50–60 percent of the gross domestic product of Afghanistan was generated by the heroin trade alone. (Note that in the United States, nearly all clandestine laboratories are devoted solely to the manufacture of METHAMPHETAMINE.) In past years, heroin was actually used as a form of currency.

Background
Although drugs were produced in Afghanistan in the past, the large-scale growth and production of drugs did not occur until the late 20th century, when farmers experienced poverty that was related to years of war, starting with the Soviet invasion in Afghanistan in 1979, and the subsequent conditions of anarchy. Many Russian soldiers who had invaded Afghanistan became addicted to heroin, and they returned to their country with an addiction problem.

According to a Congressional Research Service Report, "Following the Soviet invasion of 1979 and during the civil war that ensued in the aftermath of the Soviet withdrawal, opium poppy cultivation expanded in parallel with the gradual collapse of state authority across Afghanistan. As the country's formal economy succumbed to violence and disorder, opium became one of the few available commodities capable of both storing economic value and generating revenue for local administration and military supplies."

The Taliban movement also affected the escalation of the production of heroin from the mid- to late 1990s, when Taliban officials collected taxes from the increasing output of poppies grown to produce heroin.

Political Implications of Heroin Exports from Afghanistan

Although few Americans use heroin that originates in Afghanistan, this drug trafficking has political implications for the United States and other countries. According to a report on narcotics and U.S. policy in Afghanistan, "The trafficking of Afghan drugs also appears to provide financial and logistical support to a range of extremist groups that continue to operate in and around Afghanistan, including remnants of the Taliban regime and some Al Qaeda operatives."

Some officials are concerned that the heavy dependence on heroin exports will impede or even prevent the growth of democracy in Afghanistan.

According to a 2005 report from the United Nations Office on Drugs and Crime, there was a decline in the cultivation of opium poppies in Afghanistan in 2005, because farmers refrained from growing poppies at the urging of the president of Afghanistan as well as law enforcement and religious authorities. In addition, the government ordered provincial governors to destroy opium fields. However, the weather was excellent for poppy growing in 2005, and as a result, the average productivity increased by about 22 percent. The result was only a decrease of 2 percent over the harvest in 2004.

The report urges officials not to limit their targeting to farmers alone, who receive only an estimated 3–4 percent of the money from illegal drugs.

Says the report, "On the other hand, fat bank accounts inflated by narco-dollars are harder to spot, whether the money remains in Afghanistan, resides

in neighbouring countries, or is stowed away in off-shore havens. Also, this money belongs to people with influence. Yet, the international community has to have *the wisdom to fight drugs, corruption, and terrorism simultaneously*. In other words, the world will not condone counter-narcotic measures that hit only the poorest of the poor, namely measures that do not target the illicit wealth belonging to corrupt officials, or to warlords seemingly engaged in the fight for democracy, or to newly elected members of the Afghan Congress who are seeking impunity through parliamentary immunity."

In addition, according to this report, "If there is another concrete measure that the Government and its coalition partners (including NATO forces) can take now to ensure the country's future, it is this: *as fields are eradicated, all other links of the drug chain, in Afghanistan and abroad, must be broken: heroin labs destroyed, trafficking disrupted, bank accounts closed, corrupt officials arrested, and warlords neutralized. Also Afghanistan's counter-narcotic efforts are more likely to succeed if supported by lower heroin demand in drug consuming countries.*"

Seeking to Curtail Heroin Production in Afghanistan

The United States has provided funds to cut back the drug trade, giving the Afghan government $780 million for this purpose in 2005, up from a total of $100 million for the period 2002–4. The *Wall Street Journal* article points out that, in comparison, the United States spent $4.5 billion from 2000 to 2006 in Colombia under the "Plan Colombia" program to stop COCAINE trafficking.

Despite the presence of U.S. and NATO troops in Afghanistan in 2007, Afghanistan continued as the world's largest producer of heroin, where the opium poppies are primarily grown in the country's mountainous areas. Commanders of U.S. troops have not increased their military mission to include drug interdiction because they reportedly do not have the resources and because such actions would antagonize local residents who are economically dependent on the drug trade.

Information on Users of Afghan Heroin

Information provided to the *Wall Street Journal* reporters indicated that heroin addicts in countries such as Tajikistan (a former republic of the Union of Soviet Socialist Republics) are as young as 14 years old. In addition, the injecting of heroin has caused an increase in the incidence of the HUMAN IMMUNODEFICIENCY VIRUS (HIV) in Tajikistan, and an estimated 5,000 people in that country have HIV. Most of the new cases (80 percent) of HIV were contracted through the use of dirty needles to inject the heroin. Heroin addiction is also a problem in other Asian countries, such as in Kazakhstan and Russia.

See also CANADA; COLOMBIA; CRIME AND CRIMINALS; GANGS; MEXICO; NARCOTICS; ORGANIZED CRIME.

Blanchard, Christopher M. *Afghanistan: Narcotics and U.S. Policy,* Washington, DC: Congressional Research Service, updated May 26, 2005. Available online. URL: http://www.usembassy.at/en/download/pdf/afgh_ narcs.pdf. Downloaded on January 19, 2006.

Shiskin, Philip, and David Crawford. "In Afghanistan, Heroin Trade Soars Despite U.S. Aid." *Wall Street Journal,* 18 January 2006, A1, A8.

United Nations Office on Drugs and Crime. *The Opium Situation in Afghanistan as of 29 August 2005.* Available online. URL: http://www.unodc.org/pdf/afghanistan_ 2005/opium-afghanistan_2005-08-26.pdf. Downloaded January 19, 2006.

United Nations Office on Drugs and Crime. *World Drug Report 2006.* Vol. 1 *Analysis.* United Nations, June 2006. Available online. URL: http://www.unodc.org/pdf/ WDR_2006/wdr2006_volume1.pdf. Downloaded July 28, 2006.

alcohol   An intoxicating drug whose use can lead to ABUSE or dependence (ALCOHOLISM) in some individuals. Alcohol does not cause a problem of abuse or dependence for many people; however, some individuals experience severe problems with their frequency and quantity of alcohol use, which in turn lead to health problems, family problems, and issues where these individuals work or attend school.

In the United States, it is legal for individuals age 21 and older to purchase alcohol. Although it is illegal for younger individuals to purchase alcohol, it is sometimes possible. The most common method is through the use of "helpful" adults who will purchase alcohol for minors. The use of false identification can be effective in some settings, because of inattentive service staff or the quality of the identification. Some younger individuals are able to purchase alcohol in situations where their fake identification is not requested. It is illegal to sell alcohol to minors. It is also a requirement of law to check identification for individuals except among those who are clearly middle-aged or older. (State law varies on identification policies.)

In other cases, parents either allow minors to consume their own alcohol in their homes or fail to supervise minors, who then may consume alcohol in the parents' unlocked liquor cabinet. Whether in or out of the home, it is still illegal for minors to consume liquor, although very small amounts of alcohol consumed for religious purposes may not be regarded as a problem by law enforcement authorities.

Alcohol Content

Some forms of alcohol are measured by the "proof" of the alcohol, which is an indication of its alcoholic content; for example, a form of alcohol that is 80 proof is actually composed of 40 percent ethyl alcohol. Distilled beverages are generally in the range of 80 proof or higher and are often referred to as "hard liquor."

In general, beer and wine manufacturers do not provide information on the containers that includes the proof of the alcohol. Nonetheless, their alcohol content is usually noted on the container in terms of percentage by volume. Wine is usually in the 12–15 percent range, and beer and other fermented beverages such as hard cider are generally in the 3 to 6 percent range. Some states have specific requirements regarding the allowable percentage of alcohol in various beverages.

When considering different types of alcohol and the alcohol content of major forms of alcoholic beverages, in general, 12 ounces of beer is equivalent to five ounces of wine and to 1.5 ounces of 80-proof distilled spirits. As a result, a smaller absolute quantity of distilled spirits is needed in order for a person to become intoxicated than if the individual were drinking beer or wine.

One common myth about alcohol is that it is not possible for beer or wine drinkers to become alcoholics, because of the lower alcohol content of beer or wine compared to spirits (also known as "hard liquor"). This is not true; some individuals who exclusively or primarily drink beer or wine may also become alcoholics.

Per Capita Consumption of Alcohol

In the United States, beer is the most popular alcoholic beverage, and the per capita consumption in gallons of beer for individuals ages 14 and older was 1.22 gallons in 2003, according to the National Institute on Alcohol Abuse and Alcoholism (NIAAA). States varied widely in their per capita consumption of beer, from a low of 0.77 per capita gallon in Utah to a high of 1.69 in Wyoming.

When considering the per capita consumption of spirits, the percentage of consumption in 2003 was the lowest in Utah (0.39 gallons per year) and the highest in New Hampshire (1.61 gallons).

In considering all forms of alcohol, the national per capita (per person) average was 2.22 gallons, with a low of 1.31 gallons in Utah to a high of 4.03 gallons in New Hampshire. (See Table I for state-by-state per capita consumption of beer, wine, spirits, and all alcoholic beverages.)

Information is also available on the per capita assumption of alcohol by region. In considering beer consumption, the Midwest led slightly at 1.28 gallons of beer per capita, followed closely by the South at 1.27 gallons. The Northeast had the lowest per capita beer consumption of 1.11 gallons in 2003. In considering only the per capita consumption of wine, the West led at 0.46 gallon, followed by the Northeast at 0.41. Individuals in the Midwest (0.26 gallon) and the South (0.27 gallon) consumed significantly less wine. See Table I for further information.

TABLE I: PER CAPITA ALCOHOL CONSUMPTION FOR STATES, CENSUS REGIONS, AND THE UNITED STATES, 2003 (PER CAPITA CONSUMPTION IN GALLONS, BASED ON POPULATION AGE 14 AND OLDER)

State or Other Geographic Area	Beer, per Capita	Wine, per Capita	Spirits, per Capita	All Beverages, per Capita
Alabama	1.18	0.19	0.52	1.89
Alaska	1.27	0.37	0.79	2.43
Arizona	1.41	0.37	0.71	2.48
Arkansas	1.06	0.14	0.56	1.76
California	1.06	0.50	0.65	2.22
Colorado	1.34	0.40	0.87	2.60
Connecticut	0.93	0.52	0.77	2.22
Delaware	1.37	0.56	1.17	3.11
District of Columbia	1.40	0.90	1.54	3.84
Florida	1.32	0.44	0.86	2.63
Georgia	1.19	0.26	0.66	2.11
Hawaii	1.30	0.42	0.67	2.39
Idaho	1.14	0.64	0.54	2.33
Illinois	1.25	0.35	0.74	2.34
Indiana	1.11	0.21	0.64	1.96
Iowa	1.37	0.15	0.53	2.05
Kansas	1.15	0.17	0.56	1.88
Kentucky	1.03	0.15	0.56	1.74
Louisiana	1.42	0.25	0.73	2.39
Maine	1.24	0.39	0.73	2.36
Maryland	1.02	0.32	0.77	2.11
Massachusetts	1.10	0.56	0.82	2.48
Michigan	1.17	0.26	0.70	2.13
Minnesota	1.21	0.29	0.90	2.41

State or Other Geographic Area	Beer, per Capita	Wine, per Capita	Spirits, per Capita	All Beverages, per Capita
Mississippi	1.40	0.12	0.62	2.14
Missouri	1.33	0.25	0.68	2.26
Montana	1.55	0.33	0.72	2.59
Nebraska	1.42	0.18	0.63	2.23
Nevada	1.76	0.62	1.25	3.63
New Hampshire	1.72	0.70	1.61	4.03
New Jersey	0.95	0.50	0.79	2.24
New Mexico	1.52	0.27	0.61	2.40
New York	0.93	0.40	0.61	1.93
North Carolina	1.21	0.27	0.52	2.00
North Dakota	1.53	0.17	0.86	2.56
Ohio	1.33	0.22	0.48	2.03
Oklahoma	1.06	0.13	0.73	1.93
Oregon	1.20	0.47	0.68	2.35
Pennsylvania	1.46	0.23	0.51	2.20
Rhode Island	1.12	0.51	0.79	2.42
South Carolina	1.38	0.23	0.74	2.35
South Dakota	1.51	0.16	0.73	2.40
Tennessee	1.26	0.18	0.52	1.96
Texas	1.46	0.23	0.51	2.19
Utah	0.77	0.15	0.39	1.31
Vermont	1.32	0.51	0.64	2.47
Virginia	1.14	0.36	0.53	2.03
Washington	1.05	0.46	0.67	2.19
West Virginia	1.23	0.10	0.38	1.71
Wisconsin	1.52	0.29	1.00	2.81
Wyoming	1.69	0.23	0.90	2.82
Regions				
Northeast	1.11	0.41	0.68	2.20
Midwest	1.28	0.26	0.69	2.22
South	1.27	0.27	0.64	2.18
West	1.16	0.46	0.69	2.31

Source: Adapted from Lakins, Nekisha, et al. "Apparent per Capita Alcohol Consumption, National State and Regional Trends, 1977–2003." Surveillance Report # 73. Bethesda, Md.: National Institute of Alcohol Abuse and Alcoholism, August 2005, pp. 13–14.

Blood Alcohol Levels

In past years, the states set different levels of alcohol in the bloodstream as a measure beyond which the person was considered to be legally intoxicated under state law. Today, because of federal requirements, all states in the United States use 0.08 as the blood alcohol level above which a person is legally intoxicated. In addition, all states have *zero tolerance laws* that apply to individuals below 21 years, which mean that if those younger than age 21 have *any* measurable amount of alcohol in their blood, they are considered to be legally intoxicated under the law.

A person driving a vehicle who has a proven blood alcohol level that exceeds the legal limit is legally intoxicated and may be charged with "driving while intoxicated" (DWI) or "driving under the influence" (DUI) as well as other offenses that are defined by law enforcement. Punishments may be severe for such crimes, particularly if a car crash

TABLE II: THE INCREASED RISK OF DEATH AS BLOOD ALCOHOL LEVELS RISE

Multiplies the Chance of Being Killed in a Single-Vehicle Crash Increase By:

Driver's Blood Alcohol (BAC) In This Range	Males			Females		
	Ages 16–20	21–34	35+	16–20	21–34	35+
0.02–0.049	5	3	3	3	3	3
0.05–0.079	17	7	6	7	7	6
0.08–0.099	52	13	11	15	13	11
0.10–0.149	241	37	29	43	37	29
0.15+	15,560	572	382	738	572	382

Source: Hingson, Ralph, and Michael Winter. "Epidemiology and Consequences of Drinking and Driving." *Alcohol Research & Health* 27, no. 1 (2003): 63–70.

occurs and/or if others are injured by the intoxicated person. The punishment may be a fine, suspension, or revocation of a driver's license; in some cases it may include a jail or prison sentence.

Breath, blood, or urine tests can determine whether a person is legally intoxicated under the laws of the state. In many states, if the apparently intoxicated person refuses to take a test for intoxication, then he or she is automatically regarded as intoxicated, regardless of the reason for the refusal.

Driving While Intoxicated and the Risk for Death   The risk for death dramatically increases with a rising blood alcohol level. For example, according to a 2003 article in *Alcohol Research & Health*, young men ages 16–20, who drive with a blood alcohol level of 0.15 or greater carry a risk of death in a car crash that is 15,560 times greater than males who do not drink. (See Table II for the risk ratios of death from car crashes for males and females.)

See also ABUSE, ALCOHOL; ADDICTION/DEPENDENCE; ADOLESCENTS AND SUBSTANCE ABUSE; ALCOHOL ABUSE AND DEPENDENCE AND HEALTH PROBLEMS; ALCOHOL ABUSE/DEPENDENCE; ALCOHOLISM; BINGE DRINKING; DELIRIUM TREMENS; YOUNG ADULTS.

Gwinnell, Esther, M.D., and Christine Adamec. *The Encyclopedia of Addictions and Addictive Behaviors.* New York: Facts On File, 2006.

Hingson, Ralph, and Michael Winter. "Epidemiology and Consequences of Drinking and Driving." *Alcohol Research & Health* 27, no. 1 (2003): 63–70.

Lakins, Nekisha, et al., "Apparent Per Capita Alcohol Consumption, National State and Regional Trends, 1977–2003," Surveillance Report # 73. Bethesda, Md.: National Institute of Alcohol Abuse and Alcoholism, August 2005.

alcohol abuse   See ABUSE, ALCOHOL.

alcohol abuse and dependence and health problems   Both chronic alcohol abuse as well as alcohol dependence (alcoholism) cause or contribute to many health problems, including increased risks to the liver, kidneys, heart, and other organs. Alcohol use disorders (which include both alcohol abuse and alcohol dependence) are also linked to psychiatric problems, such as depression and anxiety disorders. Alcoholism is linked to an increased risk for some psychotic disorders, such as SCHIZOPHRENIA. In addition, if a pregnant woman drinks even small amounts of alcohol, her fetus may develop FETAL ALCOHOL SYNDROME, a significant developmental disability.

Alcohol Abuse versus Alcohol Dependence and Health Risks

Alcohol abusers fit at least one of the following criteria that are directly caused by their excessive drinking:

• They fail to fulfill their personal responsibilities at work, school, or home.

• They drive or operate dangerous equipment while they are under the influence of alcohol.

- They have been arrested for an alcohol-related problem, such as driving while intoxicated or assaulting another person while under the influence of alcohol.

- They drink despite family or personal relationship problems that are either created or worsened by the excessive drinking.

In contrast, those who are alcohol-dependent (or alcoholics), drink more heavily and are more chronic drinkers who fit the following criteria:

- They have a TOLERANCE to alcohol (more alcohol is needed to achieve intoxication than in the past).

- They experience WITHDRAWAL symptoms (when alcohol is not consumed, physical symptoms occur, such as nausea, sweating, and shakiness).

- There is use of the substance in a larger quantity than intended.

- There is the persistent desire to cut down or to control the use of alcohol.

- A significant amount of time is spent on obtaining, using, or recovering from alcohol.

- Drinking occurs in order to prevent the symptoms of withdrawal.

- There is neglect of the individual's normal social, occupational, or recreational tasks.

- There is a continued use of alcohol despite the physical and psychological problems of the user.

In general, alcoholics have a greater risk for health problems than do alcohol abusers. For example, with regard to the rate per 1,000 of those who have cirrhosis of the liver, based on data provided in 2006 from the National Institute of Alcohol Abuse and Alcoholism (NIAAA), among alcohol abusers, the rate in 2001–2 was 0.75 per 100,000 people. However, among alcoholics, the rate was a much more dramatic 11.07 per 100,000. Alcoholics had about double the rate of chest pain, or angina pectoris: 19.86 per 100,000 among alcohol abusers and 37.24 per 100,000 among alcoholics.

Alcoholics had a dramatically higher incidence of SCHIZOPHRENIA or other psychotic illnesses, or 2.38 per 100,000 for alcohol abusers versus 18.46 per 100,000 for alcoholics. Only with arthritis did the alcoholics

TABLE I: RATE PER 100,000 POPULATION OF SELECTED HEALTH CONDITIONS, AMONG ALCOHOL ABUSERS AND ALCOHOLICS, UNITED STATES, 2001–2002

	Alcohol Abuse	Alcohol Dependence
Hardening of the arteries, or arteriosclerosis	4.65	5.47
Cirrhosis of the liver	0.75	11.07
Any other form of liver disease	3.92	12.57
Hypertension	108.65	116.69
Chest pain, or angina pectoris	19.86	37.24
Rapid heartbeat, or tachycardia	17.00	51.54
Heart attack or myocardial infarction	3.17	6.83
Any other form of heart disease	12.75	18.47
Stomach ulcer	12.18	38.69
Gastritis	26.76	45.13
Arthritis	111.18	76.47
Schizophrenia or psychotic illness	2.38	18.46

Source: Adapted from the National Institute on Alcohol Abuse and Alcoholism. *Alcohol Use and Alcohol Use Disorders in the United States: Main Findings from the 2001–2002 National Epidemiologic Survey on Alcohol and Related Conditions (NESARC).* U.S. Alcohol Epidemiologic Data Reference Manual 8, number 1. Bethesda, Md.: National Institutes of Health, January 2006, p. 189.

fare better than the alcohol abusers, or 111.88 per 100,000 for the alcohol abusers compared to 76.47 for the alcoholics. The reasons for this disparity are unknown. (See Table I for further comparisons.)

Emotional Health

People who abuse or who are dependent on alcohol are more likely than others to suffer from DEPRESSION, ANXIETY DISORDERS, and other psychiatric diagnoses. It is not known whether people who have psychiatric problems are more likely to drink heavily or whether excessive alcohol use may trigger these emotional problems in some people. Genetics also often clearly plays a role in alcoholism, and there is usually more than one alcoholic in an extended family.

As can be seen from Table II, studies have shown that the prevalence of psychiatric disorders is much

TABLE II: PREVALENCE OF PSYCHIATRIC DISORDERS IN PEOPLE WITH ALCOHOL ABUSE AND ALCOHOL DEPENDENCE, ONE-YEAR RATE

	Alcohol Abuse	Alcohol Dependence
Mood disorders	12.3 percent	29.2 percent
Major depressive disorder	11.3 percent	27.9 percent
Bipolar disorder	0.3 percent	1.9 percent
Anxiety disorders	29.1 percent	36.9 percent
Generalized anxiety disorder (GAD)	1.4 percent	11.6 percent
Panic disorder	1.3 percent	3.9 percent
Post-traumatic stress disorder	5.6 percent	7.7 percent

Note: The one-year rate is the percentage of people who met the criteria for the disorder during the year prior to the survey.
Source: Petrakis, Ismene L., M.D., et al., "Comorbidity of Alcoholism and Psychiatric Disorders." *Alcohol Research & Health* 26, no. 2 (2002), p. 82.

higher among those individuals who are alcohol-dependent. For example, among alcohol abusers, 11.3 percent have major depressive disorders, while among alcoholics, the rate is 27.9 percent. Anxiety disorders are common among those who have alcohol disorders, and 29.1 percent of alcohol abusers and 36.9 percent of alcoholics have an anxiety disorder.

Alcohol Combined with Other Drugs in Underage Drinking

Many people who abuse alcohol also abuse other drugs, and the combination that is abused can be very dangerous or even fatal. This pattern of combination drug and alcohol use is especially likely to occur among young people, ages 12 to 20 years. According to the Drug Abuse Warning Network (DAWN), when a combination of alcohol and drugs was found in emergency room visits in 2004 among patients ages 12–20 years, such patients were nearly twice as likely to be admitted to the hospital (19 percent) than when alcohol alone was present (10 percent). Of patients treated in hospital emergency rooms who used other drugs in conjunction with alcohol, most (49 percent) used MARIJUANA, followed by COCAINE (22 percent). (See Table III.) Patients may have used more than one type of drug other than alcohol.

Some drugs that were combined with alcohol were over-the-counter (OTC) drugs, such as acet-

TABLE III: TOP TEN OTHER DRUGS IN ALCOHOL-RELATED EMERGENCY DEPARTMENT VISITS AMONG PATIENTS AGES 12–20 YEARS, 2004

Rank		Drug Visits	Percentage of Visits
Total alcohol with other drug(s)		45,282	100
1	Marijuana	22,244	49
2	Cocaine	10,066	22
3	Stimulants (amphetamine/methamphetamine)	3,805	8
4	Alpazolam (Xanax)	3,057	7
5	Drug unknown	1,835	4
6	Ibuprofen	1,585	3
7	Acetaminophen	1,524	3
8	Methylenedioxymethamphetamine (MDMA)/Ecstasy	1,502	3
9	Acetaminophen-hydrocodone	1,436	3
10	Heroin	1,323	3

Source: Office of Applied Studies. "Emergency Department Visits Involving Underage Drinking." *The DAWN Report* 1 (2006), p. 3.

aminophen or ibuprofen. Many people believe that all OTC drugs are inherently safe, and they do not realize that chronic use of such drugs can be harmful; for example, acetaminophen (Tylenol) can damage the liver and when alcohol is abused, liver damage is more likely to occur because the liver metabolizes alcohol and becomes overworked by the excessive consumption of alcohol.

Alcohol and the Systems of the Body

Alcohol abuse and alcoholism can have major effects on the various systems of the body, particularly if the abuse continues for years. However, sometimes even short-term alcohol use, as with only one or more bouts of BINGE DRINKING, is extremely dangerous and can be fatal.

The Brain Alcohol consumption over a period of years may lead to brain damage, causing such disorders as Wernicke's encephalopathy. However, experts Marlene Oscar-Berman and Ksenija Marinkovic have reported that about half of those who have ALCOHOLISM in the United States are apparently free of permanent cognitive impairments. The other half of all alcoholics have mild to severe brain impairment. As many as 2 million alcoholics need full-time care by others. Some have dementia. This situation is likely to increase as the baby boomers become ELDERLY individuals.

The Heart and Circulatory System Heavy and chronic alcohol consumption increases the risk of a heart attack, and this risk is exacerbated by high blood cholesterol levels. Individuals who are heavy drinkers have a much higher risk of having high blood pressure. (See Table IV.) As can be seen from this table, heavy female drinkers (Category III) have an elevated risk of having hypertensive

TABLE IV: RELATIVE RISK FOR MAJOR CHRONIC DISEASE CATEGORIES BY GENDER AND AVERAGE DRINKING CATEGORY

	Females			Males		
	I	II	III	I	II	III
Disease						
Malignant cancers						
Mouth and oropharynx cancers	1.45	1.85	5.39	1.45	1.85	5.39
Esophagus cancers	1.80	2.38	4.36	1.80	2.38	4.36
Liver cancer	1.45	3.03	3.60	1.45	3.03	3.60
Breast cancer	1.14	1.41	1.59	—	—	—
Other cancers	1.10	1.30	1.70	1.10	1.30	1.70
Cardiovascular diseases						
Hypertensive disease	1.40	2.00	2.00	1.40	2.00	2.00
Ischemic stroke	0.52	0.64	1.06	0.94	1.33	1.65
Hemorrhagic stroke	0.59	0.65	7.98	1.27	2.19	2.20
Other cardiovascular causes	1.50	2.20	2.20	1.50	2.20	2.20
Digestive disease						
Cirrhosis of the liver*	1.26	9.54	9.54	1.26	9.54	9.54

Note: Relative risk estimates are shown to quantify the effect size of the risk relationships. For example, females in drinking category I have a relative risk of 1.14 compared with female abstainers, of breast cancer. A relative risk of 1.14 corresponds to a 14 percent higher risk. For females in drinking category III, the relative risk is 1.59, a risk increase of 59 percent compared to that female abstainers.
Definition of drinking categories:
Category I: for females, 0–19.99 grams pure alcohol daily; for males, 0–39.99 g pure alcohol daily
Category II: for females, 20–39.99 g pure alcohol daily; for males, 40–59.99 g pure alcohol daily
Category III: for females, 40 g or more pure alcohol; for males 60 g or more pure alcohol
* For liver cirrhosis, a combined estimate was derived for drinking categories II and III.
Note: A standard drink is generally considered to be equal to either 12 ounces of beer, 5 ounces of wine, or 1.5 ounces of distilled spirits. Each of these amounts is also equivalent to 0.5 ounce or 12 grams of alcohol. As a result, individuals in Category I drink from 0 to 1.67 standard drinks per day. Individuals in Category II drink 1.67 drinks to 3.3 drinks per day. Those in Category III drink from 3.33 drinks per day to 5 or more drinks per day.
Source: Adapted from Rehm, Jurgen, et al. "Alcohol-Related Morbidity and Mortality." *Alcohol Research & Health* 27, no. 1 (2002): p. 41.

disease compared to those who drink much less (Category I).

The risk for ischemic stroke and especially hemorrhagic stroke is much greater among heavy drinkers than light drinkers or nondrinkers; for example, among women, heavy drinkers have nearly an eight times greater risk of having a hemorrhagic stroke. This is also a higher rate than among heavy drinkers who are male, who have more than twice the risk of a stroke.

The Reproductive System Menstruation is affected by alcoholism, and these effects can cause infertility in women. The male reproductive system may also be affected by alcoholism, not only in incidents of impotence (due to drunkenness) but also in penile dysfunction caused by alcoholic-induced neuropathy.

The Digestive System Alcoholism may severely harm the liver and the pancreas, causing alcoholic HEPATITIS, pancreatitis, and even liver failure. As can be seen from Table IV, both male and female drinkers who are at levels II and III drinking have a much greater risk of development of cirrhosis of the liver than those at Level I. They have a significantly elevated risk of cirrhosis (9.54) compared to drinkers at level I, who have a risk of 1.26.

Abnormal clotting of the blood that is caused by liver damage may lead to excessive bleeding. The damaged liver may decrease the blood flow through the liver, causing swollen veins in the esophagus. These veins may rupture in response to only minor trauma. When combined with the problem of abnormal clotting, bleeding from these veins can lead to rapid death through blood loss.

The Immune System Chronic alcoholism appears to harm the immune system, causing alcoholics to contract more infections than others. According to Elizabeth J. Kovacs and Kelly A. N. Messingham in their article in *Alcohol Research & Health*:

Taken together, these studies show clearly that there are dramatic suppressive effects of both acute and chronic alcohol exposure on inflammation and immunity, regardless of gender. This results in decreased ability of the immune system to fight infections and tumors. The decrease in immunity after consumption of larger quantities of alcohol is

in marked contrast to the effects of very low levels of some alcoholic beverages (such as a single glass of red wine), which contain immunosuppressive antioxidants. By depressing estrogen levels, chronic or acute alcohol exposure may cause females to lose the important boost to the immune system that estrogen normally provides. This could act additively or synergistically with an elevation in immunosuppressive glucocorticoids (through activation of the HPA axis) to attenuate immune response, thus leading to a weakened ability to fight infections and tumors.

Finally, although chronic alcohol exposure causes liver damage in both males and females, it takes less alcohol and shorter periods of consumption to raise the risk of liver damage for females than for males. Like the observed gender differences in alcohol-induced immune suppression, this effect may involve the combined effect of stimulating glucocorticoid production and inhibiting estrogen production.

Cancer Colorectal cancer, esophageal cancer, and stomach cancer are all forms of cancer that have been directly linked to alcoholism, and there also appears to be a relationship between alcohol consumption and the incidence of breast cancer. As can be seen from Table IV, heavy drinkers have an increased risk for the development of mouth cancer, esophageal cancer, liver cancer, breast cancer, and other cancers. Note that when individuals both drink and smoke, they have an even further elevated risk of the development of digestive cancers and cancer of the respiratory tract.

The Bones Bone density is reduced by chronic alcoholism; as a result, the risk for osteoporosis among both men and women increases.

The Effects of Alcohol in Adolescents In addition to the effects that alcohol may have on all humans, alcohol has an array of additional insidious effects on adolescents; for example, alcohol can lower the estrogen levels in girls and the testosterone levels in boys. Acute alcohol intoxication affects the growth hormones in both males and females and thus may impede growth. Increased alcohol consumption can affect the bone mineral density in adolescent males; however, it does not appear to have this effect in females.

Studies of alcohol abuse and dependence in adolescents have shown that alcohol consumption is linked to reduced hippocampal volumes in the brain as well as with subtle abnormalities in the corpus callosum of the brain.

See also ADOLESCENTS AND SUBSTANCE ABUSE; ALCOHOL; ALCOHOL ABUSE/DEPENDENCE; BINGE DRINKING; COLLEGE STUDENTS; DELIRIUM TREMENS; DRIVING; INJURIES, CAUSED BY ALCOHOL AND/OR ILLICIT DRUGS; GENETIC PREDISPOSITIONS AND ENVIRONMENTAL EFFECTS IN SUBSTANCE USE DISORDERS; PSYCHIATRIC PROBLEMS; YOUNG ADULTS.

Bagnardi, Vincenzo, et al. "Alcohol Consumption and the Risk of Cancer: A Meta-Analysis." *Alcohol Research & Health* 25, no. 4 (2001): 263–270.

Emanuele, Mary Ann, M.D., Frederick Wezeman, and Nicholas V. Emanuele, M.D. "Alcohol's Effects on Female Reproductive Function." *Alcohol Research & Health* 26, no. 4 (2002): 274–281.

Kovacs, Elizabeth J., and Kelly, A. N. Messingham. "Influence of Alcohol and Gender on Immune Response." *Alcohol Research & Health* 26, no. 4 (2002): 257–263.

National Institute on Alcohol Abuse and Alcoholism, *Alcohol Use and Alcohol Use Disorders in the United States: Main Findings from the 2001–2002 National Epidemiologic Survey on Alcohol and Related Conditions (NESARC).* U.S. Alcohol Epidemiologic Data Reference Manual 8, no. 1 (January 2006), Bethesda, Md.: National Institutes of Health, January 2006.

Office of Applied Studies. "Emergency Department Visits Involving Underage Drinking." *The DAWN Report* 1 (2006): 3.

Oscar-Berman, Marlene, and Ksenija Marinkovic. "Alcoholism and the Brain: An Overview." *Alcohol Research & Health* 27, no. 3 (2003): 125–133.

Petrakis, Ismene L., M.D., et al. "Comorbidity of Alcoholism and Psychiatric Disorders." *Alcohol Research & Health* 26, no. 2 (2002): 81–89.

Rehm, Jürgen, et al., "Alcohol-Related Morbidity and Mortality." *Alcohol Research & Health* 27, no. 1 (2002): 39–51.

Tapert, Susan F., Lisa Caldwell, and Christina Burke. "Alcohol and the Adolescent Brain: Human Studies." *Alcohol Research & Health* 28, no. 4 (2004/2005): 205–212.

alcohol abuse/dependence Frequent need to use alcohol or addiction to alcohol. (See ALCOHOL ABUSE; ALCOHOLISM.) Some studies report combined statistics for alcohol abuse and dependence. For example, according to a 2006 *NSDUH Report,* 18.2 million people, or 7.6 percent of the population, in the United States met the criteria for alcohol abuse or dependence in 2004. (The statistic did not distinguish between alcohol abuse and alcohol dependence.) Alcohol abuse or dependence was found more commonly among adults ages 18 and older who were never married (16 percent) than among adults who were divorced or separated (10 percent), married (4.5 percent), or widowed (1.3 percent).

In considering age groups, the largest percentage of alcohol abuse or dependence was found among young adults ages 18 to 25 years (17.4 percent), followed by those who were ages 26 to 34 years (11.4 percent). In considering race and ethnicity, American Indians or Alaska Natives had the highest percentage of alcohol abuse or dependence (14 percent), followed by Native Hawaiian or other Pacific Islanders (8.5 percent) and Hispanics (8.2 percent).

With regard to gender, males were more likely to be alcohol abusers or alcohol dependent (10.6 percent) than females (4.9 percent). In addition, adults living with children were *less* likely (6.5 percent) to be alcohol abusers or dependent on alcohol than those who did not have children living in the home (8.5 percent).

Those who had alcohol abuse/dependence were more likely (34.2 percent) to have been treated in an emergency room or hospital in the past year than those who were not abusers or dependent (27.9 percent). However, both groups perceived that they had very good or excellent health; 61.8 percent of those who were alcohol abusers and dependent responded that they had good health and 62.6 percent of the other group also reported good health.

See also ADDICTION/DEPENDENCE.

Office of Applied Studies. "Alcohol Dependence or Abuse: 2002, 2003, and 2004," *The NSDUH Report* 16, 2006. Available online. URL: http://oas.samhsa.gov/2k6/AlcDepend/alcDepend.pdf. Downloaded June 27, 2006.

alcoholism   An addiction to and dependence on the consumption of alcohol. Also known as *alcohol dependence*. Alcoholism is a major and severe problem in the United States and CANADA as well as in many countries around the globe. It not only negatively affects the lives of the alcoholics themselves but also has an extended and even lifelong effect on the lives of their family members. Alcoholism affects individuals in the workplace, where the alcoholic's work performance is usually impaired, and in the general economy, where the overall work productivity is shortchanged when all alcoholics are considered. Yet according to the National Institute on Alcohol Abuse and Alcoholism (NIAAA), some studies of primary care practices have shown that alcoholics receive an assessment by a medical professional and a referral to treatment only about 10 percent of the time.

According to a study released by the Substance Abuse and Mental Health Services Administration in 2004, in considering the state averages of the percentages of people with alcohol dependence, the nationwide average statewide percentage for individuals ages 12 years and older for 2002 was 3.5 percent of the population, with the highest nationwide percentage seen among young adults ages 18–25 years, or 7 percent. In considering alcohol dependence on a state-by-state basis, the highest percentage of alcohol dependence was in the District of Columbia (5.20 percent) and the lowest rate in Pennsylvania: 2.79 percent. (See Table I for further information.)

TABLE I: PERCENTAGES REPORTING PAST YEAR ALCOHOL DEPENDENCE AMONG PERSONS AGES 12 YEARS AND OLDER, BY AGE GROUP AND STATE IN THE UNITED STATES: 2002

State	Estimate	Age 12–17	Age 18–25	26 or Older
Total	3.50	2.13	7.00	3.08
Alabama	3.20	2.08	5.61	2.92
Alaska	4.01	2.14	7.98	3.74
Arizona	3.75	2.82	7.31	3.25
Arkansas	3.33	2.78	6.27	2.89
California	3.47	1.59	6.09	3.27
Colorado	4.22	2.38	8.37	3.75
Connecticut	3.16	1.73	6.68	2.85
Delaware	3.65	1.23	8.70	3.09
District of Columbia	5.20	2.24	7.80	4.95
Florida	2.97	1.84	6.61	2.60
Georgia	3.88	1.86	5.42	3.89
Hawaii	3.44	1.99	7.43	2.98
Idaho	3.82	3.42	7.22	3.19
Illinois	3.57	2.53	6.79	3.15
Indiana	3.33	2.36	7.27	2.74
Iowa	3.25	3.26	7.24	2.50
Kansas	3.24	2.43	6.80	2.68
Kentucky	3.16	2.50	6.07	2.73
Louisiana	4.20	2.56	7.70	3.75
Maine	2.95	2.17	7.41	2.39
Maryland	3.60	1.59	6.19	3.48
Massachusetts	3.75	2.36	7.68	3.29
Michigan	4.26	2.28	7.92	3.91
Minnesota	3.47	2.48	7.83	2.83
Mississippi	3.77	1.54	5.09	3.84
Missouri	3.13	1.93	7.92	2.45
Montana	3.99	4.76	9.42	2.92
Nebraska	4.21	2.81	8.91	3.52
Nevada	3.35	2.66	5.72	3.07
New Hampshire	3.74	2.62	8.67	3.13
New Jersey	3.06	1.82	7.32	2.62
New Mexico	4.35	2.77	10.23	3.51
New York	3.84	2.31	6.64	3.57
North Carolina	3.69	2.10	6.43	3.43
North Dakota	4.20	4.52	8.88	3.19
Ohio	3.46	1.62	8.31	2.88
Oklahoma	3.07	2.12	6.92	2.46
Oregon	3.12	1.83	7.60	2.53
Pennsylvania	2.79	2.16	6.76	2.23
Rhode Island	4.13	2.59	11.96	2.90
South Carolina	4.07	1.85	7.31	3.79
South Dakota	4.22	3.90	9.19	3.31
Tennessee	3.12	2.37	6.39	2.67
Texas	3.32	1.85	6.73	2.89
Utah	3.62	1.88	7.03	2.94
Vermont	3.38	2.96	7.90	2.68
Virginia	3.95	2.91	7.96	3.44
Washington	3.05	1.73	7.19	2.54
West Virginia	2.83	3.20	5.62	2.34
Wisconsin	3.82	2.98	9.39	2.94
Wyoming	4.00	2.81	9.30	3.19

Source: Wright, D. *State Estimates of Substance Use from the 2002 National Survey on Drug Use and Health.* Department of Health and Human Services Publication No. SMA 04-3907, NSDUH Series H-23. Rockville, Md.: Substance Abuse and Mental Health Services Administration, Office of Applied Studies, July 2004.

Genetic Issues

There is a family history of alcoholism among many alcoholics and this may be due at least in part to a genetic predisposition. (See GENETIC PREDISPOSITIONS AND ENVIRONMENTAL EFFECTS IN SUBSTANCE USE DISORDERS.) Studies of adoptees and their adoptive parents, with no genetic relationship to each other, have indicated that adopted adults (especially males) who have birth parents who are alcoholics have an increased risk for the development of alcoholism themselves.

According to a 2002 article in *Alcohol Research & Health*, studies of adopted individuals showed that males whose birth parents were alcoholics had a 1.6 to 3.6 times greater risk for alcoholism compared to adopted men with no birth family history of alcoholism. The results were not clear-cut for adopted females. Some studies of adopted females showed an increased risk for alcoholism among women with a family history of alcoholism, and others did not.

In another study of about 1,000 alcoholic subjects and their families, described in 2002 in *Alcohol Research & Health*, the researchers found a genetic linkage in sibling pairs on the traits of alcoholism and depression, located on chromosome 1. They also found possible evidence of a genetic link to alcohol dependence on chromosome 4.

Psychiatric Problems and Alcoholism

Many alcoholics also have psychiatric problems, such as DEPRESSION, ANXIETY DISORDERS, and other disorders; for example, alcoholics have nearly four times the risk of experiencing depression of nonalcoholics, nearly four times the risk of SCHIZOPHRENIA, and more than twice the risk for an anxiety disorder. (See Table II.)

Other studies have shown that 15–20 percent of alcoholic males and 10 percent of alcoholic females have ANTISOCIAL PERSONALITY DISORDER. In addition, EATING DISORDERS are often associated with ALCOHOLISM, particularly anorexia nervosa or bulimia nervosa, according to research discussed in 2002 in *Alcohol Research & Health*.

This does not mean that alcoholism *causes* these disorders, although it may trigger disorders in those with genetic predispositions toward them. It may also mean that individuals who have these dis-

TABLE II: PREVALENCE OF PSYCHIATRIC DISORDERS IN PEOPLE WITH ALCOHOL DEPENDENCE (ALCOHOLISM)

Comorbid Disorder	1-Year Rate (Percent)	Odds Ratio
Mood disorders	29.2	3.6
Major depressive disorder	27.9	3.9
Bipolar disorder	1.9	6.3
Anxiety disorders	36.9	2.6
Generalized anxiety disorder (GAD)	11.6	4.6
Panic disorder	3.9	1.7
PTSD	7.7	2.2
Schizophrenia	24	3.8

Source: Ismene L. Petrakis, M.D., et al. "Comorbidity of Alcoholism and Psychiatric Disorders." *Alcohol Research & Health* 26, no. 2 (2002), pp. 81–89.

orders, particularly those who are untreated, are more likely to become alcoholics, perhaps in an attempt to self-medicate. Researchers continue to argue over cause and effect when both alcoholism and psychiatric disorders are present in an individual, but the one point that they agree upon is that psychiatric disorders are more common among those who are alcoholics.

Symptoms and Diagnostic Path

There are several classic symptoms of alcoholism, particularly when the individual is undergoing WITHDRAWAL and/or suffering from DELIRIUM TREMENS.

According to the NIAAA, alcoholism is characterized in individuals by the presence of three or more of the following indicators:

- a TOLERANCE to alcohol (more alcohol is needed to achieve intoxication than in the past)
- WITHDRAWAL symptoms (when alcohol is not consumed, physical symptoms occur, such as nausea, sweating, and shakiness)
- use of the substance in a larger quantity than was intended
- the persistent desire to cut down or to control the use of alcohol
- a significant amount of time spent on obtaining, using, or recovering from alcohol

- drinking that occurs to prevent the symptoms of withdrawal
- neglect of an individual's normal social, occupational, or recreational tasks
- continued use of alcohol despite the physical and psychological problems of the user

In addition to the NIAAA criteria, the following criteria may also be used for individuals to self-evaluate: the CAGE questionnaire. The individual is to ask himself or herself the following questions:

- Have you ever felt the need to Cut down on your drinking? **(C)**
- Have you ever felt Annoyed by criticism of your drinking? **(A)**
- Have you ever had Guilty feelings about your drinking? **(G)**
- Have you ever taken a morning Eye opener? **(E)**

If a person answers yes to one or more of the CAGE criteria, this suggests that he or she should be evaluated for alcoholism. If the person answers yes to two or more questions, it is likely the individual is an alcoholic. However, one major problem with the CAGE questions is that they do not distinguish between the past and current use of alcohol, and thus a recovering alcoholic could also respond positively to two or more questions.

There are other means to evaluate whether alcohol abuse or dependence is a problem. According to the NIAAA, physicians can assess patients for alcohol dependence by using the following guidelines provided in *Helping Patients Who Drink Too Much: A Clinician's Guide* in 2005.

Determine whether, in the past 12 months, your patient's drinking has **repeatedly** caused or contributed to

- **role failure** (interference with home, work, or school obligations
- **risk** of bodily harm (drinking and driving, operating machinery, swimming)
- **run-ins** with the law (arrests or other legal problems)

- **relationship** trouble (family or friends)

If yes to one or more → your patient has alcohol abuse.

In either case, proceed to assess for dependence symptoms.

Determine whether, in the past 12 months, your patient has

- shown tolerance (needed to drink a lot more to get the same effect)
- shown signs of withdrawal (tremors, sweating, nausea, or insomnia when trying to quit or cut down)
- not been able to stick to drinking limits (repeatedly gone over them)
- not been able to cut down or stop (repeated failed attempts)
- spent a lot of time drinking (or anticipating or recovering from drinking)
- spent less time on other matters (activities that had been important or pleasurable)
- kept drinking despite problems (recurrent physical or psychological problems)

If yes to three or more → your patient has alcohol dependence.

Treatment Options and Outlook

Some individuals are treated for their alcoholism on an outpatient basis, while others receive treatment in a rehabilitative facility. Of course many patients who have alcoholism are not treated at all, because they do not acknowledge that they have alcoholism, do not wish to receive treatment, or are not referred for treatment.

According to information from the Treatment Episode Data Set (TEDS) on individuals receiving substance abuse treatment in the United States, 42 percent of patients admitted into treatment facilities had alcohol as their primary substance of abuse. Of those admitted for alcohol abuse, in about 75 percent of the cases, alcohol was the sole substance that was the individual's problem. In 74 percent of the cases, the admitted patients were males.

Treatment may include medications, such as ACAMPROSATE (CAMPRAL), NALTREXONE (REVIA), or DISULFIRAM (ANTABUSE). In addition, BENZODIAZEPINES may be used to help alcoholics who are suffering from the symptoms of withdrawal. Behavioral therapy is also used effectively to treat alcoholism. Many patients benefit from self-help groups, such as Alcoholics Anonymous.

Risk Factors and Preventive Measures

As discussed, many studies indicate that there are genetic predispositions to alcohol abuse and alcoholism; however, it is important to note that the children of alcoholics are not doomed to become alcoholics themselves. Some children of alcoholics choose never to drink, lest they risk developing the problem. Some others are able to drink in moderation without developing a problem with alcohol abuse or dependence. However, the best way to avoid alcoholism is to avoid alcohol altogether or to drink in moderation only.

See also ADDICTION/DEPENDENCE; ALCOHOL ABUSE AND DEPENDENCE AND HEALTH PROBLEMS; BINGE DRINKING; COLLEGE STUDENTS; DELIRIUM TREMENS; FAMILY, EFFECT ON; IMPAIRED DRIVING INVOLVEMENT OF ALCOHOL AND/OR DRUGS; YOUNG ADULTS.

Adamec, Christine, and Laurie C. Miller, M.D. *The Encyclopedia of Adoption.* 3rd ed. New York: Facts On File, 2007.

Bierut, Laura Jean, M.D. "Defining Alcohol-Related Phenotypes in Humans: The Collaborative Study on the Genetics of Alcoholism," *Alcohol Research & Health* 26, no. 3 (2002): 208–213.

Grilo, Carlos M., Rajita Sinha, and Stephanie S. O'Malley. "Eating Disorders and Alcohol Use Disorders." *Alcohol Research & Health* 26, no. 2 (2002): 51–160.

National Institute on Alcohol Abuse and Alcoholism. *Helping Patients Who Drink Too Much: A Clinician's Guide.* Rockville, Md.: National Institutes of Health, 2005.

Petrakis, Ismene L., M.D., et al. "Comorbidity of Alcoholism and Psychiatric Disorders." *Alcohol Research & Health* 26, no. 2 (2002): 81–89.

Prescott, Carol A. "Sex Differences in the Genetic Risk for Alcoholism." *Alcohol Research & Health* 26, no. 2 (2002): 264–273.

Wright, D. *State Estimates of Substance Use from the 2002 National Survey on Drug Use and Health.* Department of Health and Human Services Publication no. SMA 04-3907, NSDUH Series H-23. Rockville, Md.: Substance Abuse and Mental Health Services Administration, Office of Applied Studies, July 2004.

alprazolam/alprazolam XR (Xanax/Xanax XR) An antianxiety medication in the category of BENZODIAZEPINES. Alprazolam is the immediate-acting form of the drug, while alprazolam XR (generally short for *extended release*) is longer-acting. Alprazolam is approved by the Food and Drug Administration (FDA) to treat such ANXIETY DISORDERS as generalized anxiety disorder (GAD) and panic disorder. Some physicians prescribe the drug for other psychiatric or medical problems, such as anxiety that is associated with DEPRESSION, irritable bowel syndrome, or insomnia. Alprazolam is also a drug of abuse and dependence for some individuals.

Alprazolam is a Schedule III drug under the CONTROLLED SUBSTANCES ACT. When combined with alcohol, alprazolam is a dangerous drug and abusers may require emergency room services.

Some patients may experience euphoria with alprazolam, which may increase the risk for abuse among those who are at risk for abuse (such as those with a past or current history of substance abuse). Some doctors prescribe alprazolam in addition to antidepressants. Immediate-release alprazolam may be more sedating than alprazolam XR.

Side Effects

When alprazolam is used as prescribed, it may cause some side effects, which include fatigue, sedation (although alprazolam is less sedating than other benzodiazepines), and depression. Paradoxically, alprazolam may alleviate depression in some patients.

Other side effects may include slurred speech, dizziness, confusion, and forgetfulness. Rarely, the drug may cause liver or kidney dysfunction or blood diseases. Alprazolam should be prescribed only very cautiously to patients who have any known liver or kidney diseases, as well as those who have hepatic impairment (liver dysfunction), who should be started on below-normal dosages.

Elderly individuals should also be given dosages lower than the standard starting dosage.

If alprazolam is taken with another central nervous system DEPRESSANT, it may lower respiration to a dangerous level.

According to Stephen Stahl in *Essential Psychopharmacology: The Prescriber's Guide,* there is a risk for dependence with alprazolam, especially if the drug is used for more than 12 weeks. The risk is further increased if patients have had or currently have a substance abuse problem.

Abuse of Alprazolam

In 2004, according to the National Survey on Drug Use and Health, alprazolam and the related drug lorazepam (Ativan) together (these drugs were reported together as one statistic) were abused by 3.9 percent of the population, with the highest abuse seen among those who were ages 18–25 (7.7 percent of that population).

Some individuals abuse other drugs at the same time as they abuse alprazolam, an extremely risky practice. According to the Drug Abuse Warning Network (DAWN), in a 2004 report of patients who abused OXYCODONE or HYDROCODONE and who had drug abuse–related emergency visits in 2002, alprazolam was the most commonly abused benzodiazepine, found in 7 percent of the cases of patients who took oxycodone and had a drug-related emergency visit and 12 percent of the cases of patients who took hydrocodone. The next most commonly abused benzodiazepine was DIAZEPAM (VALIUM), which was present in 6 percent of the cases of oxycodone abuse and 7 percent of the case of hydrocodone abuse.

Alprazolam was the seventh most frequently mentioned drug in emergency room visits in 2000. It was also the seventh most abused drug among female patients and the 10th most commonly abused drug among male patients.

See also ADDICTION/DEPENDENCE; ANXIETY DISORDERS; PRESCRIPTION DRUG ABUSE.

Drug Abuse Warning Network, "Oxycodone, Hydrocodone, and Polydrug Use, 2002," *The DAWN Report,* (July 2004): p. 3.

Stahl, Stephen M. *Essential Psychopharmacology: The Prescriber's Guide.* Cambridge: Cambridge University Press, 2005.

amphetamines A form of central nervous system STIMULANTS that may be prescribed by a physician and that are sometimes obtained illegally for the purpose of abuse or addiction. When they are lawfully prescribed, amphetamines may be used to treat ATTENTION DEFICIT HYPERACTIVITY DISORDER (ADHD), narcolepsy, and treatment-resistant DEPRESSION. In the past, amphetamines were used by physicians for appetite suppression among overweight and obese individuals, but with the exception of phentermine (Fastin), this use is no longer medically recognized.

In addition, METHYLENEDIOXYMETHAMPETAMINE (MDMA/ECSTASY), an illegal drug, is sometimes classified as a form of amphetamine by experts.

The current brand names of amphetamine that are legally prescribed as of this writing are Adderall, Adderall XR, Dexedrine, Dextrostat, and Desoxyn.

Amphetamines increase the level of dopamine as well as that of norephinephrine, two key brain chemicals.

When abused, amphetamines are usually used to produce a state of euphoria. Once an individual develops an addiction to the amphetamine, the drug is needed to avoid the symptoms of WITHDRAWAL. According to the United Nations Office on Drugs and Crime, an estimated 29.6 million people worldwide abused amphetamines in 2003, primarily amphetamine and METHAMPHETAMINE, a form of amphetamine that is an illegal drug that is usually produced in CLANDESTINE LABORATORIES. (This entry concentrates on nonmethamphetamine drugs that are amphetamines.)

Amphetamines are Schedule II drugs under the CONTROLLED SUBSTANCES ACT. They are taken orally or through injection.

Because of their considerable addictive potential, most physicians do not prescribe amphetamines to those patients who have a current or past history of substance abuse. In addition, amphetamine should not be prescribed to patients who have BIPOLAR DISORDER because the drug could exacerbate or trigger a manic state. Patients who have Tourette's syndrome or other tic disorders should not use amphetamines because the drug may worsen their existing tics. Patients who are highly anxious should also avoid amphetamines. Excessive stimulation may occur if amphetamine is taken with large doses of

PROPOXYPHENE (Darvon, Darvocet), a medication given for pain.

Amphetamines have also been shown to worsen the psychotic symptoms in individuals diagnosed with delusional disorders and SCHIZOPHRENIA. (See PSYCHOTIC BEHAVIOR.)

According to Charles Levinthal, author of *Drugs, Society, and Criminal Justice*, the origin of amphetamines can be traced back to *ma huang*, a medicinal herb that was used by the Chinese 5,000 years ago to treat respiratory disorders. In 1887, German chemists isolated the active ingredient in *ma huang*, naming it *ephedrine*. Then in 1927, Los Angeles, California, research chemist Gordon Alles created a synthetic form of ephedrine, which he named *amphetamine*.

Amphetamine was first sold in 1932 as Benzedrine, a brand name product that was included in over-the-counter inhalers that were used to treat asthma. In 1937, amphetamine was available in a prescription tablet that was used to treat narcolepsy, excessive sleeping, and "minimal brain dysfunction" (now called ATTENTION DEFICIT HYPERACTIVITY DISORDER). The drug was also included in an inhaler to treat nasal congestion.

Amphetamine was often given to military service members in both the United States and Germany during World War II in the form of dextroamphetamine (Dexedrine) and methamphetamine (Methedrine) so that they could stay awake under battle conditions. Suicide pilots (kamikaze) in Japan also used amphetamines.

According to the Drug Enforcement Administration (DEA), amphetamines have been used for multiple purposes through the years; for example, in the 1960s, truckers used amphetamines to stay awake over long hauls. The drug was also used to treat DEPRESSION and to help athletes improve their performance. In the case of inhalers used for nasal congestion and asthma, some individuals abused the drug by withdrawing the amphetamine from the inhaler and injecting it or drinking it.

This abuse potential of amphetamines was eventually discovered and noted by federal and state authorities, and in 1965, federal food and drug laws were amended to limit the supply of amphetamine. However, abuse of the drug continued, and amphetamine abuse reached a peak in the early 1980s. Abuse fell off after that time among all age levels, as COCAINE and CRACK COCAINE became the dominant drugs of abuse.

Amphetamine abuse is no longer a major problem today, with the glaring exception of the illegal manufacture and use of methamphetamine, which is an increasing problem in the United States. However, some data suggest that with the restriction of access to pseudoephedrine, an ingredient in the manufacture of methamphetamine that is available in over-the-counter drugs, abuse of this drug is beginning to decrease.

Today, amphetamines are legally prescribed by physicians to treat some patients who have attention deficit hyperactivity disorder (ADHD) or to treat narcolepsy. However, if there is a recent past history or current history of substance abuse, most physicians will avoid prescribing amphetamines or other stimulants to individuals with ADHD, preferring to prescribe nonstimulants such as atomoxetine (Strattera), a medication that is specifically approved for the treatment of ADHD, or bupropion (Wellbutrin), an antidepressant medication with some psychostimulant effects.

Even under the care of a physician, the termination of amphetamine use may lead to the development of (or the unmasking of an existing) depression. Additionally, excessive fatigue is almost always noted during amphetamine withdrawal. Nonetheless, there are no clear life-threatening consequences of the abrupt discontinuation of amphetamines, so tapering and slow discontinuation are not usually done.

Side Effects of Amphetamines

Common side effects that may occur with the lawful use of amphetamine may include the following:

- dry mouth
- constipation
- weight loss
- insomnia
- headache
- dizziness

In some cases, beta blocker medications may be used to counteract these side effects of amphetamines.

Serious side effects from abuse Amphetamines can cause serious side effects when they are abused, including such symptoms as a rapid heartbeat, hyperthermia (high fever), high blood pressure, seizures, mania, and suicidal thoughts. In the most extreme cases, the user can experience an *amphetamine psychosis,* and ACCIDENTAL OVERDOSE DEATHS have occurred. (See PSYCHOTIC BEHAVIOR.)

Amphetamine psychosis Symptoms of amphetamine psychosis, a condition that is difficult to distinguish from SCHIZOPHRENIA, may include both auditory (heard) and visual (seen) HALLUCINATIONS, paranoid ideas, and picking at the skin. These psychotic symptoms may resolve eventually, but they may also persist for months or years, well after the drug was abused and the use was discontinued. Patients who have amphetamine psychosis may also exhibit violent behavior.

Abusers of Amphetamines

According to the Monitoring the Future study for 2004, high school seniors had a prevalence rate of 15.0 percent of having ever used amphetamines, compared to young adults (15.9 percent). The highest rate was 18.0 percent for non-college students.

TABLE I: LIFETIME PREVALENCE, ANNUAL PREVALENCE, AND CURRENT USE OF AMPHETAMINE IN 2004 IN CERTAIN POPULATIONS, PERCENTAGES

	Lifetime Prevalence	Annual Prevalence	30-Day Prevalence
8th Graders	7.5	4.9	2.3
10th Graders	11.9	8.5	4.0
High School Seniors	15.0	19.0	4.6
Young Adults Ages 19–28	15.9	6.2	2.4
College Students	12.7	7.0	3.2
Same-age Non College Students	18.0	8.5	3.4

Source: Adapted from Johnston, Lloyd D., et al. *Monitoring the Future: National Survey Results on Drug Use, 1975–2004.* Vol. 2, *College Students and Adults Ages 19–45.* Bethesda, Md.: National Institute on Drug Abuse, National Institutes of Health, 2005, pp. 37, 44.

Treatment for Amphetamine Abuse

Of those individuals who were admitted for treatment for abuse of an amphetamine (not METHAMPHETAMINE), 1.0 percent, or 19,133 individuals, reported amphetamine as their primary substance of abuse in 2004 in the United States, according to information from the Office of Applied Studies of the Substance Abuse and Mental Health Services Administration (SAMHSA).

Individuals who are dependent on amphetamines should undergo DETOXIFICATION in a treatment facility. Withdrawal from amphetamines can be difficult and is best undertaken in a treatment facility that has experience working with withdrawal procedures or treatment should occur under the care of a physician. In the first hours of withdrawal, the addict may feel depressed, anxious, and agitated. Withdrawal from amphetamines can take from six to 18 weeks.

See also ADDICTION/DEPENDENCE; CANADA; PRESCRIPTION DRUG ABUSE; PRESCRIPTION DRUG MONITORING PROGRAMS, STATES WITH; PSYCHIATRIC DISORDERS; STIMULANTS; YOUNG ADULTS.

Johnston, Lloyd D., et al. *Monitoring the Future: National Survey Results on Drug Use, 1975–2004.* Vol. 2, *College Students and Adults Ages 19–45.* Bethesda, Md.: National Institute on Drug Abuse, National Institutes of Health, 2005.

Joseph, Donald E., et al., eds. Drug *Drugs of Abuse.* Washington, D.C.: U.S. Department of Justice, 2005.

Levinthal, Charles F. *Drugs, Society, and Criminal Justice.* New York: Pearson Education, 2006.

Office of Applied Studies, Substance Abuse and Mental Health Services Administration. *Treatment Episode Data Set (TEDS) Highlights–2003: National Admissions to Substance Abuse Treatment Services.* Rockville, Md.: Department of Health and Human Services, June 2005.

Stahl, Stephen M. *Essential Psychopharmacology: The Prescriber's Guide.* Cambridge: Cambridge University Press, 2005.

anabolic steroids Prescribed drugs that are synthesized from male hormones, primarily testosterone. The full name of anabolic steroids is *androgenic anabolic steroids.* According to the Drug Enforcement Administration, the most frequently abused anabolic steroids are Deca-Durabolin, Durabolin, Equipoise, and Winstrol.

These drugs were used in the past to treat DEPRESSION, but it is known now that they may induce depression. They are sometimes prescribed by physicians to treat children or adolescents who have growth problems. However, anabolic steroids are more commonly known for their illegal use by bodybuilders, athletes, and others who wish to improve their athletic performance and achieve greater muscle development at a much faster pace than exercise alone could provide. Sometimes law enforcement officers abuse these drugs, as do bodyguards and construction workers.

Most anabolic steroids are Schedule III drugs under the CONTROLLED SUBSTANCES ACT. Federal law labeled anabolic steroids as scheduled drugs in 1991.

Some individuals who abuse anabolic steroids take different brands of steroids in complicated regimens, a practice that is known as "stacking." They may take very high doses of drugs for four to 18 weeks and then refrain from using all drugs for one to 12 months. In some cases, trainers create these detailed regimens for the steroid abuser. Some users use a method that they call "pyramiding," which means that they slowly escalate the number of drugs that are used as well as the frequency of use, after which they taper off the drugs until the next cycle.

Those who abuse anabolic steroids may take up to 100 times the therapeutic dose of the drug. Clearly this is a highly risky choice, and one that is extremely unsafe. Many abusers use at least two different steroids.

According to Timothy D. Noakes, M.D., in his 2004 article for the *New England Journal of Medicine* on steroid drug use among athletes, Testoviron (testosterone propionate) was first synthesized in 1936 and used by athletes in the 1948 Olympic Games. Subsequent drugs such as methandrostenolone (Dianabol), synthesized in 1958, and oral chlordehydromethyltestosterone (Turinabol), synthesized in 1966, were also used by athletes.

Says Noakes, "By increasing muscle size, these drugs increase strength, power, and sprinting speed; they also alter mood and speed the rate of recovery, permitting more intensive training and hence superior training adaptation." Noakes asserts that athletes using performance-enhancing drugs have "moved off the natural bell-shaped curve of normal human performance."

Anabolic steroids may be taken orally or by injection. They are also available in transdermal skin patches and gels. Examples of oral steroids are Anadrol (oxymetholone), Dianabol (methandrostenolone), Oxandrin (oxandrolone), and Winstrol (stanozolol). Examples of injectable steroids are Deca-Durabolin (nandrolone decanoate), Durabolin (nandrolone phenpropionate), Depo-Testosterone (testosterone cypionate), and Equipoise (bodenone undecylenate), which is a veterinary product sometimes abused by humans.

Short-Term and Long-Term Effects of Anabolic Steroid Use In the short term, the side effects of anabolic steroid abuse include severe acne, sexual and reproductive disorders, and fluid retention. Men who abuse these drugs may experience gynecomastia (the enlargement of a man's breasts) and atrophy of the testicles. They may also experience painful erections, decreased sperm production, and sterility.

Women who abuse anabolic steroids will experience masculinizing effects, such as an increased production of facial and body hair, enlargement of the clitoris, a deepening voice, and baldness; these effects are *not* reversible once they have occurred. In contrast, the short-term physical effects in men are mostly reversible. Women who abuse steroids will also experience menstrual irregularities.

Both men and women who abuse steroids may experience high blood pressure and liver disorders. They may have jaundice (yellowed skin) and an increase in cholesterol levels. They may also experience severe psychological side effects, such as mood swings that resemble the mania of bipolar DISORDER, DEPRESSION, DELUSIONS, extreme irritability, aggression and impaired judgment stemming from a perception of invulnerability, and even psychosis. They are at risk for blood clotting disorders and heart disease.

Adolescents who abuse anabolic steroids may prematurely halt their growth cycle, resulting in the attainment of a shorter height than they would have attained had they not abused these drugs.

Psychiatric effects Violent and even murderous behavior has been noted among those who abuse anabolic steroids because of the rage and aggression that these drugs can induce when they are abused. Hall, Hall, and Chapman in their 2005 article in *Psychosomatics* on the psychiatric effects of the use of anabolic steroids, report that they have seen six cases of criminal behavior among individuals using anabolic steroids, including three homicides and three violent assaults. In half of these cases, there was some evidence of criminal behavior or violence before the steroid-induced violent episode occurred. Two of the three homicides were not premeditated, and they happened during a psychotic episode.

Say the authors, "In each case, an irrational thought of the patient or a minor deed of an unknown individual promoted a violent attack. The mental status of all six perpetrators cleared within weeks to 2 months, and they had specific memory of the act and of their delusional thinking at the time the act was committed."

Abusers of Anabolic Steroids

Dr. Hall and his colleagues offer a profile of the typical abuser of anabolic steroids. They say that the abuser is often a person who abuses multiple substances and who performs poorly in school. Most steroid abusers are males, and males are two to three times more likely to abuse anabolic steroids than females. About 60–70 percent of steroid abusers participate in organized sports.

Say the authors, "Other factors that correlate with AAS [anabolic-androgenic steroids] abuse include higher socioeconomic status, a family history of drug abuse, higher rates of self-reported violence and aggression, lower-self-esteem, and poor body image before AAS use."

Some studies indicate that the anabolic steroid abuser has a higher risk of childhood physical or sexual abuse. Other studies indicate that the girlfriends or wives of anabolic steroid abusers are at risk for physical abuse.

Among adolescents, it is estimated that about 2 percent of 8th and 10th graders have ever tried anabolic steroids; the percentage increases to 3 percent for 12th graders.

Steroid abusers may share needles with others, increasing their risk for contracting HEPATITIS, the HUMAN IMMUNODEFICIENCY VIRUS, and other diseases.

Abusers Often Use Other Drugs Abusers of anabolic steroids often use other drugs, such as MARIJUANA and COCAINE. Some take NARCOTICS in an attempt to control the side effects of anabolic steroids, such as the insomnia and irritability that they

cause. Others take diuretics to counter the water retention steroids cause, and they may also use tamoxifen to counteract the gynecomastia. Some abusers use antibiotics or antiacne medications to prevent the acne that is induced by the steroid.

Purchases through the Internet

Many abusers of anabolic steroids buy them illegally over the Internet. A General Accounting Office report published in 2005 discussed the experience of investigators who bought drugs from Web sites advertising anabolic steroids for sale, both to determine the ease of purchases and to analyze the products that were purchased. They received 14 shipments of drugs that were purportedly anabolic steroids; however, analysis of four of the shipments revealed that they contained no steroids. Of the shipments that did contain anabolic steroids, the investigators found that the shipments originated in three countries, Italy, China, and Greece.

According to this report, anabolic steroids may be sold without a prescription in many countries worldwide; for that reason they are readily available to be ordered over the Internet.

It is often difficult for investigators to detect anabolic steroids that are transported in packages by the U.S. Postal Service, in part because the Postal Service processes a huge volume of mail and in part because some drug dealers very carefully conceal the drugs in other items, such as hollowed-out sections of books or with small electronic equipment, such as blenders, radios, or alarm clocks.

Symptoms and Diagnostic Path

Males under the influence of anabolic steroids may exhibit aggressive or even psychotic behavior, as well as other symptoms of abuse, such as gynecomastia. Females may exhibit virilizing symptoms, although there are other hormonal disorders that may also cause hirsuteness (hairiness) in females, such as polycystic ovarian syndrome, and thus, other disorders should be ruled out before it is assumed that a woman is abusing anabolic steroids. If the woman also has a deepened voice and enlarged clitoris, however, these signs make the diagnosis more likely.

Treatment Options and Outlook

Individuals abusing anabolic steroids should cease this use, before any further damage is done. There may be some symptoms of withdrawal, and thus withdrawal should be performed under the care of a physician. Symptoms of withdrawal may include fatigue, depression, sleep disturbance, and weight loss.

Risk Factors and Preventive Measures

Individuals in career fields that require intense physical actions and endurance, such as athletes and bodybuilders, should be warned away from anabolic steroids. Education about this problem in high schools and junior high schools could help warn young men away from using anabolic steroids. Female bodybuilders and other females who are considering the use of these drugs should also be alerted to their dangers. Parents should pay attention to the appearance of rapid muscle gain in their adolescent children and be aware that some athletic coaches promote the use of these drugs to improve the competitive edge of a team or an individual athlete with whom they are working.

See also PSYCHIATRIC DISORDERS; SCHEDULED DRUGS; YOUNG ADULTS.

Drug Enforcement Administration. *Steroid Abuse in Today's Society: A Guide to Understanding Steroids and Related Substances.* Washington, D.C.: U.S. Department of Justice, March 2004.

General Accounting Office Report, "Anabolic Steroids Are Easily Purchased without a Prescription and Present Significant Challenges to Law Enforcement Officials." Washington, D.C.: General Accounting Office, GAO-06-243R, November 5, 2005.

Hall, Ryan C. W., M.D., Richard C. W. Hall, M.D., and Marcia J. Chapman. "Psychiatric Complications of Anabolic Steroid Abuse." *Psychosomatics* 46, no. 4 (July–August 2005): 285–290.

Noakes, Timothy D., M.D. "Tainted Glory—Doping and Athletic Performance." *New England Journal of Medicine* 359, no. 9 (August 26, 2004): 847–849.

Antabuse See DISULFIRAM.

antidepressants Medications used to treat DEPRESSION. Many individuals who have substance-induced disorders are also clinically depressed and may benefit from treatment with antidepressants. However, it is very important that the treating physician be aware of all drugs that the patient takes, including illicit substances and the chronic use of alcohol, in order to prevent an interaction. For example, if patients frequently drink alcohol, they should generally not be given an antidepressant that is sedating. Conversely, if patients abuse a drug that is a stimulant, they generally should not be given a stimulating medication.

There are several primary categories of antidepressants. Tricyclics are antidepressant medications that have been available for many years. They often have a sedating effect and may cause weight gain. Selective serotonin reuptake inhibitors (SSRIs) are newer medications that may be helpful to depressed patients. They are generally not sedating; nor do they cause weight gain. The newest form of antidepressant is the serotonin norepinephrine reuptake inhibitor (SNRI), such as duloxetine (Cymbalta) or venlafaxine (Effexor, Effexor XR). SNRIs may be sedating and may also increase the blood pressure slightly. Some patients report weight loss with SNRIs.

Bupropion (Wellbutrin) is an atypical antidepressant, which is effective in some individuals who have depression. It does not cause weight gain.

Some physicians prescribe monoamine oxidase inhibitors (MAO inhibitors) to treat depression; however, MAOIs interact with many different foods, and it may be difficult to comply with the necessary dietary regimen. They also cause weight gain. As a result, they are infrequently prescribed by most doctors.

Early in treatment, and with *any* antidepressant, there is still a risk for SUICIDE. Any mention of suicidal thoughts or plans should be reported immediately to the treating physician, whether the person is taking antidepressants or not.

Physicians usually initially prescribe the lowest possible dose of an antidepressant and increase the dosage as needed. Sometimes more than one antidepressant is needed to resolve depression.

See also BENZODIAZEPINES.

antisocial personality disorder A psychiatric disorder that is diagnosed in those older than 15 years and who have a pattern of behavior that is characterized by criminal acts, a lack of empathy, a resistance to working, attempts to manipulate others, and an intense resistance to authority. These individuals are also more likely to have a substance abuse problem than others. According to the National Institute of Mental Health (NIMH), individuals who have antisocial personality disorder have a 15.5 percent greater risk than those without psychiatric disorders for having a drug abuse problem. (See PSYCHIATRIC DISORDERS.) They are also more likely to abuse alcohol than those who do not have the disorder.

According to a study of a large population reported in the *Journal of Clinical Psychiatry* in 2004, an estimated 7.6 million individuals in the United States have antisocial personality disorder.

Many individuals who have antisocial personality disorder (ASPD) are eventually imprisoned for criminal acts, and an estimated 50–60 percent of all prison inmates have this disorder. However, some high-functioning individuals who have ASPD are able to succeed in society.

Some studies have shown that men who have ALCOHOLISM are four to eight times more likely to have ASPD than others. In addition, the prevalence of ASPD among alcoholic women is even greater than among alcoholic men: Alcoholic women have ASPD 12–17 times more than nonalcoholic women. (This is a striking finding, because in the general population, men are about three times more likely to have ASPD than women.) An estimated 15–20 percent of alcoholic males and 10 percent of alcoholic females have ASPD.

Symptoms and Diagnostic Path

By definition, individuals who have antisocial personality disorder exhibited problem behavior as children or adolescents, such as stealing items and frequently being in trouble. Such behavior is called CONDUCT DISORDER when it occurs in a child or adolescent. However, some children who have problem behavior may have been diagnosed with *oppositional defiant disorder,* primarily because of their refusal to follow the rules that are set by others, including their parents.

In adulthood, the behavior continues or escalates, and the individual is usually arrested and

incarcerated in jail or prison. The adult who has ASPD may tend to get many traffic tickets for offenses such as speeding. He or she may refuse to pay traffic fines and continue to drive, even after the driver's license is suspended for failure to pay fines, and ultimately the individual may be jailed for driving with a suspended driver's license.

Some individuals who have ASPD are very effective at manipulating others. They usually lack empathy, however, and although they understand how other people think, they have considerable contempt for them, particularly for those who willingly follow the laws, rules, and regulations of society.

Treatment Options and Outlook

The prognosis for ASPD is poor, and many individuals who have this disorder will be imprisoned, often for years, because of their criminal acts and their repeated refusal to follow the laws of society. The peak of antisocial behavior often occurs in the late teens and early 20s. Some research indicates that the behavior of males who have ASPD may improve when they are in their 40s. It is unknown whether this finding also applies to women who have ASPD.

Most individuals who have antisocial personality disorder do not acknowledge that they have a problem and will not seek treatment unless they are compelled, such as with a court order. Even when individuals who have ASPD accept treatment, it is difficult for most clinicians to treat the disorder. However, psychiatrists may treat concurrent disorders that are common among individuals with ASPD, such as substance abuse and depression. There are no known medications or reliably effective psychotherapies as of this writing to treat antisocial personality disorder.

Risk Factors and Preventive Measures

Studies have indicated that males have a three times greater risk of having antisocial personality disorder than females. A study on personality disorders in the United States based on a very large population of over 43,000 respondents and reported in the *Journal of Clinical Psychiatry* in 2004 found that 5.5 percent of the males met the criteria for antisocial personality disorder, as did 1.9 percent of the females.

They also found that the risks of this disorder were highest among Native Americans and lowest among Asians. Those ages 18–29 years had the greatest proportion of antisocial personality disorder in comparison to individuals of other ages. In terms of income, the risks were greatest among individuals earning less than $35,000. Individuals who had never married had a higher risk than those who had been (or were) married. Individuals living in the West had a significantly greater risk of having antisocial personality disorder than individuals in other parts of the country.

See also ADOLESCENTS AND SUBSTANCE ABUSE; ANXIETY DISORDERS; ATTENTION DEFICIT HYPERACTIVITY DISORDER; BIPOLAR DISORDER; CONDUCT DISORDER; CRIME AND CRIMINALS; DEPRESSION; DUAL DIAGNOSIS; JAIL INMATES; PSYCHIATRIC DISORDERS; YOUNG ADULTS.

Compton III, William M., M.D, et al. "The Role of Psychiatric Disorders in Predicting Drug Dependence Treatment Outcomes." *American Journal of Psychiatry* 160, no. 5 (May 2003): 890–895.

Grant, Bridget, F., et al. "Prevalence, Correlates and Disability of Personality Disorders in the United States: Results from the National Epidemiologic Survey on Alcohol and Related Conditions." *Journal of Clinical Psychiatry* 65 (2004): 948–958.

Shivani, Ramesh, M.D., R. Jeffrey Goldsmith, M.D., and Robert M. Anthenelli, M.D. "Alcoholism and Psychiatric Disorders: Diagnostic Challenges." *Alcohol, Research & Health* 26, no. 2 (2002): 90–98.

anxiety disorders   A group of serious emotional disorders that can cripple an individual's life, including generalized anxiety disorder (GAD), panic disorder, OBSESSIVE COMPULSIVE DISORDER (OCD), and post-traumatic stress disorder (PTSD). In addition, phobias are a form of anxiety disorder, including such phobias as social phobia (extreme fear of social situations), agoraphobia (fear of being in a situation from which escape appears difficult or impossible), and many specific phobias, such as a fear of spiders or of elevators.

According to the National Institute of Mental Health (NIMH), about 40 million adults in the United States ages 18 and older, or about 18 percent of the population, suffer from some sort of an anxiety disorder. About 75 percent of people who have anxiety disorders experience their first anxiety episode by age 21. Most people who have one anxiety disorder also have another anxiety disorder. In addition, depressive disorders and EATING DISORDERS are also often present in individuals who have anxiety disorders.

According to NIMH, about 2.2 million adults in the United States have OCD, or about 1 percent of the population age 18 and older. Generally the first symptoms of OCD occur in childhood or adolescence; however, the median age of onset is 19 years. OCD is now believed to have significant genetic patterns and to run in families.

An estimated 6.8 million adults in the United States suffer from GAD according to NIMH, or 3.1 percent of people ages 18 and older. GAD can occur at any age; the median age of onset is 31 years.

According to the NIMH, about 6 million adults in the United States, or 2.7 percent of the population, suffer from panic disorder. The age of onset is usually in early adulthood (with a median age of onset of 24 years), but it can occur at any time. An estimated one in three adults who have panic disorders develop agoraphobia. About 1.8 million adults ages 18 and older in the United States have agoraphobia, and the median age of the onset of the disorder is age 20.

About 7.7 million adults ages 18 and older in the United States have PTSD according to the NIMH, or about 3.5 percent of adults. PTSD can develop at any age; the median age of onset is 23 years. An estimated 30 percent of Vietnam War veterans experienced PTSD after the war. Other adults and children may develop PTSD after an extremely traumatic event, such as a natural disaster or a kidnapping.

An estimated 19.2 million adults ages 18 and older in the United States have specific phobias, according to NIMH, or about 9 percent of the adult population. The onset is usually in childhood and the median age of onset is seven years.

With regard to social phobia, about 15 million Americans ages 18 and older suffer from this form of anxiety disorder, or about 6.8 percent of the adult population. The onset of social phobia is usually in childhood or adolescence, typically at about age 13.

TABLE I: PREVALENCE OF PSYCHIATRIC DISORDERS IN PEOPLE WITH ALCOHOL ABUSE AND
ALCOHOL DEPENDENCE, ONE YEAR RATE[1]

	Alcohol Abuse	Alcohol Dependence
Anxiety disorders	29.1 percent	36.9 percent
Generalized anxiety disorder (GAD)	1.4 percent	11.6 percent
Panic disorder	1.3 percent	3.9 percent
Post-traumatic stress disorder	5.6 percent	7.7 percent

[1] The one-year rate is the percentage of people who met the criteria for the disorder during the year prior to the survey.
Source: Petrakis, Ismene L., M.D., et al. "Comorbidity of Alcoholism and Psychiatric Disorders." *Alcohol Research & Health* 26, no. 2 (2002), p. 82.

Individuals who have anxiety disorders have an increased risk for substance abuse and dependence. For example, according to the NIMH, individuals who have panic disorder have a 4.3 percent greater risk for substance abuse than those who do not have panic disorder. The rates are also elevated for those who have obsessive compulsive disorder (OCD), or 3.4 percent, and for those who have phobias (2.4 percent).

In addition, of those who *are* diagnosed with alcohol abuse or dependence, there is a high rate of anxiety disorders, particularly for the development of generalized anxiety disorder (GAD), post-traumatic stress disorder, or panic disorder. (See Table I.) For example, of those who were diagnosed with alcohol dependence (alcoholism), nearly 37 percent had some form of an anxiety disorder and nearly 12 percent suffered from GAD. Of those who were diagnosed with alcohol abuse, 29.1 percent also had an anxiety disorder. Post-traumatic stress disorder was present in 5.6 percent of those who were alcohol abusers.

Symptoms and Diagnostic Path

The symptoms of each individual anxiety disorder depend upon the particular disorder, as described in the following.

Generalized anxiety disorder (GAD)   In generalized anxiety disorder, the key symptoms are an uncontrollable and unrealistic worry about at least several issues, accompanied by physical symptoms such as insomnia, fatigue, and irritability. Somatic symptoms such as muscle tension are common with GAD. The anxiety and the physical symptoms significantly impair the person's life, both at work and at home.

Panic disorder   A panic disorder is an intense feeling of terror that occurs for no apparent reason. Many people who experience their first panic attack are convinced that they are having a heart attack because of their shortness of breath and an overwhelming feeling of fear and dread.

With panic disorder, the key symptoms are

- repeated panic attacks
- distress and concern about having more panic attacks
- behavioral changes related to the attacks
- fear of what these attacks may mean, such as that the person may be losing sanity, having a heart attack, or losing control

Obsessive compulsive disorder (OCD)   Obsessive compulsive disorder (OCD) is an anxiety disorder that involves obsessive and distressing thoughts or compulsive behavior undertaken to deal with anxiety. This behavior may increase when the person is under severe stress. It is unknown what is the initial trigger for the development of OCD, although there appears to be a genetic component.

In OCD, the key symptoms may include excessive checking, such as repeatedly checking to see whether the stove is turned off or the door is locked. Counting behavior and compulsive touching are common, as are preoccupations with cleanliness or germs. Repeated hand washing is common, along with avoidance of perceived dirty areas or activities. Meaningless actions, such as walking in a particular pattern, or taking particular routes to and from locations, are also OCD symptoms. Individuals who have OCD know that their unwanted thoughts and their compulsive rituals are abnormal, yet they are compelled to repeat them despite this knowledge. (See OBSESSIVE COMPULSIVE DISORDER.) Attempts to stop compulsive behavior cause in severe anxiety.

Post-traumatic stress disorder (PTSD) Some studies have shown that adults who were placed as abused children in foster care have a high rate of PTSD in adulthood, even higher than that of soldiers who have experienced combat conditions. (See POST-TRAUMATIC STRESS DISORDER [PTSD]). However, this disorder is frequently noted in combat veterans, victims of violent crime, and survivors of natural disasters, such as hurricanes or major floods.

The symptoms of post-traumatic stress disorder may include being hypervigilant and being easily startled, as well as experiencing sleep disorders and other symptoms.

Phobias A phobia is an extreme dread of a feared object, situation, or activity. Individuals who have phobias actively go to extreme lengths to avoid the feared thing; for example, those who fear flying will drive a thousand miles by car or travel by train rather than travel by airplane.

Social phobia, which typically begins in childhood or adolescence, is a disorder in which the individual is fearful of interacting with others or of doing something embarrassing in front of other people. This can include a multitude of ordinary activities, such as writing a check, using a public restroom, talking to a stranger, or paying for something.

Specific phobia is a fear of a particular situation or an object, and there are many different types of specific phobias, ranging from a fear of flying to a fear of spiders to a fear of cats.

Treatment Options and Outlook

Many people find relief from their anxiety disorders with antianxiety medications (BENZODIAZEPINES) or ANTIDEPRESSANTS. Many patients need treatment with two or more medications, in part because it is common for those who have anxiety disorder to suffer from more than one type. Psychotherapy is often beneficial for individuals with anxiety disorders. Most people who have them benefit from a combination of medications and psychotherapy.

The medication that is used to treat the anxiety disorder depends on the type of disorder as well as its severity.

Psychotherapy may also be beneficial to the patient; for example, phobic patients may benefit from systematic desensitization to the situation or item feared, such as when the person who is fearful of heights steps up a shorter distance than is comfortable and gradually the distance from the ground is increased. Computer simulations are also used to help people overcome phobias. There are many different treatments for anxiety disorders, depending upon the particular form of the disorder.

Risk Factors and Preventive Measures

Individuals who have a family history of anxiety disorders may be at risk for the development of an anxiety disorder. In addition, under severe stress an anxiety disorder may develop. If the stress is very extreme, the individual is at risk for the development of post-traumatic stress disorder.

See also ANTISOCIAL PERSONALITY DISORDER; ATTENTION DEFICIT HYPERACTIVITY DISORDER; BIPOLAR DISORDER; CONDUCT DISORDER; DEPRESSION; DUAL DIAGNOSIS; PRESCRIPTION DRUG ABUSE; PSYCHIATRIC DISORDERS; SCHIZOPHRENIA.

Doctor, Ronald M., and Ada P. Kahn. *The Encyclopedia of Phobias, Fears, and Anxieties.* 3rd ed. New York: Facts On File, 2008.
Fricchione, Gregory, M.D. "Generalized Anxiety Disorder." *New England Journal of Medicine* 351, no. 17 (August 12, 2004): 675–682.
National Institute of Mental Health. "The Numbers Count: Mental Disorders in America." 2006. Rockville, Md.: National Institutes of Health Available online. URL: http://www.nimh.nih.gov/publicat/numbers.cfm#readNow. Downloaded April 22, 2006.
Petrakis, Ismene, L., M.D., et al. "Comorbidity of Alcoholism and Psychiatric Disorders." *Alcohol Research & Health* 26, no. 2 (2002):

athletes Individuals who participate and compete in organized sports or in individual feats against each other. Some athletes, especially professional athletes, have an increased risk for becoming substance abusers, and some may become addicted to alcohol and/or drugs.

Some athletes may not be addicted to drugs, but use them for the specific purpose of enhancing their athletic performance, for example, using ANABOLIC STEROIDS for rapid increase in muscle mass and strength. Steroid use among athletes began sometime after the 1948 Olympic Games. Steroid users often convince themselves that these drugs are necessary in order for them to compete effectively, and they may also rationalize that other athletes also use drugs and that they therefore need them to be competitive.

Some experts say that even when professional athletes are identified as drug abusers and they admit their fault, they are still admired by others (especially adolescents and young adults) who may emulate them, including emulating their abuse of drugs.

Some high school athletes, primarily males, abuse drugs because they believe that these drugs will improve their athletic performance and increase their odds of attaining a professional sports career or an athletic scholarship to a college. In some cases, the drugs actually do enhance their athletic performance; however, the side effects of the drug abuse can be severe and even fatal.

According to Dr. Timothy J. Noakes in his 2004 article in the *New England Journal of Medicine* on drugs and athletic performance, athletes have misused drugs for many years. For example, in the 1950s, many athletes used AMPHETAMINES to improve their physical performance. Amphetamines minimized their fatigue and are still popular among some cyclists in competitions. Some athletes also use cortisone at abusive levels to limit their inflammation and pain. Dr. Noakes says that many professional cyclists abuse cortisone.

Some athletes abuse growth hormone, a very dangerous practice.

Another type of drug that is abused by athletes is erythropoietin, a hormone that regulates the red blood cell mass and is believed to increase athletic performance for a period of minutes to hours. Some professional cyclists have abused erythropoietin and in one case, the cyclist Marco Pantani, who won the 1998 Tour de France, was later banned from cycling after testing positive for erythropoietin.

Noakes says the extent of the use of performance-enhancing drugs by athletes is often difficult to determine:

The true extent of the use of performance-enhancing drugs is uncertain for a variety of reasons: athletes avoid detection by using scheduled testing for illicit drugs to plan their drug use; those conducting "out-of-competition" testing of athletes may intentionally avoid testing known drug users; hormones such as testosterone and insulin are initially undetectable, since they are so similar to the naturally produced substances, and designer drugs such as tetrahydrogestrinone (THG) are initially developed specifically to elude detection by all the current testing protocols; and positive tests are often not reported, and even proven drug users are generally not prosecuted.

Drug testing may identify the presence of drugs in some athletes, but many individuals have found ways to "beat the system."

Another problem that commonly occurs, especially among adolescents, is that they are skeptical of those who caution them that the abuse of these drugs is dangerous and that they should avoid them. Says Tracy Hampton in an article for the *Journal of the American Medical Association*, "Because most adolescents feel a sense of invincibility, convincing individuals in this age group to avoid or cease using these substances is another challenge."

See also YOUNG ADULTS.

Hampton, Tracy. "Researchers Address Use of Performance-Enhancing Drugs in Nonelite Athletes," *Journal of the American Medical Association* 295, no. 6 (February 8, 2006): 607–608.
Noakes, Timothy D., M.D. "Tainted Glory—Doping and Athletic Performance." *New England Journal of Medicine* 351, no. 9 (August 26, 2004): 847–849.

attention deficit hyperactivity disorder (ADHD)
A common psychiatric disorder that is characterized by impulsivity, distractibility, and inattentiveness, and if present, it is usually diagnosed in childhood or adolescence. However, adults may also have ADHD.

In the past, it was commonly believed that ADHD was a disorder of some children that was outgrown in puberty. However, researchers realized in the late 20th century that most children and adolescents who had ADHD did *not* outgrow the problem, and consequently, these individuals continue to need medication and therapy into adulthood. The median age of onset for ADHD is seven years; however, ADHD in affected individuals is not always diagnosed in childhood.

According to the National Institute of Mental Health (NIMH), ADHD is a common disorder in children and adolescents in the United States and is present among 3–5 percent of all schoolchildren; it is also affects an estimated 4 percent of adults ages 18–44.

A study on the prevalence of adult ADHD, based on more than 3,000 respondents from the National Comorbidity Survey Replication and reported in 2006 in the *American Journal of Psychiatry*, estimated the prevalence of adult ADHD at 4.4 percent.

The researchers for this study found that risks for an ADHD diagnosis were significantly greater among unemployed males who were non-Hispanic whites. In addition, adult ADHD was significantly associated with substance abuse problems; for example, 15 percent had a substance use disorder, compared to about 6 percent of respondents who did not have ADHD. About 4 percent of the respondents who had ADHD were dependent on drugs, compared to less than 1 percent of the respondents who did not. About 6 percent of the respondents who had ADHD were alcoholics, compared to 2 percent of the respondents who did not have ADHD.

Other psychiatric disorders were also more common among the adult respondents who had ADHD; for example, 47 percent of the respondents who had ADHD had an ANXIETY DISORDER, compared to about 20 percent of those without ADHD. In addition, about 19 percent of those who had ADHD had major depressive disorder (DEPRESSION), compared to 8 percent of the respondents who did not have ADHD. In considering IMPULSE CONTROL DISORDER, 20 percent of the group who had ADHD had this diagnosis, compared to only 6 percent of the respondents in the non-ADHD group.

Some, but not all individuals who have ADHD are also hyperactive. Individuals who have ADHD have an increased risk for the development of a substance abuse disorder or for substance dependence (addiction). This risk may relate to decreased impulse control that is also associated with ADHD. Adolescents also have an increased risk for "drug diversion," or giving or selling their prescribed stimulant medication to others.

It is important to note that research on adolescents who have received stimulants for their ADHD has demonstrated that medicated adolescents who have ADHD may have a significantly lower risk for substance abuse than unmedicated adolescents who have ADHD. Unmedicated adolescents who have ADHD may consciously or unconsciously use alcohol and/or drugs in an attempt to self-treat their symptoms.

Symptoms and Diagnostic Path

If ADHD is suspected, clinicians consider the individual's behavior and whether distractibility, hyperactivity, and impulsivity significantly interfere with functioning at home and at school or work. For example, many people lose items occasionally; individuals who have ADHD may lose items on a regular basis. Many people daydream or fail to pay attention sometimes, whereas the individual who has ADHD has a chronic problem with attending to what is going on.

According to the *Diagnostic and Statistical Manual of Mental Disorders*, which is published by the American Psychiatric Association, there are three major types of ADHD: including attention deficit hyperactivity disorder, combined type; attention deficit hyperactivity disorder, predominantly inattentive type; and attention deficit hyperactivity disorder, predominantly hyperactive-impulsive type.

Hyperactivity may be observed in children who are constantly in motion; however, hyperactivity in adults may be displayed in excessive talking. Most experts agree that girls who have ADHD are more likely to exhibit inattentive behavior than hyperactivity, and that adults with ADHD in general are more likely to be inattentive than hyperactive.

Treatment Options and Outlook

Individuals diagnosed with ADHD are usually treated with a combination of medication and therapy.

Many individuals who have ADHD are treated with stimulant medications, such as methylphenidate (Ritalin, Focalin XR, etc.) or AMPHETAMINE (Adderall, Dexedrine, etc.). Atomoxetine (Strattera) is specifically approved by the FDA for the treatment of ADHD in adolescents and adults. Some individuals who have ADHD are treated with other medications; for example, studies have shown that some patients improve with bupropion (Wellbutrin, Wellbutrin SR, Wellbutrin XL), an antidepressant. However, bupropion is not specifically approved by the FDA to treat ADHD.

As mentioned earlier, many individuals who have ADHD have other psychiatric diagnoses, such as anxiety disorders, depression, and substance use disorders. These problems should also be treated with medication and therapy.

Risk Factors and Preventive Measures

Studies have indicated that there is an apparent genetic risk for ADHD. In general, boys are more likely to be diagnosed with ADHD than girls, but it is unclear whether this is due to gender bias or the actual greater occurrence of ADHD in boys.

Some studies indicate that children who were adopted have a greater risk for an ADHD diagnosis than nonadopted children, although this topic continues to be debated and some experts insist that adopted children are more likely to be taken to clinicians because of the higher economic status of their adoptive parents compared to others.

There are no known preventive measures against ADHD.

Controversies with ADHD and Its Treatment

A continuing controversy in the United States and other developed countries surrounds whether children and adolescents (as well as adults) who have ADHD should be given medications that are stimulants. Opponents of the use of stimulant medication see the prescribing of stimulants as an unnecessary and even harmful "drugging" of children and adolescents, and some groups who take this position issue dire warnings that the children or teenagers who are treated with stimulants will grow up to be drug abusers or even addicts.

Yet the research actually indicates that the opposite finding is true: When adolescents have ADHD, stimulant medications apparently may *decrease* the likelihood that they will become substance abusers.

For example, a study of adolescents who had ADHD, reported in *Pediatrics* in 1999, demonstrated that teenage boys who had ADHD and who were treated with stimulant medications for their ADHD had about the same rate of substance abuse as adolescent boys who did not have ADHD. However, among those who were *not* taking medication, the rate of substance abuse was significantly higher.

Researchers at Massachusetts General Hospital, the Harvard School of Public Health, and Harvard Medical School performed a joint study in which they examined the records of 56 adolescent boys who were diagnosed with ADHD and who had also received stimulant medication for more than four years. They also looked at these boys' record of substance abuse. In addition, the researchers viewed the records of 19 boys who had ADHD who did *not* take medication and their substance abuse records. Finally, the researchers looked at 137 boys who did not have ADHD and considered the presence or absence of substance abuse in these boys.

The researchers found that 75 percent of the *unmedicated* boys who had ADHD had a substance abuse problem, versus only 25 percent of the medicated boys who had ADHD. The substance abuse rate for the boys who did not have ADHD was 18 percent, more similar to the abuse statistic for the medicated boys who had ADHD. As a result, it appears that for many adolescent ADHD patients, stimulant medication may protect *against* substance abuse. Of course it is important that a mental health professional, such as a psychiatrist, first determine whether ADHD is present in a particular patient. The psychiatrist (or another medical doctor, such as a pediatrician) also needs to determine which medication (if any) is indicated.

Note that stimulant medications are not the only drugs that are used to treat ADHD. Wellbutrin (bupropion) is an antidepressant that some physicians find effective in treating the symptoms of ADHD, especially in adults, although it is not specifically approved by the Food and Drug Administration (FDA) for this purpose. Strattera (atomoxetine) is another drug used to treat ADHD, and it is a nonstimulant that is specifically approved by the FDA to treat ADHD. Clonidine, an alpha-agonist medication that is used most commonly to treat high blood pressure, is also used as an adjunct medication to treat ADHD in individuals who do not respond adequately to the standard medication regimens.

Another controversy centers on whether ADHD is a valid diagnosis. Because ADHD is more prevalent in some populations, there is a question of whether it may represent a version of normal brain function. However, ADHD has been studied in many clinical studies, and it is clear that it represents a type of brain function that seriously limits educational function, social development, and psychological health for many children and adolescents.

Substance Abusers Who Have ADHD

Some physicians believe that if a patient was *ever* an abuser of any drugs, then he or she should never be treated with stimulants. However, other experts believe that stimulants can be safely prescribed if the patient is not currently a substance abuser and the medication is carefully monitored by the doctor.

In a study by Wilens and colleagues reported in the *Journal of the American Academy of Child & Adolescent Psychiatry* in 2005, the researchers studied drug diversion among 98 adolescents and young adults with an average age of 20.8 years. The study included 55 subjects who had ADHD and were taking stimulants (96 percent). The ADHD group also took other medications such as antidepressants and benzodiazepines. The non-ADHD group was taking antidepressants (80 percent), as well as benzodiazepines, stimulants (10 percent), lithium (10 percent), and other medications.

The researchers found that 11 percent of the group taking ADHD medication admitted selling their medications to others, while none of the non-ADHD group said they had sold their medication. In addition, 22 percent of the ADHD group said they had taken too much of their medication, compared to 5 percent of the non-ADHD group.

Those most likely to divert their medications were individuals in the ADHD group who had substance abuse problems as well as those who had the diagnosis of CONDUCT DISORDER. (Conduct disorder is characterized by breaking the laws of society.)

Report the researchers, "Our findings suggest that clinicians should closely monitor the appropriate use of medication in older adolescent and young adult ADHD patients with CD [conduct disorder] and/or SUD [substance use disorder]."

The Wilens and associates study found that only immediate-release medications were sold or abused; that finding is an indication for physicians concerned about abuse to prescribe extended-release medications when possible.

It may not be the adolescent who has ADHD who initiates the misuse of his or her medication. Studies have indicated that adolescents who have ADHD and who take stimulants are often approached by their peers, who want to be given or sold stimulants such as METHYLPHENIDATE (RITALIN/CONCERTA/FOCALIN, ETC.) or AMPHETAMINES. Such drug diversion is illegal.

To investigate this issue, researcher Christiane Poulin undertook a study, published in 2001 in the *Canadian Medical Association Journal*, based on a survey of more than 13,000 students in grades 7 through 12. Among the students, 5.3 percent reported taking stimulant medications within the 12 months before the survey. About 15 percent of students who were prescribed stimulants said that they had given away some of their medication. In addition, 7 percent said that they had sold their medication to others. In addition, 80 percent of the students who said that they had sold their stimulants also reported giving some of the drugs to others.

Other Cases of Diversion Poulin also reports that 4 percent of the students said that their ADHD medication was stolen from them (it was missing and presumed stolen), and 3 percent said the medication was forcibly taken from them. According to Poulin, "From a clinical perspective, physicians prescribing stimulant medication should be vigilant concerning potential abuse, particularly among adolescent patients known or thought to be using other substances. Physicians and parents should keep track of stimulant medication, especially when several months' supply is prescribed."

This research was further validated by a study reported in a 2004 issue of *Substance Use & Misuse*, in which the researchers surveyed 1,723 students in grades 6 to 11 in the Detroit, Michigan, area.

They found that among the students who were taking prescribed stimulants, 23 percent had been approached by others to give or sell them the stimulants or to trade them for other drugs.

As a result, parents of adolescents who are prescribed stimulants for their ADHD should carefully monitor the drug to ensure that their children are not manipulated or compelled into giving the medication to others. Parents should also tell their children that such drug diversion is illegal and grounds for arrest. It should never be assumed that adolescents already realize that giving away or selling their ADHD drugs is illegal.

If physicians are concerned that there is a moderate to high risk of drug diversion, they may wish to prescribe one of the nonstimulant drugs, for which there is little or no risk of diversion.

Patterns among Abusers of ADHD Drugs

Adolescents who abuse or misuse stimulants that are prescribed for ADHD patients are more likely to be male and to have other substance abuse problems, such as alcohol abuse and/or the abuse of other drugs, such as MARIJUANA and COCAINE. Some abusers mix the stimulant with other drugs. Drugs such as methylphenidate can be taken orally, intranasally ("snorting"), or by injection. Abusers seek to attain a state of euphoria from the drug.

Possible Interventions to Monitor or Prevent Diversion of Stimulants

Evans and her colleagues suggest several practical interventions for physicians who suspect that ADHD patients are diverting their medication to others. One suggestion is to use a random drug screening for the stimulant. The drug should show up in the urine, and if it does not, the patient may be diverting the drug to others rather than taking it him- or herself. In some cases, asking the school to control the administration of the drug is a solution, rather than allowing an adolescent to take the drug at home.

Physicians (and parents) may also wish to do random pill counts of the number of the pills left in the container from the pharmacy, to determine whether the number of pills that remains in the container is equivalent to the number that *should* be left. For example, if a drug was to be taken once a day starting on March 1, and the patient was given 30 pills on the first of the month, there should be 15 pills left on March 15 if the drug was taken as directed. If there are significantly fewer drugs in the container (such as only five or six pills or fewer, in this example), this may indicate that the patient either is taking too many pills or may be giving or selling them to others. If there are too many pills, this indicates the patient is noncompliant; this is also important information for parents and physicians.

Some physicians who are concerned about the diversion of stimulants will circumspectly view the arms of the patient's parents to see whether there are needle marks, indicating possible diversion of the stimulants, which can also be injected when used illegally. However, it is more likely that diverted drugs are going to other adolescents.

It is also important for physicians to advise children who take stimulants, as well as their parents, teachers, and others, to avoid talking openly about the child's stimulant therapy because interested parties may often overhear and may then seek to obtain the child's drugs through whatever route they consider most effective. Say Evans, and associates, "If this information ends up in the wrong hands, patients' homes may become targets for break-ins or children may become targets on the playground."

See also ADOLESCENTS AND SUBSTANCE ABUSE; AMPHETAMINES; ANXIETY DISORDERS; BIPOLAR DISORDER; CRIME AND CRIMINALS; DEPRESSION; DIVERSION, DRUG; PRESCRIPTION DRUG ABUSE; PSYCHIATRIC DISORDERS.

American Psychiatric Association. *Diagnostic and Statistical Manual of Mental Disorders.* 4th ed. Washington, D.C.: American Psychiatric Association, 2000.

Evans, Charity, et al. "Use and Abuse of Methylphenidate in Attention-Deficit/Hyperactivity Disorder." *Canadian Pharmacists Journal* 137, no. 6 (July–August 2004): 30–35.

Kessler, Ronald C., et al. "The Prevalence and Correlates of Adult ADHD in the United States: Results from the National Comorbidity Survey Replication." *American Journal of Psychiatry* 163, no. 4 (April 2006): 716–723.

McCabe, S. E., C. J. Teter, and C. J. Boyd. "The Use, Misuse and Diversion of Prescription Stimulants among

Middle and High School Students." *Substance Use and Misuse* 39, no. 7 (2004): 1,095–1,116.

National Institute of Mental Health. "The Numbers Count: Mental Disorders in America." Rockville, Md.: National Institutes of Health, 2006. Available online. URL: http://www.nimh.nih.gov/publicat/numbers.cfm#readNow. Downloaded April 22, 2006.

Poulin, Christiane. "Medical and Nonmedical Stimulant Use among Adolescents: From Sanctioned to Unsanctioned Use." *Canadian Medical Association Journal* 165, no. 8 (2001): 1,039–1,044.

Wilens, Timothy E., M.D. "Attention-Deficit/Hyperactivity Disorder and the Substance Use Disorders: The Nature of the Relationship, Subtypes at Risk, and Treatment Issues." *Psychiatric Clinics of North America* 27 (2004): 283–301.

Wilens, Timothy E., et al. "Characteristics of Adolescents and Young Adults with ADHD Who Divert or Misuse Their Prescribed Medications." *Journal of the American Academy of Child & Adolescent Psychiatry* 45, no. 4 (2006): 408–414.

Wilens, Timothy E., M.D., et al. "Does Stimulant Therapy of Attention-Deficit/Hyperactivity Disorder Beget Later Substance Abuse? A Meta-Analytic Review of the Literature." *Pediatrics* 111, no. 1 (2003): 179–185.

barbiturates A category of sedating drugs that are derived from barbituric acid. Barbiturates were introduced in the United States in 1903 and became very popular drugs of abuse in the middle of the 20th century. Barbiturates are DEPRESSANTS, or drugs that depress the central nervous system, and medications in this category represent about 10 percent of all the prescribed depressant medications in the United States. Some other categories of depressant drugs are BENZODIAZEPINES, FLUNITRAZEPAM (ROHYPNOL), and some medications prescribed for the treatment of insomnia, such as zolpidem (Ambien) and zaleplon (Sonata). (See SLEEP REMEDIES, ADDICTIVE.)

In past years, barbiturates were often used to commit SUICIDE. In addition, the use of barbiturates was associated with an increased frequency of accidental overdose and death, which led to a decrease in their popularity among physicians. According to Levinthal in his book *Drugs, Society, and Criminal Justice,* between the years 1973 and 1976, barbiturates were used in more than half of drug-related suicides. It is not that barbiturates themselves lead to increased attempts at suicide, but rather that the lethal dose of barbiturate is close to the therapeutic dose. As a result, an overdose of barbiturates in a suicide attempt is more likely to be successful than an overdose of many other drugs.

Barbiturates are sometimes used for patients who have ALCOHOLISM, to help them tolerate the effects of withdrawal; however, individuals who abuse barbiturates should not combine these drugs with alcohol because coma and ACCIDENTAL OVERDOSE DEATHS often result from their combination.

Barbiturates are also used to treat epilepsy patients and to treat insomnia. They are also sometimes used as a surgical anesthetic. Barbiturates are sometimes abused because they may cause euphoria at the same time as relaxation, because of the effects on the cerebral cortex. Barbiturates should not be used by individuals who will be driving or operating machinery because they can impede performance.

In general, barbiturates may cause such side effects as impaired judgment, poor motor coordination, and slurred speech. Some individuals develop a TOLERANCE to barbiturates, and they may also develop a PHYSICAL DEPENDENCE and a PSYCHOLOGICAL DEPENDENCE on these drugs. When used frequently, barbiturates can suppress rapid eye movement (REM) sleep, during which dreaming occurs. When the drug is stopped, REM periods are extended and the person may experience distressing nightmares. This condition is called the REM-sleep rebound effect (also called "rebound dreaming"). In addition, the day after REM-sleep rebound, the individual usually feels irritable and tired.

There are about 12 barbiturates used in the United States, and they are classified as ultrashort-, short-, intermediate-, and long-acting barbiturates. Ultrashort barbiturates act within about a minute of the intravenous administration of the drug. The most commonly used ultrashort drugs are methohexital (Brevital), a Schedule IV drug under the CONTROLLED SUBSTANCES ACT, and thiamyl (Surital) and thiopental (Pentothal).

Short-acting or intermediate-acting barbiturates include such Schedule II drugs as amobarbital (Amytal), pentobarbital (Nembutal), secobarbital (Seconal), and Tuinal (a combination of amobarbital and secobarbital). Other short-acting or intermediate-acting barbiturates that are Schedule III drugs include butalbital (Fiornal), butabarbital (Butisol), talbutal (Lotusate), and aprobarbital (Alurate). These drugs act within 15 to 40 minutes after taking them orally and are used for headaches, preoperative sedation, or insomnia. They last for about six hours.

Phenobarbital (Luminal) and mephobarbital (Mebaral) are Schedule IV drugs that are long-acting. They take effect in about an hour and last for as long as 12 hours. They are used for the treatment of seizures or daytime sedation.

Abusers of Barbiturates

Among 12th graders, about 9.9 percent had ever abused barbiturates in 2004, according to the Monitoring the Future reports. This usage was up 1 percent from 2003. In considering high school seniors in the United States who had abused barbiturates in the past month, 2.9 percent fit this category, the same percentage seen in 2003.

Among college students and their same-age peers in 2004, according to data from the Monitoring the Future study of adults, among those who abused barbiturates, there was a lifetime prevalence of 7.2 percent for college students and 12.2 percent for their same-age peers. In considering the 30-day prevalence of barbiturate abuse, however, college students had a lower abuse rate than adolescents, or 1.5 percent, while their same-age peers had a slightly higher rate than adolescents, at 3.2 percent.

In considering the annual prevalence of the use of barbiturates by high school seniors as well as individuals up to 45 years, the greatest percentages of abuse occurred among high school seniors (6.5 percent), followed by individuals 19–20 years (6.0 percent), and those 23–24 years (5.0 percent). Among those 40–45 years, the abuse rate was only 1.0 percent.

Withdrawal from Barbiturates

If the individual has developed a tolerance of or an addiction to barbiturates, then withdrawal of the drug often causes anxiety and insomnia, at the least.

If the dependence is severe, the individual may experience delirium and seizures, HALLUCINATIONS, high fever, elevated body temperature, and, in some rare cases, withdrawal may be life-threatening. When individuals are dependent on barbiturates, physicians may choose to taper them off the drugs. Barbiturate withdrawal syndrome often resembles that of alcohol withdrawal.

See also CONTROLLED SUBSTANCES ACT; DEPRESSANTS; DETOXIFICATION; SCHEDULED DRUGS; YOUNG ADULTS.

Johnston, Lloyd D., et al. *Monitoring the Future: National Results on Adolescent Drug Use: Overview of Key Findings 2004.* Bethesda, Md.: National Institute of Drug Abuse, April 2005.
Johnston, Lloyd D., et al. *Monitoring the Future: National Survey Results on Drug Use, 1975–2004.* Vol. 2, *College Students and Adults Ages 19–45.* Bethesda, Md.: National Institute on Drug Abuse, National Institutes of Health, 2005.
Joseph, Donald E., et al., eds. *Drugs of Abuse.* Washington, D.C.: U.S. Department of Justice, 2005.
Levinthal, Charles F. *Drugs, Society, and Criminal Justice.* New York: Pearson Education, 2006.

benzodiazepines Central nervous system DEPRESSANTS that are usually prescribed to help individuals cope with severe ANXIETY DISORDERS and may also be used on a short-term basis to treat insomnia. They are also sometimes called *tranquilizers*. The CONTROLLED SUBSTANCES ACT classifies benzodiazepines as depressants, and they are Schedule IV drugs. These medications may be offered orally or by injection.

Some benzodiazepines, particularly chlordiazepoxide hydrochloride (Librium), clorazepate (Tranxene), DIAZEPAM (VALIUM), and oxazepam (Serax), are used to help individuals who are undergoing WITHDRAWAL from alcohol or drugs. Some benzodiazepines, such as ALPRAZOLAM (XANAX) and clonazepam (Klonopin), are used to treat panic disorder. In some cases, benzodiazepines such as clonazepam, diazepam, and lorazepam (Ativan) are used to treat seizure disorders, such as epilepsy.

Note that benzodiazepines should not be taken with alcohol or with any other sedating drugs because the combination of these substances could become dangerous or even fatal to the consumer.

Leo Sternbach, a Polish chemist who fled to the United States in 1941 during the Nazi occupation, is credited with discovering the formulation for the first two benzodiazepine medications, Valium and Librium, for Roche, a global pharmaceutical company. These medications were first marketed to the public in the 1960s, Librium in 1960 and diazepam in 1963. These medications were extremely popular around the world during the 1960s and 1970s. However, concern about the potentially addictive qualities of benzodiazepines when the drugs were abused eventually developed.

Benzodiazepines are cross-tolerant with alcohol; that means that the chronic use of alcohol can create a greater tolerance for benzodiazepines, and vice versa. In addition, this cross-tolerance is the reason that benzodiazepines are used in the treatment of acute alcohol withdrawal, as carefully chosen doses of benzodiazepines in a tapering schedule can treat or prevent severe alcohol withdrawal symptoms. The withdrawal from an addiction to benzodiazepines is extremely similar to alcohol withdrawal, and it can also be life-threatening.

Abuse of and Dependence on Benzodiazepines

According to the National Survey on Drug Use and Health, in 2004, 11.2 percent of YOUNG ADULTS ages 18–25 used benzodiazepines illegally, as with PRE-SCRIPTION DRUG ABUSE. The single most commonly abused benzodiazepine was diazepam (Valium), and 6.1 percent of individuals of all ages had ever abused Valium in 2004. Another commonly prescribed benzodiazepine, alprozalam (Xanax), was also a drug of abuse.

Other benzodiazepine drugs are abused, especially among abusers of HEROIN and COCAINE, who usually use benzodiazepines to counteract the side effects of the use of heroin or cocaine.

There are about 15 brand names of benzodiazepines that are prescribed in the United States, according to the Drug Enforcement Administration.

Signs of dependence on benzodiazepines include the following:

- a strong desire or need to continue taking the medicine
- a need to increase the dose of the medication to receive the same effects (PHYSICAL TOLERANCE)
- withdrawal effects (such as irritability, nervousness, insomnia, abdominal cramps, and/or shaking) if the drug is not taken

Individuals who are dependent on a benzodiazepine should be tapered off the drug under medi-cal supervision. Stopping the drug immediately could lead to serious side effects, such as seizures or DELIRIUM TREMENS.

In one study reported in the *Archives of Internal Medicine* in 1999, researchers tapered the subjects off benzodiazepines, testing the efficacy of melatonin supplements to cope with problems of insomnia. The researchers found that of the 24 elderly patients who received controlled-release melatonin and discontinued benzodiazepines, 19 reported good sleep quality with melatonin.

Short- and Long-Acting Benzodiazepines   There are both short- and long-acting benzodiazepines, and benzodiazepines with rapid and slow onset of action. Short-acting benzodiazepines have a short half-life: that is, the body breaks them down rapidly and clears them from the system. They are often prescribed to treat insomnia or for short-term acute use, such as in panic attacks or fear of flying.

Benzodiazepines that are used to treat insomnia include estazolam (ProSom), temazepam (Restoril), and triazolam (Halcion). Another short-acting benzodiazepine is midazolam (Versed), a drug that is used primarily for surgical sedation. Alprazolam (Xanax), a short-acting drug with a half-life of approximately 2.5 hours, can, however, be a long-acting drug in a preparation that allows the medication to dissolve more slowly.

Benzodiazepines that have a rapid onset include alprazolam and diazepam. These drugs are rapidly absorbed into the system and reach peak blood levels quickly. In the special case of diazepam, it may be viewed as both a long- and a short-acting medication because of its rapid absorption into body fat. After several weeks of use, however, the amount of diazepam in the body fat reaches equilibrium with the amount in the bloodstream. This means that in the initial weeks of using diazepam, the drug appears to "wear off" within two to four hours, but after reaching equilibrium, it can last for 12 to 24 hours. In individuals who have decreased liver function, the half-life of diazepam can be upward of 100 hours.

Some benzodiazepines are long-acting drugs, and they can be used to treat insomnia among patients who also have daytime anxiety. Examples of long-acting benzodiazepines include Tranxene, diazepam, halazepam (Paxipam), Ativan, prazepam (Centrax), and quazepam (Doral). Some longer-acting benzodiazepines, such as Klonopin, Valium, and Tranxene, are used as antiseizure drugs.

A particular concern in treatment with long-acting benzodiazepines is that withdrawal can occur days after abrupt ceasing of use of the medication, and misdiagnosis and incorrect treatment can result. An initial false sense of security can also be created as individuals taking the drug believe that they were able to stop the medication without difficulty, only to have withdrawal symptoms days later.

Side Effects

The effects of benzodiazepines are analogous to alcohol effects. Thus, benzodiazepines can cause drowsiness, slowed reaction times, poor judgment, and decreased impulse control. In higher doses, significant intoxication can occur, with clumsiness, amnesiac episodes (blackouts), and confusion. The excessive use and abuse of benzodiazepines can lead to withdrawal symptoms up to and including delirium tremens, as is also seen with the excessive chronic use of alcohol.

Benzodiazepinelike Drugs

There are several central nervous system depressant drugs that are similar to benzodiazepine and, as are benzodiazepines, used over the short term to treat insomnia. These drugs include zolpidem (Ambien), zaleplon (Sonata), and eszopiclone (Lunesta). They are Schedule IV drugs.

See also ANTIDEPRESSANTS; ANXIETY DISORDERS; DEPRESSION; DIVERSION, DRUG; PRESCRIPTION DRUG ABUSE; PSYCHIATRIC DISORDERS; SCHEDULED DRUGS; SLEEP REMEDIES, ADDICTIVE.

Garfinkel, Doron, M.D., et al. "Facilitation of Benzodiazepine Discontinuation by Melatonin." *Archives of Internal Medicine* 159 (November 8, 1999): 2,456–2,460.
Joseph, Donald E., et al., eds. *Drugs of Abuse.* Washington, D.C.: U.S. Department of Justice. 2005.
Longo, Lance P., M.D., and Brian Johnson, M.D. "Addiction: Part I, Benzodiazepines—Side Effects, Abuse Risk and Alternatives." *American Family Physician* 61 (2000): 2,121–2,128. Available online. URL: http://www.aafp.org/afp/2000401/2121.html. Downloaded January 15, 2006.
Substance Abuse and Mental Health Services Administration. *Results from the 2004 National Survey on Drug Use and Health: National Findings.* Rockville, Md.: U.S. Department of Health and Human Services, September 2005.

binge drinking Excessive consumption of alcohol over a short period, also known as heavy episodic drinking. In many cases, binge drinking has led to alcohol poisoning, which causes death because the liver cannot process the amount of alcohol that has been consumed quickly enough, and consequently, the body shuts down. A person who has alcohol poisoning may have a blood alcohol level of 0.4, which is at least five times the legal limit for operating a motor vehicle in any state in the United States. This blood alcohol level does not necessarily represent drinking five times as much alcohol in the same period; rather, this level can be achieved through the speed of drinking a lesser amount of alcohol.

Binge drinking is usually defined, for men, as the consumption of five or more drinks on one occasion in the past two weeks, and for women, the consumption of four or more drinks in the same time frame. Binge drinking most commonly occurs among adolescents and YOUNG ADULTS, and it is often done under the influence of intense PEER PRESSURE. It may also be perceived as a necessary part of joining a fraternity or sorority among COLLEGE STUDENTS, although such drinking practices are actively discouraged by the administration on most college campuses. Some misguided individuals still believe that binge drinking is a sort of rite of passage to adulthood.

Some colleges have instituted programs to educate their students about the high risks of binge drinking, not only in terms of health risks but also in terms of the increased risk for engaging in unsafe sex and causing or being victimized by physical or SEXUAL ASSAULTS. (See Table I.)

For example, according to the Substance Abuse and Mental Health Administration, 8 percent of nonbinge drinkers had unplanned sex, compared to 20 percent of bingers, and 41 percent of frequent bingers. The risk for unprotected sex was greater with binge drinking, or 4 percent among nonbinge drinkers, which increased to 10 percent among bin-

TABLE I: PERCENT OF COLLEGE STUDENTS REPORTING ALCOHOL-RELATED PROBLEMS AS A RESULT OF THEIR OWN DRINKING, UNITED STATES

	Non-binge Drinkers	Binge Drinkers	Frequent Bingers
Forgot where they were or what they did	8 percent	26 percent	54 percent
Got behind in school work	6 percent	21 percent	46 percent
Argued with friends	8 percent	22 percent	42 percent
Engaged in unplanned sexual activity	8 percent	20 percent	41 percent
Had unprotected sex	4 percent	10 percent	22 percent
Got hurt or injured	2 percent	9 percent	23 percent
Damaged property	2 percent	8 percent	22 percent
Got into trouble with campus/local police	1 percent	4 percent	11 percent

Source: Rouse, Beatrice A. *Substance Abuse and Mental Health Services Administration (SAMHSA) Statistics Source Book.* Rockville, Md.: Office of Applied Studies, 1998, p. 262.

gers and 22 percent of frequent bingers. In addition, bingers and frequent bingers had a markedly higher rate of alcohol-induced memory lapses (blackouts), which were present among 8 percent of bingers, 26 percent of binge drinkers, and 54 percent (nearly seven times greater than the rate among nonbingers) of frequent bingers.

According to Robert D. Brewer and Monica H. Swahn in their article on binge drinking and violence in a 2005 issue of the *Journal of the American Medical Association,* about 75,000 deaths in the United States were caused by excessive drinking in 2001, and of these deaths, binge drinking accounted for more than half.

Binge Drinkers

Researchers have found some clear patterns among those who engage in binge drinking, as described in the following.

High school students and college students   On the basis of data from the Monitoring the Future survey, released in 2005, 29 percent of high school seniors had engaged in binge drinking at least once in the two weeks before the survey, and nearly half (49 percent) of college students (particularly males) had engaged in binge drinking.

Some people began their binge drinking in college; however, about 85 percent of college student drinkers have reported that their alcohol abuse began in high school.

According to the National Center for Health Statistics in their annual *Chartbook on Trends in the Health of Americans,* released in 2005, an estimated 10.6 percent of adolescents engaged in binge drinking in 2003, including 11.1 percent of males and 10.1 percent of females in this age range.

Race and ethnic differences   According to the National Survey on Drug Use and Health, there were some racial and ethnic differences among binge drinkers among adolescents in 2004. For example, the rate of binge drinking in 2004 in the United States was the highest among American Indians/Alaska Natives (25.8 percent), followed by Hispanics (24.0 percent), whites (23.8 percent), and African Americans (18.3 percent). The lowest rate of binge drinking was found in Asians (12.4 percent).

Male arrestees   There is a high level of binge drinking among a particular population: males who are arrested for crimes. For example, according to the Arrestee Drug Abuse Monitoring (ADAM) report for 2000, based on data from cities throughout the country and released in 2003, about 53 percent of arrestees who are older than age 35 years, and 45 percent of those below age 21 years, had engaged in binge drinking at least once in the month before they were arrested. In most areas for which data were collected (32 of 35), white arrestees surpassed black arrestees in the percentage of those who had engaged in binge drinking. In addition, homeless arrestees were more likely to have engaged in binge drinking than those who were not homeless.

Binge drinking rates varied considerably among the city location of the arrestees. For example, among the arrestees below age 21 years, the rates of binge drinking ranged from a low of 17 percent

Source: National Institute of Justice, Office of Justice Programs.
2000 Arrestee Drug Abuse Monitoring: Annual Report, NCJ 193013.
Washington, D.C.: U.S. Department of Justice, April 2003, p. 49.

TABLE II: BINGE DRINKING IN PAST YEAR AND PAST MONTH BY SITE, ADULT MALE ARRESTEES, 2000

Primary City	Percentage Who Said They Binged	
	In Past Year	In Past Month
Albany/Capital Area, NY	65.1	53.2
Albuquerque, NM	82.0	70.2
Anchorage, AK	78.5	69.5
Atlanta, GA	52.3	42.5
Birmingham, AL	55.6	48.5
Charlotte-Metro, NC	56.4	47.6
Chicago, IL	51.0	44.2
Cleveland, OH	59.3	54.1
Dallas, TX	56.7	46.1
Denver, CO	71.2	62.9
Des Moines, IA	69.3	56.1
Detroit, MI	47.2	38.4
Fort Lauderdale, FL	60.6	52.6
Honolulu, HI	59.9	46.4
Houston, TX	50.7	41.0
Indianapolis, IN	6.10	50.6
Laredo, TX	75.2	64.6
Las Vegas, NV	65.7	53.6
Miami, FL	50.6	40.2
Minneapolis, MN	64.9	54.3
New Orleans, LA	52.7	36.0
New York, NY	55.5	39.8
Oklahoma City, OK	72.1	61.3
Omaha, NE	61.4	51.0
Philadelphia, PA	47.0	35.4
Phoenix, AZ	64.3	54.2
Portland, OR	57.5	40.5
Sacramento, CA	60.7	51.7
Salt Lake City, UT	61.9	48.6
San Antonio, TX	54.7	43.5
San Diego, CA	67.0	54.5
San Jose, CA	72.1	61.0
Seattle, WA	63.2	52.1
Spokane, WA	67.5	55.9
Tucson, AZ	70.5	59.2
Median	**61.0**	**51.7**

75 percent in Albuquerque. The reasons for these disparities in arrests are unknown. It may be that police in some cities are more vigilant with arrests than others, although only research can determine the probable causes for this broad variation.

In considering arrestees of all ages, they ranged from a low of 35.4 percent of arrestees in Philadelphia who had engaged in past-month binge drinking to a high of 70.2 percent in Albuquerque. (See Table II for further information.)

Binge Drinking around the World
The World Health Organization has provided data on the percentage of heavy episodic drinkers (binge drinkers) among adults in countries around the world in 2004. For example, 49.1 percent of males in Finland were binge drinkers. The highest rate of binge drinking among males only was in Nigeria, or 52 percent of the male population. Rates of binge drinking among males were also high in Mexico (46.9 percent) and Uganda (46 percent).

Among females who binge drank in 2004, the highest rates were seen in Nigeria (39.6 percent), Uganda (17.6 percent), and Iceland (20 percent). Other high rates of binge drinking among females were noted in Finland (14.1 percent), Germany (12.7 percent), and Australia and the Netherlands (both at 11.6 percent).

Psychiatric Problems among Binge Drinkers
According to the National Institute of Alcohol Abuse and Alcoholism in their study released in 2006, in their survey of more than 43,000 subjects, binge drinkers had a higher rate of DEPRESSION, ANTISOCIAL PERSONALITY DISORDER, and many other diagnoses, compared to those who had not binged in the past year. For example, among nonbingers, the rate of depression was 6.6 percent, compared to 9.8 percent among bingers. The percent of nonbingers with antisocial personality disorder was 2.6 percent, whereas it was 5.9 percent among bingers, more than a doubling of the rate of nonbingers.

In considering alcoholism (alcohol dependence), the rate among nonbingers was less than 1 percent, or 0.72 percent, while among bingers, the rate was 4.43 percent, more than quadruple the rate of the nonbingers. Bingers also had higher rates of ANXIETY DISORDERS than nonbingers, including panic disor-

in New Orleans, Louisiana, to a high of 66 percent in Albuquerque, New Mexico. Among arrestees ages 21 to 25 years, the rate ranged from 24 percent who binge drank in New Orleans to a high of

TABLE III: PERCENTAGE OF SELECTED PSYCHIATRIC DISORDERS, BY SEX, ACCORDING TO FREQUENCY OF DRINKING FIVE OR MORE DRINKS FOR MEN OR FOUR OR MORE DRINKS FOR WOMEN IN A SINGLE DAY IN THE PAST YEAR, AMONG CURRENT DRINKERS, UNITED STATES, 2001–2002

	Both Sexes, Age 18 and Older	Males	Females
Never Binged in the Past Year			
Alcohol abuse	2.0	2.8	1.3
Alcohol dependence (alcoholism)	.72	1.0	.43
Drug abuse/dependence	.30	.44	.17
Major depression	6.6	4.1	8.7
Manic disorder	1.3	1.2	1.4
Panic disorder without agoraphobia	1.3	.86	1.68
Panic disorder with agoraphobia	.42	.14	.67
Social phobia	2.5	1.8	3.1
Specific phobia	6.8	3.8	9.4
Generalized anxiety disorder	1.9	1.1	2.5
Antisocial personality disorder	2.6	3.8	1.4
Binged 1 to 11 Times in the Past Year			
Alcohol abuse	11.2	13.7	8.3
Alcohol dependence (alcoholism)	4.4	4.0	5.0
Drug abuse/dependence	.72	.72	.73
Major depression	9.8	5.8	14.7
Manic disorder	2.6	1.7	3.6
Panic disorder without agoraphobia	2.1	1.0	3.4
Panic disorder with agoraphobia	.74	.32	1.24
Social phobia	3.7	2.7	4.8
Specific phobia	10.0	6.4	14.4
Generalized anxiety disorder	2.9	1.3	4.7
Antisocial personality disorder	5.9	7.4	4.1

Note: Note that the per-100,000 rate was converted to 1 in 100 rate, or a percentage, and percentages were rounded off.
Source: Adapted from National Institute on Alcohol Abuse and Alcoholism. *Alcohol Use and Alcohol Use Disorders in the United States: Main Findings from the 2001–2002 National Epidemiologic Survey on Alcohol and Related Conditions (NESARC).* U.S. Alcohol Epidemiologic Data Reference Manual 8, number 1 (January 2006). Bethesda, Md.: National Institutes of Health, January 2006, p. 213.

der, social phobia, specific phobia, and generalized anxiety disorder. Bingers also had a significantly higher percentage of drug abuse/dependence than nonbingers.

In general, male nonbingers and bingers had a higher rate of alcohol dependence and drug abuse/dependence, while women (including nonbingers and bingers) had a higher rate of psychiatric problems, such as major depression, which was about twice as common among female nonbingers compared to male nonbingers and nearly three times as common among female bingers compared to male bingers.

Males have a much higher rate of antisocial personality disorder than females. The general rate for males was 3.8 percent among nonbingers, compared to 7.4 percent among the bingers, a dramatic difference. (See Table III for further details.)

When males and female bingers are contrasted, it can be seen that the female bingers had a *higher* rate of alcoholism than the males: 4.0 percent of the male bingers were alcoholic versus 5.0 percent of the female bingers. In comparing females to females, the women bingers had a much higher rate of psychiatric disorders compared to the female nonbingers. For example, 8.7 percent of the nonbinger females had major depression, compared to 14.7 percent of the female bingers.

On the basis of this information, it is clear that both male and female bingers have more serious psychiatric problems than those who do not engage in binge drinking.

Effects on Those Prenatally Exposed to Binge Drinking

According to Beth Nordstrom Bailey and colleagues in their 2004 article in the *American Journal of Obstetrics and Gynecology,* prenatal exposure to binge drinking can have a profound impact on the children born to binge drinkers. It is already known that even moderate or light drinking may lead to FETAL ALCOHOL SYNDROME in infants born to drinking mothers. However, Nordstrom Bailey and her colleagues specifically looked at the effects of binge drinking alone on the children born to bingers. They found that the children exposed to binge drinking had nearly twice the risk (1.7) of having intelligence quotient (IQ) scores in the mentally retarded range. In addition, at age seven, the children were 2.5 times more likely to exhibit significant levels of acting out behavior than children born to nonbingers.

Say the researchers, "Results of the current study support the findings of other researchers who suggest that exposure to binge drinking has more deleterious consequences than the overall amount of exposure to alcohol during pregnancy. Binge drinking, which produces higher blood alcohol content, produces a higher threshold of exposure and exposes the fetus to alcohol for a longer period of time, both of which are likely to have a more profound effect on developing structures."

The researchers also expressed concern that pregnant women need to understand that "cutting back" on alcohol consumption is insufficient if the woman engages in drinking binges:

Pregnant women who drink heavily are routinely advised of the potential consequences and encouraged strongly to cease or at least to cut back intake. However, if cutting back involves drinking less often, but still consuming large amounts when intake occurs, [the] offspring may not experience improved outcomes. Understanding the conse-

quences of prenatal exposure to binge drinking is especially important because surveys indicate that women of childbearing age who consume alcohol are more likely to binge than drink in a chronic heavy pattern.

See also ABUSE, ALCOHOL; ALCOHOL ABUSE/DEPENDENCE; ADOLESCENTS AND SUBSTANCE ABUSE; ALCOHOLISM; COLLEGE STUDENTS; GENETIC PREDISPOSITIONS AND ENVIRONMENTAL EFFECTS IN SUBSTANCE USE DISORDERS; JAIL INMATES; YOUNG ADULTS.

Brewer, Robert D., M.D., and Monica H. Swahn. "Binge Drinking and Violence." *Journal of the American Medical Association* 294, no. 5 (August 3, 2005): 616–618.
Department of Mental Health and Substance Abuse. *Global Status Report on Alcohol 2004.* Geneva: World Health Organization, 2004.
Johnston, Lloyd D., et al. *Monitoring the Future: National Survey Results on Drug Use, 1975–2004.* Vol. 2, *College Students and Adults Ages 19–45.* Bethesda, Md.: National Institute on Drug Abuse, National Institutes of Health, 2005.
National Center for Health Statistics. *Health United States, 2005 with Chartbook on Trends in the Health of Americans.* Hyattsville, Md.: National Center for Health Statistics, 2005.
National Institute of Justice, Office of Justice Programs. *2000 Arrestee Drug Abuse Monitoring: Annual Report,* NCJ 193013. Washington, D.C.: U.S. Department of Justice, April 2003.
National Institute on Alcohol Abuse and Alcoholism. *Alcohol Use and Alcohol Use Disorders in the United States: Main Findings from the 2001–2002 National Epidemiologic Survey on Alcohol and Related Conditions (NESARC).* U.S. Alcohol Epidemiologic Data Reference Manual 8, no. 1 (January 2006). Bethesda, Md.: National Institutes of Health, January 2006.
Nordstrom Bailey, Beth, et al. "Prenatal Exposure to Binge Drinking and Cognitive and Behavioral Outcomes at Age 7 Years." *American Journal of Obstetrics and Gynecology* 191 (2004): 1,037–1,043.

bipolar disorder A severe psychiatric disorder that is usually characterized by periods of mania that alternate with periods of depression. It was formerly known as manic depression. Studies have shown that many patients who have bipolar disorder were not diagnosed for as long as 10 years from the time of the onset of the disorder. It is a difficult disorder to diagnose, and patients may have been diagnosed with DEPRESSION or ANXIETY DISORDERS, or with ATTENTION DEFICIT HYPERACTIVITY DISORDER (ADHD), because the highs and lows of bipolar disorder were not observed by physicians and/or reported by patients or others.

According to the National Institute of Mental Health, bipolar disorder affects about 5.7 million Americans, or 2.6 percent of the adult population ages 18 and older. The median age of onset for bipolar disorder is 25 years. Bipolar disorder occurs in people of all ages and races, both males and females, socioeconomic status affecting every and other demographic characteristics.

Patients who have bipolar disorder are more likely to abuse alcohol or drugs than patients who do not have this psychiatric disorder; for example, according to the National Institute of Mental Health (NIMH), individuals who are in a manic episode have a 14.5 percent increased risk of abusing drugs compared to others. This risk is surpassed only by individuals who have ANTISOCIAL PERSONALITY DISORDER (15.5 percent).

Substance abuse may worsen the course of bipolar disorder; for example, some studies have shown that bipolar disorder patients who are also substance abusers have more frequent hospitalizations than those without substance abuse. They also often have an earlier onset of the disorder. However, other researchers report that bipolar disorder patients are more likely to succeed at substance abuse treatment than alcoholic patients who have other psychiatric problems.

The abuse of alcohol and/or drugs may be an unconscious attempt to treat the symptoms of bipolar disorder or it may be that individuals who have bipolar disorder are more prone to exhibit addictive tendencies. Experts are divided on this issue.

There are two forms of bipolar disorder: bipolar I and bipolar II disorder. In bipolar I disorder, manic episodes may last for at least a week. They are then followed by depressive periods that may last for about two weeks. Some patients become so manic that they require hospitalization in order to avoid causing harm to themselves or others. Patients may also experience both a mania and a depression simultaneously, a condition referred to as mixed mania. These patients are at risk for SUICIDE.

The National Institute of Mental Health's Epidemiologic Catchment Area (ECA) study revealed that about 61 percent of those who had bipolar I disorder had a lifetime diagnosis of a substance abuse disorder (an alcohol or drug use disorder). In addition, 39 percent of patients who had bipolar II disorder had an alcohol use disorder.

Bipolar II disorder is typified by a predominance of depression with less well-defined episodes of hypomania, which is a less severe form of mania than seen in bipolar I disorder. This diagnosis has become more common as more treatments for this disorder are becoming available.

Symptoms and Diagnostic Path

Some individuals are alternately depressed and manic over a short period, with many ups and downs, while others have longer periods of depression or mania.

Bipolar disorder may be evidenced by the following signs and symptoms, although a psychiatric evaluation is in order before a diagnosis can be made:

- grandiose ideas
- very rapid speech, which is sometimes unintelligible to others or difficult to follow
- hypersexuality and promiscuity
- extremely poor judgment, such as impulsively making an expensive purchase far beyond the individual's means
- in the depressive cycle, extreme lethargy and despondency

Treatment Options and Outlook

Bipolar disorder is usually treated with medications known as MOOD STABILIZERS, such as lithium or mood stabilizer/antiseizure drugs such as valproate (Depakote, Depakene, Depakote ER). Some patients are treated with NALTREXONE (ReVia), a drug that was developed to treat alcoholism. In some cases, both lithium and an antiseizure drug such as valproate may be given to treat bipolar disorder.

Some patients may not comply with the medication regimen, particularly because weight gain is common with lithium and valproate, and it may be a significant weight gain for some individuals. In addition, lethargy and sedation may also be a major problem with mood stabilizers. Naltrexone does not cause a weight gain; however, Sonne and Brady found that some bipolar women experienced side effects with naltrexone that were similar to those found with withdrawal from OPIATES.

The primary medication(s) given to treat bipolar disorder may be supplemented with treatment with antidepressants or other medications, on an as-needed basis. (Many patients who have bipolar disorder have other psychiatric diagnoses, such as DEPRESSION and ANXIETY DISORDERS.) Some experts believe that individuals who have bipolar disorder should avoid antidepressants, but it is not yet clearly established that this is necessary.

Antiseizure medications that have been used to treat bipolar disorder include carbamazapine (Tegretol), topiramate (Topamax), and lamotrigine (Lamictal). In the past, gabapentin (Neurotin) was widely prescribed for bipolar disorder, but it has been shown to have a limited to no effect on the prevention of manic episodes.

Antipsychotic medications are sometimes used by bipolar disorder I patients, such as olanzapine (Zyprexa), resperidone (Resperdal), and ziprasidone (Geodon).

If the patient also has a substance use disorder, the particular drugs of abuse need to be taken into account carefully by the prescribing physician; for example, patients who have bipolar disorder should avoid stimulants, particularly AMPHETAMINES, which may trigger a manic episode.

Risk Factors and Preventive Measures

Individuals who have a family history of bipolar disorder have an increased risk of developing this psychiatric problem. There are no known preventive measures for bipolar disorder, which may develop in some family members and yet not appear in others. However, it is preferable to avoid the abuse of alcohol and illegal drugs because in some cases, substance abuse may trigger other psychiatric disorders in some individuals who have bipolar disorder.

See also ANTISOCIAL PERSONALITY DISORDER; ATTENTION DEFICIT HYPERACTIVITY DISORDER; CONDUCT DISORDER; PRESCRIPTION DRUG ABUSE; PSYCHIATRIC DISORDERS.

Belmaker, R. H., M.D. "Bipolar Disorder." *New England Journal of Medicine* 351, no. 5 (July 29, 2004): 476–486.

Gwinnell, Esther, M.D., and Christine Adamec. *The Encyclopedia of Addictions and Addictive Behaviors.* New York: Facts On File, 2005.

Kupfner, David. "The Increasing Medical Burden in Bipolar Disorder." *Journal of the American Medical Association* 293, no. 20 (May 25, 2005): 2,528–2,530.

National Institute of Mental Health. "The Numbers Count: Mental Disorders in America." Rockville, Md.: National Institutes of Health, 2006. Available online. URL: http://www.nimh.nih.gov/publicat/numbers.cfm#readNow. Downloaded April 22, 2006.

Sonne, Susan C., and Kathleen T. Brady, M.D. "Bipolar Disorder and Alcoholism." National Institute on Alcohol Abuse and Alcoholism. Available online. URL: http://www.niaaa.nih.gov/publicatons/arh26-2/103-108.htm. Downloaded March 25, 2006.

Stahl, Stephen M. *Essential Psychopharmacology: The Prescriber's Guide.* Cambridge: Cambridge University Press, 2005.

buprenorphine A semisynthetic narcotic medication that is derived from THEBAINE, which is itself an alkaloid of the opium poppy. Buprenorphine is a Schedule III drug under the CONTROLLED SUBSTANCES ACT. The drug is used to help individuals with DETOXIFICATION from narcotics.

It was first synthesized as an analgesic (painkiller) in England in 1969. The National Institute of Drug Abuse (NIDA) in the United States researched its possible efficacy as a treatment for opiate addiction in the 1970s. It was ultimately found to be effective in treating HEROIN addiction, and it was also found to produce a lower level of PHYSICAL TOLERANCE than METHADONE, another treatment for opiate addiction. Thus, patients who stop taking buprenorphine will experience fewer withdrawal symptoms than patients who stop taking methadone.

In 2002, two new brand names of buprenorphine, Subutex and Suboxone, were approved by the Food and Drug Administration (FDA) as a treatment for narcotic addiction. (Suboxone also includes another treatment drug, naloxone.) These drugs are sublingual (under the tongue) medications. A transdermal (skin patch) delivery system has been approved for use in Europe but has not been approved as of this writing in the United States.

According to the Substance Abuse and Mental Health Services Administration, about 5 percent of treatment facilities in the United States use buprenorphine.

Physicians who wish to treat addicted patients with buprenorphine must obtain a special waiver from the federal government, and as of 2004, there were about 4,000 physicians in the United States who had been approved to use buprenorphine for treating addiction. These physicians must meet specific criteria; for example, they must have a board certification in addiction psychiatry, and they must also be certified in addiction medicine, among other criteria.

According to Welsh and Valadez-Meltzer in their article on buprenorphine in *Psychiatry*, it has three primary medical uses: DETOXIFICATION from narcotics, opioid maintenance, and PAIN MANAGEMENT. The goal of detoxification is to help patients rid themselves of the addiction; in opioid maintenance buprenorphine is given instead of the narcotic to which the patient is addicted, in a similar manner to the way METHADONE is often used. In pain management the drug is used as an analgesic for chronic severe pain.

Some patients taking buprenorphine have experienced elevated levels of liver enzymes, and such patients should be monitored carefully.

See also DETOXIFICATION; SCHEDULED DRUGS; WITHDRAWAL.

Welsh, Christopher, M.D., and Adela Valadez-Meltzer, M.D. "Buprenorphine: A (Relatively) New Treatment for Opioid Dependence." *Psychiatry* 2, no. 12 (December 2005): 29–39.

caffeine A legal STIMULANT that is found in many common products, such as coffee, soft drinks, chocolate, and tea. Caffeine is not a problem for many people but it is mildly addictive, such that if the person is a heavy consumer of caffeinated products and suddenly stops using them, mild WITHDRAWAL effects, such as vascular headaches, tiredness, and irritability, often occur for several days. Individuals also build up a tolerance to caffeine so that the dose required for the stimulant effect can increase over time.

The amount of caffeine in individual foods or drinks varies. In general, a cup of brewed coffee (eight ounces) has about 85 mg of caffeine, while the same amount of iced tea has 25 mg. A can of a caffeinated soft drink usually has about 24 mg of caffeine. One ounce of milk chocolate has about six milligrams of caffeine, and dark chocolate has about 20 mg. Most adults receive two-thirds of their daily consumption of caffeine from coffee, and children receive about half their daily caffeine consumption from soft drinks.

As much as 80 percent of the world population consumes some form of caffeine. Many COLLEGE STUDENTS use caffeinated beverages to remain awake and study all night, such as before taking examinations. Some people think giving an intoxicated person a large quantity of coffee to drink will counteract the effect of alcohol. It will not.

Health Effects

Many people can tolerate about 300 mg of caffeine per day; however, some people greatly exceed this amount. In one study of 36 children and adolescents in Israel who suffered from chronic or near-daily headaches, reported in a 2003 issue of *Cephalgia*, the researchers discovered that all of the children were heavy consumers of caffeinated cola. The chil-

dren consumed up to 385 mg per day. The parents were advised to taper their children slowly off cola. They did so, and as a result, 33 of the 36 children reported a complete remission of their headaches.

Sleep can be affected by as low a dose as 200 mg of caffeine per day. Caffeinated beverages and foods containing caffeine should not be consumed within three or four hours before the time when an individual wishes to sleep. Heavy caffeine users should avoid caffeine after about noon if they are having difficulty sleeping.

Excessive caffeine consumption can also be dangerous for the fetuses of pregnant women. In a study of 562 women in Sweden who had miscarriages in the first trimester of pregnancy, discussed in the *New England Journal of Medicine* in 2000, more pregnancy losses occurred in women who ingested at least 100 mg of caffeine per day than in women who consumed lower amounts.

Positive and Protective Aspects of Caffeine

In addition to the negative effects of caffeine, it has been shown to have some positive effects, and it has often been combined with acetaminophen or aspirin in over-the-counter preparations to treat patients who have migraine or tension-type headaches. However, regular use of over-the-counter or prescribed medications that include caffeine, such as butalbital (Fiorcet), can lead to rebound headaches, or headaches that are actually caused by the medication as it wears off. People who have such problems are usually slowly tapered off the drug.

In a study reported on Finnish middle-aged men and women and the relationship between caffeine consumption and the incidence of type 2 diabetes, published in 2004 in the *Journal of the American Medical Association*, the researchers found that there was a lower incidence of type 2 diabetes among the coffee drinkers, although the reason for this lower incidence was unknown.

In a study reported in a 1999 issue of the *Journal of the American Medical Association* of 46,000 men ranging from age 40 to age 75 years, with no prior history of gallstone disease, the men who had significantly higher consumption of coffee had a lower risk of development of gallstones than the other subjects. (The study did not address caffeine consumption and gallstones among women.)

In one study on coffee consumption, whose findings were discussed in 2000 in the *Journal of the American Medical Association*, data were analyzed on the use of coffee among 8,000 Japanese American men, ages 45 to 68 years old. The researchers found higher coffee and caffeine intake among the subjects was associated with a lower risk for the development of Parkinson's disease. The researchers suggested that it was probably the caffeine, rather than any other substance that was present in the coffee, that was responsible for these favorable results.

One study has indicated that habitual tea consumption may decrease the risk for hypertension. In a study of tea drinking for the past year among patients ages 20 and older in China, described in 2004 in the *Archives of Internal Medicine*, the researchers found that the risk of the development of hypertension *decreased* by 46 percent among those subjects who drank 120 to 599 mL per day of either green tea or oolong tea.

Although it seems counterintuitive, the risk for the development of hypertension was further reduced by 65 percent among those who drank 600 mL/day or more of these teas. It is unknown why this effect occurred. It is possible that some other component of the tea beyond the caffeine itself was responsible for this effect.

Cnattingius, Sven, M.D., et al. "Caffeine Intake and the Risk of First-Trimester Spontaneous Abortion." *New England Journal of Medicine* 343, no. 25 (December 21, 2000): 1,839–1,945.

Hering-Hanit, R., and Gadoth, N. "Caffeine-Induced Headache in Children and Adolescents." *Cephalgia* 23, no. 5 (June 2003): 332–335.

Leitzmann, Michael F., M.D., et al. "A Prospective Study of Coffee Consumption and the Risk of Symptomatic Gallstone Disease in Men." *Journal of the American Medical Association* 281, no. 22 (June 9, 1999): 2,106–2,112.

Ross, G. Webster, M.D. "Association of Coffee and Caffeine Intake with the Risk of Parkinson Disease." *Journal of the American Medical Association* 283, no. 20 (May 24/31, 2000): 2,674–2,679.

Tuomilehto, Jaako, M.D. "Coffee Consumption and Risk of Type 2 Diabetes Mellitus among Middle-Aged Finnish Men and Women." *Journal of the American Medical Association* 291, no. 10 (March 10, 2004): 1,213–1,219.

Yang, Yi-Chang, et al. "The Protective Effect of Habitual Tea Consumption." *Archives of Internal Medicine* 164 (July 26, 2004): 1,534–1,540.

Canada   According to the 2006 *International Narcotics Control Strategy Report*, released by the Bureau for International Narcotics and Law Enforcement Affairs of the U.S. State Department, Canada is a significant producer of high-quality MARIJUANA. It is an area from which PRECURSOR chemicals and over-the-counter pharmaceuticals that are used to produce drugs such as METHAMPHETAMINE are sent. Marijuana is smuggled from British Columbia, Ontario, and Quebec into the United States. In addition, drugs such as METHYLENEDIOXYMETH-AMPHETAMINE (MDMA/ECSTASY) and methamphetamine are also smuggled into the United States. As of September 30, 2005, 54,194 doses of MDMA were seized at the U.S./Canadian border.

Canada has a federal policy opposed to the harmful use of substances, Canada's Renewed Drug Strategy of 2003. In addition, in 2005, the government created counternarcotics legislation and expanded their law enforcement programs against the illegal use of NARCOTICS. In 2005, Health Canada, the national health organization, released the first edition of the *National Framework for Action to Reduce the Harms Associated with Alcohol and Other Drugs and Substances in Canada*.

Law enforcement authorities in Canada are concerned about ORGANIZED CRIME, and there are reports that foreign organized crime is active in all aspects of illegal drugs in Canada. In 2005, four Royal Canadian Mounted Police (RCMP) officials were killed when assisting local police when a marijuana farm was discovered in Alberta.

The United States and Canada cooperate at the federal, state, and local levels and have collaborated on joint cross-border drug threat assessments. In addition, Canada has expanded its collaboration with the United States in fighting illegal drug trafficking from South America to North America by using Maritime Patrol Assets.

Canadian Campus Survey

In 2004, the Centre for Addiction and Mental Health made a countrywide survey of Canadian undergraduate college students on their substance use, surveying 6,282 full-time students drawn from 40 universities. They found that a majority of students used alcohol, and 85.7 percent had used alcohol in the past year and 77.1 percent had used alcohol in the past month. Interestingly, female students were slightly more likely to have used alcohol than male students: of the female students 87.1 percent had used alcohol in the past year, compared to 84 percent of the male students. In addition, 77.7 percent of the females had used alcohol in the past month, compared to 76.5 percent of the male students.

The most commonly abused illicit drug was CANNABIS (MARIJUANA), which had been ever used by 51.4 percent, as well as by 32.1 percent of the students in the past 12 months and 16.7 percent in the 30 days before the survey. (The lifetime use of marijuana by U.S. college students was comparable, at 49.1 percent.)

After cannabis, the most commonly used illicit drugs were HALLUCINOGENIC DRUGS, such as magic mushrooms, MESCALINE, and PHENCYCLIDINE; 16.9 percent of the students had ever used this type of drug, and 5.6 percent of the students had used this type of drug in the past year. The lifetime usage of the Canadian students was higher than the lifetime use of U.S. college students, or 12 percent. (See COLLEGE STUDENTS.)

Opiates were also used, and 13.7 percent of the students had ever abused this type of drug, 5 percent of the students had abused opiates in the past year, and 1 percent had abused this type of drug in the past month.

Some of the students reported alcohol-related sexual harassment, including 14.3 percent of the females and 4.2 percent of the males. In addition, 43.9 percent of the students reported at least one indicator of harmful drinking, such as experiencing memory loss, feeling guilty, having an injury, or having other concerns related to drinking.

2004 Canadian Addiction Survey

In 2004, the Canadian Centre on Substance Abuse performed a nationwide survey of 13,909 respondents, including 5,721 males and 8,188 females, ages 15 to older than 75 years, on their alcohol and drug use.

With regard to alcohol use, the researchers found that 79.3 percent of the respondents consumed alcohol in the 12 months before the survey. The lowest rate of past-year drinking was on Prince Edward Island (70.2 percent) and the highest was in Quebec (82.3 percent). They also found that males were more likely to report drinking alcohol at least once a week (55.2 percent of males compared to 32.8 percent of females) and to have five or more drinks at a sitting (23.2 percent of males versus 8.8 percent of females). They also found that most Canadians drank in moderation, or one or two drinks per drinking day, with a higher proportion of female moderate drinkers (74.2 percent) than males, who were at 53.4 percent.

With regard to the use of cannabis, the researchers found that 44.5 percent of Canadians reported ever using the drug, while 14.1 percent said they had used marijuana in the 12 months before the survey. Males were more likely to use marijuana in their lifetime (50.1 percent) and in the past year (39.2 percent) than females, who had a lifetime use of 18.2 percent and a past-year use of 10.2 percent.

Cannabis usage was more common among younger people, and nearly 70 percent of the young adults between the ages of 18 and 24 had used marijuana at least once. In addition, 47 percent of those who were 18–19 years old had used the drug in the past year. According to the researchers one in 20 Canadians reported a concern about marijuana, such as the failure to control use of the drug (4.8 percent), the strong desire to use it (4.5 percent), and their friends' concern about their use of it (2.2. percent).

With regard to the illicit use of drugs, the most commonly abused drugs in the lifetime of Canadians were HALLUCINOGENIC DRUGS (11.4 percent), followed by cocaine (10.6 percent), AMPHETAMINES (6.4 percent), and Ecstasy (4.1 percent). The lifetime use of heroin and inhalants and lifetime INJECTION DRUG USE was about 1 percent or less. Men were more likely to report use of these drugs. However, most Canadians had not used drugs in the past year and the use was 1 percent or less except for the past-year usage of cocaine (1.9 percent).

As with other drugs, the highest use was among Canadians ages 18–19 years, after which the usage declined.

See also AFGHANISTAN; COLLEGE STUDENTS; COLOMBIA; MEXICO.

Adlaf, E. M, P. Begin, and E. Swaka, eds. *Canadian Addiction Survey (CAS): A National Survey of Canadians' Use of Alcohol and Other Drugs: Prevalence of Use and Related Harms: Detailed Report.* Ottawa: Canadian Centre on Substance Abuse, 2005. Available online. URL: http://www.ccsa.ca/NR/reonlyres/6806130B-C314-4C96-95CC-075D14CD83DE/0/ccsa0040 282005.pdf. Downloaded June 27, 2006.

Adlaf, Edward M., André Demers, and Louis Gliksman, eds. *Canadian Campus Survey 2004.* Toronto, Canada: Centre for Addiction and Mental Health, 2005. Available online. URL: http://www.camh.net/Research/Areas_of_research/Population_Life_Course_Studies/CCS_200 4_report.pdf. Downloaded June 27, 2006.

International Narcotics and Law Enforcement Affairs. "Canada, Mexico and Central America." *International Narcotics Control Strategy Report.* March 2006. Available online. URL: http://www.state.gov/p/inl/rls/nrcrpt/2006/vol1/html/62107.htm. Downloaded May 3, 2006.

cannabis An alternative name for MARIJUANA. Europeans are more likely to use this term than Americans. Sometimes LAW ENFORCEMENT authorities prefer it to *marijuana.*

child abuse Physical, sexual, or emotional harm to children as well as the neglect of children. Child abuse and neglect together are known as child maltreatment. Substance abuse is a major risk factor for child abuse. As many as one-third to two-thirds of all the substantiated cases of child abuse in the

United States involve substance abuse by parents or other caretakers.

About 5 million parents in the United States who abuse alcohol have at least one child in the home younger than 18 years. Victims of childhood abuse often develop lifelong problems, such as substance abuse as well as psychiatric problems, such as ANXIETY DISORDERS or DEPRESSION. They are also at greater risk for SUICIDE than adults who were not abused as children. They have a greater risk of abusing their own children as adults than those who were not abused as children.

Children of all ages may also be exposed to passive smoke from adults using MARIJUANA or CRACK COCAINE. In addition, children are also directly affected before birth by the mother's use of drugs and alcohol.

Child Victims and Perpetrators of Maltreatment

Small children from birth to age three years had the highest victimization rate of all ages in 2003, according to *Child Maltreatment 2003,* an annual report published by the Department of Health and Human Services in the United States (published in 2005). The rate of abuse for infants and young children in 2003 was 16.4 per 1,000 children. This rate steadily decreased with age: the rate was 13.8 for children ages four to seven, 11.7 for children age eight to 11, 10.7 for children ages 12 to 15, and 5.9 for children ages 15 to 17. Girls were slightly less likely to be victimized than boys, with the exception of SEXUAL ABUSE, in which most victims are girls.

Most perpetrators of child maltreatment (84 percent) are parents, with the exception of the perpetrators of sexual abuse, in which parents represented less than 3 percent of all perpetrators. Instead, nearly 76 percent of the perpetrators of sexual abuse were friends or neighbors.

Some children die of abuse or neglect, and in 2003, 78 percent of the fatalities were caused by one or both parents. The form of maltreatment that most often resulted in death was neglect.

The most common forms of child maltreatment in 2003 were neglect only (35.6 percent), followed by multiple maltreatment (28.9 percent) and physical abuse only (28.4 percent).

In 2003, 61 percent of the child victims were neglected by their parents or other caretakers, while

19 percent were physically abused, 10 percent were sexually abused, and 5 percent were emotionally abused. In addition, 2 percent were medically neglected, receiving insufficient or no needed medical treatment. Seventeen percent were victimized by "other" types of maltreatment, according to state laws. (Children may suffer more than one type of maltreatment.)

Substance-Abusing Perpetrators of Child Abuse

Adults who abuse alcohol and/or drugs have an increased risk of abusing and/or neglecting their children. Mothers who have undergone treatment for substance abuse may have also experienced DOMESTIC VIOLENCE or abuse in their own childhood, and they have an increased risk for committing child abuse. However, it is *not* true that all children who are abused in childhood will invariably become abusive to their own children. Studies indicate that about 40 percent of all abused children may become abusive to their own children in adulthood.

In general, as pointed out by David Howe in *Child Abuse and Neglect: Attachment, Development and Intervention,* substance abusers have such traits as impulsivity, feelings of inadequacy, self-centeredness, DEPRESSION, emotional deprivation, and a low frustration tolerance, which probably contribute to their addiction and/or abuse of substances. Together, these personality traits are risk factors for child abuse as well.

Howe describes the viewpoint of the child of a substance-abusing parent.

> The more the parent becomes lost in his or her own substance-altered state of mind, the less contingently accurate or relevant is his or her behaviour with the child. From the child's point of view, it feels as if the parent is no longer able to recognize and read his or her attachment needs and emotional states. Emotional availability and understanding disappear. So not only might the parent's behaviour and manner be odd, confusing and frightening, but also the carer is unavailable to deal with that confusion and fear. The carer causes the distress, does not see it, and fails to repair the relationship that is now under growing stress. In these conditions, the young child's distress is likely

to escalate and go unregulated. The child can find no behavioural strategy that increases his or her security. Her attachment behaviour is therefore likely to be disorganized. In the presence of a drunk or drugged parent, the child feels emotionally abandoned and frightened. So long as the parent remains "out of his or her mind," the child is psychologically alone, feeling bewildered and unsafe, and unable to manage.

Abusers often misread the emotions of their children, misperceiving the child's expressed surprise as resentment and acting on that erroneous misperception. This risk for misinterpretation increases further with the mental haze that often descends with the use of alcohol or drugs.

Neglect and substance abuse Neglect is the most common form of child maltreatment among substance abusers. Neglect can be very serious and may cause fatalities in infants and young children because of their survival needs for food, shelter, and medical care. In addition, if toddlers or young children are ignored when the caretaker is present or they are left alone while the parent seeks alcohol and/or drugs, small children are at risk for harm from others who may know that they are alone.

They are also at risk from their own exposure to dangers about which they are curious; they may explore, for example, exposed electrical wiring that they either touch or mouth, or ingest alcohol or drugs that are left about carelessly. Small children may also ingest toxic household products or may handle sharp objects or even firearms, sometimes leading to a tragedy. A parent who is impaired by alcohol or drugs when a child is harmed may fail to take action in sufficient time (or at all) to help the child. As a result, accidents that an emergency room doctor could readily resolve are not treated, leading to permanent damage and even to death.

There are some studies that suggest that children whose parents abuse substances are at a greater risk themselves for ingesting toxic substances or household medications than children in other family settings. This may be related to a desire to mimic the parental use of medications or substances.

Clandestine laboratories and abuse Parents who operate a clandestine laboratory in their home to create METHAMPHETAMINE create an extremely dangerous and toxic environment for children of all ages. It is an environment that may lead to harm or death for several reasons; for example, children are at risk for harm because of the often-negligent handling of the dangerous chemicals that are needed to create the drug, which are made more dangerous by heating them to a very high temperature as part of the drug manufacturing process. Sometimes these chemicals spill, or they may explode with nearby children present, who are harmed or killed.

According to Kathryn Wells in her chapter on substance abuse in *Understanding the Medical Diagnosis of Child Maltreatment: A Guide for Nonmedical Professionals,* in about 35 percent of these environments, children are present in the home. Not only are the substances used to create methamphetamine extremely dangerous, but the vapors that are released in the making of methamphetamine permeate the entire house.

Even when the laboratory has been closed down, there is still a long-term effect of the manufacture of methamphetamine within the buildings where the drug was made. Says Wells, "These homes need to be considered contaminated until they have undergone extensive cleanup and have been released for safe occupancy by building inspectors."

Wells cites the case of Lilah (age four) and Omar (age two), who were removed from a home that was a methamphetamine laboratory. Although the children were doing well in foster care, they suffered from developmental delays, severe dental problems, and respiratory problems. Their doctors were unable to determine the cause of these conditions, but they speculated they were probably caused by both a toxic environment and the chronic neglect that the children suffered.

Physical abuse   Incidents of beating, assaulting, burning, immersion, and other forms of physical abuse are increased when parents are substance abusers. Infants and small children cry when they need something, and this crying may increase the irritability level of the substance abuser to the point that he or she decides to "teach" the child (including an infant) a lesson by abusing him or her. The drugs that these parents take, particularly methamphetamine and cocaine, often lower their frustration threshold. When the child cries, the parent

may take more drugs, which further reduce their ability to meet the needs of the child, causing the child to cry more, in a vicious circle of an escalating risk for abuse.

Sexual abuse   Because drugs may lower the inhibitions of users, substance-abusing parents are at risk for sexually abusing their children. Methamphetamine use in particular, as well as cocaine, often increases the individual's sex drive to the point of hypersexuality, although if these same parents were not impaired by drugs, they would never sexually abuse their children.

Methamphetamine-abusing parents are also likely to use pornography. Often young children are exposed to this pornography and may suffer from sexual abuse by the parent and others whom the parents allow to abuse the child sexually. In such cases, the child is at risk for contracting sexually transmitted diseases, as well as suffering physical and emotional harm that is often lifelong. Although parental sexual abuse is statistically rare, the risk is greater among parents who abuse methamphetamines.

Emotional maltreatment   Substance-abusing parents are more likely than nonabusers to make cruel statements to their children, telling them they are unwanted or even evil children no one would ever want. Often emotional maltreatment may accompany physical abuse, and the combination of physical and psychological abuse causes severe psychological damage in the long term.

Investigations of Child Abuse

The protective services division of the state child social services department investigates allegations of abuse and/or neglect. The finding of the investigator and whether the allegations are substantiated or not will affect whether the parents or other caretakers are allowed to continue to care for their children. If the caretaker is found to have a substance abuse problem, then the child is usually placed in FOSTER CARE or with relatives while the parent or caretaker is given a chance to undergo rehabilitation.

The parents (or other caretakers) will be given a service plan to comply with and substance abusers are expected to seek rehabilitation and to make significant progress before their children may be

TABLE I: ALCOHOL AND DRUG USE CONTINUUM AND IMPLICATIONS FOR RISKS FOR CHILD MALTREATMENT

Alcohol and Drug Use Continuum	Implications for Child Welfare/Examples of Risk to Children
Use of alcohol or drugs to socialize and feel effects; use may not appear abusive and may not lead to dependence; however, the circumstance under which a parent uses can put children at risk of harm.	• Use during pregnancy can harm the fetus • Use of prescription pain medication per the instructions from a prescribing physician can sometimes have unintended or unexpected effects—a parent caring for children may find that he or she is more drowsy than expected and cannot respond to the needs of children in his or her care
Abuse of alcohol or drugs includes at least one of these factors in the last 12 months: • Recurrent substance use resulting in failure to fulfill obligations at work, home, or school • Recurrent substance use in situations that are physically hazardous • Recurrent substance-related legal problems • Continued substance use despite having persistent or recurrent social or interpersonal problems caused by or exacerbated by the substance	• Driving with children in the car while under the influence • Children may be left in unsafe care—with an inappropriate caretaker or unattended—while parent is partying • Parent may neglect or sporadically address the children's needs for regular meals, clothing, and cleanliness • Even when the parent is in the home, the parents' use may leave children unsupervised • Behavior toward children may be inconsistent, such as a pattern of violence followed by remorse
Dependence, also known as addiction, is a pattern of use that results in three or more of the following symptoms in a 12-month period: • Tolerance—needing more of the drug or alcohol to get "high" • Withdrawal—physical symptoms when alcohol or other drugs are not used, such as tremors, nausea, sweating, and shakiness • Substance is taken in larger amounts and over a longer period than intended • Persistent desire or unsuccessful efforts to cut down or control substance use • A great deal of time is spent in activities related to obtaining the substance, use of the substance, or recovering from its effects • Important social, occupational, or recreational activities are given up or reduced because of substance use • Substance use is continued despite knowledge of persistent or recurrent physical or psychological problems caused or exacerbated by the substance	• Despite a clear danger to children, the parent may engage in addiction-related behaviors, such as leaving children unattended while seeking drugs • Funds are used to buy alcohol or other drugs, while other necessities, such as buying food, are neglected • A parent may not be able to think logically or make rational decisions regarding children's needs or care • A parent may not be able to prioritize children's needs over his or her own need for the substance

Source: Adapted from Breshears, E. M., S. Yeah, and N. K. Young. *Understanding Substance Abuse and Facilitating Recovery: A Guide for Child Welfare Workers.* Rockville, Md.: U.S. Department of Health and Human Services, Substance Abuse and Mental Health Services Administration, 2004, p. 3.

returned to them. They may also be required to seek counseling and to take anger management and/or parenting classes, as well as performing other actions in order to reunite with their children, such as attending Alcoholics Anonymous or Narcotics Anonymous self-help meetings. If the substance abuser either does not or cannot recover from the substance abuse problem within about one year (depending on state law), then his or her custody rights may be involuntarily terminated by the state. The child will then usually be placed with relatives or may be adopted by nonrelatives, such as foster parents or other individuals.

Risks for Reabuse

Some factors are predictive for the future maltreatment of children. For example, in one study of 95 parents who were substance abusers and who had maltreated their children in the past, as described in 2003 in *Children & Youth Services Review,* when substance abuse was identified as a factor in child abuse, these abusers where 13 times more likely to maltreat their children again compared to those who were not substance abusers. In addition, if criminal activity was present among those who abused substances, and this factor was noted by protective services workers in their initial reports, these individuals were 770 times more likely to reabuse their children.

The level of drug or alcohol use, abuse, and addiction may affect the risks for child maltreatment, as seen in the table from *Understanding Substance Abuse and Facilitating Recovery.*

Indicators of Drug and Alcohol Abuse for Protective Service Workers

Child welfare experts recommend that important indicators of drug or alcohol use should be checked in any allegation and/or investigation for child abuse. Most of these indicators require an in-home examination of the parent or caretaker.

A checklist of indicators of substance abuse that protective services workers should consider from *Understanding Substance Abuse and Facilitating Recovery: A Guide for Child Welfare Workers* follows:

- A report of substance use is included in the child protective services report

- Drug paraphernalia is found in the home (syringe kit [and the parent is not a diabetic], or there are pipes, charred spoon, foils, or a large number of liquor or beer bottles)
- The home or the parent may smell of alcohol, marijuana, or drugs
- A child reports alcohol and/or other drug use by the parent(s) or other adults in the home
- A parent appears to be actively under the influence of alcohol or drugs (slurred speech, inability to focus mentally, physical balance affected, extremely lethargic or hyperactive)
- A parent shows signs of addiction (needle tracks, skin abscesses, burns on inside of lips)
- A parent shows or reports experiencing physical effects of addiction or being under the influence, including withdrawal (nausea, euphoria, slowed thinking, or hallucinations are other symptoms)

Lifelong Effects of Child Abuse

Many studies have found a correlation between children who have lived with substance-abusing parents and/or children who were abused in childhood who later developed serious problems in their own adulthood. For example, childhood abuse is a risk factor for adult substance abuse, marital problems, psychiatric problems (such as anxiety disorders or depression), suicide, problems with work, abuse of their own children, and many other problems.

In a study of the relationship of childhood adverse events and later serious problems in adulthood, the Adverse Childhood Experiences (ACE) Study, discussed by Valerie Edwards and colleagues in their chapter in *Child Victimization,* the researchers questioned adults on their adverse experiences in childhood, such as physical abuse, sexual abuse, witnessing of violence between parents, household alcohol/drug abuse, parental separation/divorce, household mental illness, household criminal activity, and emotional abuse. They found that the number of ACE events in childhood was directly linked to adult problems.

The prevalence of some ACE events was high; for example, 28 percent of the adults had experienced physical abuse in childhood and 27 percent had experienced household alcohol/drug abuse.

Adults who experienced one or more ACEs in childhood had an increased risk of alcohol problems in adulthood, such as heavy drinking, alcoholism, or marrying an alcoholic person. Other childhood problems were linked to adult problems. Women who reported four or more ACEs in childhood had about six times the risk of initiating sexual activity by age 15 and were 5.5 times more likely to state that they had had 30 or more sexual partners. They were 2.4 times more likely than those without ACEs to perceive themselves as at risk for acquired immune deficiency syndrome (AIDS).

Parental Substance Abuse and Childhood Mental Illness

Studies have shown a link between parental substance abuse and psychiatric disorders in their children. In one study of psychiatric disorders in children among drug-abusing, alcohol-abusing, and non-substance-abusing fathers reported in the *Journal of the American Academy of Child & Adolescent Psychiatry* in 2004, researchers Michelle L. Kelley and William Fals-Stewart found that the children of substance-abusing fathers had a significantly greater risk for psychiatric illness than the children of non-abusing fathers, with the children of drug abusers having the greatest risk for psychiatric disorders.

The researchers studied 120 biological fathers: 40 fathers who met the American Psychiatric Association's criteria for alcohol dependence (alcoholism), 40 fathers who met the criteria for a cocaine or opiate use disorder, and 40 fathers who had no substance abuse problems.

In these groups, 62.5 percent of the fathers in the drug-abusing group had legal or criminal problems, compared to 55 percent of the fathers in the alcoholism group and 5 percent of the fathers in the non-substance-abusing group.

In considering the children of these fathers, 53 percent of the children of the drug-using fathers had a psychiatric diagnosis, compared to 25 percent of the children of alcoholic fathers and 10 percent of children of the non-substance-abusing fathers. With regard to depression alone, among the children, 38 percent of the children of drug-using fathers had depression, as did 13 percent of the children of alcoholic fathers and 3 percent of the children of the non-substance-abusing fathers.

See also DOMESTIC VIOLENCE; FAMILY, EFFECT ON; GENETIC PREDISPOSITIONS AND ENVIRONMENTAL EFFECTS ON SUBSTANCE USE DISORDERS; PREGNANCY; PSYCHIATRIC DISORDERS.

Administration on Children Youth, and Families. *Child Maltreatment 2003.* Washington, D.C.: Children's Bureau, U.S. Department of Health and Human Services, 2005.

Breshears, E. M., S. Yeah, and N. K. Young. *Understanding Substance Abuse and Facilitating Recovery: A Guide for Child Welfare Workers.* Rockville, Md.: U.S. Department of Health and Human Services, Substance Abuse and Mental Health Services Administration, 2004.

Clark, Robin E., Judith Freeman Clark, and Christine Adamec. *The Encyclopedia of Child Abuse.* New York: Facts On File, 2006.

Edwards, Valerie, et al. "The Wide-Ranging Health Outcomes of Adverse Childhood Experiences. In *Child Victimization.* Kingston, N.J.: Civic Research Institute, 2005.

Fuller, Tamara L., and Susan J. Wells. "Predicting Maltreatment Recurrence among CPS Cases with Alcohol and Other Drug Involvement." *Children and Youth Services Review* 25, no. 7 (2003): 553–569.

Howe, David. *Child Abuse and Neglect: Attachment, Development and Intervention.* New York: Palgrave Macmillan, 2005.

Kelley, Michelle L., and William Fals-Stewart. "Psychiatric Disorders of Children Living with Drug-Abusing, Alcohol-Abusing, and Non-Substance-Abusing Fathers." *Journal of the American Academy of Child & Adolescent Psychiatry* 43, no. 5 (May 2004): 621–628.

Wells, Kathryn M. "Substance Abuse and Child Maltreatment." In *Understanding the Medical Diagnosis of Child Maltreatment: A Guide for Nonmedical Professionals.* New York: Oxford University Press, 2006.

clandestine laboratories Illicit places used to manufacture illegal drugs, particularly METHAMPHETAMINE. In other countries, however, clandestine laboratories are often primarily devoted to the production of HEROIN and other drugs. However, MEXICO has numerous clandestine laboratories that are dedicated to the production of methamphetamine, which is subsequently trafficked into the United States. Since the United States has cracked down on methamphetamine production, a great deal of production has moved to Mexico, according to law-enforcement authorities.

Individuals use a variety of common household chemicals to manufacture illegal drugs such as methamphetamine. As a result, federal laws limit the amounts of common household products that can be sold to individuals, and when individuals seek to buy large amounts of these chemicals, law enforcement authorities are alerted.

The manufacture of drugs such as methamphetamine in the home or other location is very dangerous because the chemicals are volatile. Individuals have been harmed or killed when the chemicals spilled or exploded. In some states, if an individual operates a clandestine laboratory, it is specifically considered a form of CHILD ABUSE, and the child is removed from the family for his or her safety.

Some experts believe there is an environmental risk to the home when illegal drugs are created there and report that the chemicals used may linger within the walls of the home or other site for extended periods before they dissipate.

Despite the health and safety risks, as well as the risk of losing their children to state control, some individuals persist in creating drugs in clandestine laboratories because they consider it financially profitable. They may not factor in the high risk of being caught by federal and state authorities and the risk of prosecution and INCARCERATION.

Indicators of a Clandestine Methamphetamine Laboratory

Most clandestine laboratories in the United States operate solely to create methamphetamine, in large part because it is a highly profitable business, albeit an illegal one.

The following signs may indicate the presence of a clandestine laboratory that is used to create methamphetamine:

- strange smells emanating from the home, similar to the odors of cat urine or nail polish removers
- a large supply of toxic chemicals in the house, such as drain cleaner, antifreeze, and fertilizers

- large quantities of cold medicine with pseudo-ephedrine or ephedrine (beyond what would be needed in a normal household)
- many empty pill bottles throughout the house, with no apparent lawful reason for their presence
- excessive amounts of matches, lithium batteries, and plastic bags
- the constant presence of many people in the house, at all times of the day and night
- individuals in the home who are irritable, have mood swings, and may exhibit aggressive or repetitious behavior
- many visitors at unusual times, especially in the evening or late evening
- blackened windows or windows that are covered with aluminum foil, obscuring a view into the interior of the home

Danger from Methamphetamine Laboratories

It should also be noted that the clandestine laboratories that produce methamphetamine are extremely dangerous, not only to those who produce the drug but also to any others who may reside in the home or be present during the manufacture of the drug, such as children and other family members. The fumes from methamphetamine are so toxic that they can cause brain damage.

Methamphetamine must be produced at very high temperatures, and it is extremely volatile during manufacture. As a result, there is a high risk of fires and explosions, as well as a risk for unusually severe chemical burns that are usually difficult for physicians to treat. Methamphetamine abusers who create the drug may be impaired because they are using the drug, and thus, they have a greater risk of accidents and injuries from its manufacture. However, even those who are *not* abusers of methamphetamine or other drugs but who operate clandestine laboratories find the manufacture of methamphetamine to be difficult and dangerous.

The vapors that emanate from the production of methamphetamine will seep into the carpet and walls of the homes where methamphetamine is produced, and some experts have estimated that the cost is at least $2,000 per site to make a home fit to live in again after a laboratory has been removed. The restoration work must be performed by experienced specialists.

Methamphetamine production is also bad for the environment because it produces a considerable amount of toxic waste, and experts estimate that for each pound of methamphetamine that is produced, there are about five or six pounds of hazardous chemicals created. Since the individuals who create methamphetamine in clandestine laboratories are operating illegally, they are unlikely to have any concern about protecting the environment, and thus, they will often empty their waste material from the drug manufacture into fields and rivers, which may then contaminate the water that is available to both humans and animals.

See also CRIME AND CRIMINALS; LAW ENFORCEMENT; ORGANIZED CRIME; SCHEDULED DRUGS; STIMULANTS.

club drugs   Generally refers to illegal drugs that are used at all-night parties that are sometimes known as raves. Common club drugs include METHYLENEDIOXYMETHAMPHETAMINE (MDMA/ECSTASY), FLUNITRAZEPAM (ROHYPNOL), GAMMA-HYDROXYBUTYRATE (GHB), and KETAMINE, as well as MARIJUANA and COCAINE. Many adolescents and young adults may combine alcohol with another drug, a dangerous practice that can cause ACCIDENTAL OVERDOSE DEATHS.

The abuse of club drugs can be extremely dangerous and even fatal. In her article for the *New England Journal of Medicine* in 2005, McGinn describes a case in which the girlfriend of a man noticed that he and a friend had disappeared. She discovered them unconscious in the basement of a building where a party they had attended had been held, and she immediately called for help. These men, both college seniors, were extremely fortunate that the woman acted as she had, rather than leaving them to "sleep it off," because both were nonresponsive to all stimuli when treated by emergency medical personnel and would have died without treatment.

Says McGinn, "Had these men been left in the basement, they would have been brain-dead within about six minutes after they had stopped breathing, and their hearts would have stopped shortly there-

after. As it was, both required mechanical ventilation for the rest of the night." The men made a full recovery and left the hospital the next day.

McGinn was unable to confirm what drug the men took that caused such an extreme problem, but she suspected it was GHB combined with alcohol. Says McGinn, "In combination with alcohol, GHB can cause decreased respiratory drive, coma, and death."

See also CRIME AND CRIMINALS; DATE RAPE DRUGS; MALICIOUS POISONING; SEXUAL ASSAULTS; YOUNG ADULTS.

McGinn, Cynthia G., M.D. "Close Calls with Club Drugs." *New England Journal of Medicine* 352, no. 26 (June 30, 2005): 2,671–2,672.

cocaine   A powerful central nervous system STIMULANT that is extracted from the leaves of the *Erythroxylum coca* plant, which is located primarily in the South American countries of Bolivia and Peru and is primarily trafficked to the United States through COLOMBIA. Cocaine is highly addictive, and for this reason, it is a Schedule II drug under the CONTROLLED SUBSTANCES ACT. There are some limited legal medical uses of powdered cocaine, which may only be used by a physician, usually to treat a patient who has a medical problem that is related to the eyes or the nose.

The powdered form of cocaine is a hydrochloride salt. It dissolves in water and can be injected intravenously. This form of cocaine can also be taken orally or inhaled (snorted). Drug dealers often dilute cocaine with other substances that resemble cocaine, such as talcum powder, cornstarch, or sugar. They may also dilute the drug with procaine (an anesthetic) or other stimulants, such as AMPHETAMINES. Some users of cocaine combine the drug with HEROIN.

In contrast to powdered cocaine, CRACK COCAINE is a compound that has *not* been neutralized by an acid. In this form, the drug is *freebased:* processed with baking soda or ammonia and water and subsequently heated to remove the hydrochloride so that it can be smoked by the person abusing the drug.

Cocaine (whether powdered cocaine or crack cocaine) acts on dopamine, a brain chemical, by preventing the existing dopamine from being carried away and thus by causing a buildup of dopamine. It is believed that it is this buildup that causes the euphoria that is associated with cocaine abuse. In addition, cocaine prevents the reuptake of other neurotransmitters, such as serotonin and noradrenaline, and it causes the release of extra adrenalin by the adrenal glands.

Cocaine has been used by the Indians in Peru and Bolivia for about 1,200 years. They chew the coca leaves. Initially, the leaves were reserved for Incan priests, who used them in religious ceremonies, and they were also given as rewards. When Pizarro conquered the Inca in 1533, the Indians chewed coca leaves to stave off hunger and fatigue.

A Corsican, Angel Mariani, imported massive quantities of cocaine in the mid-1800s, mixing it with wine and selling his concoction as Vin Mariani. It was an extremely popular drink in both Europe and the United States, and Mariani received a gold medal achievement award in 1860 from Pope Leo XII for creating his invigorating drink.

According to Steven Karch in his 1999 article in the *Journal of the Royal Society of Medicine*, two glasses of Vin Mariani contained less than 59 mg of cocaine, which is roughly equal to one "line" of cocaine that is snorted today by cocaine abusers. However, when a better method to transport coca leaves from South America was developed, there were many competitors and Karch says that problems with toxicity and some deaths occurred as many producers included large amounts of cocaine in their products. Says Karch, "Vin Mariani may have contained only 6 mg cocaine per ounce, but competitors' products contained hundreds of milligrams per ounce."

An Atlanta, Georgia, pharmacist, John Pemberton, later developed his cocaine-containing drink Coca Cola in 1885, selling the first drink at Jacob's Pharmacy in Atlanta in 1886, according to the Library of Congress. Pemberton, a morphine addict who had serious financial and medical problems, sold his formula and his wife died impoverished. In 1905, the cocaine was completely removed from the soft drink.

Karl Koller, an Austrian ophthalmologist and friend of Sigmund Freud, discovered that cocaine could be isolated and used as a local anesthetic in 1884, and it was used in this manner for individuals having surgery of the eyes and nose. (This use continues in the 21st century, although many doctors rely on other anesthetics.) Cocaine was popular among physicians in the late 19th and early 20th centuries, because they were seeking an effective anesthetic.

Dr. Freud wrote a monograph on the beneficial effects of cocaine as a miracle drug in 1884. He used the drug to treat opium addiction, although later he realized cocaine itself was addicting.

President Taft proclaimed cocaine to be "Public Enemy Number One" in 1913 and in 1914, the Harrison Act was passed, which banned the nonmedical use of cocaine. Its usage declined. Prior to that time, cocaine was readily available in numerous elixirs, tobacco products, liquors, and wines and no prescription was required. According to Shanti and Lucas in their article on cocaine in *Critical Care Medicine*, "Cocaine was promoted for the treatment of opiate and alcohol addiction, runny nose, sore throat, headaches, fatigue, hay fever, high blood pressure, nervous disorders, and even tuberculosis."

Because cocaine abuse began to rise again in the 1960s, cocaine was classified as a Schedule II drug by Congress in 1970 and it could be used by a physician only for medical purposes. This restriction still applies.

Cocaine Abusers

According to the National Survey on Drug Use and Health, an estimated 1 million people had used cocaine for the first time in 2004, which was the same level of new users in 2002 and 2003. Most of the new users (66 percent) were ages 18 and older, and the average age for new users was 20 years. The number of people receiving treatment for a cocaine abuse problem at a specialty facility increased significantly from 276,000 in 2003 to 466,000 in 2004.

In considering the lifetime use of cocaine, about 34 million Americans (14.2 percent of the population) ages 12 and older had ever used cocaine in 2004. When the population was limited to adolescents who were ages 12–17 years, lower percentages were reported: 3.4 percent of eighth graders had ever used cocaine in 2004 and that percentage increased slightly to 3.7 percent in 2005. The percentages were higher among college students and young adults; for

TABLE I: LIFETIME PREVALENCE, ANNUAL PREVALENCE, AND CURRENT USE OF COCAINE (NOT INCLUDING CRACK COCAINE), 2004, IN CERTAIN POPULATIONS, PERCENTAGES

	Lifetime Prevalence	Annual Prevalence	30-Day Prevalence
8th Graders	3.4	2.0	0.9
10th Graders	5.4	3.7	1.7
High School Seniors	8.1	5.3	2.3
Young Adults Ages 19–28	15.2	7.1	2.2
College Students	9.5	6.6	2.4
Same-Age Non College Students	16.5	8.5	2.4

Source: Adapted from Johnston, Lloyd D., et al. *Monitoring the Future: National Survey Results on Drug Use, 1975–2004.* Vol. 2, *College Students and Adults Ages 19–45.* Bethesda, Md.: National Institute on Drug Abuse, National Institutes of Health, 2005, pp. 36, 43, 49, 230.

example, in 2004, 9.5 percent of college students had ever used cocaine, and 15.2 percent of young adults had ever abused this drug. (See Table I.)

According to the National Survey on Drug Use and Health, there were 2.0 million current users of cocaine in the United States in 2004. Of these users, 467,000 used crack cocaine. According to the *Monitoring the Future* study for 2004, 16 percent of all Americans have tried cocaine by the age of 30, and of these 8 percent have tried cocaine by their senior year in high school.

See Table I for a comparison of cocaine abuse among specific populations, including students in the eighth, 10th, and 12th grades, as well as college students and their same-age noncollege peers and young adults ages 19–28 years old. The table includes the lifetime prevalence for each group (having ever used cocaine), the annual prevalence (having used the drug in the past year), and the 30-day prevalence (having used the drug in the past month).

In considering the lifetime prevalence of the abuse of cocaine, the highest rates were seen among the noncollege age peers of college students and young adults, and the lowest rates were seen among eighth graders.

In considering the annual prevalence of the abuse of cocaine, the highest rates were again seen among the noncollege age peers of college students and among young adults.

Last, in considering the 30-day prevalence of the abuse of cocaine, the rates were very similar (or identical) for high school seniors, college students, and their noncollege age peers and young adults.

According to the United Nations Office on Drugs and Crime, an estimated 13.3 million people world-wide abused cocaine in 2003. In the United States, 20 percent of all drug-related emergency room visits involved cocaine in 2003, or 125,921 cases.

Cocaine Abuse in Selected Cities and States Nationwide

The Community Epidemiology Work Group reports on 21 areas in the United States on drug abuse patterns, and in their 2005 report, cocaine abuse continued to dominate in many areas of the country and to have serious consequences for users, service providers, and law enforcement officials. High levels of violence and GANG activity were associated with the trafficking (sale) of cocaine. Crack cocaine was also a major problem in many areas.

The Work Group found cocaine/crack to be a primary drug of abuse in Atlanta, Georgia, in 2004, as well as in Boston, Massachusetts; New Orleans, Louisiana (especially crack cocaine); Philadelphia, Pennsylvania; South Florida; and Washington, D.C. (especially crack).

As can be seen from Table II, many cities have seen a decline in the percentage of treatment admissions due to cocaine since 2002, while some have stayed at about the same level. Cocaine/crack cocaine also represents a large percentage of treatment admissions in some areas of the country. For example, in Atlanta, Georgia, more than half (52.5 percent) of treatment admissions in 2004 were for cocaine (down from 68.1 percent in 2001). Of these admissions, most cases (77.2 percent) were for crack cocaine.

The prevalence of cocaine also varies greatly from city to city in terms of the highest percentage of total drug items, from a high of Miami in

TABLE II: PRIMARY COCAINE TREATMENT ADMISSIONS (EXCLUDING ALCOHOL) BY MAJOR CITIES AND PERCENTAGE, 2001–2004

City/State	2001	2002	2003	2004	Percentage Crack, 2003–2004
Atlanta	68.1	60.8	57.6	52.5	77.2
Baltimore	15.1	15.7	15.5	16.0	79.4
Boston	16.0	15.0	12.7	11.3	58.0
Chicago	NR	NR	NR	32.7	90.5
Denver	21.8	23.0	22.4	23.2	60.8
Detroit	38.7	38.6	38.5	35.6	89.8
Los Angeles	22.9	23.3	23.0	22.0	88.2
Minneapolis/St. Paul	26.6	27.2	26.3	26.1	74.8
New Orleans	40.0	42.7	43.1	38.9	NR
New York	29.3	28.5	28.9	29.5	61.7
Newark	7.0	6.8	6.8	7.2	49.6
Philadelphia	39.6	40.3	36.4	33.8	77.1
St. Louis	44.3	41.9	40.2	40.9	91.7
San Francisco	24.1	24.0	25.9	29.7	85.0
Seattle	21.9	19.8	22.6	21.8	NR
Washington, D.C.	41.4	41.9	34.9	NR	66.2
Arizona	19.0	16.7	16.2	16.1	NR
Hawaii	8.0	8.5	6.3	6.3	41.2
Texas	38.9	38.7	38.2	35.7	68.7

Note: NR: Not reported.
Source: National Institute of Drug Abuse. *Epidemiologic Trends in Drug Abuse.* Vol.1, *Proceeding of the Community Epidemiology Work Group. Highlights and Executive Summary.* Bethesda, Md.: National Institutes of Health, June 2005, p. 8.

2004 (69.1 percent) to a low of 14.3 percent in San Diego. (See Table III.)

Predictive and Protective Factors for Heavy Cocaine Use in Adulthood

Some researchers have studied the relationship of a variety of factors to heavy cocaine use among adults and found predictive factors as well as protective factors against heavy use. These results were reported by the Office of National Drug Control Policy in 2004. The data were drawn from the Department of Labor's National Longitudinal Survey of Youth, from 1984 to 1998. A longitudinal study resurveys former respondents and provides an opportunity to observe behavior over time.

The researchers found many relationships between the early use of drugs and a later heavy cocaine use. For example, adolescents and young adults who were heavy marijuana users, and especially those who had started smoking marijuana by the age of 12 years, were also more likely to become heavy cocaine abusers. These early abusers of mar-

ijuana were more than four times more likely to become heavy cocaine abusers than those who did not start smoking marijuana at this early age. In addition, adolescents who had smoked marijuana more than 50 times were more than six times more likely than others to become heavy cocaine users in adulthood.

Another factor was the age when the individual first began using cocaine, with an early age being predictive for heavy use in adulthood. Those who began abusing cocaine before age 15 were found more likely to become heavy cocaine abusers than others; for example, youths who had used cocaine by the age of 15 years were nearly six times more likely to become heavy cocaine abusers than others.

Alcohol use at an early age was also associated with heavy cocaine use, and the heaviest rate of cocaine abuse was found among individuals who began drinking alcohol twice a week by the age of 12 years. They were about three times as likely to become heavy cocaine users as those who did not start drinking before age 12.

TABLE III: COCAINE ITEMS ANALYZED BY FORENSIC LABORATORIES IN 20 AREAS, ORDERED BY HIGHEST PERCENTAGE OF TOTAL ITEMS IN 2004: 2003–2004

Area	2003	2004
Miami	66.7	69.1
New York City	51.3	48.9
Denver	50.3	48.8
Newark	48.3	45.5
Washington, D.C.	39.5	44.7
Baltimore	46.9	44.3
Philadelphia	43.7	44.3
Atlanta	39.7	44.2
Detroit	45.2	41.9
St. Louis	45.1	41.5
New Orleans	38.4	40.8
Los Angeles	32.7	38.3
Seattle	40.5	38.1
Chicago	33.8	32.6
Phoenix	NR	32.2
Texas	30.6	31.8
Boston	27.6	30.7
Minneapolis/St. Paul	21.3	21.4
Honolulu	12.2	14.8
San Diego	13.1	14.3

Note: NR: Not reported.
Source: National Institute of Drug Abuse. *Epidemiologic Trends in Drug Abuse.* Vol. 1, *Proceeding of the Community Epidemiology Work Group: Highlights and Executive Summary.* Bethesda, Md.: National Institutes of Health, June 2005, p. 7.

The researchers found other predictive factors for heavy cocaine use. Young men who were drug users were about twice as likely as young women drug users to become heavy users of cocaine. Students suspended from school were one to one and one-half times more likely to become heavy users of cocaine in adulthood. Adolescents and adults who obtained a significant portion of their income from illegal activities were twice as likely to become heavy cocaine users as those for whom none or little income was generated by illegal activities. Those who sold drugs in adolescence were twice as likely to become heavy cocaine abusers in adulthood.

Some factors mitigated *against* heavy cocaine use in adulthood. For example, adolescents and young adults who had attended religious services at least twice each month were one-third *less* likely to become heavy cocaine users than those who attended no religious services. Individuals who expected to be married within the next five years were significantly less likely to become heavy cocaine users. Those who expected to go to college or finish high school were also lower risks for becoming heavy cocaine abusers. In addition, those who reported feeling satisfied with themselves were at lower risk for heavy cocaine use.

Effects of Cocaine Use

Physical effects of cocaine may include

- dilated pupils
- rapid heartbeat
- hyperthermia (high body temperature)
- reduced fatigue
- euphoria
- increased energy

Chronic use of cocaine can lead to a variety of health effects; for example, if the drug is snorted on a regular basis, the individual may suffer from nosebleeds and a chronically runny nose, as well as the loss of the sense of smell. An oral intake of cocaine on a regular basis can lead to severe bowel gangrene caused by reduced blood flow. Frequent injections of cocaine can sometimes cause severe allergic reactions. If shared needles are used, the individual is at risk for contracting the HUMAN IMMUNODEFICIENCY VIRUS (HIV), HEPATITIS, and other bloodborne infections.

Possible serious health effects of the use of cocaine may include

- strokes
- heart attack
- acute kidney failure
- respiratory failure
- seizures
- tardive dyskinesia

Psychological effects of the long-term abuse of cocaine may include the following symptoms:

- paranoia
- auditory hallucinations

- restlessness
- delusions
- irritability and mood disturbances
- addiction
- suicidal or homicidal behavior
- panic attacks

In large amounts, cocaine can induce a psychotic state that is similar to and sometimes indistinguishable from SCHIZOPHRENIA. Some users become aggressive and violent and may harm others.

According to Nnadi and his colleagues in 2005 in the *Journal of the National Medical Association,* if patients overdose on cocaine, special care should be taken:

> Acute agitation in cocaine overdose can manifest as garrulousness, excitement, restlessness, and confusion. Patients with suspected overdose of cocaine should be transported urgently to the nearest emergency department using advanced life-support ambulance, when possible. The patients' family, ambulance service personnel, law enforcement officers and physicians need to be aware that attempts to control cocaine agitation with physical restraints and neck hold can result in lethal complications.

They also note that suicide is a high-risk complication in cases of patients who abuse cocaine: "Cocaine exacerbates suicidal and omnipotent fantasies, making the prevention of self-harm an important treatment focus. Suicidal intent is a common psychiatric complaint related to cocaine presentation in the emergency room."

According to Dr. Karch, most deaths (60 percent) of cocaine abuse among long-term users are a direct result of chronic toxicity, while homicides represent about 20 percent of the deaths of cocaine abusers, and suicide represents less than 10 percent of deaths. The other cocaine-related deaths are caused by stroke, excited delirium, myocardial infarction (heart attack), and sudden cardiac death.

Karch describes *excited delirium* in this manner: "This syndrome is comprised of four elements that occur in sequence—hyperthermia, psychotic agitation, respiratory arrest, and death." He adds that "hyperthermia is the result of dopamine receptor changes in the brainstem, while the psychotic behaviour results from up-regulation of kappa-2 receptors in the amygdala."

Deaths from strokes and excited delirium are relatively rare among cocaine abusers, but deaths that result from cardiac causes are common and may constitute the majority of all cocaine-related deaths.

Cocaine and Alcohol Abuse

Many individuals who abuse or are dependent on cocaine are also heavy users of alcohol, particularly those who are users of powdered cocaine. In one study in the United Kingdom that compared the users of powdered cocaine to those who abused crack cocaine, reported in *Alcohol and Alcoholism* in 2006, the researchers found that although heavy drinking was common among both groups, there were more frequent occurrences of heavy drinking among the powdered cocaine users. In contrast, the users of crack cocaine were more likely to have problems with other illicit drugs and to have both psychological and physical health problems, as well as criminal issues.

Said the researchers, "The differences in alcohol consumption patterns confirm the importance of differentiating between use of cocaine powder and crack cocaine."

The use of alcohol and cocaine at the same time presents a health risk because the two drugs together cause the formation of the substance *cocaethylene* in the body. This substance increases the euphoric qualities of cocaine, while it also escalates the risk for sudden death.

Cocaine and Crime

Because of its addicting effects, cocaine is often associated with crimes, including drug dealing, burglary, and PROSTITUTION. In a report on those inmates who tested positive for powdered cocaine in 2003, researchers found that 30 percent of all the male arrestees and more than one-third of females (35.3 percent) tested positive. The inmates were also asked about their use of cocaine in the past week, month, and year, as well as the average number of days they had used cocaine in the past 30 days. Males were somewhat heavier abusers of cocaine than females; for example, 9.6 percent of the males reported using cocaine in the past 30 days, compared to 7.2 percent of the females.

Treatment for Cocaine Abuse and Dependence

Significantly more people who are addicted to cocaine are receiving treatment than in past years. According to the Substance Abuse and Mental Health Services Administration, the number of admissions into substance abuse treatment centers for powder cocaine increased from 62,405 admissions in 2001 to 68,705 in 2003.

Individuals dependent on cocaine may be treated with medication and therapy. Research released in 2005 by the National Institute on Drug Abuse indicated that modafinil (Provigil), a narcolepsy drug, has been found to be effective in treating patients addicted to cocaine. This study was discussed in *NIDA Notes* in 2005.

In a study of 62 individuals (44 men, 18 women) who sought treatment for cocaine addiction, the patients were given either modafinil (30 patients) or an identical-appearing placebo (32 patients). The researchers found that the subjects in the modafinil group were more able (33 percent) to be abstinent from cocaine for three or more weeks than were the subjects in the placebo group (13 percent). This is significant because cocaine is a binge type of drug, and consequently many patients relapse shortly after treatment.

Charles Dackis concludes of this study, "The long continuous abstinence we saw with modafinil is a strong and encouraging signal that this medication can help patients avoid relapse during the critical first weeks of treatment."

Dackis also states that patients taking modafinil reported that if they *did* use cocaine, they did not experience an irresistible urge to use more of the drug, a problem they said that they had always experienced in the past. This may be because modafinil increases the level of glutamate, a chemical that is depleted by an addiction to cocaine. Says Dackis, "Some of the patients told me they had flushed cocaine away. In 25 years of treating addiction, no one ever told me they threw away cocaine."

Some studies have also found that DISULFIRAM (ANTABUSE), an aversive drug that is sometimes used to treat ALCOHOLISM, has also been shown to be effective in treating cocaine dependence.

Prevention of Cocaine Abuse and Dependence

The best prevention against cocaine abuse and the development of cocaine addiction is to avoid using the drug at all, unless it is needed for a medical procedure and is administered by a medical doctor. In such a case, the drug is carefully administered and there is no risk for addiction. In addition, it is best to avoid individuals who are users of cocaine.

See also ADDICTION/DEPENDENCE; CRIMES AND CRIMINALS; IMPAIRED DRIVING, INVOLVEMENT OF ALCOHOL AND/OR DRUGS; JAIL INMATES; NARCOTICS; PROSTITUTION; SCHEDULED DRUGS; YOUNG ADULTS.

Gossop, Michael, Victoria Manning, and Gayle Ridge. "Concurrent Use of Alcohol and Cocaine: Differences in Patterns of Use and Problems among Users of Crack Cocaine and Cocaine Powder." *Alcohol and Alcoholism* 41, no. 2 (2006): 121–125.

Johnston, Lloyd D., et al. *Monitoring the Future: National Survey Results on Drug Use, 1975–2004.* Vol. 2, *College Students and Adults Ages 19–45.* Bethesda, Md.: National Institute on Drug Abuse. National Institutes of Health, 2005.

Karch, Steven B., M.D. "Cocaine: History, Use, Abuse." *Journal of the Royal Society of Medicine* 92 (August 1999): 393–397.

Library of Congress. "Today in History: May 8: Coca Cola." Available online. URL: http://memory.loc.gov/ammem/today/may08.html. Downloaded July 3, 2006.

National Institute of Justice. *Drug and Alcohol Use and Related Matters among Arrestees, 2003.* 2004. Available online. URL: http:www.ncjrs.gove/nij/adam/ADM2003.pdf. Downloaded May 19, 2006.

National Institute on Drug Abuse. *Epidemiologic Trends in Drug Abuse.* Vol. 1, *Proceeding of the Community Epidemiology Work Group: Highlights and Executive Summary.* Bethesda, Md.: National Institutes of Health, June 2005.

Nnadi, Charles U., et al. "Neuropsychiatric Effects of Cocaine Use Disorders." *Journal of the National Medical Association* 97, no. 11 (November 2005): 1,504–1,515.

Office of Applied Studies, Substance Abuse and Mental Health Services Administration. *Treatment Episode Data Set (TEDS) Highlights—2003: National Admissions to Substance Abuse Treatment Services.* Rockville, Md.: Department of Health and Human Services, June 2005.

Office of National Drug Control Policy, *Predicting Heavy Drug Use.* Publication no. NCJ 208382. Washington, D.C.: Executive Office of the President, 2004.

Shanti, Christina M., M.D., and Charles E. Lucas, M.D. "Cocaine and the Critical Care Challenge." *Critical Care Medicine* 31, no. 6 (2003): 1,851–1,859.

Spillane, Joseph F. *Cocaine: From Medical Marvel to Modern Menace in the United States, 1884–1920.* Baltimore, Md.: Johns Hopkins University Press, 2000.

Substance Abuse and Mental Health Services Administration. *Overview of Findings from the 2004 National Survey on Drug Use and Health.* Washington, D.C.: Department of Health and Human Services, September 2005.

Zickler, Patricia. "Modafinil Improves Behavioral Therapy Results in Cocaine Addiction." *NIDA Notes* 20, no. 5 (2005): 1, 11.

codeine   A mild NARCOTIC that is derived from opium and is found in some cough syrups and cold remedies and included in some analgesics, such as Tylenol 3 and other drugs. When taken alone, which rarely occurs in the United States, codeine is a Schedule II drug under the CONTROLLED SUBSTANCES ACT. When it is combined with aspirin or acetaminophen (as with a medication that includes Tylenol with codeine) the drug is a Schedule IIII drug. When it is included in a cough medication, the drug is categorized as a Schedule V drug. (See SCHEDULED DRUGS.)

In addition, codeine is a starter material for the production of HYDROCODONE. Codeine is sedating, and it can be addicting with regular use.

Codeine is usually found in tablet form but it may also be injected to treat pain.

According to a study reported in a 1999 issue of the *Journal of Clinical Psychopharmacology,* of 339 users of codeine-containing products, codeine dependence (addiction) was found in close to half (41 percent) of these respondents. In addition, the researchers noted that two-thirds of the respondents had received help for their serious mental-health problems, particularly depression. The researchers speculated that depressive mood states could be a factor in maintaining codeine dependence.

It should also be noted that excessive codeine ingestion can be very dangerous and even may be fatal. In a report in 1998 in *Travel Medicine,* medical researchers described the case of a 42-year-old man who had traveled to Nepal and was found unconscious by his female friend upon her return to the hotel. The man was hospitalized and nonresponsive to deep pain, and the physicians felt that they needed to act like the fictional detective Sherlock Holmes in order to determine what was wrong with this patient.

His female friend showed the doctors the man's diary, which said that he had "sneaked out to get some C," and they deduced that the man may have taken some illicit codeine on his vacation, possibly because of a problem with impotence, which had depressed him. The man was administered naloxone to counteract the effects of the codeine, and shortly thereafter, woke up, admitting that he had taken many codeine pills as well as diazepam (Valium). A phone call to his brother revealed that the man had a history of codeine abuse in the past. The man recovered completely within five days, and he was advised to see his psychiatrist upon his return home. This man was fortunate that his drug abuse was uncovered. He could have suffered long-term ill effects or even death from his codeine abuse.

See also COUGH SYRUP; PRESCRIPTION DRUG ABUSE.

Basnyat, Buddha and Yogesh Shreshtha, "Travel Medicine and Sherlock Holmes." *Journal of Travel Medicine* 5 (1998): 42–43.

Joseph, Donald E., et al., eds. *Drugs of Abuse.* Washington, D.C.: U.S. Department of Justice, 2005.

Romach, Myroslava K., M.D., et al. "Long-Term Codeine Use Is Associated with Depressive Symptoms." *Journal of Clinical Psychopharmacology* 19, no. 4 (August 1999): 373–376.

codependency   An unhealthy relationship in which a person closely related to and/or involved with a person who abuses or is addicted to drugs or alcohol, such as a parent, spouse, lover, or friend, behaves in a way that makes it much easier for the addict to continue the abusive or addictive behavior.

Rather than the addict's suffering for his or her own actions, the codependent person assumes responsibility for many of the acts of the addicted person. For example, an addicted person may be sick or unconscious from the effects of drugs or alcohol and the codependent person may attempt to hide the behavior from others. The codependent person may call in sick to work for the addicted individual or may invent illnesses to account for withdrawal or hangover symptoms, such as saying that the person has the flu or a cold. It is said that the codependent person "enables" the addiction to continue by his or her actions and may be described as an "enabler."

People who are codependent usually are convinced that their behavior is good and helpful, and they do not realize how harmful it is to them, the addict, or others, such as other family members. They may feel that they are proving their love by giving up their time, money, and even personal integrity for the addicted person. They may find it difficult or impossible to believe that their behavior is not helpful to them or the addict. They may fear a loss of the relationship if they change their behavior. They may also reasonably fear that the substance users will lose a job, or even that the substance user will become ill or die if the codependent partner stops caretaking.

Often, there are boundary issues, and the codependent person struggles to differentiate what is best for her or him from what is best for the addicted individual. If there is a conflict, the codependent person usually defaults to what he or she believes is best for the addict, subordinating personal needs.

Codependent individuals may have several primary conscious or unconscious fears; for example, they may fear that if the addict recovered, the codependent person would then have to deal with new demands with which he or she may be uncomfortable, such as demands for sex, companionship, or greater control of the children or of the household. In some situations, the codependent partner also has an addictive problem, such as to food or gambling; there may be an unspoken contract between the partners to enable each other's addiction.

Organizations like Al-Anon and related organizations teach people who are codependent to give up their codependency and to let the addicted person face the responsibility for his or her actions. Such organizations can offer ongoing support and advice to help codependent people to avoid assuming that role in the future.

See also DENIAL.

Gwinnell, Esther, M.D., and Christine Adamec. *The Encyclopedia of Addictions and Addictive Behaviors.* New York: Facts On File, 2006.

college students Students in postsecondary schools. College students are more likely to have problems with alcohol abuse or with ALCOHOLISM rather than with drug abuse or dependence; however, drug abuse is also a problem for many students. Some students are illicit abusers of prescription drugs, while others use illegal drugs: MARIJUANA, COCAINE, METHAMPHETAMINE, and other drugs. PEER PRESSURE and/or loneliness or other factors may lead college students to substance abuse, although some students had previously abused alcohol and/or drugs in high school.

Drug Abuse

In general, college students have a *lower* risk of using illicit substances than their peers who do not attend college; for example, as seen in Table I, college students were much *less* likely to abuse COCAINE than their same-age peers, and only 9.5 percent of college students have ever abused cocaine, compared to 16.5 percent of their same-age peers. Among college students, the next most frequently abused drug after alcohol was marijuana, which was abused by 49.1 percent of college students and 57.8 percent of their same-age peers not in college.

However, research from the annual Monitoring the Future study, released in 2005, reveals that college students have *higher* rates of abuse than their age peers for some specific drugs, such as FLUNITRAZEPAM, GAMMA-HYDROXYBUTYRIC ACID (GHB), and KETAMINE. These drugs are all considered DATE RAPE DRUGS, or drugs that are administered to others without their knowledge or permission for nefarious purposes; however, these drugs are sometimes used voluntarily and knowingly by students.

In addition, college students are more likely to abuse methylphenidate (Ritalin) than their non-college peers; about 5 percent of college students abuse methylphenidate compared to less than 2 percent of their peers not attending college.

TABLE I: LIFETIME PREVALENCE OF USE FOR VARIOUS TYPES OF DRUGS, 2004: FULL-TIME COLLEGE STUDENTS VERSUS OTHERS, AMONG RESPONDENTS ONE TO FOUR YEARS BEYOND HIGH SCHOOL, BY PERCENTAGE

	Total		Males		Females	
	Full-Time College	Others	Full-Time College	Others	Full-Time College	Others
Any Illicit Drug[1]	52.2	60.0	54.9	59.4	50.6	60.6
Any Illicit Drug Other Than Marijuana	28.0	35.5	31.1	35.6	26.2	35.3
Marijuana	49.1	57.8	53.7	58.4	46.5	57.3
Inhalants	8.5	11.4	12.3	13.1	6.1	10.1
Hallucinogens	12.0	17.9	16.1	20.5	9.6	15.8
LSD	5.6	11.4	6.9	12.3	4.9	10.7
Cocaine	9.5	16.5	12.5	17.5	7.8	15.6
Crack cocaine	2.0	5.5	2.4	5.8	1.7	5.2
MDMA (Ecstasy)	10.2	15.4	9.2	16.1	10.9	14.9
Heroin	0.9	1.7	1.2	1.6	0.7	1.8
Other Narcotics	13.8	20.2	18.2	20.8	11.2	19.6
Amphetamines	12.7	18.0	13.8	16.7	12.1	19.0
Ice (crystal methamphetamine)	2.2	8.3	3.5	9.8	1.5	7.1
Sedatives (Barbiturates)	7.2	12.2	8.4	12.4	6.5	12.0
Tranquilizers	10.6	16.6	13.5	17.4	8.8	16.1
Alcohol	84.6	85.8	83.2	85.3	85.3	86.2
Flavored alcoholic beverages	79.0	76.3	73.9	74.3	82.3	77.6

[1] Use of "any illicit drug" includes any use of marijuana, hallucinogens, cocaine, or heroin, or any use of other narcotics, amphetamines, sedatives (barbiturates), or tranquilizers not under a doctor's orders.
Source: Johnston, Lloyd D., et al. Monitoring the Future: National Survey Results on Drug Use, 1975–2004. Vol. 2, College Students and Adults Ages 19–45. Bethesda, Md.: National Institute on Drug Abuse, National Institutes of Health, 2005, p. 230.

Gender Differences

In most cases, males, whether in college or not, were more likely to abuse drugs than females. However, females were slightly more likely to abuse alcohol than males, whether the women were in college or not. (See Table II.)

In general, male college students consume larger amounts of both alcohol and illicit drugs than female students; for example, in 2004, 6.8 percent of male college students abused MARIJUANA on a daily basis, compared to 3.1 percent of females, according to the Monitoring the Future study. In addition, nearly half (49 percent) of college males reported having five or more drinks in a row over the previous two weeks, versus 38 percent of college females who reported this type of BINGE DRINKING behavior. (See GENDER DIFFERENCES.)

There were also some other gender differences in consumption of marijuana; for example, male college students were more likely to use marijuana than were their noncollege male peers, while female college students were less likely to abuse marijuana than their female peers.

In considering the 30-day prevalence of the abuse of illicit drugs, prescribed drugs, and alcohol in 2004, as shown in Table II, male college students were slightly more likely to abuse illicit drugs (26.1 percent) than their noncollege male peers of the same age (25.3 percent). In contrast, female college students were less likely to abuse illicit substances than noncollege females.

Male college students were also more likely than their same-age male peers to abuse marijuana over 30 days, although again, this finding was not true for female college students, who had a lower abuse rate than their noncollege female peers. Surprisingly, when considering the 30-day prevalence, male college students were more likely than the noncollege male peers to abuse both cocaine and crack cocaine. (See Table II.)

TABLE II: THIRTY-DAY PREVALENCE OF USE FOR VARIOUS TYPES OF DRUGS, 2004: FULL-TIME COLLEGE STUDENTS VERSUS OTHERS AMONG RESPONDENTS ONE TO FOUR YEARS BEYOND HIGH SCHOOL (IN PERCENTAGES)

	Total		Males		Females	
	Full-Time College	Others	Full-Time College	Others	Full-Time College	Others
Any illicit drug	21.2	23.2	26.1	25.3	18.4	21.5
Any illicit drug other than marijuana	9.1	11.6	11.3	13.8	7.8	9.7
Marijuana	18.9	20.3	24.6	22.1	15.6	18.9
Inhalants	0.4	0.7	0.5	0.4	0.4	0.9
Hallucinogens	1.3	1.8	1.9	2.7	1.0	1.2
LSD	0.2	0.4	0.2	0.6	0.2	0.1
Cocaine	2.4	2.4	3.6	3.1	1.8	1.9
Crack cocaine	0.4	0.3	0.5	0.2	0.4	0.3
MCMA (Ecstasy)	0.7	1.2	1.0	1.5	0.5	1.0
Heroin	0.1	0.1	0.3	0.0	0.1	0.2
Other Narcotics	3.0	4.3	3.8	5.0	2.5	3.7
Amphetamines	3.2	3.4	3.6	3.6	3.1	3.2
Ice (crystal methamphetamine)	0.1	1.4	0.3	2.1	0.0	0.8
Sedatives (Barbiturates)	1.5	3.2	1.5	3.7	1.5	2.8
Alcohol	67.7	59.3	66.7	62.8	68.2	56.3
Flavored alcoholic beverages	34.0	30.0	27.4	22.3	21.1	34.4

Source: Johnston, Lloyd D., et al. *Monitoring the Future: National Survey Results on Drug Use, 1975–2004.* Vol. 2, *College Students and Adults Ages 19–45.* Bethesda, Md.: National Institute on Drug Abuse, National Institutes of Health, 2005, 232.

Prescription Drug Abuse

Some college students abuse prescription drugs. (See PRESCRIPTION DRUG ABUSE.) Studies have shown that college students were also less likely to use other drugs than their age peers, such as METHYLENEDIOXYMETHAMPHETAMINE (MDMA/ECSTASY), as well as prescription drugs such as Vicodin, a form of hydrocodone. In addition, college students were much less likely to use crystal METHAMPHETAMINE ("ice"); or 2.2 percent of the college students abused this drug compared to 8.3 percent of their noncollege same-age peers.

In one random sample of more than 9,000 undergraduate students, reported in *Drug and Alcohol Dependence* in 2005, the researchers found that the illicit use of prescription painkiller drugs in the past year was a greater problem among undergraduate students with a prior prescription for pain medication. For example, only 4.4 percent of women who had had no painkillers prescribed used pain medications illicitly in the past year, compared to 9.4 percent who had been previously prescribed painkillers in college.

With regard to prescription drug abuse, the abuse rates were higher for men; 6.3 percent of the male college students who had not previously used prescription painkillers had abused these drugs in the past year, compared to 15.4 percent of the male college students who had been prescribed a painkiller in college.

The researchers also found that college students who had been prescribed a prescription painkiller while in elementary school were more likely than others to abuse painkillers in college; for example, about 14 percent of the men and 16 percent of the women who reported past year illicit use of pain medications had been prescribed painkillers in elementary school. The researchers state:

Of greatest significance is our finding regarding early exposure to pain medication. Interestingly, those exposed earlier to prescription pain medications reported higher rates of illicit use of prescription pain medications and this positive relationship was apparent across every age of exposure and was particularly evident among women. In other words, the earlier the initiation of prescribed pain medication, the higher the reported use of illicit pain medication both lifetime and in the past year and this indicated that this was not merely a cumulative effect of illicit use. Furthermore, this positive relationship remained across every age of exposure after controlling for other important variables such as race, class year, among others.

For both male and female college students, prescription painkiller drug abuse in the past year was more common among those who lived outside the city in which the university was located or lived in a house or an apartment, compared to those students who lived in a residence hall (dormitory).

College students who had lower grade point averages (GPAs), such as below a 2.5 GPA, were more likely to have used painkillers illicitly in the past year.

The researchers also found that most of the students had obtained the prescription pain medication illicitly from their peers, and the next most common source were family members (and most often their mothers). In some cases, the family members were medical professionals, such as nurses, who gave the drug to their child to alleviate pain rather than to induce intoxication.

Often when they had obtained the drug from a friend, abusers combined the prescription painkiller with alcohol. Those users who obtained the drugs from their peers had significantly higher rates of other forms of substance abuse than those who obtained the drugs from their family members.

In a more recently reported study on college students and prescription drug abuse, reported in 2005 in *Addiction,* the researchers sampled nearly 11,000 college students in 2001 on their abuse of prescribed stimulants, such as Adderall, Dexedrine, and Ritalin. They found higher rates of prescription drug abuse among students in northeastern colleges with competitive admission standards. Members of fraternities and sororities were more likely to abuse stimulants than other students. Abusers were more likely to report that they also abused alcohol, cocaine, marijuana, and Ecstasy in addition to the prescription drugs.

Alcohol Abuse

The Monitoring the Future study revealed that college students were about as likely to abuse alcohol as their same-age peers, with a lifetime prevalence of 84.6 percent of the college students compared to 85.8 percent of their peers, which is a minor difference. The college students were also slightly more likely to choose flavored alcoholic beverages than their noncollegiate peers; 79 percent versus 76.3 percent. (Most of this difference was accounted for by female college students, among whom 82.3 percent had used flavored alcoholic beverages compared to 77.6 percent of the noncollege women; see Table I.)

When considering the 30-day prevalence of various drugs (as shown in Table II), it is clear that the college students had a higher rate of abuse: 67.7 percent had used alcohol in the past 30 days compared to 59.3 percent of their noncollege peers. The difference was particularly striking among females: 68.2 percent of the female college students had used alcohol in the past 30 days, compared to 56.3 percent of the noncollege females.

In considering binge drinking (Table III), college students were more likely to binge drink than their noncollege peers, particularly the female students.

In general, research has shown that students at four-year colleges are more likely to abuse alcohol than are students at two-year colleges. Alcohol abuse is also strongly associated with membership in Greek organizations. In one study, 86 percent of the fraternity members reported that they were heavy drinkers versus 45 percent of the students who were not fraternity members. Surprisingly, the situation was even *more* pronounced for female members of sororities: 80 percent of sorority residents reported heavy alcohol abuse compared to only 17 percent among nonsorority members.

Life satisfaction and drinking　The researchers James G. Murphy and Meghan E. McDevitt-Murphy studied the impact of alcohol use and abuse on 353 college students and various life satisfaction variables, such as general satisfaction, social satisfaction, and school satisfaction. The majority of the subjects in the sample were females (78.2 percent). The results were reported in *Psychology of Addictive Behaviors* in 2005.

TABLE III: THIRTY-DAY PREVALENCE OF DAILY USE OF ALCOHOL AND BINGE DRINKING, 2004: FULL-TIME COLLEGE STUDENTS VERSUS OTHERS AMONG RESPONDENTS ONE TO FOUR YEARS BEYOND HIGH SCHOOL (IN PERCENTAGES)

	Total		Males		Females	
	Full-Time College	Others	Full-Time College	Others	Full-Time College	Others
Daily Alcohol Consumption	3.7	5.8	7.2	9.0	1.8	3.1
Drinking 5+ Drinks in a Row in Past 2 Weeks (Binge drinking)	41.7	33.7	48.9	41.7	37.7	27.0

Source: Johnston, Lloyd D., et al. *Monitoring the Future: National Survey Results on Drug Use, 1975–2004.* Vol. 2, *College Students & Adults Ages 19–45.* Bethesda, Md.: National Institute on Drug Abuse, National Institutes of Health, 2005, p. 233.

The researchers found that female abstainers had higher levels of life satisfaction than moderate or heavy drinkers. Abstainers also had higher anticipated future satisfaction than heavy drinkers. (There were an insufficient number of male subjects to draw statistically valid conclusions about the differences between abstainers and moderate and heavy drinkers.) They also found that the male college students had significantly more alcohol-related problems than the female students; for example, the men drank nearly twice as much as the women and had a higher frequency of heavy drinking.

Most of the sample (91 percent) were white but there were sufficient numbers of African Americans to make some comparisons, and the researchers found that the white students were heavier weekly drinkers than the African-American students. They also found that the white students reported higher levels of school and social satisfaction than the African-American students.

Say the authors, "The present findings suggest that college student alcohol consumption (among women) and alcohol-related problems (among both men and women) are associated with diminished LS [life satisfaction] which is yet another reason why prevention and treatment of young adult alcohol abuse should be a priority."

Psychiatric problems and drinking College students who have DEPRESSION and/or poor mental health have a greater risk of some problems that are related to alcohol consumption, according to a variety of studies. One study by Elissa R. Weitzman reported in the *Journal of Nervous and Mental Disease* in 2004 was a survey of more than 27,000 students at 119 colleges in the United States. She found that

about 5 percent of the students had poor mental health/depression (PMHD). These students were more likely to be female, nonwhite, and members of families in which their parents had not attended college.

Of the PMHD students, Weitzman found that about 82 percent consumed alcohol: "Compared with their peers, students with PMHD were less likely to report lifetime abstinence; more likely to report drinking but not heavy episodic drinking [binge drinking]; and more likely to report drinking to get drunk."

Perhaps not surprisingly, Weitzman also found that drinking itself was causing problems in the lives of the students who had poor mental health/depression. She states, "Drinkers with PMHD were more likely than drinkers without PMHD to report drinking-related problems, including academic troubles, unplanned and unsafe sex, alcohol overdosing, and experiencing five or more problems from alcohol."

Other studies of general populations have shown a significant relationship between depression and ALCOHOLISM or BINGE DRINKING, such as a study of more than 43,000 subjects published by the National Institute of Alcohol Abuse and Alcoholism. Among nonbingers, the rate of depression was 6.6 percent. Among binge drinkers, the rate of depression was 9.8 percent.

Drinking as a way of life on the college campus In their report *High Risk Drinking in College; What We Know and What We Need to Learn*, the National Institute on Alcohol Abuse and the Alcoholism National Advisory Council on Alcohol Abuse and Alcoholism Task Force on College Drinking discuss the problem of the general acceptance of heavy drinking as a normal and accepted condition among many college students.

They state, "The Panel found that on many college campuses, heavy drinking is interwoven overtly or subtly throughout the culture of the institution. As a result, students perceive this drinking pattern as the social norm rather than as unhealthy and potentially destructive behavior."

According to the National Institute on Alcohol Abuse and Alcoholism in their report on the culture of campus drinking in their 2002 *Alcohol Alert* article, "Traditions and beliefs handed down through generations of college drinkers serve to reinforce students' expectations that alcohol is a necessary component of social success." Yet the report also notes that more than 600,000 students are assaulted each year by other students who have been drinking and alcohol consumption is linked to at least 1,400 student deaths and a half-million unintentional injuries each year.

Key factors that the Task Force on College Drinking found to be related to drinking problems were as follows:

- the students' value systems and personalities
- the family background and peers
- the students' expectations regarding alcohol's effects (good or bad)
- a genetic predisposition, often reflected in a family history of alcoholism
- the social integration of drinking into college life
- the context in which drinking occurs (on- or off-campus parties, on- or off-campus bars)
- the economic availability of alcohol (lower prices or two-for-one drinks are linked to higher levels of alcohol use)
- the level of law enforcement

Being Away from Home May Have an Effect on Substance Abuse

Some college students are away from their home for the first time, and as a result of loneliness, boredom, and other emotions, they may exhibit behavior that they think is daring and exciting, including abusing alcohol and drugs. They may also try to impress or fit in with their new peers by using alcohol and/or drugs. However, many individuals who abuse alcohol and drugs actually began their abuse during high school, and they continue to do so into their college years (and beyond).

See also ADOLESCENTS; ANXIETY DISORDERS; BINGE DRINKING; GENDER DIFFERENCES, ABUSE OF DRUGS AND ALCOHOL; GENETIC PREDISPOSITIONS AND ENVIRONMENTAL EFFECTS IN SUBSTANCE USE DISORDERS; PSYCHIATRIC PROBLEMS; YOUNG ADULTS.

Johnston, Lloyd D., et al. *Monitoring the Future: National Survey Results on Drug Use, 1975–2004*. Vol. 2, *College Students and Adults Ages 19–45*. Bethesda, Md.: National Institute on Drug Abuse, National Institutes of Health, 2005.

McCabe, Sean Esteban, Christian J. Teter, and Carol J. Boyd. "Illicit Use of Prescription Pain Medication among College Students." *Drug and Alcohol Dependence* 77 (2005): 37–47.

McCabe, Sean Esteban, et al. "Non-Medical Use of Prescription Stimulants among U.S. College Students: Prevalence and Correlates from a National Study." *Addiction* 100, no. 1 (January 2005): 96–106.

Murphy, James G., Meghan E. McDevitt-Murphy, and Nancy P. Barnett. "Drink and Be Merry? Gender, Life Satisfaction, and Alcohol Consumption among College Students." *Psychology of Addictive Behaviors* 19, no. 2 (2005): 184–191.

National Institute on Alcohol Abuse and Alcoholism. *Alcohol Use and Alcohol Use Disorders in the United States: Main Findings from the 2001–2002 National Epidemiologic Survey on Alcohol and Related Conditions (NESARC)*. U.S. Alcohol Epidemiologic Data Reference Manual 8, no. 1 (January 2006). Bethesda, Md.: National Institutes of Health, January 2006.

National Institute on Alcohol Abuse and Alcoholism. "Changing the Culture of Campus Drinking," *Alcohol Alert* 58 (October 2002).

National Institute on Alcohol Abuse and Alcoholism, National Advisory Council on Alcohol Abuse and Alcoholism Task Force on College Drinking. *High-Risk Drinking in College: What We Know and What We Need to Learn: Final Report of the Panel on Contexts and Consequences*. April 2002.

Weitzman, Elissa R. "Poor Mental Health, Depression, and Associations with Alcohol Consumption, Harm, and Abuse in a National Sample of Young Adults in

College." *Journal of Nervous and Mental Disease* 192, no. 4 (April 2004): 269–277.

Colombia A source country in South America for many illegal drugs that are trafficked into the United States and other countries, such as COCAINE, MARIJUANA, and HEROIN. Working with officials in the United States, Colombia, and other countries, law enforcement agencies such as the U.S. Drug Enforcement Administration actively seek to prevent the flow of illegal drugs into the United States.

According to the 2006 *National Drug Control Strategy* from the White House, expanded aerial eradication efforts have succeeded in causing major damage to opium poppy cultivation in Colombia, and a 68 percent reduction occurred from 2001 to 2004. In addition, increased airport security in the United States has led to increased seizures of heroin and other drugs from Colombia.

According to this report, Colombian President Uribe and the government in Colombia are committed to fighting drugs and are working together with the United States to eradicate and interdict illegal drugs. For example, in 2004 Colombia sprayed more than 131,000 hectares of coca (from which cocaine is produced) and manually destroyed another 10,279 hectares. In 2005, the government increased their efforts, spraying more than 138,000 hectares of coca and manually eradicating plants on more than 31,000 hectares.

Attacks on opium poppies have also been aggressive, and in 2005, Colombia sprayed more than 1,600 hectares of poppy and manually eradicated 496 hectares. These efforts have been effective in decreasing illegal heroin sales in the United States.

The Department of State in the United States received authorization for $30 million in fiscal year 2006 to buy and refurbish spray aircraft for Colombia. With training from U.S. law enforcement personnel, police efforts have become more successful; for example, more than 200 metric tons of cocaine and coca base were seized in Colombia in 2005.

The government of Colombia has also taken action against drug traffickers in their country and extradited 131 Colombia nationals to the United States for prosecution, up from 11 in 2000.

See also AFGHANISTAN; COCAINE; CRIME AND CRIMINALS; FOREIGN JAILS/RIGHTS; GANGS; INCARCERATION; LAW ENFORCEMENT; MEXICO; ORGANIZED CRIME.

conduct disorder A psychiatric diagnosis that is recognized by the American Psychiatric Association and is based on particular types of *behaviors* of some children and adolescents (and some adults), rather than on the way they feel, as with DEPRESSION or an ANXIETY DISORDER. Conduct disorder may appear early, before the age of 10 years, or it may appear in adolescence. Conduct disorder may also be diagnosed in some individuals older than 18 years if they are not diagnosed with ANTISOCIAL PERSONALITY DISORDER.

Boys are significantly more likely to be diagnosed with conduct disorder than girls. In addition, individuals who have conduct disorder are more likely to abuse alcohol and/or drugs than are those who do not have the disorder. Some studies indicate that if an individual has both ATTENTION DEFICIT HYPERACTIVITY DISORDER (ADHD) and conduct disorder, then the risk for the development of a substance use disorder is greatly increased.

In a retrospective study of the national prevalence of conduct disorder in the United States, based on data from over 3,000 respondents in the National Comorbidity Survey Replication study, researcher Matthew K. Nock and his colleagues determined a lifetime prevalence (of ever being diagnosed) of conduct disorder. They found a lifetime prevalence of 9.5 percent of the population with conduct disorder, or 12 percent of males and 7.1 percent of females. The researchers also found that conduct disorder was strongly associated with IMPULSE CONTROL DISORDERS (such as compulsive gambling or fire setting), which the researchers found usually appeared *before* the conduct disorder was diagnosed.

In addition, the researchers found that substance-induced disorders were common among individuals who had conduct disorder, although they were typically preceded by the conduct disorder. The researchers also found that a diagnosis of conduct disorder was most commonly associated with specific demographic factors, such as low educational achievement, non-Hispanic white race, marital failure, residing in an urban setting, and living in the western part of the United States.

Symptoms and Diagnostic Path

According to the American Psychiatric Association in the *Diagnostic and Statistical Manual—IV-TR (DSM-IV-TR)*, "The essential feature of Conduct Disorder is a repetitive and persistent pattern of behavior in which the basic rights of others or major age-appropriate societal norms or rules are violated."

There are four primary types of conduct disorder:

1. aggressive conduct that harms or threatens people or animals
2. nonaggressive conduct that causes the loss of or damage to property
3. theft or deceitfulness
4. serious violation of rules

The disruptive behavior has been present for the past six months and impairs the individual at home and at school or work. Such children may exhibit bullying and threatening of others. They may be physically cruel and the violence may escalate to rape and even homicide.

If the person who has conduct disorder primarily violates the property rights of others, he or she may set fires on purpose or damage property, such as by smashing mailboxes or car windows.

Acts of deceitfulness or theft by an individual who has conduct disorder may include chronic lying and failing to fulfill promises to others, as well as breaking into homes in a nonviolent manner to steal.

Children and adolescents who have conduct disorder may be frequently truant from school, while older individuals may have many unexplained absences from work (and eventually lose the job). Some individuals who have conduct disorder stay out all night or run away from home for an extended period.

Conduct disorder may be mild, moderate, or severe. In severe cases individuals use weapons, force others into sex, or use physical cruelty.

Treatment Options and Outlook

Some studies, such as one published in 2000 in the *Journal of the American Academy of Child & Adolescent Psychiatry,* have shown that resperidone (Resperdal), an antipsychotic medication, is effective in reducing the aggressive behavior of youths who have conduct disorder. Other studies have shown success at curtailing aggression with other antipsychotics, such as olanzapine (Zyprexa).

Many individuals who have conduct disorder have other psychiatric disorders, such as ADHD, depression, and/or anxiety disorders; when such problems are present, they should be treated as well.

Psychotherapy may be helpful for individuals who have conduct disorder, and anger management classes may help them to manage feelings of anger and rage more effectively.

Many children who have conduct disorder are known to juvenile justice authorities because of the crimes they commit. For serious crimes they may be incarcerated in a juvenile justice facility. Individuals older than age 18 who have conduct disorder may be incarcerated in jail or prison for their offenses.

Risk Factors and Prevention

Individuals who have a family history of conduct disorder have an increased risk for the disorder. Early diagnosis and treatment are the best methods to prevent the many problems that are associated with conduct disorder, although preventing conduct disorder itself may not be possible.

See also ANTISOCIAL PERSONALITY DISORDER; ANXIETY DISORDERS; ATTENTION DEFICIT HYPERACTIVITY DISORDER; BIPOLAR DISORDER; CRIME AND CRIMINALS; DEPRESSION; PSYCHIATRIC DISORDERS.

American Psychiatric Association. *Diagnostic and Statistical Manual of Mental Disorders.* 4th ed. DSM-IV-TR. Washington, D.C.: American Psychiatric Association, 2000.

Findling, Robert L., M.D., et al. "A Double-Blind Pilot Study of Resperidone in the Treatment of Conduct Disorder." *Journal of the American Academy of Child & Adolescent Psychiatry* 39, no. 4 (April 2000): 509–516.

Nock, Matthew K., et al. "Prevalence, Subtypes, and Correlates of DSM-IV Conduct Disorder in the National Comorbidity Survey Replication." *Psychological Medicine* 36 (2006): 688–710.

Controlled Substances Act (CSA) A law passed in 1970 in the United States that determines the drugs that are classified as SCHEDULED DRUGS, as well as their specific classification. The drugs that are regulated by the act are those drugs that are also regulated by federal law. The drugs are placed into one of five schedules based on the medical use of the substance, its abuse potential, and the risk for dependence (addiction). In addition, the CSA discusses the method by which drugs may be added to or removed from a schedule or transferred from one schedule to another. The Comprehensive Crime Control Act of 1984 amended the CSA, such that the drug enforcement administrator may place a substance that has no approved medical use under Schedule I (which includes only illegal drugs with addictive potential) on a temporary emergency basis for up to one year. This time frame may be extended a further six months.

Organizations that may add, delete, or change a schedule include the Drug Enforcement Administration (DEA) and the Department of Health and Human Services (HHS). In addition to these organizations, a petition to change a drug schedule can be made by a drug manufacturer, a medical association, a pharmacy association, a public group, and even an individual U.S. citizen. At one point, there was an effort by some individuals to move METHYLPHENIDATE (RITALIN/CONCERTA/FOCALIN, ETC.) to classification as a Schedule III drug; however, this attempt was disapproved.

The CSA regulates NARCOTICS, DEPRESSANTS, STIMULANTS, HALLUCINOGENIC DRUGS, and ANABOLIC STEROIDS. It also requires strict record keeping of all controlled substances, and each substance must also be inventoried every two years. These requirements were made to help to trace the flow of drugs from the point of manufacture or importation to distribution, then to the pharmacy and hospital and finally, to the patient who received the drug. Such requirements help to prevent DRUG DIVERSION. Records for Schedule I and II drugs must be kept separate and in a more secure place than for drugs that fall into Schedules III, IV, and V.

Schedule I drugs, which include MARIJUANA, HEROIN, LYSERGIC ACID DIETHYLAMIDE (LSD), and CRACK COCAINE, are considered highly addictive and may only be used lawfully in government-approved research. Schedule II, III, IV, and V drugs may be prescribed by or directly administered by a doctor. Some states require multiple-copy prescriptions of Schedule II drugs.

Under the CSA, refills may not be prescribed for Schedule II drugs. If the patient continues to need the drug, he or she must receive a new prescription every 30 days, which is also not refillable. The doctor may not call in the prescription over the phone to a pharmacist. In contrast, if the doctor prescribes drugs from Schedules III through V, he or she may give the patient a written prescription or call in the drug to the pharmacy. Refills of drugs in those categories may be authorized.

With Schedule V drugs, which are primarily cough medicines with codeine and some antidiarrhea drugs, the law requires that the patient be at least 18 years old and show the pharmacist personal identification, and his or her name must be entered into the pharmacist's special log.

States have the option to schedule a drug at a *higher* scheduled level than that which has been conferred by the federal government, but they may not schedule drugs at a *lower* level. Thus, states may be more punitive than the federal government but may not be less punitive.

This is one of the reasons why when states have passed laws legalizing marijuana (primarily for medical purposes for patients who have severe illnesses), the federal government has expressed its adamant opposition to these laws, since marijuana is classified as a Schedule I drug under the Controlled Substances Act. They argue that only Congress can make laws that assign a lower rating to a drug, and that this is not an act that is within the powers of any individual state. Those who wish to decriminalize the use of marijuana, for medical or recreational use, do not regard marijuana as a dangerous and addictive drug. This controversy is likely to continue, as of this writing.

Since 1970 when the Controlled Substances Act was enacted, many drugs have been added to the scheduled drugs list, such as METHYLENEDIOXY METHAMPHETAMINE (MDMA/ECSTASY) and ANABOLIC STEROIDS.

See also AMPHETAMINES; COCAINE; CRACK COCAINE; DEPRESSANTS; DIAZEPAM (VALIUM); FLUNITRAZ-

EPAM (ROHYPNOL); HALLUCINOGENIC DRUGS; HASH-ISH/HASHISH OIL; HEROIN; HYDROCODONE; INHALANTS; MARIJUANA; MEPERIDINE (DEMEROL); MESCALINE; METHAMPHETAMINE; METHYLPHENIDATE (RITALIN/CON-CERTA/FOCALIN, ETC.); NARCOTICS; OXYCODONE; OXY-CONTIN; PHENCYCLIDINE (PCP); PRESCRIPTION DRUG ABUSE; PROPOXYPHENE; PSILOCYBIN; SCHEDULED DRUGS; STIMULANTS.

Joseph, Donald E. *Drugs of Abuse.* Washington, D.C.: U.S. Department of Justice, 2005.

cough syrup   Medication that is used as a cold and cough remedy. However, some individuals abuse cough syrup, especially cough syrup that contains the substance CODEINE or DEXTROMETHORPHAN. Some pharmacies maintain special control over such drugs, refusing to sell them to minors. Excessive amounts of dextromethorphan may induce HALLU-CINATIONS as well as dissociative effects (a feeling of not being really present). These symptoms are also similar to the symptoms that may be experienced by individuals who abuse KETAMINE.

Dextromethorphan is often an adulterant found in drugs such as METHYLENEDIOXYMETHAMPHETAMINE (MDMA/ECSTACY).

Excessive dosages of cough syrup with codeine can, in rare cases, be lethal. Robert Earl Davis, Jr., also known as DJ Screw, was a popular Houston, Texas, disk jockey and a producer of slowed down mixes of hit rap and hip hop music and songs. He died in 2000 at the age of 29 from an overdose of Promethazine, a cough syrup with codeine.

See CONTROLLED SUBSTANCES ACT; DEXTROMETHO-RPHAN; SCHEDULED DRUGS.

crack cocaine   A highly concentrated and extremely addictive form of COCAINE that is smoked and can be injected. It is available in a rock crystal form that is heated to very high temperatures or *freebased.* The drug is called *crack* cocaine because of the crackling sound that it makes when it is heated. There is no legal medical use in the United States for this form of cocaine, and consequently, crack cocaine is an illegal Schedule I drug under the CONTROLLED SUB-STANCES ACT.

Crack cocaine addicts frequently use other drugs in conjunction with crack, such as MARIJUANA, HER-OIN, and METHAMPHETAMINE. Many crack cocaine users also abuse alcohol as well.

Users of Crack Cocaine

According to the National Survey on Drug Use and Health, there were 467,000 current users of crack cocaine in 2004. Usage of crack is lower among high school students (see Table I); how-ever, about 25 percent of adolescents have stated that it would be easy for them to obtain the drug if they wanted it.

According to information from the Monitor-ing the Future data in 2005, a minority of COLLEGE STUDENTS (2 percent) have abused crack in their lifetime, less than half the rate for their same-age noncollege peers, which is 5.5 percent.

In considering the annual prevalence (use in the past year) and the 30-day prevalence (use in the past month) the rates are much lower for all age groups than the lifetime prevalence. (See Table I.) As can be seen from the table, the highest 30-day prevalence abuse rates were among young adults ages 19–28 years, or 2.1 percent.

Crack and Crime

Crack cocaine is used much more frequently by individuals who are convicted of crimes than by noncriminals. Crack cocaine addicts often turn to crimes, such as stealing, drug dealing, and PROSTI-TUTION, in order to obtain the money that they need to purchase the drug. Many addicts are subject to arrest and INCARCERATION. They are also often neglectful of their children and may also abuse them, acts that can lead to the removal of their chil-dren from their custody and their placement in the FOSTER CARE system. (See CHILD ABUSE.)

Information from the National Institute of Jus-tice indicates that among individuals arrested for crimes in major cities throughout the United States, nearly a third of the males (30 percent) and more than a third of the females (35 percent) tested posi-tive for crack cocaine abuse. Significant percentages of inmates in jail have reported using crack cocaine within the past week, month, and year.

As can be seen from Table II, the abuse rate of females was *higher* than that of arrested males,

TABLE I: LIFETIME PREVALENCE AND CURRENT USE OF CRACK COCAINE, 2004, PERCENTAGES

	Lifetime Prevalence	Annual Prevalence	30-Day Prevalence
8th Graders	2.4	1.3	0.6
10th Graders	2.6	1.7	0.8
High School Seniors	3.9	2.3	1.0
Young Adults Ages 19–28	4.2	6.4	2.1
College Students	2.0	1.3	0.4
Same-Age Noncollege Students	5.5	2.3	0.3

Source: Adapted from Johnston, Lloyd D., et al. *Monitoring the Future: National Survey Results on Drug Use, 1975–2004.* Vol. 2, *College Students and Adults Ages 19–45.* Bethesda, Md.: National Institute on Drug Abuse, National Institutes of Health, 2005, pp. 36, 43, 44, 49, 230, 231, 232.

although in the general population, the rate of drug abuse of crack cocaine is usually higher among males; for example, 12.9 percent of the male arrestees reported using crack cocaine in the past seven days compared to 20 percent of the female arrestees. (See Table II.) The abuse rate among female arrestees may be due in part to their higher level of crime and violence than is common among adult females in the general population.

Treatment for Crack Cocaine Addiction

It is very difficult for individuals addicted to crack cocaine to recover. Many of those who are treated for their drug dependence eventually experience RELAPSES. According to the National Institute on Drug Abuse in a 2005 issue of *NIDA Notes,* a small pilot study has revealed that some patients who were treated for dependence on crack cocaine had success with topiramate (Topamax), a drug that is usually used to treat individuals for seizure dis-

orders. The drug enabled the patients to stay off cocaine for three to four weeks, which is the time frame during which many patients relapse.

The patients who were tested were mostly African-American males who were addicted to crack cocaine. They were long-term abusers, having abused cocaine for an average of 10 years. Further research is needed to determine whether topiramate may also help others who are addicted to crack cocaine as well as to ascertain whether individuals who have succeeded with topiramate are at risk for a later relapse or can continue to stay off crack cocaine.

See also CRIME AND CRIMINALS; GANGS; JAIL INMATES; LAW ENFORCMENT; NARCOTICS; ORGANIZED CRIME; PROSTITUTION; SCHEDULED DRUGS.

Johnston, Lloyd D., et al. *Monitoring the Future: National Survey Results on Drug Use, 1975–2004.* Vol. 2, *College Students and Adults Ages 19–45.* Bethesda, Md.: National Institute on Drug Abuse, National Institutes of Health, 2005.

National Institute of Justice. *Drug and Alcohol Use and Related Matters among Arrestees, 2003.* 2004. Available online. URL: http:www.ncjrs.gove/nij/adam/ADM2003.pdf. Downloaded May 19, 2006.

Substance Abuse and Mental Health Services Administration. *Overview of Findings from the 2004 National Survey on Drug Use and Health.* Washington, D.C.: Department of Health and Human Services, September 2005.

Whitten, Lori. "Topiramate Shows Promise in Cocaine Addiction," *NIDA Notes* 19, no. 6 (May 2005): 1, 6.

TABLE II: MALE AND FEMALE ARRESTEES REPORTING USE AND ACQUISITION OF CRACK COCAINE IN THE PAST WEEK, MONTH, AND YEAR, 2003

Past Crack Cocaine Use by Arrestees	Male	Female
Used in past 7 days	12.9%	20.0%
Used in past 30 days	13.8%	20.5%
Used in past year	17.2%	24.5%
Average number of days used in past 30 days	8.1 days	10.1 days

Source: National Institute of Justice. *Drug and Alcohol Use and Related Matters among Arrestees, 2003.* 2004. Available online. URL: http:www.ncjrs.gove/nij/adam/ADM2003.pdf. Downloaded May 19, 2006.

craving An intense and sometimes overwhelming desire to consume the item to which a person is addicted, whether it is drugs and/or alcohol.

Craving is also an essential aspect of an addiction (also known as dependence) to drugs or alcohol.

When an individual is addicted to a substance, the craving builds up to a high level until the substance is consumed, after which the craving temporarily abates, only to return and increase in intensity again until the substance is consumed yet again. Even after a person has undergone DETOXIFICATION in a rehabilitation program and has successfully ended the addiction, often the cravings for drugs or alcohol return and persist, and this is why many individuals RELAPSE into using addictive substances.

Self-help programs such as Alcoholics Anonymous and Narcotics Anonymous are very helpful to many individuals who are combating their craving for alcohol and drugs. However, some individuals need medication as well.

Anticraving Medications

Some physicians use medications to combat the craving for drugs or alcohol. For example, NALTREXONE is a medication approved by the Food and Drug Administration to treat alcoholism, and it helps to reduce the craving for alcohol. According to Charles O'Brien in his 2005 article in the *American Journal of Psychiatry* on anticraving medications, studies have shown that subjects who received naltrexone had lower craving levels than those who took a placebo. Alcohol was also made available to the subjects in one study. The study subjects were given either naltrexone or a placebo as well as one "priming drink" of alcohol.

O'Brien reports:

Participants had the choice of more alcoholic drinks or money instead of each drink after the priming drink. The placebo group chose to drink significantly more than the naltrexone group, resulting in a progressively increasing blood alcohol level, whereas the naltrexone group reported less craving during alcohol availability, consumed fewer drinks, and drank them more slowly when they did drink. This human laboratory study was remarkable in that it produced results consistent with both animal models and clinical trials.

Other drugs have been tested for their efficacy in reducing the craving for illegal drugs. BUPRENORPHINE (Subutex, Suboxone) is approved by the FDA to treat drug cravings for HEROIN, and in some cases, to treat narcotic addiction, such as an addiction to HYDROCODONE (Vicodin), OXYCODONE/acetaminophen (Percocet), or oxycodone controlled release (OXYCONTIN). METHADONE is also commonly used to treat patients addicted to narcotics.

Other anticraving drugs are being studied. For example, modafinil (Provigil), a drug that is approved by the FDA to treat narcolepsy, has also been found to be effective at reducing both the euphoria from COCAINE as well as the craving for this drug. It also reportedly reduces the WITHDRAWAL symptoms from cocaine dependence. Modafinil is under further study for the treatment of cocaine addiction as of this writing.

Other drugs are under study to treat cocaine addiction, such as DISULFIRAM (ANTABUSE), a drug used to treat ALCOHOLISM that causes violent vomiting if any alcohol is consumed. Topiramate (Topamax), propranolol (Inderal), and baclofen (Lioresal) are also under study for the treatment of cocaine addition. Rimonabant (Acomplia) is under study to treat both alcoholism and cocaine addiction. In addition, ondansetron (Zofran) is being studied for the treatment of alcohol addiction.

ACAMPROSATE (CAMPRAL) is a delayed-released medication that is used to treat alcoholism, first used in the United States in 2005 after its FDA approval in 2004. Campral was the first new antialcoholism drug to be introduced into the United States in about 10 years. It is used to decrease the CRAVING for alcohol and helps to reduce the risk for RELAPSE.

Another medication, vigabatrin (Sabril), which is an antiseizure medication, has been shown to reduce craving in a preliminary study of cocaine addicts. However, trials have been suspended in the United States because the medication may cause visual problems. Some research has shown that topiramate, another antiseizure medication, can help individuals addicted to CRACK COCAINE.

See also ADDICTION/DEPENDENCE; DENIAL; PSYCHOLOGICAL DEPENDENCE; RELAPSE.

O'Brien, Charles P., M.D. "Anticraving Medications for Relapse Prevention: A Possible New Class of Psychoactive Medications." *American Journal of Psychiatry* 162 (2005): 1,423–1,431.

crime and criminals and substance abuse   Crimes are illegal acts and those who perpetrate them are criminals. Many criminals are involved in the use and/or the sale of illegal drugs and alcohol or the misuse of prescription drugs, or DRUG DIVERSION. The use of all drugs in Schedule I of the CONTROLLED SUBSTANCES ACT are prohibited, including such drugs as MARIJUANA, HEROIN, and CRACK COCAINE. It is also illegal to buy or sell drugs that are prescribed to others. (See PRESCRIPTION DRUG ABUSE.)

According to the U.S. Department of Justice, there were 1,745,712 drug law violation arrests in the United States in 2004, the highest number of arrests from 1980 to 2004. Of these arrests, 1,426,200 were for possession of drugs and 319,500 were for the sale and/or manufacture of drugs. In considering the type of drug the individual was arrested for possessing or selling, the greatest number of arrests were for marijuana (771,600), followed by heroin/cocaine (530,700).

There are many types of crimes that involve drugs. Trafficking (selling) drugs is a felony (serious crime). Possession of a small amount of drugs (particularly marijuana) is often a misdemeanor, depending on state law. Drugs are also often associated with other crimes, such as PROSTITUTION, as well as crimes of violence. Some children are victims of CHILD ABUSE because the abuser was under the influence of alcohol and/or drugs at the time the abuse was committed. In addition, the manufacture of some drugs in a household with a child, particularly METHAMPHETAMINE manufactured in CLANDESTINE LABORATORIES, is considered a form of child abuse in some states.

Individuals who are using illegal drugs and/or excessive amounts of alcohol are more likely to have car crashes and other types of accidents that may harm them and others. When the use of alcohol and/or illegal drugs is detected in relation to a car crash or another accident, this may be a criminal act.

Most Jail Inmates Either Are Dependent on or Abuse Alcohol or Drugs

Many inmates are substance abusers. According to a special report from the Bureau of Justice Statistics in 2005 on substance dependence and abuse among jail inmates in 2002 in the United States, more than two-thirds (68 percent) of all inmates in jail either were dependent on or had abused alcohol or drugs. In contrast, about 9 percent of the general noncriminal public either abuse or are dependent on alcohol and/or drugs.

Forty-five percent of the inmates were dependent on (addicted to) alcohol or drugs, and 23 percent were abusers of alcohol or drugs, although they were not dependent on them. (The minority of the inmates, 32 percent, had neither abuse of nor a dependence on either alcohol or drugs.)

Table I illustrates the percentage of inmates who met symptomatic indicators for either abuse or dependence. According to the study, "Abuse symptoms included repeated use of alcohol or drugs in hazardous situations or recurrent occupational, educational, legal or social problems related to alcohol or drug use. The most common abuse criteria reported by jail inmates were recurrent social problems because of alcohol (40%), drugs (43%), and the combination of alcohol or drugs (58%)."

They add, "The dependence criteria covered a range of symptoms, including behavioral, cognitive, and physiological problems. The criteria most often cited by inmates were impaired control (44%) and continued use despite problems (45%)."

Substance Abuse and the Commission of Crimes

Drug and/or alcohol abuse and dependence were also factors in the actual commission of the crime, as indicated by the study of the inmates. An estimated 50 percent of all the convicted jail inmates were influenced by alcohol or drugs when they committed their crimes. It was also noted in the report that substance abuse was related to recidivism (committing crimes again at a later date). For example, of those inmates who met the criteria for substance abuse or dependence, they had twice the risk of having had three or more past probations or incarcerations.

TABLE I: PREVALENCE OF SUBSTANCE DEPENDENCE OR ABUSE SYMPTOMS AMONG JAIL INMATES, 2002

Abuse symptoms	Percentage of Jail Inmates		
	Alcohol	Drugs	Alcohol or Drugs
Failure to fulfill major role obligations	15.9	26.7	33.1
Lose job; job/school problems, such as missing too much work/school, being demoted at work, dropping out of school; not taking care of children			
Continued use [of substances] in hazardous situation	30.0	29.7	43.0
Get in situations that increases chances of getting hurt, like driving, swimming, using machinery, or walking in unsafe area			
Alcohol-drug-related legal problems	20.9	25.0	37.7
Arrested or held by police due to drinking or drug use			
Recurrent social or interpersonal problems	39.8	43.3	57.8
Arguments, problems with spouse, intimate, family, or friends or get into physical fights			
Dependence symptoms			
Tolerance	21.0	33.4	42.1
Usual drinks/drugs had less effect; or drank more or used more drugs to get the wanted effect			
Withdrawal	19.5	27.8	36.4
Bad aftereffects from cutting down or stopping alcohol/drugs, such as shaking, feeling nervous, anxious, sick to stomach; or taking a drink/drugs to get over any bad aftereffects			
Compulsive use	23.6	30.9	42.7
More alcohol/drug use or using for longer periods than intended			
Impaired control	20.1	34.8	44.4
More than once wanted to cut down/tried to cut down but couldn't			
Time spent obtaining, using, recovering	18.4	30.5	39.0
Spent a lot of time using alcohol/drugs or getting over the bad aftereffects			
Neglect of activities	13.2	25.7	30.8
Gave up on activities of interest/importance, like work, school, hobbies, or associating with family and friends			
Continued use despite problems	22.3	35.6	44.8
Continued to drink/use drugs even though it was causing emotional or psychological problems			

Source: Adapted from Karberg, Jennifer C., and Doris J. James, *Substance Dependence, Abuse, and Treatment of Jail Inmates, 2002.* Washington, D.C., U.S. Department of Justice, 2005, p. 2.

Alcohol and drug abuse also contributed to violent crimes; for example, among those who committed homicide, nearly half (47.2 percent) had used alcohol or drugs. In considering SEXUAL ASSAULT, including rape and other forms of sexual assault, nearly half (47.4 percent) had used alcohol or drugs when they committed the crime. The rate was highest among those who used weapons: 55.7 percent had used alcohol or drugs when they used a weapon. (See Table II for more data.)

Those who were dependent on drugs or alcohol also had a higher rate of violent, property, drug, and

TABLE II: PRIOR ALCOHOL OR DRUG USE AT TIME OF OFFENSE AMONG CONVICTED JAIL INMATES, BY TYPE OF OFFENSE, 2002, NUMBERS AND PERCENTAGE

Most Serious Offense	Estimated Number of Inmates	Used at time of offense, by Percentage		
		Alcohol	Drugs	Alcohol or Drugs
Total[1]	440,570	33.3	28.8	49.7
Violent offenses	96,359	37.6	21.8	47.2
Homicide	5,967	41.6	20.0	47.4
Sexual assault[2]	13,252	37.2	13.5	42.2
Robbery	18,826	37.6	39.9	55.8
Assault	50,226	39.7	18.2	47.5
Property offenses	112,895	28.5	32.5	46.8
Burglary	29,767	32.6	40.8	55.1
Larceny/theft	33,691	29.0	32.0	47.3
Motor vehicle theft	9,414	35.4	39.8	54.5
Fraud	22,817	21.5	27.9	38.6
Drug offenses	112,447	22.4	43.2	51.7
Possession	48,823	19.9	45.9	51.4
Trafficking	56,574	24.8	40.7	51.8
Public-order offenses	83,193	26.2	19.5	37.7
Weapons	9,128	35.3	36.8	55.7
Other public-order[3]	73,975	25.1	17.4	34.6

[1] Includes some offenses not shown.
[2] Includes rape and other sexual assault.
[3] Excludes driving while under the influence (DWI)/driving under the influence (DUI).
Source: Adapted from Karberg, Jennifer C., and Doris J. James, *Substance Dependence, Abuse, and Treatment of Jail Inmates, 2002.* Washington, D.C., U.S. Department of Justice, 2005, p. 6.

public-order crimes than those who abused but were not dependent on substances. For example, 40.8 percent of those who were alcohol- and/or drug-dependent had committed violent crimes as their most serious offense, compared to 22.3 percent who were substance abusers. Together, they represented 63.1 percent of the violent crime offenders. Most of the offenders, however, had committed drug crimes (72.1 percent), property crimes (71.7 percent), or public-order offenses (67.0 percent). (See Table II.)

Demographics of Inmates with Substance Abuse Issues

The researchers who studied the inmates and their substance abuse found that females had a *higher* rate of drug or alcohol dependence than the male inmates; for example, 51.8 percent of the female inmates were substance-dependent, compared to only 44.3 percent of male inmates. In considering both substance abuse and dependence, the males (67.9 percent) and females (69.2 percent) were nearly equal. However, this finding is in sharp contrast to that for males and females in the general public, where the abuse and dependence rate of men (13 percent) is more than twice the rate for women (6 percent).

In considering race, white prisoners had the highest rate of dependence (55.4 percent), followed by the race known as "others," which included Asians, American Indians, Alaska Native, Native Hawaiians, other Pacific Islanders, and inmates who specified more than one race. Among those inmates, the dependence rate was 45.4 percent. In considering both dependence and abuse, whites had the highest proportion in this category among all races: 77.1 percent. (See Table II.)

In considering the age of inmates, those who were ages 35–44 years had the highest rate of dependence (50.4 percent) followed closely by those inmates who were ages 25–34 (48.1 percent).

TABLE III: SUBSTANCE DEPENDENCE AND ABUSE AMONG JAIL INMATES, BY SELECTED CHARACTERISTICS, 2002

Characteristic	Percentage of Jail Inmates		
	All	Dependence	Abuse only
Percentage of all jail inmates	68.0	45.2	22.9
Gender			
Male	67.9	44.3	23.6
Female	69.2	51.8	17.4
Race/Hispanic origin			
White[1]	77.7	55.4	22.3
Black[1]	64.1	40.4	23.7
Hispanic	58.7	35.7	23.0
Other[2]	66.0	45.4	20.7
Age			
24 or younger	66.1	40.3	25.8
25–34	70.5	48.1	22.4
35–44	71.4	50.4	21.0
45–54	61.9	41.7	20.3
55 or older	46.2	23.1	23.1
Most serious offense			
Violent	63.1	40.8	22.3
Property	71.7	50.6	21.1
Drug	72.1	49.6	22.4
Public-order	67.0	41.3	25.7

[1] Excludes persons of Hispanic origin.
[2] Includes Asians, American Indians, Alaska Natives, Native Hawaiians, other Pacific Islanders, and inmates who specified more than one race.
Source: Adapted from Karberg, Jennifer C., and Doris J. James, Substance Dependence, Abuse, and Treatment of Jail Inmates, 2002. Washington, D.C., U.S. Department of Justice, 2005, p. 3.

Family Background

The inmates who had a substance abuse or dependence problem also had a much higher rate of past problems in their background, such as physical abuse, sexual abuse, parents who used drugs, and family members who were incarcerated, than inmates who did not have a substance abuse problem. (See Table IV.) The substance abusers in jail were more than twice as likely to have grown up with a parent who had a drug or alcohol abuse problem (37 percent) compared to the nonabusers (17 percent).

Of the inmates who abused or were dependent on alcohol and/or drugs, 17.6 percent had been sexually abused, compared to 9.8 percent of the inmates who were not substance abusers or dependent on substances. In addition, more than half (50.3 percent) of those who were substance abusers or substance-dependent had a family member who had ever been incarcerated (most often a brother, for both groups), compared to 37.9 percent of the inmates who were not substance abusers or dependent on substances.

Those who abused or were dependent on substances were twice as likely (13.9 percent) to have ever lived in a foster home, agency, or institution as the inmates who were not substance abusers or substance-dependent (6.6 percent).

Treatment Is Essential

According to a report released in 2006 by the National Institute on Drug Abuse (NIDA), *Principles of Drug Abuse Treatment for Criminal Justice Populations*, it is important to identify those incarcerated individuals who are dependent on drugs to break the family cycle of drugs (in their children and grandchildren) and to reduce the risk of recidivism (repeated crimes).

It would also be cost-effective to do so, according to NIDA; for example, the Office of National Drug Control Policy estimated that the societal cost of drug abuse was nearly $181 billion, while the cost of treating drug abuse (including research, training, and prevention) was estimated to be $15.8 million. Drug abuse treatment would also reduce the rate of crimes and subsequent incarcerations, since drug users are more likely to perform repeated crimes compared to nonusers.

Some individuals who are drug abusers or drug-dependent may not willingly obtain treatment, but legal pressure may be a successful inducement for treatment. In fact, according to NIDA, a large percentage of individuals admitted to drug abuse treatment did so because of legal inducements (such as either going to treatment or going to jail).

See also ANTISOCIAL PERSONALITY DISORDER; CRIME AND CRIMINALS; DRUG DEALERS; GANGS; INCARCERATION; JAIL INMATES; LAW ENFORCEMENT; NARCOTICS; ORGANIZED CRIME; PRESCRIPTION DRUG ABUSE; PROSTITUTION; PSYCHIATRIC DISORDERS; TRAFFICKING.

Dorsey, Tina L., Marianne W. Zawitz, and Priscilla Middleton. *Drugs and Crime Facts*. Washington, D.C.: U.S.

TABLE IV: FAMILY BACKGROUND OF JAIL INMATES, BY SUBSTANCE DEPENDENCE OR ABUSE, 2002

Characteristic	Percentage of Jail Inmates	
	Dependence on or Abuse of Substances	Other Inmates
Homeless in past year	16.5	9.1
Employed in month before admission to jail	71.1	72.5
Ever physically or sexually abused	21.1	12.5
Physically abused	17.6	9.8
Sexually abused	9.0	5.2
While growing up:		
Ever received public assistance[1]	50.8	33.2
Ever lived in foster home, agency, or institution	13.9	6.6
Lived most of the time with:		
Both parents	42.1	48.5
One parent	46.4	40.3
Someone else	11.5	11.1
Parents or guardians ever abused:	36.8	17.4
Alcohol	23.6	11.8
Drugs	2.3	1.7
Both alcohol and drugs	10.9	3.9
Neither	63.2	82.6
Family member ever incarcerated:	50.3	37.9
Mother	8.0	5.6
Father	20.7	13.9
Brother	33.9	26.6
Sister	10.6	5.7
Spouse	2.1	1.4
Number of jail inmates	415,242	195,054

[1] Public assistance includes public housing, Aid to Families with Dependent Children (AFDC), food stamps, Medicaid, Women, Infants and Children (WIC), and Temporary Aid to Needy Families (TANF), other welfare programs.
Source: Adapted from Karberg, Jennifer C., and Doris J. James, *Substance Dependence, Abuse, and Treatment of Jail Inmates, 2002.* Washington, D.C., U.S. Department of Justice, 2005, p. 4.

Department of Justice, Office of Justice Programs, Bureau of Justice Statistics. Available online. URL: http://www.ojp.usdoj.gov/bjs/pub/pdf/dcf.pdf. Downloaded July 16, 2006.

Karberg, Jennifer C., and Doris J. James. *Substance Dependence, Abuse, and Treatment of Jail Inmates, 2002.* Bureau of Justice Statistics Special Report. Washington, D.C.: U.S. Department of Justice, July 2005.

National Institute on Drug Abuse. *Principles of Drug Abuse Treatment for Criminal Justice Populations: A Research-Based Guide.* Rockville, Md.: National Institutes of Health, U.S. Department of Health and Human Services, July 2006. Available online. URL: http://www.drugabuse.gov/PODAT_CJ/PODAT_CJ.pdf. Downloaded August 6, 2006.

cross-tolerance The abuse of or dependence on one drug that affects the use of another drug, such that the dosage of the second drug needs to be higher to be effective; for example, a cross-tolerance is found between alcohol and BENZODIAZEPINES. There is also a cross-tolerance among METHADONE and HEROIN as with OXYCODONE and HYDROCODONE. HEROIN abusers can become extremely tolerant of and resistant to all opiate pain medication, and alcoholics can become very tolerant of BENZODIAZEPINES and related drugs.

It is very important for patients to tell their doctors whether they are taking other drugs than those the doctor already knows about, including illegal drugs or even supplements, so that the doctor can make adjustments of medications he or she prescribes, as needed. This can be particularly important if the patient needs anesthesia for surgical treatment but is already taking a narcotic painkiller for pain management. In this case, the patient may need higher than normal doses of the anesthetic.

crystal methamphetamine   See METHAMPHETAMINE.

date rape drugs Sedating drugs that are usually illegally administered to individuals without their knowledge or consent, often added to the unknowing victim's drink at a bar, restaurant, or the site of a party. This practice is also known as a form of MALICIOUS POISONING. In most cases, date rape drugs are controlled substances under the CONTROLLED SUBSTANCES ACT. Date rape drugs cause sedation as well as a retrograde amnesia (memory loss) of what has occurred during the time that the victim was sedated and sexually assaulted. Not all date rape drugs are unknowingly used; some individuals self-administer them.

In a study reported by the National Criminal Justice Service of 144 sexual assault victims, nearly 5 percent of the victims were administered date rape drugs without their knowledge or permission. (See SEXUAL ASSAULTS.)

Some examples of date rape drugs are FENTANYL, FLUNITRAZEPAM (ROHYPNOL), GAMMA-HYDROXYBUTYRATE (GHB), carisoprodol (Soma), and KETAMINE. It is unknown how many individuals are sexually assaulted after they are given date rape drugs each year, and it is likely that many such rapes are never reported because of the confusion of the victim and the short time frame in which the drug remains in the body.

Date rape drugs enable the perpetrator to commit a sexual assault with no resistance. Often after the drug is administered, the perpetrator may appear to others as if he is assisting an individual intoxicated with alcohol. If the victim has ingested any alcohol prior to unknowingly consuming the date rape drug, then the drug often acts more quickly than otherwise. The perpetrator then removes the victim to a private location, where he or she is sexually molested. When victims regain consciousness, they may not know where they are. They may be naked or show signs of having been molested. Perpetrators may tell victims that they had agreed to have sex, or perpetrators may have left the scene altogether.

Under the Drug-Induced Rape Prevention Act of 1996 in the United States, individuals who use date rape drugs in order to facilitate a rape and/or a violent crime may be imprisoned for up to 20 years and be fined.

Most date rape victims are young adult females, but some males have been assaulted with date rape drugs, usually by other males.

Date rape drugs are generally odorless and colorless, and they will not show up on a toxicology screening unless the particular drug is tested for and within a short period. Often individuals who have been date raped do not report the assault to the police because they are embarrassed and fearful. They may mistakenly believe that they somehow bear some responsibility for what has happened to them. In some cases, they may be uncertain of what has happened and may not know whether they gave consent to sexual contact or not.

Say Fitzgerald and Riley in their article on date rape in the *National Institute of Justice Journal,* "Even when victims do suspect a drug-facilitated rape and seek help immediately, law enforcement agencies may not know how to collect evidence appropriately or how to test urine using the sensitive method required." As a result, often valuable evidence of the assault is lost with the passage of time.

Whenever possible, toxicology tests should be administered. Experts report that date rape drugs are more likely to show up in the urine than in the blood. The urine collection can occur prior to interviews by law enforcement officials and the forensic medical examination. Evidence of the crime should be sought.

Say Fitzgerald and Riley, "Drug-related evidence may be found in the glasses from which the victim drank, containers used to mix drinks, and trash cans where these items were discarded. In one case, traces of GHB were found in the box of salt that was used to make margaritas. GHB is often carried in small bottles, such as eyedrop bottles. It is often administered in sweet drinks, such as fruit nectars and liqueurs, to mask its salty taste." In addition, the offender may have a recipe for making GHB on a computer. Sometimes perpetrators videotape or photograph their victims while they were under the influence of the drug. Such evidence can also lead to other victims who have been similarly sexually assaulted.

Victims of date rapes report that they feel angry and powerless. They may feel that they have also suffered a form of "mind rape," in addition to the actual sexual assault. It can also be difficult for victims of date rape to hear others say that they think that it is better when the victim does not remember what happened, as opposed to being conscious and aware while the rape is occurring.

Sometimes, memories of the sexual assault may occur at a later time. But they may never come back. According to Gail Abarbanel in her article in *National Institute of Justice Journal,* victims of sexual assaults who were not administered date rape drugs may experience memory fragments or flashbacks.

She says, "For victims of drug-facilitated rapes, this aspect of the aftermath may be experienced differently. Because they cannot recall what happened during a significant time period, they have to cope with a gap in their memory. They experience the horror, powerlessness, and humiliation of not knowing what was done to them. They can only imagine what happened. One victim said, 'I would rather have the nightmare.'" (She means that she would rather have experienced the actual rape.)

See also COLLEGE STUDENTS; CRIME AND CRIMINALS; MALICIOUS POISONING; SEXUAL ASSAULTS; VIOLENCE.

Abarbanel, Gail. "Learning from Victims." *National Institute of Justice Journal,* April 2000, 11–12.
Fitzgerald, Nora, and K. Jack Riley. "Drug Facilitated Rape: Looking for the Missing Pieces." *National Institute of Justice Journal,* April 2000, 8–15. Available online. URL: http://www.ncjrs.gov/pdffiles1/jr000243c.pdf. Downloaded on March 16, 2006.
National Drug Intelligence Center. "Drug-Facilitated Sexual Assault Fast Facts: Questions and Answers." Johnston, Pa.: National Drug Intelligence Center, 2004. Available online. URL: http://www.usdoj.gov/ndic/pubs/8/8872/8872p.pdf. Downloaded on March 16, 2006.

death   Cessation of life. Drug abuse, drug dependence, alcohol abuse, and ALCOHOLISM may all lead directly or indirectly to the death of the user. ACCIDENTAL OVERDOSE DEATHS may be caused directly; there are also many indirect causes of deaths that involve alcohol and drugs, such as car crashes and health problems. According to a study reported in 2004 in the *Journal of the American Medical Association,* an estimated 17,000 people died of the use of illicit drugs in 2000 (less than 1 percent of all deaths), compared to 435,000 people who died of the use of tobacco (18 percent of all deaths), and 85,000 people who died as a result of alcohol consumption (3.5 percent of all deaths). According to the Drug Enforcement Administration, most people who die of narcotic overdoses had trouble breathing.

Some individuals who are alcoholic or drug-addicted commit SUICIDE, usually because of the severe DEPRESSION or anxiety that accompanies these addictions, but sometimes because of psychiatric symptoms such as DELUSIONS, HALLUCINATIONS, or other psychotic symptoms that may be induced by some drugs, particularly with high doses of AMPHETAMINE, COCAINE, METHAMPHETAMINE, or HALLUCINOGENIC DRUGS.

Death may be caused by individuals who are substance abusers because of an increased level of aggression or because of psychotic behavior induced by drugs. The more illegal drugs that were taken, the greater the likelihood of violent behavior. These individuals are also more likely to become involved in car crashes and other accidents, which may injure them and others. Studies indicate that drug and alcohol abusers are more prone to violent acts than others, including murder.

Death and Drugs
Some drugs are particularly risky and may lead to death if abused, including such drugs as cocaine,

MDMA, and methamphetamine, in addition to the chronic abuse of anabolic-androgenic steroids. The individual who abuses these drugs may die of respiratory failure, a stroke or a heart attack, or by other means.

Some drugs also increase the individual's level of aggression and may increase the risk of the commission of a homicide of a child or adult, as with methamphetamine and anabolic steroids.

Cocaine is also a drug that is associated with death among long-time users. According to Dr. Karch in his 1999 article for the *Journal of the Royal Society of Medicine,* 60 percent of deaths from cocaine abuse among long-term users are caused by an individual using a chronic and toxic dosage of cocaine. In 20 percent of the cases of those who abuse or are dependent on cocaine, the victims are murdered. Suicide accounts for about 10 percent of the deaths of cocaine abusers. The other cocaine-related deaths are caused by stroke, excited delirium, myocardial infarction (heart attack), and sudden cardiac death.

The abuse of METHYLENEDIOXYMETHAMPHETAMINE (MDMA/ECSTASY) can cause a very rapid and escalating high fever, which, if untreated, can cause death.

Accidental Deaths from Illegal and Prescribed Drugs

A study in the *American Journal of Preventive Medicine* analyzed 1,906 accidental deaths from medical examiner statistics from 1994 to 2003 in New Mexico, the state which has had the highest rate of drug-induced deaths since 1990. The rate of prescription drug overdose death increased from 1.9 people per 100,000 in 1994 to 5.3 per 100,000 in 2003, a 179 percent increase.

In considering *all* drug overdose deaths, the researchers discovered that about 77 percent of the people who died were male and about 55 percent were Hispanic, 40 percent were white non-Hispanic, and 2 percent were American Indians. About a third of deaths related to drug abuse were caused by a combination of alcohol and drugs.

Opioid painkillers were involved in 77 percent of deaths caused by prescription drugs, followed by tranquilizers (34 percent), antidepressants (26 percent), and co-intoxication with over-the-counter drugs (10 percent). In many cases, however, the deceased person used more than one type of drug.

Another category of drugs that can lead to deaths are DEPRESSANTS. Abuse of depressants can slow the heart rate and decrease the body temperature (hypothermia) and, as a result, may cause death. Examples of depressants are medications in the BENZODIAZEPINE category, such as ALPRAZOLAM (Xanax) and DIAZEPAM (Valium), as well as BARBITURATES, including such drugs as pentobarbital sodium (Nembutal) and butalbital (Fiorcet).

INHALANTS are another category of drugs that may lead to death, owing to cardiac arrthymia, even the first time the substance is inhaled.

Death from Injecting Illegal Drugs

Injecting illegal drugs can also cause death. A 2004 study discussed in *Archives of Internal Medicine* found that intravenous drug users had a high risk of death, particularly IV users ages 25–34 years. Most died from an overdose; however, some contracted the human immunodeficiency virus (HIV), which then progressed to acquired immune deficiency syndrome (AIDS) and then to death.

Death from Sudden Withdrawal of Drugs

Some individuals die from drug WITHDRAWAL, whether they choose to stop taking the drug or the choice is made for them, as when they are imprisoned. Whether death occurs depends on the type of the drug and the degree of the addiction. Some people addicted to ALPRAZOLAM (Xanax) have died in jail from withdrawal symptoms.

Death and Alcohol

Some individuals die from diseases caused by chronic alcoholism; others die from car crashes or other accidents resulting from being under the influence of alcohol. For example, young men ages 16–20 who drink and drive while intoxicated are 15,560 times more likely to die in a car accident than young men who do not drink or who drink amounts insufficient to cause intoxication. In 2003 about 18,000 people died of alcohol-related fatalities, according to the National Highway and Traffic Safety Administration (NHTSA).

In addition, in non-car crash accidents, alcohol is often a factor, and about a third of all individuals in the United States who die from unintentional accidents not related to car crashes have a blood alcohol concentration above the legal limit.

The substance of alcohol itself may cause death, as when individuals (usually young men) engage in BINGE DRINKING and imbibe copious quantities of alcohol, leading to alcohol poisoning. The body is unable to metabolize the alcohol fast enough in some cases, and the individual dies.

Alcohol may also contribute to the deaths of those who do not drink, such as those who are killed by drunk drivers or who are abused by alcoholics. College students are often very heavy drinkers, and according to the National Institute on Alcohol Abuse and Alcoholism in their report on the culture of campus drinking in their article in 2002 in *Alcohol Alert,* alcohol consumption is linked to at least 1,400 student deaths each year.

See also ALCOHOL; ALCOHOLISM; BINGE DRINKING; CHILD ABUSE; DRUG ABUSE AND DEPENDENCE AND HEALTH PROBLEMS; EATING DISORDERS; INJURIES, CAUSED BY ALCOHOL AND/OR ILLICIT DRUGS; EMERGENCY TREATMENT; INHALANTS; METHAMPHETAMINE; SUICIDE.

Copeland, Lorraine, et al. "Changing Patterns in Cause of Death in a Cohort of Injecting Drug Users, 1980–2001," *Archives of Internal Medicine* 165 (June 14, 2004): 1,214–1,220.

Karch, Steven B., M.D. "Cocaine: History, Use, Abuse," *Journal of the Royal Society of Medicine* 92 (August 1999): 393–397.

Mokdad, Ali H., et al. "Actual Causes of Death in the United States, 2000." *Journal of the American Medical Association* 291, no. 10 (March 10, 2004): 1,238–1,245.

Mueller, Mark R., et al. "Unintentional Prescription Drug Overdose Deaths in New Mexico, 1994–2003," *American Journal of Preventive Medicine* 30, no. 5 (2006): 423–429.

National Institute on Alcohol Abuse and Alcoholism. "Changing the Culture of Campus Drinking," *Alcohol Alert* 58 (October 2002). Rockville, Md.: National Institutes of Health.

National Advisory Council on Alcohol Abuse and Alcoholism Task Force on College Drinking. *High-Risk Drinking in College: What We Know and What We Need to Learn: Final Report of the Panel on Contexts and Consequences.* Rockville, Md.: National Institute on Alcohol Abuse and Alcoholism, April 2002.

delirium tremens   Severe HALLUCINATIONS that are caused by an alcoholic's WITHDRAWAL from alcohol. Also known as the "DTs." This condition may also be caused by excessive overuse of BENZODIAZEPINES.

The hallucinations that accompany delirium tremens may be auditory, visual, or even tactile. One terrifying form of a tactile hallucination is FORMICATION, in which the person feels as if insects are crawling in or underneath the skin. Alcoholics experiencing delirium tremens are in urgent need of medical care, and they should be treated in a hospital or rehabilitative center staffed with physicians. Some medications, such as sedatives such as BENZODIAZEPINES, may enable the patient who has delirium tremens to be more comfortable while undergoing withdrawal from alcohol.

Individuals who have delirium tremens are extremely ill, and they can die if they are not treated by experienced physicians and nurses in an inpatient environment. They should not be treated as outpatients.

Symptoms and Diagnostic Path

The symptoms of delirium tremens are clear to most physicians. Even those who do not recognize delirium tremens clearly see that there is something wrong with the individual.

Common symptoms are

- mental confusion
- severe tremor
- hallucinations
- extreme sweating
- seizures
- nausea and vomiting
- insomnia
- fever

Treatment Options and Outlook

DETOXIFICATION from alcohol is usually best accomplished in an inpatient rehabilitative center. Delirium tremens is a relatively uncommon degree of withdrawal, and generally this problem only occurs with severe alcoholic usage: more than a fifth of hard liquor daily for lengthy periods or substantial doses of benzodiazepines far exceeding what is commonly prescribed.

If severe delirium tremens occurs, permanent brain damage may result from seizures and fever, and coma may occur. However, if it is appropriately treated, other long-term problems related to alcohol abuse may occur, but those connected specifically to delirium tremens should not.

Risk Factors and Preventive Measures

Long-term alcoholism or benzodiazepine abuse has the greatest risk for producing delirium tremens. Preventing delirium tremens involves the use of appropriate medications to manage alcohol or benzodiazepine withdrawal. Avoiding the use of excessive doses of alcohol or BENZODIZEPINES prevents the development of the tolerance and dependence that are required to develop delirium tremens.

See also ALCOHOLISM.

delusions False beliefs, such as PARANOIA, the belief that others are persecuting one. Some illegal drugs that are abused can cause delusions, especially AMPHETHAMPHETAMINE, ANABOLIC STEROIDS, COCAINE, CRACK COCAINE, LYSERGIC ACID DIETHYL-AMIDE (LDS), METHYLENEDIOXYMETHAMPHETAMINE (MDMA/ECSTASY), or METHAMPHETAMINE. Delusions are sometimes the only serious symptom of mental illness, but they are generally considered to be a feature of PSYCHOSIS, which involves delusions, HALLUCINATIONS, and some disorders of thinking.

Individuals who have SCHIZOPHRENIA usually have delusional beliefs as a part of their psychotic illness. Schizophrenia is a long-term mental illness that many believe is a genetic disorder. However, among individuals who have a predisposition to schizophrenia, drugs such as methamphetamine may trigger a psychotic episode. In addition, methamphetamine and anabolic steroids are clearly shown to cause psychosis in people who have no known predisposition to psychosis. Current imaging methods have clearly documented brain damage from cells destroyed by methamphetamine use. The causes of psychoses that are related to anabolic steroids and other drugs are not so clearly understood.

It may be extremely difficult or impossible to determine whether a person is experiencing a psychosis that was caused by an underlying psychiatric illness or by the use of a drug.

In some cases, delusions may lead to violence. Paranoid individuals may attack others to "defend" themselves, or they may hide in fear. Some drugs are more likely to induce aggression, such as anabolic steroids, amphetamines, cocaine, and MDMA (Ecstasy). Delusions may cause people to perform acts that they would not perform without the delusions, such as attack or kill their children, run naked in the streets, or attempt actions that lead to their own death.

See also ALCOHOLISM; DELIRIUM TREMENS; DRUG ABUSE AND DEPENDENCE AND HEALTH PROBLEMS; FORMICATION; HALLUCINATIONS; PSYCHIATRIC DISORDERS; PSYCHOSIS, DRUG-INDUCED; PSYCHOTIC BEHAVIOR.

denial Refusal to acknowledge or accept key aspects of life, particularly those that are difficult to accept. Many people who are substance abusers, as well as their family members and friends, are in denial that a problem with alcohol and/or drugs even exists. They may pretend that there is no problem (although they intuitively know that there is), hoping that it will go away. Although it occurs commonly, this strategy does not work.

Psychiatrists use the term *denial* to describe a defense mechanism used by individuals or family members to avoid thinking about or dealing with the likelihood that a person has a serious problem, such as substance abuse or psychiatric illness. For example, family members may not respond to the large number of empty liquor bottles in the trash, the passing out on the couch after a night (or day) of heavy drinking, and other acts that are indicative of ALCOHOLISM. The individual, his or her spouse or partner, and others may make excuses for every one of these acts, in denial that there is a real problem. (This is also called enabling behavior.) They may say that the bottles were accumulated over several weeks' time (even though it is clear that they were consumed over several days), or that the person who passed out was tired after having a hard day.

If the individual is addicted to drugs, the family may also convince themselves that there is no problem, or, if there may be a problem, that it is only a temporary one that has developed because the addicted individual is distressed by a marital failure, a job loss, or another negative life circumstance. When the situation improves, they believe, the use of drugs will cease. They fail to see that the breakup of the marriage and firing from a job may stem directly from the individual's behavior while he or she was under the influence of drugs and/or alcohol.

Denial is a normal human reaction to many problems, but the denial of the individual and/or his family members and friends can impede the recovery of an individual from substance abuse. However, even when friends and family members accept that the individual has a substance abuse problem, this is not sufficient in itself to resolve the problem. The individual who has the problem must also accept that he or she needs help and be willing to receive such help.

Sometimes family members and friends stage an INTERVENTION, with the help of a trained professional, in an attempt to compel the addicted person to accept that he or she needs help and should enter a rehabilitation facility immediately. Sometimes interventions are effective; in other cases, the addicted person adamantly denies a problem and refuses to accept treatment.

See also CODEPENDENCY; CRAVING; DELUSIONS; PSYCHIATRIC PROBLEMS.

dependence, alcohol   See ALCOHOL ABUSE/DEPENDENCE; ALCOHOLISM.

dependence, drugs   Dependence on drugs (addiction) is a chronic and relapsing brain disease, which is characterized by compulsive drug seeking and continued use, despite the many harmful consequences that inevitably ensue. The National Institute on Drug Abuse (NIDA) considers drug dependence to be a brain disease because it has been proven that chronic drug abuse actually changes the structure of the brain and how it works. These brain changes can be long-lasting; however, treatment and remission from drugs often can improve the brain.

NARCOTICS (including HYDROCODONE, OXYCODONE, and OxyCONTIN) can be addicting, as can some other types of drugs, such as stimulants (including AMPHETAMINES, COCAINE, and METHYLPHENIDATE [RITALIN/CONCERTA/FOCALIN, ETC.]), and DEPRESSANTS, such as BENZODIAZEPINES and BARBITURATES. For this reason, these drugs are SCHEDULED DRUGS under the CONTROLLED SUBSTANCES ACT.

Risk Factors for Addiction to Drugs

The NIDA estimates that 40–60 percent of the vulnerability to addiction to drugs is caused by genetic factors. (This does not, however, mean that if a parent or other relative is dependent on drugs, that others in the family are automatically susceptible to the influence of drugs. It may mean, however, that they should be even more careful than others to avoid using illegal drugs.) It is also true that adolescents and individuals with mental disorders have a greater risk for drug dependence than others in the general population.

Another factor that increases the risk for addiction is the home environment, and parents or older family members (such as older siblings) who abuse alcohol or drugs increase the risk for abuse and addiction in the younger members of the family. PEER PRESSURE is another influence, particularly in adolescence, when peer groups and friends have a profound influence. According to NIDA, "Drug-abusing peers can sway even those without risk factors to try drugs for the first time." Other risk factors for abuse that ultimately lead to addiction are poor social skills or academic failure.

The early use of drugs is another major risk factor for addiction, and the younger a person is when starting to abuse drugs, the more likely that he or she is to become addicted. According to NIDA in their 2007 report on drugs,

> Although taking drugs at any age can lead to addiction, research shows that the earlier a person begins to use drugs the more likely they are to progress to more serious abuse. This may reflect the harmful effect that drugs can have on the developing brain; it also may result from a constellation of early biological and social vulnerability factors, including genetic susceptibility, mental illness, unstable family relationships, and exposure to physical or sexual abuse. Still, the fact remains that early use is a strong indicator of problems ahead, among them, substance abuse and addiction.

The method of administering the drug also affects whether a person becomes addicted, and smoking or injecting the drug increases the risk for addiction. The intense euphoria that is generated by smoking or injecting the drug may fade within minutes, and experts believe that this plummeting of mood leads individuals to repeatedly use drugs to regain the transient state of pleasure that they experienced. (See PSYCHOLOGICAL DEPENDENCE.)

Continued drug abuse and addiction eventually results in the brain decreasing its production of dopamine, a brain chemical that is associated with pleasure. As a result, the addicted person *needs* drugs just to bring their dopamine levels up to normal. They must also take higher levels of the drug to achieve the euphoria that they experienced when they first started abusing the drug.

See also ADDICTION/DEPENDENCE; ALPRAZOLAM; ALPRAZOLAM XR (XANAX/XANAX XR); COCAINE; CRACK COCAINE; DEPRESSANTS; DETOXIFICATION; DIAZEPAM (VALIUM); HEROIN; HYDROCODONE; JAIL INMATES; METHADONE; NARCOTICS; OPIATES; OXYCODONE; OXYCONTIN; PRESCRIPTION DRUG ABUSE; PROPOXYPHENE; STIMULANTS; YOUNG ADULTS.

National Institute of Drug Abuse. *Drugs, Brains, and Behavior: The Science of Addiction.* Bethesda, Md.: National Institutes of Health, April 2007.
Substance Abuse and Mental Health Services Administration. *Overview of Findings from the 2004 National Survey on Drug Use and Health.* Washington, D.C.: Department of Health and Human Services, September 2005.

dependence, physical A physical need to use an illegal drug or to use a prescription drug nonmedically. Physical dependence is the continued need for a drug to prevent the symptoms of withdrawal.

Physical dependence alone in a person need not necessarily mean that the individual has an addiction.

According to the Drug Enforcement Administration in their 2005 publication *Drugs of Abuse,*

Contrary to common belief, physical dependence is not addiction. While addicts are usually physically dependent on the drug they are abusing, physical dependence can exist without addiction. For example, patients who take narcotics for chronic pain management or benzodiazepines to treat anxiety are likely to be physically dependent on that medication. Addiction is defined as compulsive drug-seeking behavior where acquiring and using a drug becomes the most important activity in the user's life. This definition implies a loss of control regarding drug use, and the addict will continue to use a drug despite serious medical and/or social consequences.

See also ADDICTION/DEPENDENCE; CHILDHOOD ABUSE.

Joseph, Donald E., editor. *Drugs of Abuse.* Washington, D.C.: U.S. Department of Justice, 2005.
Substance Abuse and Mental Health Services Administration. *Results from the 2004 National Survey on Drug Use and Health: National Findings.* Rockville, Md.: Department of Health and Human Services, September 2005.

dependence, psychological See PSYCHOLOGICAL DEPENDENCE.

depressants Drugs that are sedating to the central nervous system. Alcohol is the most commonly used and abused depressant in the United States. Other examples of depressants are medications that fall within the categories of BENZODIAZEPINES, such as ALPRAZOLAM/ALPRAZOLAM XR (XANAX; XANAS XR), and DIAZEPAM (VALIUM), as well as medications that are classified as BARBITURATES, such as pentobarbital sodium (Nembutal) and butalbital (Fiorcet). Depressants are sometimes referred to as "downers." Very few depressants are made illegally; one exception is GAMMA-HYDROXYBUYTRIC ACID (GHB), a depressant that is sometimes produced in CLANDESTINE LABORATORIES.

Some individuals engage in PRESCRIPTION DRUG ABUSE of products that are barbiturates or benzodiazepines. This may because they have developed a PSYCHOLOGICAL DEPENDENCE on and a physical TOLERANCE of the depressant.

Depressants can cause slowed physical coordination, slurred speech, and impaired judgment. High doses of benzodiazepines can cause memory impairment, depression, and headaches.

See also STIMULANTS.

depression/major depressive disorder A sustained mood state of a significant level of sadness and despair, which is more serious and long-lasting than normal transient periods of sadness related to outside events. Also known as clinical depression. Depression is a severe medical problem that is very different from the transient negative moods that many people experience that pass within a day or a few days in relation to a problem, such as the serious illness of a family member or the loss of a job.

Individuals who have major depressive disorder have an increased risk for substance abuse or dependence.

According to the National Institute of Mental Health (NIMH) in their 2006 report on the numbers of people with mental disorders in the United States, major depressive disorder is the leading cause of disability among individuals ages 15–44 years in the United States. NIMH estimates that 14.8 million U.S. adults ages 18 and older are affected by major depressive disorder, or about 6.7 percent of the adult population.

Depression can occur at any age, but the median age of onset is age 32. Women are about twice as likely to suffer from depression as men. Depression is highly responsive to treatment, and an estimated 80 percent of patients who have depression can improve with treatment. However, often depression is undiagnosed and untreated. Individuals may not realize that they are clinically depressed or may wrongly believe, because of their depressed mood state, that nothing and no one can help them. For this reason, it is important for others to urge a person who may have depression to seek professional help.

According to the National Survey on Drug Use and Health for 2004, individuals who have had at least one major depressive episode (MDE) in the past year are much more likely (28.8 percent) than those who have not had an MDE (13.8 percent) to have used an illicit drug in the past year. In addition, substance abuse or dependence was much more likely among people who had an MDE (22.0 percent) than those who had not had an MDE (8.6 percent).

According to the National Survey on Drug Use and Health, among those ages 12 and older in the United States with a major depressive disorder, 62.3 percent received treatment in the past 12 months.

The National Survey on Drug Use and Health also provided an estimate of persons who have serious psychological distress (SPD), which included individuals who had a high level of distress that was caused by any type of psychiatric problem. According to this report, there were 21.4 million adults ages 18 and older who had SPD in 2004. The researchers also reported that SPD was highly correlated with both substance abuse and substance dependence. In 2004, among adults who had SPD, 4.6 million people (21.3 percent) were dependent on or abused illicit drugs or alcohol. The rate among adults who did not have SPD and substance abuse or dependence was 7.9 percent.

Symptoms and Diagnostic Path

According to the National Institute of Mental Health (NIMH), individuals who have major depressive disorder may exhibit the following signs and symptoms:

- persistent sad, anxious, or empty mood
- lack of interest or pleasure in activities, including sex
- restlessness, irritability, or excessive crying
- feelings of guilt, worthlessness, helplessness, hopelessness, and pessimism
- sleep disorders, such as sleeping too much or too little, and early-morning awakenings
- change in appetite, causing weight gain or weight loss
- decreased energy, fatigue, a feeling of being "slowed down"
- thoughts of death or suicide or actual suicide attempts
- talk about suicide (such talk should always be taken seriously and further explored)
- difficulty with concentrating, remembering, or making decisions
- persistent physical symptoms that do not respond to medical treatment for these problems, such as frequent headaches, digestive disorders, and chronic pain
- inability to enjoy activities that have provided enjoyment in the past

Most physicians, such as internists, neurologists, and pediatricians, treat depression, although PSYCHIATRISTS are the most adept practitioners at the diagnosis of depression and are also the most knowledgeable about the treatment and appropriate medications. The physician who treats depression will seek to determine the severity and duration of the depressive symptoms. Individuals who are extremely depressed and are talking about a wish and a plan to die may need to be hospitalized in a psychiatric facility for their own safety, lest they attempt suicide.

Treatment Options and Outlook

Depression can be treated with antidepressants and psychotherapy, and most patients respond readily to treatment, although the initial response may not occur for weeks or longer. Sometimes the first antidepressant that is prescribed is effective; however, sometimes the medication must be changed several times, in a trial-and-error fashion, before the medication that helps an individual is identified.

However, when an individual is a substance abuser, the type of antidepressant medication that is used, as well as the type of substance that the individual abuses or is dependent upon, must be carefully considered. For example, for an individual addicted to COCAINE, it would be dangerous to prescribe a stimulating antidepressant, while for a patient addicted to a drug that is a depressant, a sedating medication could be very dangerous.

Note that it is extremely important for patients to provide information to physicians on *all* drugs that they take, including herbal remedies as well as illicit substances and alcohol. Physicians need this information to prescribe a nonharmful medication. Doctors are held to confidentiality and if they are told that a patient uses cocaine or another illicit drug, they will not contact law enforcement authorities. (The one circumstance in which doctors will contact authorities is if the patient has already or is likely to abuse children.)

Antidepressant treatment Most patients who have depression are treated with antidepressants; a variety of antidepressants are used, including the older tricyclic antidepressants (amitriptyline, imipramine, and desipramine). Tricyclics are sedating, a property that may be helpful for the depressed person suffering from insomnia, and some tricyclic antidepressants are thought to be more helpful than others in treating alcohol-related depression. However, tricyclics may be overly sedating for some people. In addition, they may also cause weight gain, constipation, or excessive dryness.

Many physicians prescribe newer medications that fall within the category of selective serotonin reuptake inhibitors (SSRIs), of which there are many different types, including fluoxetine (Prozac), escitalopram (Lexapro), and sertraline (Zoloft). In general, SSRIs appear to have fewer side effects than tricyclics. SSRIs may be sedating and may increase blood pressure slightly, as well as decreasing sexual interest or sexual function.

Some physicians treat depression with bupropion (Wellbutrin, Wellbutrin SR, Wellbutrin XL), which is an atypical antidepressant, which acts differently than the other categories of medications. Bupropion, under the name of Zyban, is also used for individuals who wish to quit smoking.

There is also a newer category of antidepressants: the serotonin norephinephrine reuptake inhibitor, or SNRI, a medication that works to retain both serotonin and norepinephrine. One example of this medication is duloxetine (Cymbalta), and others in this class are undergoing Food and Drug Administration (FDA) trials. Duloxetine is sometimes given to patients who have chronic depression, anxiety, and pain, although it is officially approved by the FDA only for the treatment of major depressive disorder.

Some physicians prescribe monoamine oxidase inhibitors (MAO inhibitors) to treat depression. MAOIs must be prescribed with extreme care because these drugs interact with many different foods and other drugs, and physicians may be concerned about dietary compliance and drug interactions. As a result, doctors often do not use them.

Note that with *any* antidepressant, there is still a risk for suicide in the depressed person, particularly in the early part of therapy. It should never be assumed that, just because the person has now begun a course of antidepressants, he or she could not or would not consider suicide. Instead, any mention of suicidal thoughts or plans should be reported immediately to the treating physician, whether the person is taking antidepressants or not.

It should also be noted that sometimes an antidepressant in one class (such as tricyclics or SSRIs) may be ineffective, but this does *not* mean that other antidepressants that are in the same class will provide no relief. Thus, one tricyclic may be ineffective while another tricyclic is very helpful, as with one SSRI to another.

Physicians usually start individuals on the lowest possible dose of an antidepressant and increase the dosage as needed. Some individuals need more than one antidepressant before they feel significantly better.

Psychotherapy sessions Psychotherapy is often very helpful to the depressed individual, particularly cognitive-behavioral therapy, in which the therapist helps the patient to reframe the way he or she views the current situation and learn to challenge negative and irrational thoughts. The therapist may also have helpful suggestions to aid patients in seeing that the outlook in their lives is not as grim as they may perceive it to be and that there are actions that they can take to improve their individual situations. Most experts believe that a combination of medication and psychotherapy is the best treatment for the depressed individual.

Risk Factors and Preventive Measures

Individuals who have a family history of depressive disorders are more likely to develop depression, although not all family members of depressed individuals will become depressed. In addition, depression can occur in an individual even when there are no other members in the family who have depression.

Individuals who have other psychiatric disorders are more likely to suffer from depression; for example, individuals who have ATTENTION DEFICIT HYPER-ACTIVITY DISORDER have a greater risk than others for developing depression.

Individuals who have certain personality traits are more likely than others to develop depression, such as those with the following traits:

- pessimistic thinking
- low self-esteem
- a sense of having little or no control over life events
- a tendency to worry to excess

There are no known measures to prevent depression from developing; however, once it is identified, depression should be treated.

See also ANTISOCIAL PERSONALITY DISORDER; ANXIETY DISORDERS; ATTENTION DEFICIT HYPERACTIVITY DISORDER; BIPOLAR DISORDER; CONDUCT DISORDER; PSYCHIATRIC DISORDERS; PSYCHOSIS, DRUG-INDUCED; PSYCHOTIC BEHAVIOR; SCHIZOPHRENIA.

Compton III, William M., M.D., et al. "The Role of Psychiatric Disorders in Predicting Drug Dependence Treatment Outcomes." *American Journal of Psychiatry* 160, no. 5 (May 2003): 890–895.

Mann, J. John, M.D. "The Medical Management of Depression." *New England Journal of Medicine* 353, no. 17 (October 27, 2005): 1,819–1,834.

National Institute of Mental Health. "The Numbers Count: Mental Disorders in America." Available online. URL: http://www.nimh.nih.gov/publicat/numbers.cfm#readNow. Downloaded April 22, 2006.

Nunes, Edward V., M.D., and Frances R. Levin, M.D. "Treatment of Depression in Patients with Alcohol or Other Drug Dependence." *Journal of the American Medical Association* 291, no. 15 (April 21, 2004): 1,887–1,896.

Stahl, Stephen M. *Essential Psychopharmacology: The Prescriber's Guide.* Cambridge: Cambridge University Press, 2005.

Substance Abuse and Mental Health Services Administration. *Results from the 2004 National Survey on Drug Use and Health: National Findings.* Rockville, Md.: Department of Health and Human Services, September 2005.

Trivedi, Madhukar H., M.D., et al. "Medication Augmentation after the Failure of SSRIs for Depression." *New England Journal of Medicine* 354, no. 12 (March 23, 2006): 1,243–1,252.

detoxification The process by which an individual seeks to overcome ALCOHOLISM or drug addiction while under the treatment of experienced addiction medicine physicians. The patient may reside in a rehabilitative facility or a hospital or be treated as an outpatient. People who are addicted to alcohol or drugs should *not* attempt to stop taking alcohol or drugs on their own, because their WITHDRAWAL symptoms may be very severe (such as HALLUCI-

NATIONS, DELUSIONS, high fevers), and even fatal. About 10 percent of all substance abuse TREATMENT FACILITIES in the United States (including inpatient and outpatient facilities) offer some form of detoxification treatment.

The time that is required for the detoxification process varies according to the drug to which the person is addicted, the degree of addiction, and other factors, but generally, detoxification takes at least several weeks. However, some physicians offer *ultrarapid* detoxification, in which the individual undergoes detoxification while under anesthesia. This process is very controversial, and it is extremely costly. It must be performed in a hospital.

Detoxification from Alcohol

Individuals who are addicted to alcohol cannot readily stop drinking if and when they decide to do so (although they and their loved ones may believe that they can). However, medications and therapy may help achieve this goal. (See DENIAL.)

Medications that can be used In the past and often in the present, DISULFIRAM (ANTABUSE) has been used to detoxify alcoholic patients on an outpatient basis. Disulfiram is used as an *aversive* form of therapy. When it is taken, if patients subsequently consume any amount of alcohol, even an extremely low amount, as with cooking sherry, they become extremely nauseous and vomit copiously. Even the alcohol in a shaving lotion can induce the severe vomiting response. Often patients actively resist taking disulfiram because of this extreme side effect. Experts disagree about the efficacy of this drug, although many treatment centers continue to use it.

Other drugs that have been successfully used to treat individuals for alcoholism are ACAMPROSATE (CAMPRAL) and NALTREXONE (REVIA). Sometimes a combination of drugs is used to detoxify patients with alcoholism.

Some experts believe that only inpatient rehabilitation for alcoholism is effective, while others believe in outpatient treatment combined with a twelve-step group, such as Alcoholics Anonymous. Many experts believe that a combination of therapies, such as medication, psychotherapy, and a support group, is the most effective means in helping patients to stop drinking.

Detoxification from Illegal Drugs

Many patients who are addicted to drugs such as COCAINE, METHAMPHETAMINE, HEROIN, as well as others, need inpatient detoxification, although some may be able to detoxify from drugs as outpatients.

Medications that may be used Some drugs are used to help patients with detoxification from illegal drugs or from PRESCRIPTION DRUG ABUSE, such as BUPRENORPHINE or naltrexone. Other drugs may be used to limit the withdrawal symptoms that accompany detoxification, such as BENZODIAZEPINES or ANTIDEPRESSANTS.

Therapies that may help Many patients who were addicted to drugs and who have undergone detoxification usually need psychotherapy to stay off drugs. The therapist can help the patient to learn new coping mechanisms to reduce the risk of a RELAPSE.

Detoxification from Nonmedical Uses of Prescription Drugs

Some individuals become addicted to prescription drugs because of the misuse of these drugs, including pain medications that are abused such as OXYCODONE, OXYCONTIN, or HYDROCODONE or ALPRAZOLAM/ALPRAZOLAM XR (XANAX/XANAX XR). They may have abused their own medications or may have abused medications that were prescribed to others. Some individuals who are addicted steal prescription pads from doctors and write their own prescriptions. They are usually caught and then charged with this crime.

See also NARCOTICS; PRESCRIPTION DRUG ABUSE; REHABILITATION; SCHEDULED DRUGS.

Collins, Eric D., M.D., et al. "Anesthesia-Assisted vs Buprenorphine- or Clonidine-Assisted Heroin Detoxification and Naltrexone Induction: A Randomized Trial." *Journal of the American Medical Association* 294, no. 8 (August 24/31, 2005): 903–913.

O'Connor, Patrick G., M.D. "Methods of Detoxification and Their Role in Treating Patients with Opioid Dependence." *Journal of the American Medical Association* 294, no. 8 (August 24/31, 2005): 961–963.

dextromethorphan A substance with cough-suppressing capabilities that is found in some COUGH

SYRUPS and cold medicines. Sometimes dextromethorphan is used as an adulterant in illegal drugs, particularly with METHYLENEDIOXYMETHAMPETAMINE (MDMA/ECSTACY).

Dextromethorphan is available to be taken orally in lozenges, tablets, capsules, and cough syrups. Medications that include this drug should not be taken by individuals who are also taking monoamine oxide inhibitors (MAOIs) or antidepressants that are selective serotonin reuptake inhibitors (SSRIs). The combination could induce serotonin syndrome, which is characterized by cardiac arrhythmia, hypertension, and fever. It should also be noted that dextromethorphan increases the action of antihistamines, ANTIPSYCHOTICS, and alcohol, and the combination should be avoided whenever possible.

At normal recommended doses, dextromethorphan does not affect the central nervous system, and few people experience any adverse effects, although some may experience a slight drowsiness or nausea. With the higher doses of drugs used "recreationally" by abusers, however, dextromethorphan *is* a central nervous system depressant, and it may induce euphoria, heightened mood, and increased perceptual awareness.

Abusive dosages may also cause visual and auditory HALLUCINATIONS, altered time perception, confusion, and decreased sexual performance. In the worst case, dextromethorphan abuse may cause brain damage and even death.

Some pharmacies will not sell drugs with dextromethorphan to minors because they are concerned about possible abuse.

Dangerous Combinations at High Dosages

Often dextromethorphan is sold with cold remedies that include other substances that can be dangerous when large dosages are ingested but are safe at the indicated dosage. For example, if the preparation includes both dextromethorphan and guaifenesin, this combination at high dosages can cause extreme nausea and vomiting. In addition, a high dosage of the combination of dextromethorphan and chlorpheniramine can cause seizures and loss of consciousness.

With regular use of abusively high levels of dextromethorphan, the individual may develop a mild PSYCHOLOGICAL DEPENDENCE to the drug. If the usage abruptly ceases, the individual may experience DEPRESSION and INSOMNIA.

See also COUGH SYRUP.

National Highway Traffic Safety Administration. *Drugs and Human Performance Fact Sheets.* Washington, D.C.: National Highway Traffic Safety Administration, 2004.

diazepam (Valium)   A sedating drug that is also used to treat ANXIETY DISORDERS. It is a drug in the category of BENZODIAZEPINE medications. Discovered by Leo Sternbach in 1963 at Roche, a large global pharmaceuticals company, it became one of the most popularly prescribed drugs ever marketed. At its peak in 1978, more than 2 billion diazepam pills were sold to consumers worldwide that year.

Diazepam is a Schedule IV drug under the CONTROLLED SUBSTANCES ACT. Some individuals who have chronic anxiety disorders may take this drug on a regular basis. Others may use it to overcome their phobias with regard to experiences that they must undergo, such as those who are claustrophobic and must have a magnetic resonance imaging (MRI) test in which they would be enclosed or those who fear flying on a plane yet who need to fly. The drug may also be given to patients who are fearful of dental treatment or other medical procedures in which the patient remains awake, albeit sedated.

In addition to the antianxiety effect, diazepam and other benzodiazepines have a significant amnesiac effect: that is, these drugs can cause a degree of amnesia. This effect is frequently thought to be desirable for surgical procedures but can create considerable difficulty for individuals who use or abuse the drug. Episodes of amnesia, similar to alcoholic blackouts, are common with high doses of benzodiazepines.

Diazepam can become addictive, particularly when it is used nonmedically as a drug of abuse.

See also ALPRAZOLAM/ALPRAZOLAM XR (XANAX/ XANAX XR); ANTIDEPRESSANTS; DEPENDENCE, DRUG; PRESCRIPTION DRUG ABUSE; SCHEDULED DRUGS.

diet drugs   Prescribed or over-the-counter (OTC) drugs that are taken to treat individuals for obesity. They are also called anorectic drugs. Some individuals abuse prescribed or OTC diet pills, often in a rush to become slender sooner than would be medically safe. Some individuals misuse laxatives in order to lose weight, using them inappropriately as diet drugs. (It is also true that some OTC drugs have laxativelike qualities.)

Many individuals who use diet drugs are not obese or even overweight, a matter of some concern to medical professionals and others. One study reported in the *Annals of Internal Medicine* found that about half of the consumers using diet drugs in 1996–98 were below the recommended minimal weight *before* they began using them. Such people may have EATING DISORDERS, such as anorexia nervosa or bulimia nervosa. Diet drugs are inappropriate for individuals who are underweight or who need to lose only a small amount of weight.

Prescribed diet drugs may be taken legally when prescribed by a physician who carefully monitors the patient; however, diet drugs that are also AMPHETAMINES have a potential for abuse or dependence; that is why they are SCHEDULED DRUGS under the CONTROLLED SUBSTANCES ACT. Despite this legal control, prescribed diet pills are actively marketed and sold on illegal Internet pharmacies, which often offer such drugs to consumers without requiring any prescription from a medical doctor. Often these drugs are purchased from individuals in other countries, and they may be adulterated with other substances. (See INTERNET DRUG TRAFFICKING/ILLEGAL PHARMACIES.)

Individuals have sought to lose weight by using medications for many years. Amphetamines were first approved by the Food and Drug Administration (FDA) as treatments for obesity in 1947; Desoxyn and Hydrin were approved. In the 1960s, a variety of amphetamines were used as weight loss drugs; however, physicians discovered that when the drugs were discontinued, individuals regained weight. In addition, amphetamines were (and are) dangerous for many individuals because of the risk for addiction.

In the 1990s, on the basis of several studies of fenfluramine and phentermine, a combination of medications (often referred to as "fen-phen") used to achieve weight loss, the numbers of prescriptions for these drugs exploded, and it is estimated that 14 million prescriptions for these drugs were written from 1995 to 1997, until fenfluramine was withdrawn from the market as dangerous to those at risk for heart disease. Phenteramine may still be prescribed as of this writing.

Common Prescribed Diet Medications

Several nonscheduled medications may be prescribed to treat obesity in addition to amphetamines. Sibutramine (Meridia) and orlistat (Xenical) are two nonamphetamine medications that have been approved by the FDA for the treatment of obesity. Sibutramine and other prescribed or over-the-counter diet drugs are used to suppress an individual's appetite, while orlistat inhibits the absorption of some fats by the digestive system. Some studies have shown that these medications may achieve moderate weight loss (about 10 pounds) over the course of a year, particularly when combined with weight loss counseling.

Other common diet pills are benzphetamine (Didrex), diethylpropion (Tenuate, Tepanil), mazindol (Sanorex, Mazanor), phedimetrazine (Bontril, Prelu-27), and phentermine (Lonamin, Fastin, Adipex). All of these drugs are either in Schedule III or Schedule IV of the CONTROLLED SUBSTANCES ACT.

New Diet Drugs May Be Effective for Those Who Need Them

New diet medications are under development as of this writing. For example, studies have shown that rimonabant, a selective blocker for the newly discovered cannabinoid CBI receptors in the central nervous system and the peripheral tissues, such as in the fatty tissue, muscle, and the liver and gastrointestinal tract, is effective for the treatment of both obesity and nicotine dependence. (CBI receptors are involved in the immune system.)

Some experts believe that the endocannibinoid system is implicated in major forms of addictive behavior, such as drug use, smoking, and excessive eating. Rimonabant (Acomplia) is under study as a possible drug therapy for individuals with drug dependence.

With regard to obesity and this system, Luc F. Van Gaal and his colleagues in a study for the *Lancet* in 2005 said, "Insights into the endocannibinoid system have been derived from studies in animals with genetic deletion of CB_1 [a cannibinoid receptor], which have a lean phenotype and are resistant to diet-induced obesity and associated insulin resistance produced by a highly palatable high-fat diet."

The *Lancet* study revealed that 20 mg of rimonabant, combined with a low-calorie diet, resulted in a significant decease of weight and waist circumference over a one-year period.

Other studies, such as reported in the *Journal of the American Medical Association* in 2006, further indicated that rimonabant was effective in decreasing weight and improving cardiometabolic risk factors among overweight and obese patients. According to this report, treatment with 20 mg per day of rimonabant plus dietary changes produced "modest but sustained reductions in weight and waist circumference and favorable changes in cardiometabolic risk factors."

See also PRESCRIPTION DRUG ABUSE; SCHEDULED DRUGS.

Colman, Eric. "Anorectics on Trial: A Half Century of Federal Regulation of Prescription Appetite Suppressants." *Annals of Internal Medicine* 143 (2005): 380–385.

Joseph, Donald E., et al., eds. *Drugs of Abuse.* Washington, D.C.: U.S. Department of Justice, 2005.

Pi-Sunyer, F. Xavier, M.D., et al. "Effect of Rimonabant, a Cannabinoid-1 Receptor Blocker, on Weight and Cardiometabolic Risk Factors in Overweight or Obese Patients." *Journal of the American Medical Association* 295, no. 7 (February 15, 2006): 761–775.

Van Gaal, Luc F., et al. "Effects of the Cannabinoid-1 Receptor Blocker Rimonabant on Weight Reduction and Cardiovascular Risk Factors in Overweight Patients: 1-Year Experience from the RIO-Europe Study." *The Lancet* 365 (April 16, 2005): 1,389–1,397.

disulfiram (Antabuse)   An oral drug that is taken once daily and has been used since about the mid-1950s to treat ALCOHOLISM. Some experts continue to use disulfiram as an aversive therapy and a form of behavior modification with the goal of causing patients to avoid alcohol altogether, and according to the Substance Abuse and Mental Health Services Administration, 17 percent of treatment facilities in the United States used disulfiram in 2003.

Alcohol consumption while on disulfiram is extremely unpleasant, causing severe nausea and vomiting. Disulfiram causes profuse vomiting even if the individual inadvertently consumes even a tiny amount of alcohol, such as alcohol that may be used in food preparation, and thus the person taking disulfiram must advise others that alcohol makes him or her violently ill. Some researchers have found that disulfiram is also effective at treating COCAINE dependence (addiction).

Disulfiram prevents the liver from metabolizing alcohol, and thus if even a tiny amount of alcohol is consumed, the drug causes a toxic buildup of acetaldehyde in the bloodstream. Some experts believe that it is this particular buildup that causes the nausea and vomiting that are the primary side effects of the drug. (Note that disulfiram administration is one of the few cases of a drug that is prescribed specifically *because of* its side effects, rather than despite them.)

Even the topical use of alcohol (alcohol placed on the skin) may induce violent vomiting in the patient who is taking disulfiram; for that reason it is very important for disulfiram users to wear a medical bracelet that emergency workers can clearly see, since often one of the first acts of an emergency worker is to rub alcohol on the skin in order to start an intravenous line. Emergency medical technicians and physicians rarely have time to search for an emergency identification card in a wallet or a purse, but they can quickly observe an emergency bracelet or necklace worn by the injured or ill person.

Some studies have shown that the alcohol in shaving lotion alone has induced the vomiting response in patients. Many household products must be avoided by the patient taking disulfiram, and even the smell of paint can induce a toxic reaction in some.

As a result of these side effects, many patients refuse to take disulfiram. Frequently disulfiram must be administered by a pharmacist or a medical worker to ensure the drug is taken. This situation may occur when the disulfiram was court-ordered as a result of a crime committed while the individual was under the influence of alcohol and was subsequently determined to be an alcoholic.

Other Side Effects In addition to severe vomiting, should patients on disulfiram also ingest alcohol, these additional side effects may occur

- blurred vision
- chest pain
- dilation (narrowing) of the blood vessels, leading to skin flushing, and a sharp drop in blood pressure
- headache (severe)
- rapid heartbeat
- weakness

Side Effects of Concern Doctors should be contacted immediately if a patient who is taking disulfiram experiences any of the following side effects:

- dark urine
- eye pain or vision changes
- numbness and tingling or pain is the hands and feet
- mood changes
- light-colored or grayish stools
- severe stomach pain
- yellowing of eyes or skin

Pros and Cons of Disulfiram

Considerable controversy surrounds the use of disulfiram; proponents believe in its efficacy and dissenters state that the drug's side effects are too severe.

Those who support the use of disulfiram say that patients will ultimately develop a lasting aversion to alcohol, and that while they use the drug, doing so helps them greatly with abstinence. Some experts believe that disulfiram may be most effective among highly motivated and high-functioning alcoholics, or it may be a useful therapy until other therapy programs can be provided.

Dissenters say that the drug is an archaic form of therapy that does not work for many patients because it does not reduce or eliminate the CRAVING for alcohol; nor does it address the underlying causes of an individual's alcoholism. Dissenters

believe that other forms of therapy are more effective, such as receiving treatment in a treatment facility and/or receiving help from self-help groups, such as Alcoholics Anonymous.

Who Should Avoid Disulfiram

Individuals who have the following medical problems should not be prescribed disulfiram:

- asthma or lung diseases
- diabetes
- heart or blood vessel diseases
- hypothyroidism (low thyroid levels)
- kidney disease
- liver disease or cirrhosis of the liver
- any seizure disorder
- a severe PSYCHIATRIC DISORDER, such as DEPRESSION
- skin allergies

Medication Interactions with Disulfiram

Patients who are taking some medications should avoid disulfiram altogether or have the dosages of their other medications changed, depending on the particular medication. For example, patients who are taking the antiseizure drug phenytoin (Dilantin) may need their dosage changed. Patients who are taking anticoagulants (blood thinners) may also need a medication dosage adjustment. Metronidazole (Flagyl) should be avoided completely by patients who are taking disulfiram.

See also ACAMPROSATE (CAMPRAL); ADDICTION/ DEPENDENCE; ALCOHOL ABUSE/DEPENDENCE; DETOXIFICATION; NALTREXONE (REVIA).

Gwinnell, Esther, M.D., and Christine Adamec. *The Encyclopedia of Addictions and Addictive Behaviors.* New York: Facts On File, 2005.

Vocci, Frank J., and Ahmed Elkasef. "Pharmacotherapy and Other Treatments for Cocaine Abuse and Dependence." *Current Opinion in Psychiatry* 18, no. 3 (May 2005): 265–270.

diversion, drug The misuse of scheduled prescription drugs, which are purchased, given to others, or stolen or received as stolen goods. Drugs such as painkilling narcotics are often diverted, as are DEPRESSANTS, STIMULANTS, and other types of medications. Drug diversion can be highly profitable, and diverted scheduled prescription drugs may sell for many times more than what pharmacies charge for a legitimate prescription. Some studies have shown that adolescents who have both ATTENTION DEFICIT HYPERACTIVITY DISORDER (ADHD) and CONDUCT DISORDER or a substance use disorder are more likely to sell or misuse prescribed drugs than other individuals. (An alternate meaning of diversion is to provide special programs such as DRUG COURTS to help drug offenders stay out of jail.)

Some specific drugs, such as OxyCONTIN, a narcotic painkiller, and METHYLPHENIDATE (RITALIN/CONCERTA/FOCALIN, ETC.), a drug that is often prescribed to children and adolescents who have ADHD, are also diverted. In addition, Darvocet and Tylenol 3, both prescribed analgesics, are drugs of diversion. ANABOLIC STEROIDS are often diverted. Antianxiety drugs such as ALPRAZOLAM/ALPRAZOLAM XR (XANAX/XANAX XR) are sometimes diverted.

According to the National Survey on Drug Use and Health, from 2003 to 2004, the nonmedical use of some SCHEDULED DRUGS increased significantly, such as specific pain relievers including Vicodin or Lorcet (HYDROCODONE with acetaminophen). Drug abuse in this category increased from a lifetime use of 15.0 percent among adult ages 18 to 25 years old to 16.5 percent in 2004. Other drugs, such as those including OXYCODONE (Percocet, Percodan, and Tylox), increased in lifetime prevalence from 7.8 percent to 8.7 percent.

Abuse of products containing hydrocodone increased from 16.3 percent to 17.4 percent, and OxyContin abuse increased from 3.6 percent to 4.3 percent. Abuse of products containing oxycodone increased from 8.9 percent to 10.1 percent.

According to the National Survey on Drug Use and Health, in 2004, 6 million people in the United States used prescribed drugs nonmedically, including 4.4 million who abused prescribed pain relievers, 1.6 million who used tranquilizers, 1.2 million who used stimulants, and 0.3 million who used sedatives. Although most street drug abuse decreased among young adults ages 18–25 years over the period 2003 to 2004, the nonmedical lifetime use of prescription drugs showed little change. It was 6.1 percent in 2004 compared to 6.0 percent in 2003 and 5.4 percent in 2002. Clearly, the demand for such drugs remains high, and thus drug diversion is likely to continue.

Some physicians are so concerned about drug diversion that they will not prescribe any scheduled medications, and some experts worry that patients in severe pain may be seriously undermedicated. (See PAIN MANAGEMENT AND NARCOTIC MEDICATIONS.)

Key Means of Prescribed Drug Diversion

Drug diversion essentially includes six primary means of transferring drugs for medical purposes to individuals who use them for abuse, including the following:

- prescription forgery or fraud
- doctor shopping
- Internet pharmacies (See INTERNET DRUG TRAFFICKING/ILLEGAL PHARMACIES)
- illicit prescribing practices of some physicians
- drug theft
- personal sales of their own legitimately prescribed drugs (often by adolescents or young adults)

Prescription forgery or fraud Most patients do not forge or alter the prescriptions that they are given for legitimate medical problems, but some patients who are addicted to prescribed drugs, particularly scheduled drugs, will take whatever action they feel is necessary to obtain the drug that they need. Patients may take the prescription that a doctor has written and then change the quantity that the doctor ordered to a greater number than the physician intended. In addition, some individuals steal blank prescription pads or even create their own prescription pads.

Fraud also plays a role in drug diversion. Some patients have attempted to call in their own prescriptions by phone to pharmacies by impersonating physicians.

Pharmacists themselves sometimes become involved in drug diversion and use their database of physicians to "write" prescriptions for drugs that they sell illegally. Pharmacists or pharmacy technicians may also skim off prescriptions, for instance, they give a patient a smaller quantity of pills than were prescribed and then pocket a portion for self-use or resale. This allows the pharmacy count to be accurate while leaving some patients in difficulty with an inadequate medication quantity. In some cases, physicians, dentists, and other health care workers who have access to scheduled drugs divert the drugs to themselves or others who should not have them.

Doctor shopping Some patients who abuse or are dependent on prescription drugs make appointments with several different physicians, seeking a prescription for the same or a similar drug from each doctor, thus obtaining multiple prescriptions. They may go from doctor to doctor seeking a prescription until they find one who will prescribe the drug that they seek. This is known as "doctor shopping."

Because of this and related problems with prescription drug abuse, about half the states in the United States have prescription drug monitoring programs, which capture data on all prescriptions for scheduled drugs. In this way, the monitoring agency can identify patients who are receiving multiple prescriptions of the same drug.

In 2005, President George W. Bush signed the National All Schedules Prescription Electronic Reporting Act of 2005, a new program offering financial grants to states that create or enhance the electronic monitoring of scheduled prescription drugs.

It should be noted that sometimes patients who experience severe pain, such as caused by cancer or chronic serious illnesses, consult two or more doctors because they are undertreated for pain and seek adequate pain relief. (See PSEUDOADDICTION.) As a result, it should not be assumed automatically that individuals who see several doctors for the same complaint are invariably seeking drugs for abuse. However, sometimes even patients who have legitimate medical complaints divert drugs. In one highly unusual case reported in Arizona, a genuinely ill patient consulted physicians in several states and was prescribed an estimated 8,000 pills in one year, which were then sold on the street in Maryland.

Internet pharmacies Although a few legitimate pharmacies offer pharmacy services over the Internet, requiring a prescription from a medical doctor, there are also many Web sites that offer virtually every drug, including Schedule II drugs such as OXYCONTIN, HYDROCODONE, and other narcotics, to consumers without a prescription. Often all these sites require to order their prescribed drugs is a valid credit card, and they then send the drugs directly to the consumer. Some adolescents have ordered illegal drugs through the Internet, usually using a parent's credit card. It is difficult to control this form of drug diversion; however, federal and state agencies are seeking solutions to this problem.

Illicit practices of some doctors Although most doctors do not overprescribe scheduled drugs to their patients, there are some physicians who will write a prescription for scheduled drugs for nearly any patient and who often fail to monitor the drug use of these patients.

This is very risky behavior for the doctor, who usually will eventually attract the notice of the Drug Enforcement Administration and/or other federal and state agencies. Doctors stand to lose their right to prescribe scheduled drugs or even to lose their medical licenses. In some cases, physicians have been jailed for prescribing very large quantities of scheduled drugs, with little or no oversight. Some physicians have been indicted for knowingly participating in Internet pharmacy sales of controlled drugs for illegal purposes.

According to data from *Under the Counter: The Diversion and Abuse of Controlled Prescription Drugs in the U.S.,* 16 percent of the pharmacists who were surveyed said that doctors who "knowingly divert controlled prescription drugs" were the primary cause of drug diversion.

Drug theft Some individuals steal scheduled drugs, whether from pharmacies, clinics, or individuals who are patients with legitimate prescriptions. Drugs are also stolen from pharmaceutical warehouses, and in some cases, replaced with counterfeit drugs, although the extent of this problem is unknown. Some drugs that have been stolen from pharmacies have been OxyContin, Darvocet, and Soma (carisprodol). Sometimes drugs are stolen from veterinarians or dentists.

Some pharmacies in supermarkets or other locations refuse to carry the medications that they believe are the most likely to be stolen, such as some narcotics.

It is also true that some individuals raid the bathroom medicine cabinets of their parents, relatives, or clients, seeking drugs that they can abuse or sell. Selling narcotics can be particularly profitable for some individuals willing to risk the high probability of arrest. Individuals who take narcotics for pain management should not keep these drugs in the medicine cabinet but should locate them elsewhere, preferably in a locked location.

Personal drug sales of legitimately prescribed drugs Some adolescents and young adults sell or trade their own scheduled drugs with others. In addition, studies have shown that some students who have ATTENTION DEFICIT HYPERACTIVITY DISORDER who take stimulants, particularly Ritalin, report that other individuals sometimes forcibly take their medications from them.

In some cases, patients receiving Medicaid, a medical program for low-income adults and children who qualify for it, may legally obtain their prescriptions at very low or no cost, then sell them on the street.

Research on Drug Diversion

The National Center on Addiction and Substance Abuse (CASA) at Columbia University performed a three-year study on the diversion and abuse of prescription drugs with the potential for abuse and addiction, publishing their findings in their 2005 report, *Under the Counter: The Diversion and Abuse of Controlled Prescription Drugs in the U.S.* The organization also surveyed physicians and pharmacists on diversion issues, incorporating the results in the report.

One finding was not surprising: that central nervous system depressants, stimulants, and opioids are abused by those who want a "mind-altering" experience, while drugs such as anabolic steroids are abused by those such as athletes who wish to become more muscular and/or improve their physical performance.

Pharmacists' responses in the CASA survey In the CASA survey of pharmacists reported in *Under the Counter: The Diversion and Abuse of Controlled Prescription Drugs in the U.S.*, 89 percent of pharmacists said that doctor shopping was the primary method of drug diversion and 75 percent said forging or altering prescriptions was a key method of diver-

sion. Patient manipulation or deception of doctors was named by 65 percent. (Pharmacists were allowed to choose more than one method of drug diversion.) In addition, 35 percent of the pharmacists said that theft of prescription pads was a method of diversion.

According to the CASA survey of pharmacists, 29 percent of the pharmacists reported theft of scheduled drugs in the past five years, and 21 percent said they did not stock some scheduled drugs because of the risk of drug diversion. When pharmacists were asked for the source of most drug diversion, 52 percent said the diversion was caused by patients, 15 percent named Internet pharmacies as the driving force, 10 percent said other pharmacies (hospital/clinic or retail) caused most of the problem, and 10 percent said most diversion was caused by physicians.

A broad majority of the respondents (89 percent) said that finding mistakes or irregularities in a prescription led to a suspicion that a prescription was forged. If they suspected a prescription was forged, 83 percent said that they would contact the prescribing doctor. The patient's own behavior was a clue to many pharmacists that drug diversion might play a role; for example, 78 percent said that a patient's nervous or unusual behavior was an indicator of possible drug diversion.

A majority also said that they noted the method of payment for the drug, and if the patient paid cash instead of using insurance, 53 percent of the pharmacists were suspicious. Many pharmacists (83 percent) reported having refused to dispense a drug in the past year because of concern or suspicion of drug diversion

When asked what they would do if they suspected drug diversion, 93 percent of the pharmacists said they would call the prescribing physician and 77 percent said they would refuse to fill the prescription. Other actions pharmacists said that they would take would be to document the incident (71 percent), contact the police (48 percent), counsel the patient on the dangers of drug abuse (34 percent), and confront the patient with their suspicions (32 percent).

The pharmacists also provided potential signs of diversion, such as the following:

- The doctor's handwriting is too good.
- The quantities or dosages of the drug are not in line with what most doctors order.
- The prescription appears photocopied rather than an original.
- The directions on the prescription include no abbreviations.

Another sign of the diversion of drugs is when a prescribing physician writes prescriptions for antagonistic drugs at the same time, such as both stimulants and depressants. Although there are some situations that require this combination, it sends a red flag for closer inspection to the pharmacist.

Doctors' responses to the CASA survey on drug diversion The CASA survey of doctors reported in *Under the Counter: The Diversion and Abuse of Controlled Prescription Drugs in the U.S.* provided valuable information based on the knowledge and perceptions of physicians. For example, 59 percent of the doctors said patients accounted for most of the drug diversion, while 12 percent said that it could be attributed to doctors, and 9 percent named Internet pharmacies as a primary problem. Two-thirds of the doctors said that they had diagnosed an adult with a prescription drug abuse problem in the past 12 months, and 15 percent reported that they had diagnosed an adolescent with such a problem.

The doctors were asked to name the three most common methods of drug diversion; an overwhelming 96 percent named doctor shopping, while 88 percent cited patient deception or manipulation of doctors, and 69 percent named forged or altered prescriptions. Theft of prescription pads from doctors' offices was a problem cited by 17 percent, while 9 percent cited physicians who knowingly diverted scheduled drugs.

Almost half of the doctors (47 percent) reported that patients have pressured them in the past to prescribe a scheduled drug, although doctors ages 50 and younger reported experiencing this problem significantly more frequently than did the older doctors. Twenty percent of the doctors said that pharmacists called them frequently to report their suspicions of drug abuse or fraud.

The surveyed doctors said there were three primary manipulative methods that patients used to try to convince the physician to prescribe a scheduled drug. One tactic was to fake medical problems. Some patients went so far as to self-induce bleeding by using blood thinners or self-inflicted wounds. Another tactic was to fake psychological symptoms, such as anxiety, fatigue, insomnia, and depression. A third tactic was to request refills sooner than should have been needed.

The doctors were asked what they would do if they suspected a patient of abusing or diverting a drug, and the physicians provided several responses. Eighty-nine percent said they would document the incident, while 80 percent said they would confront the patient, and 72 percent said they would counsel the patient. Few (11 percent) chose contacting the police as an option.

The doctors reported potential signs of diversion or drug abuse. Some of these signs included a patient's reporting textbook symptoms of a medical problem or having no regular doctor. Another indicator to the doctors of potential diversion or drug abuse was a patient's requesting a specific scheduled drug and being unwilling to try another nonscheduled drug. Other signs were patients showing no interest in their diagnosis and failing to keep appointments or to obtain the diagnostic tests that the doctor ordered. Physical signs of drug abuse were also an indicator, such as "track marks" on the skin and scars on the neck, underarm, forearm, wrist, ankle, or foot.

Reporting medications as lost is another tactic that is sometimes used by patients to obtain early refills.

Abusers of Prescription Drugs

Diversion is particularly a problem among adolescents, who are easily influenced by PEER PRESSURE. In some cases, adolescents steal drugs from their parents and give or sell them to their friends. Older individuals may also receive diverted drugs or engage in stealing, prescription tampering, and illegal purchases of drugs over the Internet. Many abusers use two or more substances; for example, diverted Ritalin is often used in combination with alcohol and/or other drugs. (See PRESCRIPTION DRUG ABUSE.)

Types of abusers   According to Zacny and colleagues in their article on opioid abusers of prescription drugs, there are four major types of abusers: (1) those who abuse or depend on *only* prescription drugs and not other drugs, (2) those who normally abuse illegal opioids such as heroin and will use prescribed opioids when they cannot obtain heroin, (3) those who primarily use other drugs but who sometimes use prescription opioids to gain an enhanced or different type of euphoria, and (4) those who have legitimate medical problems and sometimes develop a dependence on opioids. (Note that most experts agree that patients who experience severe pain and have no past history of abuse or dependence usually do *not* develop an addiction to a prescribed scheduled drug.)

College students and prescription drug abuse   In a study reported in 2005 in *Addiction*, the researchers sampled nearly 11,000 college students in 2001 on their abuse of prescribed stimulants, including Adderall, Dexedrine, and Ritalin. The researchers found that higher rates of abuse were found in students in northeastern colleges with competitive admission standards. They also discovered that abuse was more common among students who were white males. Members of fraternities and sororities were more likely to abuse stimulants than other students. In addition, abusers were more likely to report that they also abused alcohol, cocaine, marijuana and Ecstasy.

Prevention of Drug Diversion

Experts report that there are several major ways to decrease prescription drug diversion, including the implementation of state prescription drug monitoring programs; further education of health care professionals, such as doctors and nurses; and plans to prevent theft and fraud, such as preventing theft from pharmacies and also prosecution of illegal Internet pharmacies.

OxyContin, a timed-release form of oxycodone, was partly developed to reduce its abuse potential because the medication is gradually delivered over time. Unfortunately, abusers subsequently discovered that the drug could be crushed and swallowed or injected, so that the entire drug would be absorbed at once.

See also ADOLESCENTS; COLLEGE STUDENTS; HYDRO-CODONE; PRESCRIPTION DRUG ABUSE; PRESCRIPTION DRUG MONITORING PROGRAMS, STATES WITH; YOUNG ADULTS.

Kraman, Pilar. *Prescription Drug Diversion.* Lexington, Ky.: The Council of State Governments, April 2004.

McCabe, Sean Esteban, et al. "Non-Medical Use of Prescription Stimulants among US College Students: Prevalence and Correlates from a National Study." *Addiction* 100, no. 1 (January 2005): 96–106.

McCabe, S. E., C. J. Teter, and C. J. Boyd. "The Use, Misuse and Diversion of Prescription Stimulants among Middle and High School Students." *Substance Use and Misuse* 39, no. 7 (2004): 1,095–1,116.

National Center on Addiction and Substance Abuse (CASA) at Columbia University. *Under the Counter: The Diversion and Abuse of Controlled Prescription Drugs in the U.S.* New York: National Center on Addiction and Substance Abuse at Columbia University, July 2005.

Office of Applied Studies, Substance Abuse and Mental Health Services Administration. *Overview of Findings from the 2004 National Survey on Drug Use and Health.* Rockville, Md.: Department of Health and Human Services Publication Number SMA 05-4061, September 2005.

Poulin, Christiane. "Medical and Nonmedical Stimulant Use Among Adolescents: From Sanctioned to Unsanctioned Use." *Canadian Medical Association Journal* 165, no. 8 (2001): 1,039–1,044.

Zacny, James, et al. "College on Problems of Drug Dependence Taskforce on Prescription Opioid Non-Medical Use and Abuse: Position Statement." *Drug and Alcohol Dependence* 69 (2003): 215–232.

domestic violence, associated with alcohol and/or drugs   Harm caused to family members, particularly spouses and significant others, that is linked to the abuse of or dependence on alcohol and/or drugs. Sometimes the term *domestic violence* is used to refer exclusively to the victimization of adult family members, such as spouses or partners who are abused by other adult members.

Numerous studies have demonstrated that women who abuse alcohol and/or drugs are more likely to be victimized in incidents of domestic violence as well as in cases of SEXUAL ASSAULTS.

Women who have partners who abuse alcohol and/or drugs have an increased risk for being injured by acts of violence. According to a study of 256 women who were intentionally injured by others, reported in 1999 in the *New England Journal of Medicine* by Demetrios N. Kyriacou and colleagues, the researchers found characteristics that were closely associated with an increased risk for suffering from violence, including alcohol abuse among their current or former male partners (with a 3.6 times greater risk than without alcohol abuse) and drug use among their partners (a 3.5 times greater risk).

Other lesser associated factors were male partners who were unemployed, who had received less than a high school education, and who were former husbands, estranged husbands, or former boyfriends of the women.

In another study reported in the *New England Journal of Medicine* in 1999, the researchers studied 405 adolescent girls and women who had been intentionally injured by others. The researchers found that the male partners of the injured women were significantly more likely to have abused COCAINE than the male partners of the control group; however, about half of the injuries were perpetrated by individuals other than the women's partners. The researchers also found that the women's own use of illicit drugs and alcohol increased the risk of violence at the hands of their partners or others.

Say the authors, "Women in this urban, low-income community face violence from both partners and other persons. Substance abuse, particularly cocaine use, is a significant correlate of violent injuries."

See also CHILD ABUSE; CODEPENDENCY; HOMICIDE; FAMILY, EFFECT ON; INJURIES, RELATED TO ALCOHOL AND/OR DRUG ABUSE; GENETIC PREDISPOSITIONS AND ENVIRONMENTAL EFFECTS IN SUBSTANCE USE DISORDERS; HOMICIDE; VIOLENCE.

Tjaden, Patricia, and Nancy Thoennes. *Full Report of the Prevalence, Incidence, and Consequences of Violence against Women: Findings from the National Violence against Women Survey.* Washington, D.C.: Office of Justice Programs, U.S. Department of Justice, November 2000.

driving   See IMPAIRED DRIVING, INVOLVEMENT OF ALCOHOL AND/OR DRUGS.

dronabinil (Marinol)   An oral synthetic form of 9-tetrahydrocannibinol (THC), the intoxicating substance that is found in MARIJUANA. It is a Schedule III drug under the CONTROLLED SUBSTANCES ACT. Dronabinil is approved by the Food and Drug Administration (FDA) for the treatment of the anorexia and wasting away of people who have ACQUIRED IMMUNE DEFICIENCY SYNDROME (AIDS), as well as for the treatment of the nausea and vomiting associated with some forms of chemotherapy treatment for cancer. The drug is given to stimulate appetite and decrease nausea. Dronabinil was developed with the cooperation of the Drug Enforcement Administration (DEA) and was first approved by the FDA in 1985.

A related drug, Sativex, which is a liquid cannabis extract that patients spray under the tongue, was approved for use in Canada in 2005 for the neuropathic pain of multiple sclerosis, according to the *New England Journal of Medicine*. This drug includes dronabinil and cannabidiol, both ingredients in marijuana. The manufacturer is testing the drug for the pain of cancer and rheumatoid arthritis and for other uses.

Patients considering use of dronabinol should tell their doctors whether they have any allergies to marijuana or sesame oil. Studies have not been performed on pregnant women, but animal studies in which the animals were given high doses of dronabinil found the drug increased the risk of the death of a fetus. Women who are breastfeeding should know that the drug passes into human breast milk and can affect the nursing infant.

When patients first start taking dronabinil, they should avoid driving or operating equipment until they know how the drug affects them. Dronabinil may be very sedating to some patients. Patients taking the drug should avoid alcohol, marijuana, and other drugs that affect the central nervous system, such as sedatives or tricyclic antidepressants. Sedating cold medications may also interact with dronabinil.

Common side effects, which may disappear as the body adjusts to the drug, include dizziness, drowsiness, clumsiness, a false sense of well-being, nausea, trouble with thinking, and vomiting. Less common side effects are blurred vision, dryness of the mouth, restlessness, flushed face, a feeling of lightheadedness when getting up from a lying down or sitting position, and unusual fatigue or weakness.

Adverse side effects associated with toxic levels of dronabinil include DELUSIONS, HALLUCINATIONS, depression, anxiety, heart palpitations, and tachycardia (rapid heartbeat).

The drug should be used with caution by patients who have heart disease, new or worsened hypertension, or a history of substance abuse. The drug should also be used with care among patients who have DEPRESSION, SCHIZOPHRENIA, or mania, since it may exacerbate the psychiatric problem.

Advocates of smoking marijuana rather than taking dronabinil say that it is difficult to find the right dose of the drug and it may be overly sedating. However, the DEA bans all use of marijuana that is smoked, whether for medical purposes or recreational purposes. The federal ban against marijuana continues despite some state laws that allow certain patients to use marijuana for medical purposes. Federal law prevails over state law; however, enforcement by state officials may be less strict in states with medical marijuana laws.

Okie, Susan, M.D. "Medical Marijuana and the Supreme Court." *New England Journal of Medicine* 353, no. 7 (August 18, 2005): 648–651.

drug abuse   See ABUSE, DRUGS.

drug abuse and dependence and health problems Acute and chronic physical as well as psychological problems that stem from the abuse of or addiction to illegal drugs or some prescribed drugs, such as SCHEDULED DRUGS that are painkillers, sedatives, BENZODIAZEPINES, HALLUCINOGENIC DRUGS, or ANABOLIC STEROIDS. Some health problems that are caused by drug abuse and dependence are minor and transient, while others are more severe or even life-threatening. (See EMERGENCY TREATMENT.) Some individuals recover from their health problems if they discontinue use of the drug, while in other cases, the health problems will continue despite the disuse of the drug.

Many drug abusers use more than one type of drug at a time, such as a combination of alcohol and MARIJUANA or COCAINE and METHAMPHETAMINE.

Some users combine many different drugs, making it difficult for physicians to treat them when they arrive at a hospital emergency room with seizures, unconsciousness, or other serious conditions. Of course laboratory screening can be performed to detect the presence of drugs, but some patients arrive in a critical state, needing urgent attention. If others who were with the individual are aware of what drugs the ill person consumed, it is essential to tell health authorities so that they can best treat the ill patient. This information may mean the difference between life and death.

Different drugs vary greatly in their effects on the body; for example, the abuse of some categories of prescribed drugs, such as STIMULANTS like AMPHETAMINES, can cause rapid heartbeat, hyperthermia (high fever), high blood pressure, seizures, and mania. In the most extreme cases, the amphetamine abuser can experience a psychotic state known as an *amphetamine psychosis;* ACCIDENTAL OVERDOSE DEATHS have also resulted from use of amphetamines. Amphetamines are generally not prescribed to patients who have been diagnosed with BIPOLAR DISORDER because the drug may exacerbate or even cause a manic state. Amphetamine may induce anxiety or even an ANXIETY DISORDER in some individuals, and this problem is more likely to occur when the drug is abused at high dosages.

METHAMPHETAMINE, which is a lawful drug that is frequently synthesized illegally in CLANDESTINE LABORATORIES, provokes great concern among law enforcement authorities and medical personnel. This illegal form of the drug can cause the same physical effects as other forms of amphetamine, but it is far more likely to lead to aggressive behavior. Continued use of the drug may cause a heart attack, kidney failure, stroke, seizures, and lung damage.

The abuse of METHYLENEDIOXYMETHAMPHETAMINE (MDMA/ECSTASY) can cause a very rapid and escalating high fever, which, if untreated, can cause death. Other health risks with MDMA are heart attack, kidney failure, and brain damage.

In contrast, other drugs, such as DEPRESSANTS, are sedating, and abuse of these drugs may slow the heart rate and decrease the body temperature (hypothermia). Such drugs, when used illegally, can lead to unconsciousness or even coma or death when abused. Some examples of depressants are medications in the BENZODIAZEPINE category, such as ALPRAZOLAM (Xanax) and DIAZEPAM (Valium), as well as drugs in the category of BARBITURATES, including pentobarbital sodium (Nembutal) and butalbital (Fiorcet). Alcohol is also a depressant. Most narcotics act as depressants, including such drugs as HYDROCODONE, OXYCODONE, and OXYCONTIN.

Marijuana and HASHISH, both derived from the cannabis plant, are considered benign drugs by many people. However, when abused regularly, these drugs may lead to aggression and an increased risk for criminal behavior, especially among adolescents but also among YOUNG ADULTS and other users. There is also a risk for the development of paranoia and possible psychosis.

INHALANTS are another category of drugs that are very dangerous when misused. Some individuals die the first time that they abuse an inhalant, because the drug triggers erratic heart rhythms (arrhythmias) that lead to heart failure. Inhalants can also impair memory and cause vitamin deficiency and even organ damage.

Although used far more infrequently today than in past decades, HALLUCINOGENIC DRUGS continue to be dangerous to the health of users. Hallucinogens may elevate body temperature, blood pressure, and pulse. They may generate a feeling of euphoria. They may also cause convulsions, depression, and HALLUCINATIONS.

Individuals under the influence of a hallucinogenic drug, such as LYSERGIC ACID DIETHYLAMIDE (LSD), PHENCYCLIDINE, or MESCALINE, may believe themselves to have super powers and may engage in such acts as attempting to fly out of a tree or off a building, which may lead to broken bones, paralysis, or even death. They may also exhibit symptoms of paranoia. They are also more likely than others to engage in risky sexual behavior and fail to practice safe sex.

It should be noted that many people who abuse all types of drugs often also combine illicit drugs with alcohol, and this combination is dangerous and can be fatal. Some individuals use a combination of alcohol and drugs to commit SUICIDE; ACCIDENTAL OVERDOSE DEATHS also occur.

When individuals take their prescribed drugs in accordance with their physician's orders, they may experience side effects, but in most cases, they will gain a therapeutic benefit, such as pain relief, sedation, or stimulation, as with the stimulants that are prescribed to increase focus and concentration among individuals who have ATTENTION DEFICIT HYPERACTIVITY DISORDER.

In contrast, those who abuse prescription drugs or illegal drugs actively seek their intoxicating effects or, if they are addicted to the drug, seek to avoid the symptoms of WITHDRAWAL. As a result, they take higher than normal dosages of the drugs and often are not really sure of what dosage it is that they are taking, since there is little uniformity in illegal drugs. (See Table I for a description of the intoxicating effects of key categories of prescribed drugs and the side effects that may result from abuse.)

All drugs, when abused, can impair the individual's cognitive and physical abilities, thereby increasing the risk for injuries and car or motorcycle crashes. (See IMPAIRED DRIVING, INVOLVEMENT OF ALCOHOL AND/OR DRUGS; INJURIES, CAUSED BY ALCOHOL AND/OR ILLICIT DRUGS.)

Illnesses Caused or Worsened by Drug Abuse
Already existing disorders that are present, such as with the heart, kidneys, and most other organs and organ systems, can be severely exacerbated by drug abuse or dependence, depending on the particular drug. Some drugs may damage specific organs or organ systems. For example, many drugs are metabolized by the liver or the kidneys, and if these organs are already weak or impaired, then excessive and chronic drug abuse could lead to harm and even the failure of these organs.

Harmful effects to the brain Inhalant abuse may lead to brain damage, causing permanent memory loss as well as long-term or lifelong learning problems. (Psychiatric problems are discussed in a separate section of this essay.) The chronic abuse of MARIJUANA may cause deficits in short-term thinking, motivation, and memory.

Some drugs may lead to the development of neurological problems, such as seizures and memory loss or even strokes and/or brain damage. Drugs that may lead to neurological symptoms or disorders include COCAINE, GAMMA-HYDROXYBUTYRATE (GHB), INHALANTS, MARIJUANA, METHYLENEDIOXYMETHAMPHETAMINE (MDMA/ECSTASY), methamphetamine, and prescription stimulants. In addition, the

TABLE I: SELECTED DRUGS WITH POTENTIAL FOR ABUSE AND THEIR INTOXICATION EFFECTS/ POTENTIAL HEALTH CONSEQUENCES

Substances: Category and Name	DEA Schedule/ How Administered	Examples of Commercial and Street Names	Intoxication Effects/ Potential Health Consequences
Depressants			
Barbiturates	II, III, V/Injected, swallowed	Amytal, Nembutal, Seconal, Phenobarbital, butalbital; barbs, reds, red birds, phennies, tooies, yellows, yellow jackets	Reduced pain and anxiety; feeling of well-being; lowered inhibitions; slowed pulse and breathing; lowered blood pressure; poor concentration/confusion; fatigue; impaired coordination, memory, judgment; respiratory depression and arrest, addiction Also, for barbiturates: sedation, drowsiness/depression, unusual excitement, fever, irritability, poor judgment, slurred speech, dizziness
Benzodiazepines	IV/Swallowed	Ativan, Halcion, Librium, Restoril, Valium, Xanax; candy, downers, sleeping pills, tranks	
Flunitrazepam (Rohypnol)	IV/Swallowed, snorted	Rohypnol; forget-me pill, Mexican Valium, R2, Roche, roffies, rootinol, rope, rophies	For benzodiazepines: sedation, drowsiness/dizziness
Gamma-hydroxybutyric acid (GHB)	I/Oral		For flunitrazepam: visual and gastrointestinal disturbances, urinary retention, memory loss for the time under the drug's effects
			For GHB, anxiety, insomnia, tremors, delirium, convulsions, death
Dissociative anesthetic			
Ketamine	III/Injected, snorted, smoked	Ketalar, Ketaset cat Valium, K, Special K, vitamin K	Increased heart rate and blood pressure, impaired motor function/ memory loss; numbness, nausea/ vomiting
			Also for ketamine: at high doses: delirium, depression, respiratory depression, and arrest
Hallucinogens: MDMA, LSD, phencyclidine	I/Oral, smoked, snorted, injected	MDMA: Ecstasy, XTC, Adam LSD: Acid, microdot, sunshine, boomers Phencyclidine: PCP, angel dust	Increased body temperature, heightened senses; euphoria, increased pulse rate, elevated blood pressure, insomnia, loss of appetite, agitation, hallucinations, convulsions, depression, irritability, disorientation
			MDMA: teeth grinding and dehydration, muscle aches, depression, electrolyte imbalance, cardiac arrest, kidney failure, brain damage LSD and phencyclidine: inability to detect movement, feel pain, or remember events; altered perception of time and distance

Substances: Category and Name	DEA Schedule/ How Administered	Examples of Commercial and Street Names	Intoxication Effects/ Potential Health Consequences
Cannabis: marijuana, hashish and hashish oil	I/Smoked, oral	Marijuana: pot, grass, blunts, grass hashish and hashish oil: hash, hash oil	Euphoria, relaxed inhibitions, increased appetite, disorientation, fatigue, paranoia, possible psychosis
Inhalants			
Amyl and butyl nitrates	Not scheduled/ inhaled	Pearls, poppers, rush, locker room	Flushing, hypotension, headache, agitation
Nitrous oxide	Not scheduled/ inhaled	Laughing gas, balloons, whippets	Impaired memory, drunken behavior, slow-onset vitamin deficiency, organ damage, vomiting, respiratory depression, loss of consciousness, possible death
Other inhalants	Not scheduled/ inhaled	Not scheduled/adhesives, spray paint, hair spray, dry cleaning fluid, spot remover, lighter fluid	
Opioids and Morphine Derivatives (Narcotics)			
Codeine	II, III, IV/Injected, swallowed	Empirin with Codeine, Fiornal with Codeine, Robitussin A0C, Tylenol with Codeine: Captain Cody, Cody, schoolboy	Pain relief, euphoria, constricted pupils of the eyes, drowsiness/respiratory depression and arrest, slow and shallow breathing, clammy skin, nausea, confusion, constipation, sedation, unconsciousness, coma, tolerance, addiction, possible death
Fentanyl (This drug is also associated with sexual assaults)	II/Injected, smoked, snorted	Actiq, Duragesic, Sublimaze: Oralet, Innovar Apache, China girl, China white, dance fever, friend, goodfella, jackpot, murder 8, TNT, Tango and Cash	For codeine: less analgesia, sedation, and respiratory depression than morphine
Heroin	I/Injected, snorted, smoked	Horse, smack, black tar	
Morphine	II, III/Injected, swallowed, smoked	Roxanol, Duramorph; M, Ms-Contin Miss Emma, monkey, Oramorph white stuff	
Opium	II, III, V/Swallowed, smoked	Laudanum, paregoric; big O, black stuff, block, gum, hop	
Other opioid painkillers (oxycodone, meperidine, hydromorphone, hydrocodone, propoxyphene)	II, III, IV/Swallowed, injected, suppositories, chewed, crushed, snorted	Tylox, OxyContin, Percodan, Percocet; oxy 80s, oxycotton, oxycet, hillbilly heroin, percs. Demerol, meperideine hydrochloride: demmies, painkiller. Dilaudid: juice, dillies Vicodin, Lortab, Lorcet, Darvon, Darvocet	

(table continues)

TABLE I (continued)

Substances: Category and Name	DEA Schedule/ How Administered	Examples of Commercial and Street Names	Intoxication Effects/ Potential Health Consequences
Stimulants			
Amphetamines	II/Injected, swallowed, smoked, snorted	Biphetamine, Dexedrine: bennies, black beauties, crosses, hearts, LA turn-around, speed, truck drivers, uppers	Increased heart rate, blood pressure, metabolism; feelings of exhilaration, energy, increased mental alertness/ rapid or irregular heartbeat; reduced appetite; weight loss; heart failure. Also, for amphetamines: rapid breathing, hallucinations/tremor, loss of coordination; irritability, anxiousness, restlessness, delirium, panic, paranoia, impulsive behavior, aggressiveness, tolerance, addiction
Cocaine	II/Injected, smoked, snorted	Cocaine hydrochloride; blow, bump, C, candy, Charlie, coke, crack, flake, rock, show, toot	
Methamphet-amine	II/Injected, swal-lowed, smoked, snorted	Desoxyn; chalk, crank, crystal, fire, glass, go fast, ice, meth, speed	For cocaine: increased tempera-ture/chest pain, respiratory failure, nausea, abdominal pain, strokes, seizures, headaches, malnutrition
Methylpheni-date	II/Injected, swal-lowed, snorted	Ritalin; Concerta, Methylin JIF, MPH, R-ball, Skippy, the smart drug, vitamin R	For methamphetamine: aggression, violence, psychotic behavior/mem-ory loss, cardiac and neurological damage; impaired memory and learning, tolerance, kidney failure, stroke, seizures, lung damage
			For methylphenidate: increase or decrease in blood pressure, psy-chotic episodes/digestive problems, loss of appetite, weight loss
Other compounds			
Anabolic ste-roids	III/Injected, swallowed, applied to skin	Anadrol, Oxandrin Durabolin, Depo-Testoserone, Equipoise; roids, juice	No intoxication effects
			Hypertension, blood clotting and cholesterol changes, liver cysts and cancer, kidney cancer, hostility and aggression, acne; adolescents, pre-mature stoppage of growth; in males, prostate cancer, reduced sperm pro-duction, shrunken testicles, breast enlargement; in female, menstrual irregularities, development of beard and other masculine characteristics

Schedule I and II drugs have a high potential for abuse. These drugs require greater storage security, and there is a quota on manufacturing, among other restrictions. Schedule I drugs are available for research only and have no approved medical use; Schedule II drugs are available only by prescription (not refillable) and require a form for ordering. Schedule III and IV drugs are available by prescription, may have five refills in 6 months, and may be ordered by the doctor over the telephone. Most Schedule V drugs are available as over-the-counter (OTC) drugs.
Note: Taking drug by injection can increase the risk of infection through needle contamination with staphylococci, HIV, hepatitis, and other organisms.
Source: Adapted from data available from the Drug Enforcement Administration and the National Institute of Drug Abuse.

excessive abuse of barbiturates may cause delirium and seizures.

Benzodiazepines can cause drowsiness, slowed reaction times, poor judgment, and decreased impulse control. At higher doses, individuals may experience amnesiac episodes (blackouts) and confusion.

Damage to the Gastrointestinal System and the Liver The abuse of some drugs may harm the gastrointestinal system, causing inflammation of the stomach, severe chronic constipation, and ulcers. Drugs that may cause gastrointestinal harm include cocaine, GHB, HEROIN, LYSERGIC ACID DIETHYLAMIDE (LSD), MDMA, and prescription OPIATES. In addition, most NARCOTICS are severely constipating. Some individuals find that PROPOXYPHENE (Darvon, Darvocet) causes stomach pain.

Some drugs are particularly harmful to the liver and can cause serious liver damage, including heroin, inhalants, and ANABOLIC STEROIDS. The damage is accentuated if the person abuses alcohol in addition to the drug, a situation that is common. Contaminants from illegally manufactured methamphetamine may include substances that are harmful to the liver.

The Heart and Circulatory System The abuse of many drugs may have adverse effects on the heart and may cause an abnormal heart rate (abnormally low or abnormally high) as well as heart attack. The injection of illegal drugs can lead to collapsed veins and bacterial infections of the heart valves and blood vessels.

Some drugs that may harm the heart and circulatory system are cocaine, heroin, inhalants, KETAMINE, LSD, marijuana, MDMA, methamphetamine, PHENCYCLIDINE, and prescription stimulants. Regular abusers of marijuana may also develop an increased heart rate. Abusers of steroids may develop problems with hypertension and high blood cholesterol, which together put them at an increased risk for experiencing a cardiovascular event, such as a stroke and/or heart attack.

The Urinary System and Kidneys Drug abuse and dependence may be harmful to the kidneys and in the worst case can cause the destruction of the kidneys and lead to the need for kidney dialysis and, eventually, kidney transplantation. Drugs

that may harm the kidneys specifically are heroin, inhalants, MDMA, and phencyclidine.

The Respiratory System Some drugs are harmful to breathing and the respiratory system. They may slow the individual's breathing and can worsen already-existing asthma. Drugs that may be harmful to the respiratory system include cocaine, GHB, inhalants, ketamine, marijuana, phencyclidine, and prescription opiates. Heroin abuse and dependence can cause lung complications, such as tuberculosis and pneumonia.

Reproductive System The abuse of anabolic steroids may permanently impair fertility in both men and women. Steroids can also cause feminizing effects in men and masculinizing effects in women, such as the development of permanently enlarged breast tissue (gynecomastia) in men and the development of increased facial hair in women, with decreased or absent menstruation.

Drug abusers and those who are addicted to drugs have an increased risk for contracting sexually transmitted diseases, which may also impair fertility if and when individuals wish to have a child.

Skin Some drugs can cause extreme itching of the skin, such as methamphetamine. Drugs such as cocaine and amphetamines may lead to excessive scratching or more serious injuries due to the individual's delusion of parasites under the skin (FORMICATION). Chronic injections of illegal drugs may also cause skin sores, lesions, and infections that may spread throughout the body if untreated.

Immune System Some drugs increase the risk to the abuser of contracting the human immunodeficiency virus (HIV) and the later development of acquired immune deficiency syndrome (AIDS). Individuals who use contaminated shared needles to inject their drugs intravenously are at greatest risk, such as those who inject cocaine, heroin, methamphetamine, and other drugs. These individuals also face an increased risk for contracting HEPATITIS as well as HIV and other infectious diseases that can be transmitted through shared needles.

Some studies, such as reported in *Archives of Internal Medicine* in 2004, have linked intravenous (IV) drug users of illegal drugs to a high risk of death, particularly among people ages 25–34 years.

The researchers studied IV drug users from 1980 to 2001. They found that most of the subjects died of drug overdoses. Say the researchers, "In particular, young female drug users in the 15–24 year age group have a very high relative risk of dying (increased by a factor of 76.3) compared with young females in the general population, and in nearly 90% of these cases drug overdose was the principal cause."

Prenatal Effects   Drug abuse and dependence can cause serious and potentially lifelong harm to the developing fetus. Pregnant women who abuse HEROIN risk a miscarriage or a premature delivery. The newborn who survives being delivered to a woman addicted to heroin has an increased risk of sudden infant death syndrome (SIDS). Other drugs that may be particularly harmful to the fetus of a pregnant woman include COCAINE, HEROIN, INHALANTS, MARIJUANA, MDMA, and METHAMPHETAMINE.

The use of many legitimate prescription drugs used as directed can potentially be harmful to the fetus, but most doctors are very careful about the prescriptions they recommend to pregnant women and monitor side effects. Despite this, some pregnant women abuse drugs without their doctors' knowledge, and consequently, they risk harm to the babies they later bear. Of course, the most dangerous drug to the fetus is alcohol. (See ALCOHOL ABUSE AND DEPENDENCE AND HEALTH PROBLEMS; FETAL ALCOHOL SYNDROME; PREGNANCY AND SUBSTANCE ABUSE.)

Psychiatric Problems May Develop with Some Drugs

The abuse of amphetamines or cocaine may trigger suicidal thoughts or even lead to a PSYCHOTIC BREAK in some individuals, one that is similar to and often indistinguishable from the symptoms that are seen with the onset of SCHIZOPHRENIA. Not all individuals recover from this psychotic break, even when the drug is no longer abused.

The abuse of anabolic steroids may induce extreme rages leading to aggression, as well as paranoia. Steroid abusers may suffer from severe DEPRESSION.

The abuse of MDMA can induce ANXIETY DISORDERS, depression, confusion, panic attacks, and paranoia.

The abuse of GHB can cause both DELUSIONS and HALLUCINATIONS.

Hallucinogenic drugs such as LSD may cause a psychotic break in users as well as depression. Phencyclidine (PCP) can induce both auditory and visual hallucinations in users and may also trigger a PSYCHOTIC BREAK. Users may experience paranoia and disorganized thinking, symptoms that resemble those of and are difficult to distinguish from schizophrenia.

Marijuana abusers who are chronic users may experience problems with depression and panic attacks. Heavy abuse may lead to paranoia and sometimes to psychosis.

The chronic use of methamphetamine can cause both visual and auditory hallucinations. Paranoia and extreme rages may precipitate VIOLENCE among methamphetamine abusers. Some chronic users of methamphetamine suffer from formication, the terrifying delusion that insects are crawling underneath their skin.

Users of crystal methamphetamine risk psychotic symptoms that may persist for months or years.

Other drugs that may induce psychiatric symptoms are inhalants, ketamine, and prescription stimulants. At high doses, narcotics may induce psychotic symptoms in some patients.

See also ADOLESCENTS; CRACK COCAINE; DATE RAPE DRUGS; DEATH; GENETIC PREDISPOSITIONS AND ENVIRONMENTAL EFFECTS IN SUBSTANCE USE DISORDERS; NARCOTICS; PRESCRIPTION DRUG ABUSE; SCHEDULED DRUGS.

Copeland, Lorraine, et al. "Changing Patterns in Cause of Death in a Cohort of Injecting Drug Users, 1980–2001." *Archives of Internal Medicine* 165 (June 14, 2004): 1,214–1,220.

Gordon, Rachel J., M.D., and Franklin D. Lowy, M.D. "Bacterial Infections in Drug Users." *New England Journal of Medicine* 353, no. 18 (November 3, 2005): 1,945–1,954.

Gwinnell, Esther, M.D., and Christine Adamec. *The Encyclopedia of Addictions and Addictive Behaviors.* New York: Facts On File, 2005.

Lange, Richard A., M.D., and L. David Hillis, M.D. "Cardiovascular Complications of Cocaine Use." *New England Journal of Medicine* 345, no. 6 (August 2, 2001): 351–358.

drug courts Special courts that deal only with drug offenses, particularly among first-time offenders who are not DRUG DEALERS. The first drug court was established in Miami, Florida, in 1989, and numerous drug courts have been established nationwide in the United States since then. According to the Office of National Drug Control Policy, there were an estimated 1,212 drug courts nationwide in all 50 states and the District of Columbia, Puerto Rico, Guam, and 52 tribal courts as of 2004, with 476 more in the planning stages in the United States. There are drug courts for adults and for juveniles.

Generally, drug offenders who are selected for drug court are given a treatment plan to follow, and they must also submit to regular DRUG TESTING. As long as they comply with the plan that is set up for them, and do not use drugs or alcohol, they will not be jailed. If a drug test reveals the presence of illegal drugs or the individual violates the program in some other way, then he or she can be incarcerated immediately, with no second chance. There are many different types of drug courts in the United States.

Successes of Drug Courts Current evidence indicates that drug courts reduce the recidivism (repeat crimes) rate. For example, in Chester County, Pennsylvania, graduates of drug courts had a rearrest rate of about 5 percent, compared to 22 percent among the control group. In Texas, drug court graduates in Dallas had a rearrest rate of 16 percent versus 49 percent for the control group who did not attend drug courts.

Drug courts can also be cost-effective; for example, researchers in two separate studies in California found that drug courts produced annual savings of $18 million.

According to a 2004 report from the National Drug Court Institute, there are some specific reasons why drug courts succeed. Say the authors, "A drug court's coercive power is the key to admitting drug-involved offenders into treatment quickly, for a period of time that is long enough to make a difference. This proposition is unequivocally supported by the empirical data on substance abuse treatment programs."

They add:

> As an alternative to less effective interventions, drug courts quickly identify substance abusing offenders and place them under strict court monitoring and community supervision, coupled with effective, long-term treatment services. In this blending of systems, the drug court participant undergoes an intensive regimen of substance abuse and mental health treatment, case management, drug testing, and probation supervision while reporting to regularly scheduled status hearings before a judge with specialized expertise in the drug court model.

See also CRIMES AND CRIMINALS; DRUG TESTING; INCARCERATION; JAIL INMATES; LAW ENFORCEMENT.

Huddleston III, C. West, Karen Freeman-Wilson, and Daniel Boone. *Painting the Current Picture: A National Report Card on Drug Courts and Other Problem Solving Court Programs in the United States.* Alexandria, Va.: National Drug Court Institute, May 2004.

drug dealers Individuals who sell drugs to others illegally for a profit. They may sell illegal drugs such as HEROIN, COCAINE, MARIJUANA, METHAMPHETAMINE, METHYLENEDIOXYMETHAMPHETAMINE (MDMA/ECSTACY), and many others. They may also obtain and sell prescription drugs nonmedically, such as prescribed narcotics or stimulants, which they then sell to others. Many drug dealers are young adult men operating in inner cities. Drug dealers who are convicted of their crime face a far more harsh prison sentence and greater fines than the individuals to whom they sell drugs, unless those individuals are also drug dealers.

Some drug dealers are part of a large criminal network while others basically operate independently. Many drug dealers sell their drugs in open-air markets, at specific places and at specific times and in public. In general, the primary products sold in this manner are CRACK COCAINE, powdered COCAINE, HEROIN, and MARIJUANA. (See OPEN AIR MARKETS, DRUG DEALING IN.)

Most drug dealers make at least cursory attempts to avoid detection by law enforcement and may hide their drugs inside alarm clocks or hollowed-out books. They may also use prepaid cell phones, which are disposable and cannot be tracked back to the user. In addition, drug dealers may employ children as young as four years old to deliver drugs to customers.

Drug dealers often cheat their customers; for example, they cut cocaine with talcum powder and other substances. In many cases, the so-called drug contains little or even none of the substance that the customers think they are purchasing. There is no recourse for the customer who has been cheated, other than complaining to other drug dealers or customers.

Teenage Drug Dealers

Some individuals who sell drugs are only adolescents themselves. Some studies have looked at the psychosocial aspects of adolescents who are dealing drugs in the inner city, such as in a 2006 article in the *Journal of Research in Crime and Delinquency*. This study found there were five key factors that significantly increased an adolescent's frequency of drug dealing, including

- low level of parental monitoring
- poor neighborhood conditions
- low neighborhood job opportunity
- parental substance use or abuse
- high levels of peer group deviance

The researchers also noted that previous studies have established that peer influence played a major role in the decision to sell illegal drugs. Said the researchers, "Adolescents' perceptions of the acceptability and profitability of drug dealing are shaped most directly by peers and young adults within their communities. Notably, too, adolescents' perception that 'everybody is doing it' is associated with persistence of drug selling."

The researchers studied 605 male juvenile offenders from Philadelphia between the ages of 14 and 17. Most of the subjects were minority members; 73 percent were African-American, 14 percent were Hispanic, 10 percent were white non-Hispanic, and less than 1 percent comprised Native Americans, Asian Americans or those of other ethnic or racial backgrounds. Most of the subjects (54 percent) had sold marijuana, and nearly half (46 percent) had sold some kind of illicit drug in the previous year. The teenagers who sold illegal drugs reported weekly incomes of about $1,700. Higher profits were made from selling illegal drugs other than marijuana.

The researchers concluded:

The results of this study suggest that juvenile courts' emphasis on time-limited punitive restrictions (probation, detention, incarceration) to juvenile drug crimes does not provide inner-city youths with adequate psychosocial resources for redirecting their lives given that the prevalence of adolescent drug selling has risen in the historical context of diminishing employment opportunities for young minority men, judicial responses to youth drug involvement that emphasize adolescents' participation in vocational skills training would no doubt aid in youths' redirection from illicit market participation. Not surprisingly, studies have shown that community-based educational and vocational programs contribute to positive adult adjustment (e.g., lower rates of recidivism [repeat crime], higher rates of employment) among formerly incarcerated youth.

See also ADDICTION/DEPENDENCE; CRIME AND CRIMINALS; DIVERSION, DRUG; DRUG SELLING, FORCED; GANGS; HEROIN; INCARCERATION; LAW ENFORCEMENT; MARIJUANA; NARCOTICS; OPIATES; ORGANIZED CRIME; PRESCRIPTION DRUG ABUSE; PROSTITUTION; VIOLENCE.

Little, Michelle, and Laurence Steinberg. "Psychosocial Correlates of Adolescent Drug Dealing in the Inner City: Potential Roles of Opportunity, Conventional Commitments, and Maturity," *Journal of Research in Crime and Delinquency* 43, no. 4 (2006): 357–386.

drug free zones   Areas in which, if illicit drugs are sold, the penalties for this crime are more severe than if these same drugs were sold elsewhere. Drug free zones usually encompass places that are known to be frequented by children, in areas such as schools, public libraries, parks, or playgrounds. Many states have passed laws on drug free zones. Some states have expanded the concept to include colleges as well.

The passage of the federal Drug-Free School Zones Act of 1984 promoted the concept of drug-free zones. The Violent Crime Control and Law Enforcement Act, a federal law that was passed in 1994, created or increased the penalties for individuals who sold drugs within those zones, as well as the penalties for drug dealing near public housing, in prisons, and in other areas.

The first drug-free zones were created based on a federal law, the Comprehensive Drug Abuse, Prevention and Control Act of 1970, which was later amended in 1984. However, support for drug-free zones in the 21st century may be eroding for a variety of reasons. For example, those who insist that drug-free zones do not work claim that these zones fail to limit drug sales to children, as intended. According to the Institute for Metropolitan Affairs, in their 2007 report on drugs in Illinois, "The availability of drugs has increased in Illinois, and the price of many drugs, like cocaine and methamphetamine, has dropped, while purity of drugs has increased."

Further, according to the 2007 report. "Despite enactment of Drug Free Zones in 1985 [in Illinois], which increased penalties and outlawed drugs in schools and within 1,000 feet of schools, drugs appear to be easier to obtain at school in 2005, than in 1993. According to analysis of the 2005 Risk Youth Behavior Survey, children in Chicago and Illinois are much more likely to report having been offered, sold or given an illegal drug on school property than in the past decade."

Other reports back up this finding. In a report published in 2007 by the New Jersey Commission to Review Criminal Sentencing. Assistant Attorney General Ron Suswein was quoted as saying, "The purpose of drug-free school zones was to protect children and schools by insulating them from drug activity. Our intention was to create a safe harbor for children by pushing the pushers away. Unfortunately, the current, 1,000 foot zones have failed to achieve that objective."

According to *Disparity by Design,* a report by the Justice Policy Institute published in March 2006, less than 1 percent of the drug cases in drug free zones involve sales to children or youth, and 71 percent of the cases occur when school is out of session.

Dissenters also say that drug-free zones may encompass such a large area that it is difficult to go anywhere without entering such a zone; for example, some states have added nursing homes, public parks, and many other areas in addition to schools as drug-free zones. For example, according to the Justice Policy Institute report, drug free zones in Connecticut include 1,500 feet from a school, a licensed-day care center, or a public housing area. In Illinois, drug-free zones include schools, public parks, public housing, bus stops, truck and rest stops, nursing homes, and places of worship.

According to this report, "These laws effectively place much of Chicago in an enhanced penalty zone." Other states also include public swimming pools and video arcades as drug-free zones.

Drug-free zones vary considerably in size, depending on the state, and may extend 300 feet from a protected area to, for example, the greatest extent of a drug-free zone, which is Alabama's three-mile radius around a public school, college, or university. Most states have between a 1,000 and 1,500 foot drug-free radius around the zone that they seek to protect.

Penalties are very high for those convicted of drug dealing in drug-free zones. Most states limit the law to the manufacture or sale of drugs, but some include simple possession if committed within a drug free zone, and in such cases, the penalties are as severe as for drug dealing. Some experts say that the high penalties are tantamount to double jeopardy, in that the individual is convicted of a crime and then sentenced based on where the crime was committed. However, the drug-free zone laws have been upheld to date.

Another key criticism of drug-free zones is that enforcement of the laws adversely affects minorities, who are more likely to live in urban areas, disproportionately. In New Jersey, 96 percent of the prisoners who are in jail for offenses in drug-free zones are black or Hispanic. Statistics from various sources back up the contention that individuals who are members of racial minorities are more likely to be convicted and incarcerated under such laws. This is true even when whites are arrested for the same or similar drug crimes.

For example, according to a Justice Policy Institute report, in Massachusetts, "Among those caught with more than a gram and a half of cocaine, ninety-four percent of minority defendants were charged as dealers compared to just over a quarter of whites. For those caught with less than 1/8 of a gram, the likelihood of being charged with delivery or possession with intent was nearly four times as great for nonwhites as for whites. Finally, defendants with no prior records were four times more likely to be charged with eligible offenses if they were nonwhite."

See also CRIME AND CRIMINALS; DRUG DEALERS; LAW ENFORCEMENT.

Greene, J. K. Pranis, and J. Zeidenberg. *Disparity by Design: How Drug-Free Zones Laws Impact Racial Disparity—and Fail to Protect Youth.* Justice Policy Institute. March 2006. Available online at URL: http://www.justicepolicylorg/content.php?hmID=1810&smID=1545. Downloaded September 20, 2007.

Kane-Willis, Kathleen, et al. *The Illinois Consortium on Drug Policy: Through a Different Lens: Shifting the Focus on Illinois Drug Policy.* 2007. The Institute for Metropolitan Affairs. Available online at URL: http://www.roosevelt.edu/pdfs/07DifferentLens.pdf. Downloaded January 15, 2008.

The New Jersey Commission to Review Criminal Sentencing. *Supplemental Report on New Jersey's Drug Free Zone Crimes & Proposals for Reform.* April 2007. Available online at URL: http://www.roosevelt.edu/pdfs/07DifferentLens.pdf. Downloaded September 21, 2007.

drug interactions   Effects that occur when two or more drugs are taken in the same time span. Many people who abuse prescription drugs or illicit substances also abuse alcohol, and this combination can be dangerous or even fatal. In addition, the combination of COCAINE and alcohol forms a more dangerous substance known as cocaethylene. Alcohol should not be taken with other DEPRESSANTS, because a dangerous level of sedation can result.

Some drugs or herbs reduce the efficacy of medications, while others increase their bioavailability; for example, vitamin E interacts with warfarin (Coumadin), a blood thinner, to the extent that vitamin E can cause dangerous bleeding in individuals who use warfarin. The combination of PROPOXYPHENE and warfarin may also lead to dangerous blood thinning and internal bleeding. Individuals who are taking DISULFIRAM (ANTABUSE) as well as phenytoin (Dilantin), an antiseizure drug, may need their dosages changed. In some cases, two medications should not be taken together; for example, disulfiram should not be taken with metronidazole (Flagyl) and alcohol should be strictly avoided while taking metronidazole. Drugs in the category of benzodiazepines may interact with lithium (usually taken for BIPOLAR DISORDER), as well as with many ANTIDEPRESSANTS.

Many elderly people take a greater number of medications than younger individuals and are at risk for drug interactions. It is advisable to use one pharmacy to fill prescriptions so that the pharmacist can advise the patient about any possible risk for drug interactions.

See also ADVERSE REACTION; MALICIOUS POISONING; PRESCRIPTION DRUG ABUSE.

drug rehabilitation centers   See TREATMENT FACILITIES; TREATMENT PLAN; TREATMENT.

drug selling, forced   Refers to compelled selling of drugs in order to avoid feared or actual threats of harm or even murder of the person coerced or others, such as a family member. Such threats may be made by a gang member or another individual involved in crime. In addition, worldwide, there are some individuals who are illegally trafficked (sold into slavery) to others, and they are forced to engage in behavior that they would not have performed otherwise, such as prostitution and/or drug selling. Adolescents in the United States and other countries may be threatened by their peers to sell illegal drugs, as well as sell or give others their own prescribed drugs. Some individuals who have ATTENTION DEFICIT HYPERACTIVITY DISORDER have reported that others have coerced them to sell or give them their stimulant medications, such as METHYLPHENIDATE (Ritalin).

See also DRUG DEALERS; PRESCRIPTION DRUG ABUSE.

drug testing   Tests that are given to detect the presence of illegal drugs in the body, such as COCAINE, METHAMPHETAMINE, and MARIJUANA, as well as addictive prescription drugs that are used nonmedically, such as HYDROCODONE or OXYCODONE. Many employers require that an individual be screened with drug testing before that person may be hired.

Individuals who have been sentenced in a DRUG COURT are also subject to random drug tests. If they fail a drug test because an illegal substance is present in their urine, then they will be sent to jail. In addition, in many cases, individuals who are on probation for a crime, including a crime that does *not* involve drugs, are subject to random drug testing at the behest of their probation officer, and they must comply with the requirement or risk being sent to jail. If they test positive for drugs, they may be arrested and jailed. Individuals who have been released from jail or prison may also be subjected to random drug testing as a condition of their parole or probation.

If an allegation is made that a parent is neglectful of their children because of drug abuse or dependence, the protective services department of the state or county may require the parent to undergo drug testing to determine whether the allegation is true or false.

Required Drug Testing

Random drug tests (tests that are called without notice) may be required among people in some professions, such as airplane pilots and military service members. Individuals who are on probation or parole may be required to undergo random drug tests. Professional athletes as well as Olympic athletes and even high school athletes often must undergo drug testing in order to remain on a team. In addition, schools may require random testing of any student, and for any reason, in accordance with a 2002 United States Supreme Court decision, *Board of Education of Independent School District No. 92 of Pottawatomie County v. Earls.*

Forms of Drug Tests

In most cases, the drug testing is performed on the individual's urine; however, blood tests and hair tests may also be used to detect the presence of illegal drugs, as well as tests of the individual's perspiration or saliva. Hair testing can reveal the use of drugs in the past several months, while urine or blood tests usually only reveal recent drug usage. (However, marijuana METABOLITEs may stay in the fatty tissue or bloodstream for up to 30 days.) A substance that is formed by the body when a drug is ingested, for example, when marijuana is smoked, a metabolite is stored in the fatty tissue and thus a drug test of the urine can reveal the use of marijuana for up to 30 days afterward. Some metabolites still have biological effects and can have significant impact on the duration of drug effect.

False Positive Results of Drug Tests

Rarely, individuals may have a FALSE POSITIVE result of a drug test: they test positive for using drugs when in fact, they do not have any illegal drugs in their system. For example, eating items with poppy seeds may cause a false positive result of a drug test. Some antibiotics, particularly drugs in the quinolone class, including levofloxacin (Levaquin) and ofloxacin (Floxin), may also cause a false positive drug test finding. This issue was discussed in 2001 at length in the *Journal of the American Medical Association.*

If a drug test result is positive, usually a secondary set of tests is done, to determine whether illicit drugs are actually present in the person's body.

Probable Positive Results That Should Be Explained by the Person Being Tested

If the person who is taking the drug test is also legitimately taking a legal scheduled drug, such as METHYLPHENIDATE (Ritalin) for ATTENTION DEFICIT HYPERACTIVITY DISORDER, then he or she should be sure to tell the testing agency requiring the test about this fact in advance, as well as telling the laboratory that is performing the tests. The person may also need a note from the doctor that the drug is taken for a legitimate medical reason and that it could cause a positive drug test result.

Some Individuals Seek to Thwart Drug Tests

Some drug users will go to elaborate lengths to thwart the results of a drug test, whether it is because they want to obtain a specific job (and a positive drug test result would disqualify them), or a positive drug test result would violate their probation or parole and lead to their INCARCERATION, or for other reasons.

Some Internet sites advise individuals on how to "beat the system" or even sell devices that purportedly will enable the individual who has abused drugs to obtain a negative test result. For example, some sites sell devices that resemble a flaccid penis, which can be prefilled with someone else's urine and then strapped onto the body. If the male is observed in the act of (apparently) urinating, it will appear to others as a natural act.

Some sites sell drugs that are designed to thwart the drug test result. These drugs are unlawful to use and their effectiveness is unknown. Other Web sites offer advice to drug users facing a drug test, such as telling the individual to drink large quantities of water the night before a scheduled test in order to dilute the urine and increase the odds of passing the drug test. If the individual fails the test anyway, such sites recommend that the individual protest loudly that he or she has been wronged and demand another opportunity to take the test within the next few days (when the drugs are more likely to be gone from the system, especially if it is the individual's urine that is tested).

Random drug testing Because of tactics that enable some drug abusers to prevent a positive drug test result, in general, random and unannounced drug tests are preferable to planned tests for employers or others who use drug testing, because with a random test, the individual will usually not have sufficient time to make or execute a plan to thwart the testing. In contrast, individuals who know they will be taking a drug test may delay the test until they feel confident that the drug is out of their system.

Most employers cannot reasonably order a random drug test, but when it is known or believed that the individual is a drug user, as with a person who has been charged with drug possession, random drug tests are preferable. Random drug testing is also sometimes used by corporations or the military.

See also CRIME AND CRIMINALS; NARCOTICS; VIOLENCE.

Baden, Lindsey R., M.D., et al. "Quinolones and False-Positive Urine Screening for Opiates by Immunoassay Technology." *Journal of the American Medical Association* 286, no. 24 (December 26, 2001): 3,115–3,119.

dual diagnosis The presence of two or more serious psychiatric disorders, such as both ALCOHOLISM and drug dependence, or both alcoholism and BIPOLAR DISORDER, or any other combination of two or more psychiatric diagnoses. Physicians often refer to these serious concurrent illnesses as comorbidities.

Many people who are substance abusers have one or more psychiatric problems, such as ANXIETY DISORDERS or DEPRESSION. Some individuals who abuse drugs and/or alcohol have ATTENTION DEFICIT HYPERACTIVITY DISORDER, which has usually not been diagnosed or treated. A low percentage of individuals have SCHIZOPHRENIA, a serious psychiatric disorder, and individuals who have this disorder are also prone to substance abuse. In addition, individuals who have OBSESSIVE COMPULSIVE DISORDER (OCD) or EATING DISORDERS have an increased risk for substance abuse.

Some experts hypothesize that individuals who have psychiatric disorders may use drugs or alcohol in an effort to self-treat their symptoms. However, it is also true that sometimes preceding substance abuse can lead to a psychiatric disorder or even a PSYCHOSIS, particularly with drugs such as AMPHETAMINES, COCAINE, or METHAMPHETAMINE. Often it is impossible to determine which factor, the psychiatric disorder or the substance abuse, is the driving factor or the trigger of the other factor. Some individuals are also genetically predisposed to developing psychiatric problems.

Difficulty in Finding Treatment for Dual Diagnoses

It is often difficult to find a treatment center that is equipped to deal with a person with both a psychiatric problem and a drug or alcohol problem because most treatment centers concentrate on one major problem alone, such as a psychiatric disorder or substance abuse. However, according to a 2006 *DASIS Report*, published by the Drug and Alcohol Services Information System, of the 13,454 public and private substance abuse treatment centers in the United States that responded to their survey in 2004, 4,756 (35 percent) reported having programs or groups for clients with both substance abuse and mental health disorders. These facilities were more likely to accept Medicare (46 percent) than facilities that did not have such programs for patients with dual diagnosis (29 percent), and they were also more likely to accept Medicaid (64 percent) versus facilities without such programs (48 percent).

It is also true that often individuals who have substance abuse issues and psychiatric problems will not seek out or accept treatment unless they are compelled to do so by a court or as a condition to avoid jail or prison or to have a chance of regaining custody of a child who was removed from them because of neglect or abuse.

See also ANTISOCIAL PERSONALITY DISORDER; ANXIETY DISORDERS; ATTENTION DEFICIT HYPERACTIVITY DISORDER; BIPOLAR DISORDER; CONDUCT DISORDER; DELUSIONS; DEPRESSION; EATING DISORDERS; HALLUCINATIONS; PSYCHIATRIC DISORDERS; SCHIZOPHRENIA.

Office of Applied Studies. "Facilities Offering Special Programs of Groups for Clients with Co-Occurring Disorders: 2004." *The DASIS Report* 2. Rockville, Md.: Substance Abuse and Mental Health Services Administration, 2006.

eating disorders Abnormal patterns of eating, including anorexia nervosa, bulimia nervosa, and binge eating disorder. Many individuals who have eating disorders experience deep guilt and shame about their bodies. They may also feel guilty and ashamed of their eating disorder, but at the same time, may feel powerless to stop the behavior.

Often these disorders are accompanied by substance abuse; for example, eating disorders are often associated with ALCOHOLISM, particularly such eating disorders as anorexia nervosa or bulimia nervosa, according to the analysis of research published in 2002 in *Alcohol Research & Health*.

In addition, according to *Food for Thought: Substance Abuse and Eating Disorders*, a report by the National Center on Addiction and Substance Abuse at Columbia University published in 2003, teenage girls who have eating disorders have five times the risk of others of abusing alcohol or illegal drugs. For example, teenage girls who have bulimia nervosa are more likely to abuse drugs and alcohol than girls who have anorexia nervosa, although girls with anorexia nervosa may abuse COCAINE or psychostimulant drugs (such as METHYLPHENIDATE) for their appetite-suppressing qualities. They may also rely on DIET PILLS, although no responsible physician would knowingly prescribe diet pills to any individual who had anorexia nervosa or bulimia nervosa.

According to the *Food for Thought* report, individuals who have bulimia nervosa have a high risk for substance abuse. This report states, "In a study comparing anorexic women with bulimic women, women with bulimia nervosa were more likely to have abused amphetamines, barbiturates, marijuana, tranquilizers and cocaine. The heaviest illicit drug use is found among those who binge and then purge (e.g. by vomiting or taking pills) to compensate for the binge eating. Indeed, some bulimics report that they use heroin to help them vomit."

Anorexia Nervosa Anorexia nervosa is a disorder of severe undereating. Most individuals who have anorexia nervosa are female, in a ratio of about 10 to 1 or greater, but the disorder may also develop in males. Some athletes or models develop anorexia nervosa, in part because of the rigid weight control demands of their sport or profession. According to the National Institute of Mental Health, from 0.5 to 3.7 percent of females suffer from anorexia nervosa at some point in their lives.

With anorexia nervosa, the individual's body mass index (BMI), a comparative measure of height and weight, is less than or equal to 17.5 kg/m². This is less than 85 percent of the normal body weight for a person of their height. (The average healthy person has a BMI within the range of 19 to 24 kg/m².)

Bulimia Nervosa In bulimia nervosa, the individual eats to excess and then purges the food, either through forcibly vomiting or through inducing diarrhea (or both). An estimated 1 to 4 percent of females develop bulimia nervosa during their lifetime, according to the National Institute of Mental Health (NIMH). Most bulimia nervosa patients are female, but about 10 to 15 percent of all patients are males. Patients who have long-term bulimia nervosa may have developed a gag reflex such that they can cause themselves to vomit without inserting their fingers into their throats.

Binge Eating Disorder Binge eating disorder refers to eating massive quantities of food without regard to hunger or appetite; however, binge eating episodes may occur in response to stress. According to the National Institute of Mental Health, from 2 to 5 percent of Americans experience binge eating disorder in a six-month period.

The binge eater typically overeats during at least two days a week over a six-month period. An estimated 4 million people in the United States are binge eaters, and the disorder is more commonly seen among females. Binge eaters may have an underlying problem with DEPRESSION.

Symptoms and Diagnostic Path

Anorexia nervosa is generally easier to diagnose than bulimia nervosa or binge eating disorder, simply because of the extremely thin and wasted appearance of the person who has anorexia nervosa. In contrast, the person who has bulimia nervosa may maintain a normal weight. Individuals who have anorexia nervosa often have a layer of downy skin, which is not seen in the person with bulimia nervosa.

Often it is the dentist who detects bulimia nervosa first, because the constant purging of acidic stomach material into the mouth damages the enamel of the teeth.

Signs of anorexia nervosa may include the following:

* excessive weight loss
* refusal to be weighed
* excessive exercising
* amenorrhea (absence or cessation of menstruation) in females
* unexplained fatigue
* markedly reduced food intake and frequent excuses to avoid eating
* an obsessive focus on body weight

According to the National Institute of Mental Health, the symptoms of bulimia nervosa are as follows:

* binge eating of excessive food, accompanied by a feeling of no control over the eating as it occurs
* inappropriate behavior to avoid weight gain, such as inducing vomiting or abusing laxatives, diuretics, enemas, or other medications; some patients fast or exercise excessively
* binge eating at least twice a week for three months
* a self-image that is heavily influenced by the weight and shape of the individual's body

Binge eating disorder is characterized by eating very large quantities of food at a time, without purging. Most individuals who have binge eating disorder are overweight or obese. It may be difficult to diagnose this disorder because some obese individuals eat large quantities of food but not in a binge fashion; rather, their food consumption is spread out over time.

According to the National Institute of Mental Health, binge eating disorder may be indicated by at least three of the following:

* eating much faster than usual
* eating that continues after the person feels full
* eating when the person is not hungry
* eating that occurs when the person is alone, as a result of embarrassment over the large quantity of food consumed
* feelings of self-disgust, depression, or guilt after overeating

Treatment Options and Outlook

Individuals who have anorexia nervosa require treatment because they risk death from starvation or heart failure (or from other causes) without it. Death may be caused by severe electrolyte imbalances, or SUICIDE. Some studies have shown that individuals who have both anorexia nervosa and alcoholism have a high risk for suicide.

Many anorexia nervosa patients develop malnutrition and other severe medical problems, some of which may be long term even if the individual recovers, such as osteoporosis and an increased risk for bone fractures.

For anorexia nervosa patients the goal of treatment is for the patient to gain weight. Treatment often also includes the identification of other psychiatric problems, such as DEPRESSION and ANXIETY DISORDERS, and medication may be indicated, although medications that often suppress appetite, such as Prozac (fluoxetine), should be avoided. Once the patient has recovered, however, Prozac may be used as a maintenance drug for the formerly anorexic patient. If the individual relies upon DIET PILLS and/or laxatives, these drugs must be discontinued immediately and should not be used upon recovery.

If necessary, as it often is with anorexia nervosa, the patient may be hospitalized to stabilize her electrolyte levels in the likely event of malnutrition and dehydration; however, unless the anorexic patient accepts that she must change her behavior, treatment is extremely difficult and many patients are treatment-resistant.

"Refeeding" of the patient with anorexia nervosa in the hospital must be done very carefully because a small percentage of individuals may develop confusion, edema, cardiac abnormalities, weakness, and temporary metabolic abnormalities if many calories are delivered too rapidly.

According to Yager and Andersen in their 2005 article on anorexia nervosa in the *New England Journal of Medicine*, this refeeding problem is seen most frequently among those who are less than 70 percent of their ideal body weight, although it can occur among other individuals who have anorexia nervosa. The patient may experience bloating because of slowed gastric emptying stemming from the anorexia nervosa and may need metoclopramide at bedtime and before meals.

Family therapy may be beneficial among patients who are younger than 18 years old, while older patients usually benefit from individual therapy.

Individuals who have bulimia nervosa often require treatment for their underlying depression and ANXIETY DISORDERS. They are at a lower risk for death than those who have anorexia nervosa but the constant purging is dangerous to the gastrointestinal system as well as to the teeth. Often individuals who have bulimia nervosa are treated with antidepressants, such as selective serotonin reuptake inhibitors (SSRIs) like fluoxetine (Prozac). As of this writing, Prozac is the only drug that is specifically approved by the Food and Drug Administration for the treatment of bulimia nervosa. Acid reflux problems caused by the bulimia can be treated with proton pump inhibitor medications.

Binge eating disorder should be identified and treated. Because of the difficulty with diagnosis, this disorder is frequently undertreated and may simply be viewed as ordinary overeating or obesity.

Some binge eating disorder patients have been successfully treated with such drugs as sibutramine (Meridia). According to a 2003 article in the *Journal of the American Medical Association* on pharmaceutical advances in eating disorders, binge eating disorder

patients who were given sibutramine reportedly ate less and reported feeling fuller than those on placebo. The patients taking sibutramine lost an average of seven pounds while those on the placebo gained one pound.

As with other forms of eating disorders, the individual may have an underlying depression and/or anxiety disorder that contributes to the periods of binging. Nutritional counseling is also recommended for patients who have any form of an eating disorder.

Recovering from binge eating disorder will enable the person to resolve problems with overweight and obesity, which increase the risk for developing serious chronic illnesses, such as diabetes and hypertension (high blood pressure).

Strict diets are usually ineffectual for the person who has binge eating disorder and should not be recommended. The individual may follow the diet and then engage in binge eating. Individuals who have this disorder usually need to be treated by a mental health professional who is knowledgeable about and familiar with this problem.

Night-Eating Syndrome   Some individuals who eat to excess contain their binge behavior to the night, a phenomenon that some call night-eating syndrome. They get up from their bed to prepare food, often a sandwich, and as much as a third of their calories are consumed after the dinner meal.

In most cases, they do not binge or purge; however, the extra calories consumed when they should be sleeping may cause a weight problem. Some research indicates that about a quarter of those seeking bariatric surgery (weight reduction surgery) are nighttime eaters. This disorder appears to be triggered by a dysregulation in the circadian pattern. It causes problems because it disrupts sleep as well as increasing weight. In one study, individuals who had night-eating syndrome ate about four times more between dinner and bedtime than did those in the control group. Patients who have this problem have responded to Zoloft (sertraline). They may also respond to cognitive-behavioral therapy.

Risk Factors and Preventive Measures

It is unknown what causes eating disorders to develop, although genetic and environmental factors may be at work.

Say Yager and Andersen, "The causes appear to be multifactorial, with determinants including genetic influences; personality traits of perfectionism and compulsiveness; anxiety disorders; family history of depression and obesity; and peer, familial, and cultural pressures with respect to appearance. These contribute to an entrenched overvaluation of slimness, distorted perceptions of body weight, and phobic avoidance of many foods." Some experts also believe the culture may play a role, and some individuals who have anorexia nervosa internalize the goal of slimness, yet their distorted body image prevents them from recognizing that they have achieved slenderness, and thus, they continue to deny themselves food to attain an unreachable goal.

It is known, however, that substance abuse will only worsen the effects of eating disorders, particularly anorexia nervosa. The painfully thin person can ill afford to add drugs and/or alcohol to his or her already meager diet. It is best for individuals who have all forms of eating disorders to avoid alcohol and illegal drugs. In addition, diet drugs and laxatives should be avoided by anorexia nervosa patients.

See also DIET PILLS; DUAL DIAGNOSIS; PSYCHIATRIC DISORDERS.

Grilo, Carlos M., Rajita Sinha, and Stephanie S. O'Malley. "Eating Disorders and Alcohol Use Disorders." *Alcohol Research & Health* 26, no. 2 (2002): 51–160.

Gwinnell, Esther, M.D., and Christine Adamec. *The Encyclopedia of Addictions and Addictive Behaviors*. New York: Facts On File, 2005.

Lamberg, Lynne. "Advances in Eating Disorders Offer Food for Thought." *Journal of the American Medical Association* 290, no. 11 (September 17, 2003): 1,437–2,442.

Lamberg, Lynne. "All Night Diners: Researchers Take a New Look at Night Eating Syndrome." *Journal of the American Medical Association* 290, no. 11 (September 17, 2003): 1,442.

National Center on Addiction and Substance Abuse at Columbia University. *Food for Thought: Substance Abuse and Eating Disorders*. New York: National Center on Addiction and Substance Abuse at Columbia University, December 2003.

Vastag, Brian. "What's the Connection? No Easy Answers for People with Eating Disorders and Drug Abuse."

Journal of the American Medical Association 285, no. 8 (February 28, 2001): 1,006–1,007.

Yager, Joel, M.D., and Arnold E. Andersen, M.D. "Anorexia Nervosa." *New England Journal of Medicine* 353, no. 14 (October 6, 2005): 1,481–1,488.

Ecstasy See METHYLENEDIOXYMETHAMPHETAMINE (MDMA/ECSTASY).

education Providing information and acquired knowledge. Education about the risks and problems associated with alcohol and drug abuse and dependence is an important part of most school curricula in the United States. Court systems may require individuals whose conviction was associated with substance abuse to take special classes to educate them about the dangers and risks that are associated with drug and alcohol abuse and dependence.

There are many programs that have been designed to prevent children and adolescents from drinking or using drugs, and many programs start at the elementary school level. Such programs are important; for example, according to the Substance Abuse and Mental Health Services Administration (SAMHSA), children who start drinking alcohol before they reach age 15 are five times more likely to have alcohol problems later in life than are those who start drinking at age 21 or older. Yet studies have shown that the majority of students report that alcohol is fairly easy or easy to get.

SAMHSA offers a program on underage alcohol use for teachers of fifth graders to help them provide students with factual information about alcohol and its effects and risks, as well as to help students develop decision-making skills and the ability to say no when alcohol is offered to them through role-playing exercises. Students in groups are given such tasks as choosing a dangerous activity—such as a friend daring a fellow student to run across the highway, hitchhike, or drink a beer—and then the students are instructed to analyze the situation by asking such questions as How would you decide whether to do what your friend is asking?, What might happen if you said yes? and What are the best and worst things that might happen if you said No.

They are also taught strategies to say no, such as repeating, "No, I don't want to", or substituting another activity "No, let's _____", walking away from the other child and so forth. (Further information is available at URL: http://www.teach.samhsa.gov/materials).

There are numerous other educational programs designed to prevent students from drinking or using drugs and there is considerable discussion about whether various programs are effective.

See ADOLESCENTS AND SUBSTANCE ABUSE; COLLEGE STUDENTS; DRUG COURTS; DRUG TESTING; SCHOOLS AND SCHOOL POLICIES.

elderly   Usually refers to individuals ages 65 and older. Although they are not generally perceived as individuals who commonly abuse or are addicted to drugs and/or alcohol, the elderly can have major substance abuse problems or dependence issues, particularly with alcohol, sedatives, and painkilling medications. They are, however, much less likely to abuse illegal drugs, such as COCAINE or MARIJUANA, than are younger individuals.

Older people who have substance abuse or dependence problems, particularly with alcohol, may have had such problems before entering their senior years, while in some cases, the substance abuse or dependence developed later in life, in response to loneliness, DEPRESSION, or other factors.

Health Providers Need Further Education

It is also true that health care providers may fail to see coexisting problems of substance abuse and prescription drug abuse. They may misperceive cognitive difficulties that are caused by drugs or alcohol as being simply caused by the normal aging process, or they may misdiagnose the problem as early dementia, failing to identify and treat the true problem of substance abuse.

It is also true that older individuals often have problems with DEPRESSION, ANXIETY DISORDERS, and dementia, which may be related to the substance abuse or dependence and may also be undiagnosed. Most older people who have such problems are not treated by psychiatrists, either because physicians do not realize they need the patient to consult a psychiatrist or because many older people fear that consulting a psychiatrist inevitably indicates insanity and subsequent hospitalization. Physicians may need to educate older patients to understand that psychiatrists treat many people with a wide variety of problems and that it is safe and socially acceptable to see a psychiatrist as needed.

Another factor preventing physicians' discovering substance abuse is that the older person as well as the family members may not tell them about substance abuse problems, because of guilt and shame. Substance abuse may have been a closely held family secret for years; however, physicians need this information because many drugs interact with alcohol, sometimes fatally.

Older Individuals and Prescribed Drugs

According to Lantz in her article on prescription drug and alcohol abuse by older women in *Clinical Geriatrics,* some patients inadvertently develop a problem with prescription drug abuse because they may be prescribed a variety of different medications, such as analgesics and sedatives, and they may not fully (or at all) understand the instructions for the use of these different drugs.

Says Lantz, "An elderly patient who visits several physicians can easily obtain multiple prescriptions and escalate their use if he or she is seeking relief from feelings of stress, grief, bereavement, depression, and anxiety."

In addition, Lantz says that it is fairly common for elderly individuals to borrow medications from family members without checking with their physician, thinking that they are being helpful to each other. This practice is illegal and unhealthy, and in some cases, these drug exchanges can lead to the abuse of drugs. Says Lantz, "Once a habitual pattern is established, many find themselves in a pattern of escalating abuse that results in significant excess morbidity [illness] and even mortality [death]."

Preventive Actions for Patients and Doctors

It is advisable for elderly individuals to take *all* their medications (prescribed, over-the-counter, and any herbal remedies) to each physician appointment, so that the doctor can check on any potential for ADVERSE REACTION with these drugs. In addition, the doctor should also gently ask older people about any other drugs that they take and may have borrowed from others. Responses to this question will give the doctor important information as well as an opportunity to warn the patient that it is very dangerous to borrow drugs from others and even illegal.

The doctor should also recommend that patients obtain all their prescribed medications from one pharmacy, so that the pharmacist will be able to provide a second check against drug interactions. This is especially useful if the patient must see different physicians who each prescribe medications.

It is also important for patients to be honest with their physicians about alcohol use. Many medications should not be combined with alcohol, such as narcotic painkillers or BENZODIAZEPINES, because such use could be dangerous or even fatal.

Treatment of Older People

Older adults who are abusing or dependent on the nonmedical use of prescription drugs are more likely to need inpatient treatment than younger individuals with the same habits. DETOXIFICATION can be particularly dangerous for an elderly person, who may have a multitude of serious medical problems that should be considered in making the detoxification plan, such as cardiovascular problems.

On the positive side, however, experts report that many older individuals who have abused or become dependent on alcohol or drugs have a good prognosis with treatment. They may be more highly motivated than younger individuals to recover, and they may have the time to participate in counseling and educational programs. Older individuals may also benefit from twelve-step programs, such as Alcoholics Anonymous.

Aging Baby Boomers

The scale and number of substance abuse problems involving older people are likely to increase as the large number of baby boomers (born between 1946 and 1964) enter their senior years, according to Bartels and associates in their 2005 report on substance abuse and mental health among older Americans. They point out that elderly people represented about 13 percent of the population in the United States in 2005 but this percentage will increase to 20 percent by 2020. In addition it is estimated that the number of elderly people needing substance abuse treatment will more than double, from 1.7 million in 2000 to 4.4 million in 2020.

According to this report, older persons on average routinely take two to six prescribed medications as well as one to three over-the-counter (OTC) medications. Problems with combining alcohol with both prescribed and OTC drug are likely to escalate in the future with the burgeoning population of older Americans.

See also ALCOHOLISM; BENZODIAZEPINES; NARCOTICS; PAIN MANAGEMENT; PRESCRIPTION DRUG ABUSE; PSYCHIATRIC DISORDERS.

Bartels, Stephen J., M.D., et al. *Substance Abuse and Mental Health among Older Americans: The State of the Knowledge and Future Directions.* Rockville, Md.: Substance Abuse and Mental Health Services Administration, August 11, 2005. Available online. URL: http://www.samhsa.gov/aging/SA_MH_%20AMongOlderAdultsfinal102105.pdf. Downloaded January 5, 2006.
Lantz, Melinda S., M.D. "Prescription Drug and Alcohol Abuse in an Older Woman." *Clinical Geriatrics* 13, no. 1 (January 2005): 39–43.
Schneider, Jennifer P., M.D. "Chronic Pain Management in Older Adults." *Geriatrics* 60, no. 5 (May 2005): 26–31.

emergency treatment Urgent medical care, usually provided in the emergency room of a hospital. Those individuals who abuse or become dependent on alcohol and/or illegal drugs or who misuse prescription drugs have an increased risk of needing emergency treatment. In some cases, individuals consume a high dosage of drugs, causing temporary or permanent injury and sometimes resulting in ACCIDENTAL OVERDOSE DEATHS.

Some individuals also attempt to or do commit SUICIDE with drugs and/or alcohol. Sometimes it is difficult to determine whether the patient has attempted to commit suicide or has consumed an accidental overdose. In some cases, patients have been victimized by MALICIOUS POISONING, which usually occurs when they have unknowingly ingested substances that others have placed in a food or beverage. In most of those circumstances, perpetrators seek to assault victims sexually once the drug sedates, disables, or confuses them. (See

DATE RAPE DRUGS.) The most common date rape drug is alcohol.

Some patients go to emergency rooms because they are unable to obtain the drugs to which they are addicted, and they are seeking drugs, such as MEPEREDINE (Demerol), Percocet (a form of OXY-CODONE), or other medications. They lie to physicians about severe pain, in the hope of being given narcotics. Others may appear in an acute stage of WITHDRAWAL from alcohol or drugs. Hospital emergency room staff do their best to stabilize patients who are suffering from withdrawal symptoms, but alcoholics and drug addicted individuals may urgently need rehabilitative services. Some emergency rooms may be located in hospitals that offer DETOXIFICATION facilities, but most are not.

According to Gail D'Onofrio and Linda Degutis in their article on screening and brief intervention in the emergency department, published in 2004/2005 in *Alcohol Research & Health,* as many as half of the severely injured trauma patients who enter the emergency room and require hospital admission (usually in intensive care) screen positive for alcohol. The authors also report that younger individuals (age 25 and younger) who enter the emergency room are more likely to have alcohol-related problems that require treatment than older adults. The authors explain the probable causes for this finding:

> First, younger people are usually healthy and are more likely than older people to be uninsured and to use the ED as their usual source of care. Second, young adults have the highest prevalence of binge and hazardous drinking in the United States, which can easily escalate to drinking patterns that require intervention.
>
> Third, particularly in younger people, these drinking patterns often occur in conjunction with driving. . . . Motor vehicle crashes are the number one cause of death in people ages 1 to 35, and the eighth leading cause of death overall. In 2003 (the most recent data available), there were approximately 43,000 motor vehicle traffic fatalities in the United States, according to the National Highway and Traffic Safety Administration (NHTSA), of which an estimated 18,000 (40 percent) were related to the use or abuse of alcohol.

Information from DAWN

The Drug Abuse Warning Network (DAWN) in the United States tracks hospital emergency department data on the treatment of patients among whom a drug either caused or was implicated in the emergency room visit. The data were derived from 260 hospital emergency rooms nationwide, and the national information was extrapolated from those data.

Essentially, a DAWN case is any emergency department visit related to recent drug use. However, not all DAWN visits are related to the illicit use of drugs, and in some cases, patients enter the hospital with an adverse reaction to a prescribed drug. However, the DAWN data do capture a significant degree of illegal drug activity and its effects.

DAWN cases do *not* include patients in the following categories:

- There is no evidence of recent drug use.
- The patient left the emergency room without receiving any treatment.
- The patient consumed a nonpharmaceutical substance that was not inhaled.
- The patient has a history of drug use but no recent drug use.
- Alcohol is the only substance involved and the patient is age 21 or older.
- The only documentation of a drug is from toxicology test results.
- The patient's current medications are unrelated to the visit.
- The patient is being treated for undermedication (receiving an insufficient dose of a drug, such as a patient in severe pain who has received too low a dose of a pain medication).

As of 2003, DAWN began providing data on cases involving drugs and/or alcohol, including the categories that follow:

- suicide attempts
- attempts to detoxify
- alcohol only in patients younger than age 21
- adverse reaction
- overmedication

- malicious poisoning
- accidental ingestion
- other

According to the organization, most drug abuse cases fall in the miscellaneous category of "other."

There are three primary categories that DAWN uses in classifying emergency department visits that involve drug misuse and abuse. First is the use of illicit drugs, as defined by the specific drug. Drugs included in this category include COCAINE, HEROIN, MARIJUANA, major STIMULANTS (such as AMPHETAMINE and METHAMPHETAMINE), METHYLENEDIOXYMETHAMPHETAMINE (MDMA/ECSTASY), GAMMA-HYDROXYBUTYRATE (GHB), FLUNITRAZEPAM (Rohypnol), KETAMINE, LYSERGIC ACID DIETHYLAMIDE (LSD), PHENCYCLIDINE (PCP), other hallucinogens, nonpharmaceutical INHALANTS, and combinations of illegal drugs.

The second category includes patients who enter the emergency room for the misuse or abuse of alcohol, subcategories within this classification include alcohol in combination with other drugs or alcohol only in patients younger than age 21.

The third category of misuse and abuse is the nonmedical use of pharmaceuticals and other substances. There are three classes in this category: overmedication (the nonmedical use, overuse, and misuse of prescription and over-the-counter medications), malicious poisoning (in which the patient was administered a drug by another person for a malicious purpose), and "other," or cases that could not be assigned to either of the other two case types and include documented drug abuse.

DAWN findings In 2003, DAWN estimated there were a total of 627,923 drug-related emergency room visits (including all types of drugs, such as illegal drugs, alcohol, prescription drugs, over-the-counter drugs, dietary supplements, and nonpharmaceutical inhalants). Of these total visits, 305,731 drug-related emergency room visits, or nearly half of all drug-related emergency room visits nationwide, involved a major drug of abuse. About 23 percent of the visits involved alcohol, either alone or in combination with another drug. Approximately one in five of all drug-related emergency room visits involved cocaine. Marijuana was involved in about 13 percent of all drug-related visits and heroin represented about 8 percent of

all drug-related visits. Stimulants such as amphetamines and methamphetamine represented about 7 percent of all visits. Unspecified opiates (which may include some instances of abuse of heroin) accounted for about 4 percent of all visits.

With regard to visits related to alcohol in combination with another drug or alcohol abuse by a person younger than age 21, DAWN estimated there were 118,724 visits involving the use of alcohol in combination with another drug and 22,619 visits related to the use of patients younger than age 21.

DAWN further estimated that there were 332,046 cases of overmedication, malicious poisonings, and "other" cases. More than half of these cases (54 percent) involved multiple drugs. The specific drugs most commonly involved in these cases were cocaine (28 percent), alcohol (26 percent), and marijuana (20 percent). A combination of the nonmedical use of BENZODIAZEPINES (antianxiety medications) and opiates accounted for 17 percent of the visits. Heroin and major stimulants (such as amphetamines and methamphetamine) were involved in 10 percent of the visits.

Table I shows the number of visits in relation to the hospitals surveyed as well as the nationwide estimate for each category. For example, the 166 cases of malicious poisoning are a nationwide estimate

TABLE I: DRUG-RELATED EMERGENCY DEPARTMENT VISITS, BY TYPE OF CASE, 2003

Type of Case	Unweighted Data	Nationwide Estimate
Suicide attempt	3,981	40,044
Seeking detoxification	9,421	61,506
Alcohol only (below age 21)	2,894	22,522
Adverse reaction	9,319	155,066
Overmedication	9,321	105,401
Malicious poisoning	166	1,300
Accidental ingestion	1,167	16,769
Other	1,167	16,769
Total drug-related visits	67,583	627,923
Total emergency department visits (all reasons)	5,268,743	52,336,352

Source: Adapted from Office of Applied Studies, Substance Abuse and Mental Health Services Administration. *Drug Abuse Warning Network, 2003: Interim National Estimates of Drug-Related Emergency Department Visits.* DAWN Series D-26. Publication no. SMA 04-3972. Rockville, Md.: Department of Health and Human Services, 2004.

extrapolated to 1,300 individuals who were victimized in this manner in 2003. Table II shows the type of drugs used in the estimated nationwide estimates. For example, there were an estimated 305,731 nationwide emergency room visits related to illegal drugs and/or alcohol. Of these visits, there were 141,343 cases in which alcohol alone or in combination with another drug was the cause of the visit to the emergency room.

Table III shows characteristics of emergency room patients in whom drugs and/or alcohol was a factor in the visit. For example, with regard to cocaine abuse, there were 125,921 patients with cocaine abuse. Most patients were male (78,293 patients) and most were age 30 and older. In addition, most were white.

In another example, with regard to the 79,663 emergency room patients who abused marijuana, most were male (53,162), age 12 and older, and white.

Suicide attempts involving drugs and/or alcohol DAWN estimated there were 40,044 nationwide drug-related emergency department visits associated with suicide attempts in 2003. Central nervous system medications, primarily pain relievers, were involved in about half (56 percent) of these cases, and the individuals attempting suicide used both prescription and over-the-counter drugs.

BENZODIAZEPINES and ANTIDEPRESSANTS were involved in nearly half (45 percent) of the cases. (Many individuals used more than one drug in their suicide attempt.) In the majority of cases, individuals attempting suicide used two or more drugs.

See also ACCIDENTAL OVERDOSE DEATHS; ADVERSE REACTIONS; BARBITURATES; BENZODIAZEPINES; CHILD ABUSE; COCAINE; DEATH; DELIRIUM TREMENS; DETOXIFICATION; DOMESTIC VIOLENCE; DRUG TESTING; HOMICIDE; INJURIES CAUSED BY ALCOHOL AND/OR DRUGS; MALICIOUS POISONING; NARCOTICS; PRESCRIPTION DRUG ABUSE; PRESCRIPTION DRUG MONITORING PROGRAMS, STATES WITH; SUICIDE; TREATMENT; VIOLENCE.

D'Onofrio, Gail, M.D., and Linda C. Degutis. "Screening and Brief Intervention in the Emergency Department." *Alcohol Research & Health* 28, no. 2 (2004/2005): 63–72.

TABLE II: ILLICIT DRUGS AND ALCOHOL IN DRUG-RELATED EMERGENCY DEPARTMENT VISITS, 2003

Drug Category and Selected Drugs	Estimated Visits
Total drug-related emergency department visits	627,923
Major substances of abuse (includes alcohol)	305,731
Alcohol	141,343
Alcohol in combination	118,724
Alcohol alone	22,619
Cocaine	125,921
Heroin	47,604
Marijuana	79,663
Stimulants	42,538
Amphetamines	18,129
Methamphetamine	25,039
Methylenedioxymethamphetamine (MDMA/Ecstasy)	2,221
Gamma-hydroxybutyrate (GHB)	990
Ketamine	73
Lysergic acid diethylamide (LSD)	656
Phencyclidine (PCP)	4,581
Miscellaneous hallucinogens	684
Inhalants	1,681
Combinations not tabulated above	1,346

Source: Adapted from Office of Applied Studies, Substance Abuse and Mental Health Services Administration. *Drug Abuse Warning Network, 2003: Interim National Estimates of Drug-Related Emergency Department Visits.* DAWN Series D-26. Publication no. SMA 04-3972. Rockville, Md.: Department of Health and Human Services, 2004.

TABLE III: ILLICIT DRUGS, BY PATIENT CHARACTERISTICS, 2003

Patient Characteristics	Cocaine	Heroin	Marijuana	Stimulants	MDMA (Ecstasy)[2]	GHB[3]	LSD[4]	PCP[5]
Total Drug-related emergency department visits	**125,921**	**47,604**	**79,663**	**42,538**	**2,221**	**990**	**656**	**4,581**
Gender								
Male	78,293	30,205	53,162	25,389	1,523	513	616	3,377
Female	47,483	17,330	26,340	17,142	698	477	39	1,202
Unknown	145	68	—	—	—	—	—	—
Age								
0–5 years	—	7	7	—	—	—	—	—
6–11 years	—	—	15	—	1	—	—	6
12–17 years	—	411	12,202	3,739	—	—	71	—
18–20 years	7,274	2,714	11,923	4,917	688	274	57	—
21–24 years	11,892	6,200	10,230	6,096	—	65	—	934
25–29 years	14,765	7,724	8,806	5,833	—	133	—	573
30–34 years	17,922	6,216	10,017	6,818	—	60	184	901
35–44 years	46,175	14,921	17,215	10,062	77	277	—	516
45–54 years	21,030	8,151	8,128	3,617	11	5	9	—
55–64 years	2,729	1,131	957	552	—	—	—	—
65 years and older	452	452	104	—	23	—	—	—
Unknown	112	25	11	8	10	—	—	—
Race/ethnicity								
White	62,581	25,209	47,175	31,098	927	84 7	562	1,442
Black	40,184	10,194	17,644	1,193	564	9	1 8	2,331
Hispanic	11,264	4,515	7,574	3,364	—	—	—	554
Race/ethnicity NTA[1]	2/005	428	1,180	756	—	—	226	31
Unknown	9,887	7,258	6,092	6,127	185	—	32	223

[1] Not tabulated above.
[2] Methylenedioxymethamphetamine.
[3] Gamma-hydroxybutyrate.
[4] Lysergic acid diethylamide.
[5] Phencyclidine.
Source: Adapted from Office of Applied Studies, Substance Abuse and Mental Health Services Administration. *Drug Abuse Warning Network, 2003: Interim National Estimates of Drug-Related Emergency Department Visits.* DAWN Series D-26. Publication no. SMA 04-3972. Rockville, Md.: Department of Health and Human Services, 2004.

Office of Applied Studies, Substance Abuse and Mental Health Services Administration. *Drug Abuse Warning Network, 2003: Interim National Estimates of Drug-Related Emergency Department Visits.* DAWN Series D-26. Publication no. SMA 04-3972. Rockville, Md.: Department of Health and Human Services, 2004.

employee assistance programs   Assistance programs that are offered in the workplace. An employee assistance program may be managed through individuals employed by the company or through contracted services. These programs can provide assistance or refer-rals to individuals who have a wide variety of personal problems, including abuse and dependence on alcohol and/or drugs, as well as psychiatric problems.

Some employees have both substance abuse problems and psychiatric illnesses. This condition is referred to as a DUAL DIAGNOSIS. The employee may be referred to an outpatient program or to a rehabilitative facility. Generally, the employee assistance program does not treat these types of disorders internally.

Virtually all large and medium-sized corporations in the United States offer an employee assistance program.

See also ALCOHOLISM; PSYCHIATRIC DISORDERS.

false positives Results of urine, blood, or hair tests for detecting illegal drugs in the body that indicate that drugs are present when the person has not actually ingested any illegal drugs. In such a case, usually a second test is performed, often a different type of test, and this test can determine that drugs are not present. For example, if the urine test result was positive, a blood test or a hair test could be used to determine the presence of drugs.

Substances That Can Cause False Positives

Some medicines or foods can cause a false positive finding on a drug test. For example, if individuals have taken a cough syrup containing DEXTROMETHO-RPHAN, they may test positive for OPIATES, although they have not used any opiates. Some antibiotics, especially quinolones, such as levofloxacin (Leva-quin) and ofloxacin (Floxin), which are often used to treat urinary tract infections, prostate infections, or bronchitis, may cause a positive test result for opiates with some drug tests. Foods that are rich in poppy seeds may also cause a false positive result on a drug test.

Some Patients on Legally Prescribed Drugs Test Positive

Some drug tests show a positive result in a drug screen because the patient *is* using a drug; however, the drug may have been legally prescribed to the patient. For example, patients who have chronic severe pain who are taking prescribed opiates show a positive result. In addition, patients who have ATTENTION DEFICIT HYPERACTIVITY DISORDER who are taking METHYLPHENIDATE (RITALIN/CONCERTA/FOCALIN, ETC.) or prescribed AMPHETAMINES will also test positive for drugs.

As a result, it is best for such individuals to fore-warn potential or current employers about such medication use, to prevent a misinterpretation of a positive drug screen finding. Sometimes a note from the doctor that states the individual has a medical need to take the specific drug, and that this drug may show up in some drug screens, is needed.

See also DRUG TESTING.

family, effect on Drug and/or alcohol abuse and dependence (addiction) has a profound and long-term effect on an individual's family members. The effect frequently continues when their children grow up to become adults and often parents themselves. Adults who are raised in a home that has substance abuse have an increased risk of becoming substance abusers in adulthood. They also have an increased risk for suffering from DEPRESSION in adulthood and are more likely to be suicidal than adults who were not reared by parents who abused or were dependent on alcohol and/or drugs.

Effect on Adult Children of Substance Abusers

Adult children of substance abusers may continue to be affected by past incidents of CHILD ABUSE and/or neglect. Some experts have studied the impact of adverse events in childhood by comparing these self-reported childhood events to problem behavior that has occurred in adulthood (such as substance abuse, abuse of their own children or other issues).

In one major study, the Adverse Childhood Experiences (ACE) study, the researchers used thousands of subjects receiving medical care at the Health Appraisal Clinic in San Diego, California, part of Kaiser Permanente's health maintenance organization. The researchers found that 64 percent of the sample reported one or more ACEs. Two very common ACEs were physical abuse in child-hood (experienced by 28 percent of the respondents) and alcohol or substance abuse by a family member during the individual's childhood (about 27 percent).

The eight categories of ACEs that were considered in the study were:

- individuals who experienced recurrent childhood emotional abuse
- those who suffered from childhood physical abuse
- those who experienced sexual abuse
- individuals who witnessed violence against their mother in childhood
- those who lost a biological parent in childhood for any reason
- those who lived with someone in the household who had mental illness (depression, suicide, or other mental illness)
- those who lived with someone who abused substances
- those who lived in a household in which a member was incarcerated for crimes

As can be seen from these categories, children reared by a family member who had a substance abuse problem could fit into several categories; for example, they may have witnessed DOMESTIC VIOLENCE ASSOCIATED WITH ALCOHOL AND/OR DRUGS, which is common among substance abusing families, and they may also have suffered from child abuse. In addition, a family member could have been incarcerated for a crime. Many people who have drug or alcohol dependence have psychiatric problems, another category that is an adverse childhood event.

In this study, 30 percent of the women reported that household alcohol/drug abuse was present in their childhood, compared to 24 percent of the men. The researchers also considered the relationship of the number of adverse childhood events to problems later experienced by adults and found a direct relationship. The greater the number of ACEs in childhood, the more likely the individuals were to experience problems in adulthood. Women were more likely to report a greater number of ACEs than men.

The researchers also found that adults who had a past history of ACEs were more likely than those with no ACEs to

- become substance abusers of drugs and/or alcohol
- abuse their own children
- suffer from psychiatric emotional disorders, such as DEPRESSION or ANXIETY DISORDERS
- commit SUICIDE (the suicide rate for women was about three times higher than for men)
- have unintended pregnancies
- contract sexually transmitted diseases
- have marital problems

According to a study reported in *Pediatrics* in 2003, when comparing people with no adverse childhood experiences to those individuals with five or more ACEs, the individuals with the five ACEs had a seven to 10 times greater risk of using illegal drugs or being addicted to illicit drugs, as well as injecting drugs.

Say the researchers, "Because ACEs seem to account for one half to two thirds of serious problems with drug use, progress in meeting the national goals for reducing drug use will necessitate serious attention to these types of stressful and disturbing childhood experiences by pediatric practice."

It is clear from this research and many other studies that adults who have substance abuse problems need to seek recovery, not only for themselves, but also for the long-term health of their children (and their grandchildren) into adulthood.

See also CHILD ABUSE; DEPRESSION; DOMESTIC VIOLENCE; DUAL DIAGNOSIS; GENETIC PREDISPOSITIONS AND ENVIRONMENTAL EFFECTS IN SUBSTANCE USE DISORDERS; PSYCHIATRIC DISORDERS; PSYCHIATRISTS.

Dube, Shanta R., et al. "Childhood Abuse, Neglect, and Household Dysfunction and the Risk of Illicit Drug Use: The Adverse Childhood Experiences Study." *Pediatrics* 111, no. 3 (March 2003): 564–572.

Edwards, Valerie J., et al. "Relationship between Multiple Forms of Childhood Maltreatment and Adult Mental Health in Community Respondents: Results from the Adverse Childhood Experiences Study." *American*

Journal of Psychiatry 160, no. 8 (August 2003): 1,453–1,460.

Edwards, Valerie, et al. "The Wide-Ranging Health Outcomes of Adverse Childhood Experiences." In *Child Maltreatment.* Kingston, N.J.: Civic Research Institute, 2005.

fentanyl   A powerful analgesic drug that was first synthesized in Belgium in the late 1950s. It is 50 times more potent than HEROIN and thus should be used only with great caution. Some illegal users have been found dead with the needle still in their arm, and it has been determined that the intravenous fentanyl stopped the person's breathing. The drug is sometimes used as an anesthetic, but anesthesiologists use machines to help patients breathe and dosages are carefully calculated.

Fentanyl is a Schedule II drug under the CONTROLLED SUBSTANCES ACT. Fentanyl was first used as an intravenous anesthetic in the United States in the 1960s, under the name Sublimaze. Several other fentanyl analogues were subsequently introduced, including alfentanil (Alfenta), a very short-acting drug (acting within five to 10 minutes) and sufentanil (Sufenta), a strong analgesic (painkiller) that is five to 10 times more potent than fentanyl and is used in heart surgery. In the 21st century, fentanyl is primarily used as an anesthetic or an analgesic (painkiller).

There are newer delivery forms of fentanyl that are used as methods of sedation or for treatment of chronic severe pain; for example, Duragesic is a form of fentanyl that is available in a transdermal patch, while Actiq is a solid form of fentanyl citrate that resembles a lollipop that dissolves slowly in the mouth.

Actiq is used for patients who are dependent on opiates, and this drug is also used to treat cancer patients suffering from breakthrough pain. An analogue of fentanyl, carfentanil (Wildnil), is a highly potent drug that is used by some veterinarians to immobilize large animals.

Fentanyl is also abused. The illegal use of fentanyl stems back to the 1970s, and fentanyl continues to be a drug of abuse in the United States. At least 12 illicit analogues of fentanyl have been produced in CLANDESTINE LABORATORIES and have been found in the United States. These drugs are usually administered intravenously, but they may also be snorted or smoked.

Some individuals steal the drug from veterinary offices as well as from physicians for the purpose of abuse and/or sale. In addition, some patients who are legally prescribed fentanyl sell or give the drug to others. Some physicians abuse fentanyl.

See also CLUB DRUGS; DATE RAPE DRUGS; DIVERSION, DRUG; MALICIOUS POISONING; PRESCRIPTION DRUG ABUSE; SCHEDULED DRUGS; SEXUAL ASSAULTS; VIOLENCE.

Joseph, Donald E., ed. *Drugs of Abuse.* Washington, D.C.: U.S. Department of Justice, 2005.

fetal alcohol syndrome/fetal spectrum disorder (FAS)   A range of birth defects and developmental disabilities in a child whose mother abused alcohol during pregnancy. Alcohol exposure during pregnancy is the primary cause of preventable mental retardation. The mother may have been an alcoholic during the pregnancy and/or may have engaged in BINGE DRINKING (defined as consuming five or more drinks on one occasion in the past two weeks). However, physicians say that the woman need not have been an alcoholic to bear a child who had fetal alcohol syndrome (FAS), and even a small amount of alcohol can cause damage to the fetus. Damage may occur to the fetus with as little as 0.5 drink per day.

There is no known *safe* quantity of alcohol that will not affect the fetus of a pregnant woman. As a result, physicians advise pregnant women to avoid alcohol altogether. Unfortunately, some pregnant women continue to drink, despite the risks. As demonstrated in Table I, about 10 percent of women drink throughout their pregnancy, and about 2 percent are binge drinkers. In some states, if a newborn is born with indicators of fetal alcohol syndrome, then the state can place the child in foster care or even terminate the mother's parental rights altogether.

The extent of the damage to the child who has FAS varies greatly and may be mild to severe. Often it is not known what the damage is until after the child is born or even several years later.

According to the Centers for Disease Control and Prevention (CDC), about 1,000 to 6,000 babies born

TABLE I: PREVALENCE OF ALCOHOL CONSUMPTION AMONG CHILDBEARING-AGED WOMEN (18–44 YEARS) BY DRINKING PATTERN AND PREGNANCY STATUS, UNITED STATES, 2002

Pregnancy Status	Drinking Pattern	Percentage
Pregnant	Binge[1]	1.9
	Frequent use	1.9
	Any use	10.1
Might become pregnant	Binge	12.4
	Frequent use[2]	13.1
	Any use	54.9
All respondents	Binge	12.4
	Frequent use	13.2
	Any use	52.6

[1] Five or more drinks on one occasion.
[2] Seven or more drinks per week or binge drinking.
Source: Centers for Disease Control and Prevention. "Alcohol Consumption among Women Who Are Pregnant or Who Might Become Pregnant—United States, 2002." *Morbidity and Mortality Weekly Review* 53, no. 50 (December 24, 2004): 1,178–1,181.

each year in the United States have FAS. This is a rate of about 0.5 to 2.0 cases per 1,000 live births. Some groups, such as Native Americans, have FAS rates that are much higher: three to five cases per 1,000 children. Some studies indicate that African-American children have a five times greater risk of having FAS than white children, and American Indian/Alaskan Native children have an greater risk: 16 times greater risk than that of white children.

Symptoms and Diagnostic Path
It can be difficult for physicians to diagnose FAS but there are some signs to consider. They include

- prematurity
- low birth weight
- microcephaly (small head)
- seizures
- distractibility
- hyperactivity
- poor muscle coordination
- heart defects

According to the National Task Force on Fetal Alcohol Syndrome and Fetal Alcohol Effect in their 2005 booklet *Fetal Alcohol Syndrome: Guidelines for Referral and Diagnosis,* a diagnosis of FAS requires the presence of the following:

1. Documentation of all three facial abnormalities, including a smooth philtrum (the area of the face between the nose and the upper lip; the normal ridges separated by a groove are underdeveloped and flattened in children with prenatal alcohol exposure), a thin upper lip with poorly defined cupid's bow, and small palpebral fissures
2. Documentation of growth deficits
3. Documentation of central nervous system abnormalities, such as structural, neurological, functional, or a combination of abnormalities. Central nervous system dysfunctions may lead to impulsivity, memory problems, and learning disorders

Treatment Options and Outlook
FAS cannot be cured, but when it is identified, intervention and treatment can be started in order to help the child achieve to the best of his or her ability. Many children benefit from early intervention programs provided in school.

Any accompanying medical problems in the child, such as cardiac or kidney problems, should be treated. (Children who have FAS have a greater risk for such problems than children who do not.) Psychological and emotional problems that are identified should be dealt with by a professional experienced in treating children and/or adolescents who have FAS and providing support to parents. Parents may benefit from support and education in taking care of a child who has FAS; when a parent has drug and alcohol problems, treatment of the parent is as necessary as is treatment of the child.

Risk Factors and Prevention
Drinking during pregnancy is the one way to cause FAS, and the only sure way to prevent FAS altogether is for pregnant women to refrain from consuming any alcohol during their pregnancies. If a woman who drinks discovers that she is pregnant, she should immediately seek help in resolving her substance abuse problem, so that she also reduces the risk of bearing a child who has FAS.

See also ALCOHOL ABUSE AND DEPENDENCE AND HEALTH PROBLEMS; ALCOHOLISM; CHILD ABUSE; DOMESTIC VIOLENCE; FAMILY, EFFECT ON; PREGNANCY.

Centers for Disease Control and Prevention. "Alcohol Consumption among Women Who Are Pregnant or Who Might Become Pregnant—United States, 2002." *Morbidity and Mortality Weekly Review* 53, no. 50 (December 24, 2004): 1,178–1,181.

Miller, Laurie C., and Christine Adamec. *The Encyclopedia of Adoption.* New York: Facts On File, 2006.

National Task Force on Fetal Alcohol Syndrome and Fetal Alcohol Effect. *Fetal Alcohol Syndrome: Guidelines for Referral and Diagnosis.* Atlanta: Centers for Disease Control and Prevention, July 2004.

Sokol, Robert J., M.D., Virginia Delaney-Black, M.D., and Beth Nordstrom. "Fetal Alcohol Spectrum Disorder." *Journal of the American Medical Association* 290, no. 22 (December 10, 2003): 2,996–2,999.

Streissguth, Ann P., et al. "Risk Factors for Adverse Life Outcomes in Fetal Alcohol Syndrome and Fetal Alcohol Effects." *Journal of Developmental and Behavioral Pediatrics* 25, no. 4 (2004): 228–238.

flunitrazepam (Rohypnol)   A central nervous system depressant, one of the BENZODIAZEPINES. The drug is legal in the United States when it is prescribed by a physician, usually for the purposes of sedation. Flunitrazepam is a Schedule IV drug under the CONTROLLED SUBSTANCES ACT.

Flunitrazepam can be taken orally and may also be injected. It is an amnesiac; that means that those who take it have no memory of what occurs during a certain time span (depending on how much is taken).

Rohypnol is used in MALICIOUS POISONING, or given to people (primarily females) who unknowingly ingest the drug, often covertly placed by others in an alcoholic drink or a soft drink, leaving the woman vulnerable to sexual assault or molestation. This is also called "date rape," and thus flunitrazepam is considered one of the DATE RAPE DRUGS. There are no statistics on the number of individuals affected by unknowingly taking date rape drugs such as Rohypnol or other drugs. It is believed many victims fail to come forward, out of fear, guilt, and shame. Others take the drug knowingly, in order to abuse it for its sedating qualities.

Flunitrazepam is sometimes used illegally to counter the stimulating effects of such drugs as COCAINE or METHAMPHETAMINE.

Most abusers of flunitrazepam are 13–30 years old. MEXICO is a major manufacturing source for the drug.

Side Effects of Flunitrazepam   Rohypnol generally causes sedation, dizziness, memory impairment, and confusion, but the drug may also cause aggressive behavior in some users. Users experience its effect in about 15 minutes, and the effects of the drug may last as long as 12 hours or more.

See also HALLUCINOGENIC DRUGS; MALICIOUS POISONING; PRESCRIPTION DRUG ABUSE; SEXUAL ASSAULTS; VIOLENCE.

foreign jails/rights   Places of incarceration in countries that are not native to an individual. Many people mistakenly believe that other countries are far more lax than the United States or Canada in their attempts to control drug abuse and trafficking; however, some countries take a harshly punitive attitude toward individuals who use drugs, and especially against those who are believed to be DRUG DEALERS.

Some Westerners have been convicted of drug use and/or drug selling and have been placed in foreign jails for many years for crimes that might merit a brief stay in a jail in their native country or even no jail time at all. In addition, the rights that many Westerners take for granted, such as the right to an attorney, the right to a speedy trial, and the presumption of innocence, are not working premises in many other countries. Although the individual's native country may try to help a person accused of drug use or selling, the laws of the country where the crime was committed will nearly always prevail.

According to the U.S. State Department, an estimated 2,500 Americans are arrested in other countries every year, and of these arrests, more than 30 percent are for drug-related offenses. Most drug offenses (at least 70 percent) involve marijuana and cocaine. The arrested individuals are subject to the laws of the country where they are arrested, and U.S. laws do not apply. Ignorance of the laws of the foreign country is not a defense. As a result, the individual may be sentenced to many years in a foreign prison.

In many other countries, the accused must prove their innocence, in contrast to the United States, where individuals are innocent until proven guilty. A U.S. consul can provide information and offer to contact the arrested person's family or friends in the United States, as well as visit the prisoner, provide a list of attorneys, protest mistreatment, and monitor jail conditions. But a consul cannot secure the release of the prisoner.

Some other examples of differences between the U.S. penal system and that in other countries are:

- many countries do not allow for bail before trial
- few countries provide a jury trial
- prison, judicial and other officials may not speak English
- pre-trial detention and often solitary confinement can last for months
- prisons may not have minimal facilities, such as toilets, beds, and washbasins
- diets are often inadequate and require supplementation from relatives and friends
- physical abuse, confiscation of property, degrading treatment and extortion may occur

See CRIME AND CRIMINALS; GANGS; INCARCERATION; JAIL INMATES; LAW ENFORCEMENT; ORGANIZED CRIME; PROSTITUTION.

formication A terrifying tactile HALLUCINATION in which the skin feels as if it is crawling with insects or snakes, located above or even underneath the skin's surface. Such hallucinations may occur with the abuse of drugs such as METHAMPHETAMINE, COCAINE, or CRACK COCAINE. In fact, this hallucination is so common with methamphetamine abuse that the imaginary insects are called "crank bugs." (*Crank* is a slang word for methamphetamine.) In addition, a person who is undergoing alcohol withdrawal and experiencing DELIRIUM TREMENS may experience formication.

See also DELUSIONS; DUAL DIAGNOSIS; PSYCHOSIS.

foster care Temporary care of a child by a state-approved foster family or in a group home for children whose parents or other caregivers are unable or unwilling to provide needed care and/or who have abused and/or neglected them. The children may also be placed with approved relatives. It should be noted that foster care is presumed to be temporary care, but for a variety of reasons, some children remain in "the system" for years.

Many of the children in the foster care system have been neglected or abused as a result of their parents' severe problems with substance abuse, and the concomitant lack of control and ready anger caused by the abused substances, and as a result, they have been involuntarily removed from their families. If the parents or other caregivers cannot or will not resolve their problems within a specific time frame (about a year, on the basis of the provisions of the Adoption and Safe Families Act, a federal law), the state may terminate their parental rights and the children may be adopted by others.

In many cases, children who were reared by and/or abused by alcoholic or drug-dependent parents grow up to experience problems with substance abuse themselves.

See also CHILD ABUSE; DOMESTIC VIOLENCE; DRUG TESTING; FAMILY, EFFECT ON.

gamma-hydroxybutyrate (GHB) A drug of abuse that was first synthesized in the 1960s and has no current medical use. In past years, however, GHB was sold by health food stores for its alleged steroidal effects, although some establishments sold the drug as a natural sedative. GHB is colorless, odorless, and tasteless. It is a central nervous system depressant that can cause seizures and coma when abused. If GHB is combined with alcohol, the individual can experience breathing difficulties and nausea. An estimated 1,861 hospital emergency room episodes nationwide in the United States involved GHB in 2005, according to the National Institute on Drug Abuse. Few high school students use the drug, and it was estimated by the 2006 Monitoring the Future survey that fewer than 1 percent of eighth and 10th grade students and about 1 percent of high school seniors used the drug.

The Food and Drug Administration (FDA) removed GHB from the market in 1990, and currently GHB is a Schedule I drug under the CONTROLLED SUBSTANCES ACT. According to the Drug Enforcement Administration, GHB is sometimes used as a DATE RAPE DRUG. It is difficult to impossible to detect GHB in the body, and consequently, the drug may be slipped into the drink of an individual, usually for the purpose of taking sexual advantage of the person once the drug takes effect. However, Drink Safe Technology, a company in Anderson, Alabama, developed a test strip that can be used to a detect the presence of GHB in a drink, as well as the presence of KETAMINE and FLUNITRAZEPAM (ROHYPNOL), other date rape drugs. Bar coasters have also been developed that incorporate the test strip. (For more information, go to http://www.drinksafetech.com/TestKit.php.)

Individual Abusers of GHB

Some individuals abuse GHB themselves rather than inflicting the drug on unknowing victims. Abusers of GHB have three primary reasons for using this drug. First, they take GHB to gain its intoxicating effects and to induce a state of euphoria. Second, bodybuilders sometimes abuse GHB because they believe the drug will build up muscle, and they also use the drug as a sleep aid. Third, as discussed, GHB is a drug that is used for SEXUAL ASSAULT.

In 2004, according to Monitoring the Future data, the annual prevalence of GHB abuse among eighth graders and 10th graders was less than 1 percent, or 0.7 percent for eighth graders and 0.8 percent for 10th graders. Among 12th graders, the annual prevalence of GHB abuse was 2.0 percent. The annual prevalence for adults ages 19–30 who abused GHB in 2004 was less than 1 percent for all age groups, with the highest abuse rate seen among adults ages 21–24 years, or 0.9 percent.

See also ATHLETES; MALICIOUS POISONING; SCHEDULED DRUGS; YOUNG ADULTS.

Johnston, Lloyd D., et al. *Monitoring the Future: National Survey Results on Drug Use, 1975–2004.* Vol. 2, *College Students and Adults Ages 19–45.* Bethesda, Md.: National Institute on Drug Abuse, National Institutes of Health, 2005.

Johnston, Lloyd D., et al. *Monitoring the Future: National Results on Adolescent Drug Use: Overview of Key Findings 2004.* Bethesda, Md.: National Institute of Drug Abuse, April 2005.

Joseph, Donald E., et al., eds. *Drugs of Abuse.* Washington, D.C.: U.S. Department of Justice, 2005.

Snead III, O. Carter, M.D., and K. Michael Gibson. "γHydroxybutyric Acid." *New England Journal of Medicine* 353, no. 26 (June 30, 2005): 2,721–2,732.

gangs Groups of individuals, often adolescents or young adult males, who band together for the purpose of committing crimes and establishing a dominant culture. They are often associated with ORGANIZED CRIME entities. There are also some adult gangs, as well as outlaw motorcycle gangs, and some gangs that operate in the prison environment. Gangs may be associated with a particular race or ethnicity.

Gangs also use violence to establish or maintain control of the distribution of illegal drugs. In addition, government sources such as the National Drug Intelligence Center report that MARIJUANA distribution in some areas, particularly New York, are associated with violent behavior, up to and including HOMICIDE. Gangs are also associated with acts of robbery and aggravated assault.

Law enforcement agencies estimate that there are at least 21,500 gangs and about 731,500 active gang members within the United States, not including prison gangs, motorcycle gangs, and adult gangs, and these gangs operate in all states of the country. Gangs are also prevalent in other countries and often engage in the trafficking of illegal drugs as well as the commission of other crimes. Gangs typically engage in violent behavior, as a rite of passage into the gang, as a way to control individual members who do not follow the basic rules of the gang, and as a means to achieve their illegal goals. Some gangs engage in the trafficking of weapons.

Some people in neighborhoods report feeling terrorized by gangs, particularly poor neighborhoods. In these areas, gang members may openly engage in drug dealing and arranging meetings for the purpose of prostitution, without any fear that LAW ENFORCEMENT agents will take action against them. They may also openly steal items and then sell them.

Gang members may wear the tattoos of the specific gang and members may also wear similar styles of clothes and colors, in order to distinguish themselves from other gang members or nonmembers.

Gang members begin their recruitment of children as prospective new members when children are in elementary, middle, and high schools, and often schoolchildren join one gang for protection against members of another gang.

Gangs, Organized Crime, and Domestic Terrorism

According to the *2005 National Gang Threat Assessment* of the Department of Justice, gangs are the

TABLE I: PERCENTAGES OF LAW ENFORCEMENT AGENCIES REPORTING ASSOCIATION BETWEEN GANGS IN THE UNITED STATES AND ORGANIZED CRIME ENTITIES (BY TYPE OF ORGANIZATION)

Type of Organized Crime	Percentage
Mexican drug organizations	78.4
Asian organized crime	28.4
Russian/Central/East European organized crime	24.1
Colombian drug organizations	16.4
Dominican drug organizations	12.9
Middle Eastern organized crime	6.9
La Cosa Nostra organized crime	6.9
Italian organized crime	6.0
Nigerian organized crime	4.3
Albanian organized crime	3.4

Source: Adapted from Bureau of Justice Assistance. *2005 National Gang Threat Assessment.* Washington, D.C.: Department of Justice, 2005, p. 3.

primary distributors of illegal drugs in the United States. They are also often associated with organized crime entities, such as with Mexican, Asian, and Russian crime groups. An estimated 78.4 percent of surveyed law enforcement agencies said that there was an association between Mexican drug organizations and gangs; 28.4 percent of law enforcement agencies reported a link between Asian organized crime entities and gangs. (See Table I.)

Some gangs are associated with domestic terrorist groups. Most of these gangs are white supremacist groups, such as the Aryan Resistance, Ku Klux Klan, National Socialist movement, Skinheads, and other groups.

Female Gang Members

Most gang members are males, but some women are active in assisting gang members, and some are members themselves. It is also estimated that about 6 percent of gang members are females, and most female gang members are affiliated with male gangs rather than with all-female gangs. Females may assist gangs in committing crimes and carrying weapons, and they may engage in prostitution to obtain money for the gang. They may also engage in drug dealing and credit card and identity theft. In general, female gang members are less violent than male gang members.

TABLE II: MODERATE AND HIGH GANG INVOLVEMENT IN DISTRIBUTION OF ILLEGAL DRUGS
(PERCENTAGE BY REGION)

Drug Type	Northeast	South	Midwest	West
Powdered cocaine	52.9	38.7	37.5	32.9
Crack cocaine	52.9	45.7	60.2	39.2
Heroin	45.1	17.9	25.0	35.7
Marijuana	56.9	54.3	67.0	79.0
Methamphetamine	17.6	24.9	23.9	73.4
Methylenedioxymethamphetamine	31.4	19.1	18.1	30.1

Source: Adapted from Bureau of Justice Assistance. 2005 National Gang Threat Assessment. Washington, D.C.: Department of Justice, 2005, p. 1.

Outlaw Motorcycle Gangs

Members of outlaw motorcycle gangs are deeply involved in criminal activities such as murder, kidnapping, prostitution, weapons trafficking, arson, and drug production and smuggling. They also steal motorcycles and motorcycle parts and engage in other criminal acts. The primary source of income for outlaw motorcycle gangs is drug trafficking. The major outlaw motorcycle gangs in the United States are the Hells Angels, Bandidos, Outlaws, and Pagans. In the United States, it is believed that there are 62 chapters of Hells Angels, as well as 80 chapters of Bandidos, 67 chapters of Outlaws, and 41 chapters of Pagans. Often these gangs fight each other over territory.

The Hells Angels is a major producer and distributor of illegal drugs, particularly MARIJUANA, METH-AMPHETAMINE, COCAINE, HASHISH, HEROIN, LYSERGIC ACID DIETHYLAMIDE (LSD), PHENCYCLIDINE (PCP), and diverted prescription drugs. The Bandidos concentrate on the distribution of marijuana, cocaine, and methamphetamine, while the Outlaws are the primary manufacturers and distributors of methamphetamine. The Pagans distribute marijuana, methamphetamine, and PCP.

The type of drugs distributed by gangs differs according to the part of the country where the gang is located; for example, nearly two-thirds of marijuana is distributed by gangs (64.8 percent) nationwide, but the distribution of this drug by gangs is highest in the West (79 percent). In considering crack cocaine, 60.2 percent of this drug is distributed by gangs in the Midwest. (See Table II.)

Prison Gangs

Some of the inmates incarcerated in prison or jail continue to engage in gang activities, and it is estimated that at least 12 percent of the prison population is involved in such activities. These gangs engage in extortion and illicit activities that involve illegal drugs and gambling. Once gang members are released from prison, they often continue to engage in criminal activities related to their gang membership.

There are many prison gangs; some who are often identified are the Crips, Bloods, Gangster Disciples, Latin Kings, and Aryan Brotherhood. While in prison, gang members recruit new members.

See also CRIME AND CRIMINALS; DRUG DEALERS; JAIL INMATES; LAW ENFORCEMENT; VIOLENCE; YOUNG ADULTS.

Bureau of Justice Assistance. 2005 National Gang Threat Assessment. Washington, D.C.: Department of Justice, 2005.

gender differences, abuse of drugs and alcohol   In broad terms, males and females in the United States show different patterns in their abuse of drugs and alcohol. In general, males are more likely to abuse alcohol and/or illegal drugs than females. For example, according to the National Survey on Drug Use and Health, males who were ages 12 and older were more than twice as likely (12.7 percent) to be either substance abusers or substance-dependent (addicted) as were females (6.2 percent) in 2004. However, in considering only youths who were ages 12–17 years, the rate of substance abuse or dependence was virtually identical, or 8.7 percent for boys and 9.0 percent for girls.

In considering cases of MALICIOUS POISONING, such as DATE RAPE DRUGS, the majority of reported victims are females.

Adolescent Girls and Boys

Complicating the picture, when other factors are considered, adolescent girls sometimes significantly exceed teenage boys in terms of their illicit consumption of drugs. For example, 675,000 adolescent girls started using MARIJUANA in 2004, compared to 577,000 boys. In addition teenage girls exceeded teenage boys in the percentage who engaged in PRESCRIPTION DRUG ABUSE in 2004: 10.1 percent of adolescent girls had abused prescription drugs in the past year compared to 7.6 percent of adolescent boys who had abused them.

Girls are more likely than boys to suffer from DEPRESSION, and an estimated 2.4 million teenage girls had ever suffered a major depressive episode in 2004, compared to 1.1 million adolescent males. Since depression is often associated with substance abuse, this finding may partly explain some of the greater levels of prescription drug abuse and marijuana abuse among female adolescents.

Women in Substance Abuse Treatment

According to Carla A. Green in her 2006 article for *Alcohol Research & Health*, women who are substance abusers or dependent on substances are less likely to seek treatment than men, and they also face more barriers to obtaining the treatment that they need. She says that women are less likely to develop alcohol-related or drug-related problems than men, but when they develop problems, the patterns are different from those seen with men.

Says Green:

Conversely, when women do develop substance abuse problems, they tend to develop them faster than men do. For example, although women tend to be older than men, on average, when they begin a pattern of regular drunkenness, women's drinking-related problems (e.g., loss of control over drinking, negative consequences of drinking) appear to progress more quickly than those of men. This faster progression also means that women experience shorter intervals than men between onset of regular drunkenness and first encountering the negative consequences of drinking, which include physical problems, interpersonal difficulties, negative intrapersonal changes (such as in personality or self-esteem), poor impulse control, and

reduced ability to maintain normal social roles and responsibilities. Women also experience shorter intervals between first loss of control over drinking and onset of their most severe drinking-related consequences, and shorter intervals between onset of regular drunkenness and treatment-seeking.

Barriers to treatment that women may face include

- economic barriers (insufficient funds to pay for treatment)
- difficulty attending treatment because of family responsibilities
- feelings of shame or embarrassment from being in substance abuse treatment
- anxiety disorders and depressive disorders that may prevent women from seeking help
- lack of availability of transportation, housing, education, and income support
- lack of information about treatment options
- cultural barriers such as language problems
- limitations in everyday function caused by substance abuse and dependence as well as mental illness

In general, women who seek treatment for alcohol or drug abuse or dependence are younger and have lower education levels than men seeking treatment. They are also more likely to identify factors other than substance abuse as their primary problems, such as stressful life events or mental health symptoms.

Women are also different from men in their relapse pattern, according to Green, who says that women are more likely to relapse with a romantic partner than men. In addition, women are more likely than men to report experiencing interpersonal problems prior to a relapse.

Despite their differences from men, many women benefit from treatment for substance abuse or dependence. Says Green, "Consistent with findings of women's better outcomes in other domains (e.g., post-treatment abstinence, retention in treatment), women are less likely than men to relapse overall, and women tend to have better long-term recovery outcomes. Such results suggest that future research on gender differences in treatment outcomes should focus on improving the understanding of the underlying factors which differ by gender and predict better outcomes (such as better therapeutic alliances among women in treatment) and reduced relapse. Such a focus might further improve treatment outcomes for both men and women."

Percentage of women in treatment for substance abuse

Information from the 2005 report *Women in Substance Abuse Treatment: Results from the Alcohol and Drug Services Study (ADSS)* indicates that only about a third (32 percent) of all clients who receive substance abuse treatment are female. In general, the study revealed that females and males were similar in terms of their race and age. However, women in outpatient treatment or nonhospital residential treatment have had more children living with them than men. Women also had lower incomes and were less likely to have jobs than men, a finding that echoes the information provided in other stud-

ies. In addition, women were more likely than men to have lived with no other adults. This information was derived from a three-part study conducted between 1996 and 1999.

As can be seen from Table I, fewer than half (49.4) percent of the women who were admitted to outpatient nonmethadone clinics and 40.5 percent who were admitted to nonhospital residential treatment were admitted for alcohol abuse, compared to nearly two-thirds (63.4 percent) of males in outpatient clinics and 45.8 percent of males in residential treatment. In addition, the women were more likely to have received treatment for COCAINE abuse, or 19.2 percent of women in outpatient treatment compared to 11.3 percent of men in outpatient treatment for cocaine. (See Table I.)

The researchers also found that women-only facilities were much more likely to offer services to women such as child care, prenatal care, and transportation. For example, more than half (55.5 percent) of the women-only treatment facilities offered child care to their female patients, compared to only 10.6 percent of the mixed-gender facilities. In addi-

TABLE I: PERCENTAGE OF CLIENTS WITH DIFFERENT CHARACTERISTICS DISCHARGED FROM SUBSTANCE ABUSE TREATMENT, BY TREATMENT SERVICE TYPE AND GENDER: 1997–1999

	Service Type of Care			
	Outpatient Nonmethadone		Nonhospital Residential	
	Female	Male	Female	Male
Estimated Annual Number of Discharges	352,922	1,049,099	160,253	537,572
Characteristic	Percent		Percent	
Presenting Substance Abuse Problem at Admission				
Alcohol and drug abuse	53.7	53.3	60.1	63.3
Alcohol abuse only	27.2	38.5	19.4	21.3
Drug abuse only (excluding alcohol)	19.1	8.2	20.5	15.4
Substance of Choice at Admission				
Alcohol	49.4	63.4	40.5	45.8
Cocaine	19.2	11.3	32.3	23.6
Marijuana, hashish, THC	14.2	16.2	4.7	10.9
Amphetamines	4.5	2.5	4.8	4.6
Heroin	2.3	2.9	7.9	9.5
Nontreatment methadone or other opiates	4.9	0.2	—	—
Barbiturates, benzodiazepines, or other sedatives or hypnotics	0.9	—	—	—
Any other drug, multiple, or no substance of choice	4.7	3.4	3.5	4.9

Source: Adapted from Brady, Thomas M., and Olivia Silber Ashley, eds. *Women in Substance Abuse Treatment: Results from the Alcohol and Drug Services Study (ADSS).* Rockville, Md.: Substance Abuse and Mental Health Services Administration, September 2005, p. 64.

tion, more than a third (39.9 percent) of the women-only facilities offered prenatal care, compared to only 10.1 percent of the mixed-gender facilities. The large majority (92.8 percent) of the women-only facilities offered transportation to clients, compared to less than half (46.6 percent) of the mixed-gender facilities. However, mixed-gender facilities were slightly *more* likely to offer services for dual diagnosis clients, or 40.5 percent of the mixed-gender facilities compared to 37.0 percent of the women-only facilities. (See Table II for more information.)

Women in Jail and Drug Use

There are some gender variations when considering prison populations, in which women have a significantly greater rate of substance abuse than is seen among women in the general population. (See CRIME AND CRIMINALS.) In part because of this greater rate of substance abuse among female

TABLE III: SUBSTANCE DEPENDENCE OF ABUSE AMONG JAIL INMATES, BY SELECTED CHARACTERISTICS, 2002

Characteristic	Percentage of Jail Inmates		
	All	Dependence	Abuse Only
Percentage of all jail inmates	68.0	45.2	22.9
Gender			
Male	67.9	44.3	23.6
Female	69.2	51.8	17.4

Source: Adapted from Karberg, Jennifer C., and Doris J. James. *Substance Dependence, Abuse, and Treatment of Jail Inmates, 2002.* Bureau of Justice Statistics Special Report. Washington, D.C.: U.S. Department of Justice, July 2005, p. 3.

inmates, there is also a higher rate of substance dependence among female inmates than male inmates. For example, as seen in Table III, 44.3 percent of the incarcerated males were dependent on substances, compared to 51.8 percent of the female inmates. However, when considering abuse only, the rate for males was higher, or 23.6 percent for men compared to 17.4 percent for women.

See also ADOLESCENTS; BINGE DRINKING; JAIL INMATES; PRESCRIPTION DRUG ABUSE; SEXUAL ASSAULTS; YOUNG ADULTS.

Brady, Thomas M., and Olivia Silber Ashley, eds. *Women in Substance Abuse Treatment: Results from the Alcohol and Drug Services Study (ADSS).* Rockville, Md.: Substance Abuse and Mental Health Services Administration, September 2005.

Green, Carla A. "Gender and Use of Substance Abuse Treatment Services." *Alcohol Research & Health* 29, no. 1 (2006): 55–62.

Karberg, Jennifer C., and Doris J. James. *Substance Dependence, Abuse, and Treatment of Jail Inmates, 2002.* Bureau of Justice Statistics Special Report. Washington, D.C.: U.S. Department of Justice, July 2005.

Office of National Drug Control Policy. *Girls and Drugs: A New Analysis: Recent Trends, Risk Factors and Consequences.* Washington, D.C.: Executive Office of the President, February 9, 2006.

TABLE III: NATIONAL FACILITY RATES AND PERCENTAGES FOR SELECTED SUBSTANCE ABUSE TREATMENT FACILITY CHARACTERISTICS, WOMEN-ONLY FACILITIES AND MIXED-GENDER FACILITIES, 1996–1997

	Facility Clientele Composition	
	Women-Only Facilities	Mixed-Gender Facilities
	Percentage	Percentage
Characteristic		
Services Offered		
Child care	55.5	10.6
Prenatal care	39.9	10.1
Transportation	92.8	46.6
Family counseling	76.8	86.1
Combined substance abuse treatment and mental health services	41.1	55.2
Special Programs Offered		
Women	91.0	34.0
Pregnant women	54.6	17.1
Dual diagnosis clients	37.0	40.5
AIDS/HIV-positive clients[1]	30.1	21.2

[1] Acquired immune deficiency syndrome/human immunodeficiency virus.

Source: Adapted from Brady, Thomas M., and Olivia Silber Ashley, eds. *Women in Substance Abuse Treatment: Results from the Alcohol and Drug Services Study (ADSS).* Rockville, Md.: Substance Abuse and Mental Health Services Administration, September 2005, p. 72.

genetic predispositions and environmental effects in substance abuse In relation to substance abuse, *genetics* refers to an inherited tendency or an increased risk of an individual to abuse or become dependent on alcohol and/or illegal drugs, while *environmental effects* refer to the impact of the family (and sometimes of peers) that may lead to or influence the abuse or dependence on alcohol and/or drugs in relatives. Often genetic effects are referred to as *nature,* while environmental impacts are called *nurture.* Many experts believe that it is a combination of genetics and environment that causes substance abuse, and that an environmental issue may trigger a preexisting genetic predisposition.

Researchers have performed numerous twin and adoption studies to determine whether a genetic propensity to substance abuse could exist, and study after study has determined that such a predisposition does indeed appear to be present. Researchers have also studied the impact of environmental effects, such as the use of drugs and/or alcohol by an individual's peers or by family members, particularly parents. Some unique studies have discovered that older adoptive siblings who have no biological relationship to a younger child have a significant impact on the younger child's abuse of drugs or alcohol, and that if the older brother abuses substances, the younger brother is also likely to abuse them as well. This appears to reflect the impact of environmental factors.

Sometimes it is difficult to determine which effects are genetic and which may be environmental; for example, if a child born to alcoholic parents later becomes an alcoholic, it is usually impossible to determine whether the child was primarily affected by genes that were inherited or by an environment in which alcohol was commonly used. In addition, the child could have been affected by both the genes that were inherited *and* the environment in which he or she was brought up. Because of this problem, many researchers like to use identical twin or adoption studies in an attempt to differentiate genetic from environmental factors.

In twin studies, presumably if one identical twin has an alcohol or drug problem, if it is an inherited problem, then the other twin should also have the problem. If he or she does not, then researchers tend to believe that the alcohol or drug problem was caused by other factors.

In adoption studies, the child has none of the genes of the adoptive parents. If the researchers can obtain data on the genetic parents of the child, as in studies in Sweden and Denmark, then they can compare the outcome of the child to both the biological parents and the adoptive parents. Thus, if the biological parents were alcoholics but the adoptive parents were not, if the child grows up to develop alcoholism, this outcome is presumably related to an inherited risk toward ALCOHOLISM.

Many adoption studies have found a significant link between the existing alcoholism of a birth parent and the later development of alcoholism in a child who was placed for adoption. (In general, the linkage is apparently stronger for male parents who placed male children for adoption. This may be true because males are more likely to become alcoholics than are females.)

Some researchers have also found a direct genetic link that affects the development of alcoholism. For example, some individuals, particularly Asians, have a genetic mutation carrying a deficiency in aldehyde dehydrogenase 2 (ALDHZ) that converts acetaldehyde to acetate. This is the process that occurs when an individual consumes alcohol. As a result, individuals who have this gene become very ill after drinking one or two drinks and experience heart palpitations, dizziness, shortness of breath, and other symptoms.

Researcher Matt McGue studied a population of 180 Korean-born adoptees; he found that about a third of them had the ALDHZ genetic mutation. He studied these individuals and their drinking patterns from ages 15 to 18 years. (This research was described by Tracy Hampton in 2006 in the *Journal of the American Medical Association.*)

McGue found that for most of the adoptees, the gene acted as a protective factor against alcohol abuse and alcoholism. However, some of the adoptees abused alcohol anyway, *despite* the unpleasant side effects that occurred with drinking. He then studied the family environment and found that among these particular individuals, who were unrelated to either their parents or siblings, the subjects who had an older sibling who drank had increased odds of drinking. As a result, clearly, the interplay of both genetics and environment occurs in substance abuse for some individuals.

Environmental Effects

The environment in which a child is raised may increase the risk for substance use and dependence. In a study reported in *Alcoholism: Clinical and Experimental Research* in 2000, the researchers studied the risk of substance-induced disorders in 442 adult adoptees and 1,859 stepchildren when the adoptive parent or stepparent fit one of the following categories: an alcohol abuser, an alcoholic, a drug abuser, or a drug addict.

They found gender differences of effects in the adoptive parents; for example, when the adoptee was raised by an alcoholic adoptive mother, the child had an increased risk for alcohol abuse. In contrast, when the adoptee was raised by an alcoholic adoptive father, the child had an increased risk of illicit drug abuse and drug dependence rather than alcohol abuse or alcoholism.

With regard to adults raised by their stepparents, the researchers found that being reared by an alcoholic stepmother was predictive for an increased use of illicit drugs by a stepchild. Being raised by an alcoholic stepfather was predictive for alcohol abuse, illicit drug use, and drug dependence in the stepchild.

See also PSYCHIATRIC DISORDERS.

Adamec, Christine, and Laurie C. Miller, M.D. *The Encyclopedia of Adoption.* New York: Facts On File, 2007.

Bouchard, Jr., Thomas J., and Matt McGue. "Genetic and Environmental Influences on Human Psychological Differences." *Journal of Neurobiology* 54 (2003): 40–45.

Hampton, Tracy. "Interplay of Genes and Environment Found in Adolescents' Alcohol Abuse." *Journal of the American Medical Association* 295, no. 15 (April 19, 2006): 1,760, 1,762.

Newlin, David B., et al. "Environmental Transmission of DSM-IV Substance Use Disorders in Adoptive and Step Families." *Alcoholism: Clinical and Experimental Research* 24, no. 12 (December 2000): 1,785–1,794.

glue An adhesive and a volatile solvent that is a common household product and is sometimes used illegally, as are other INHALANTS, particularly by school-age children and adolescents. The goal of the abuser is to attain a temporary state of euphoria. Inhalants can be extremely hazardous to the health of users, sometimes causing brain damage and even death. About 598,000 youths ages 12–17 years abused inhalants in 2004, and of these adolescents, 30 percent abused glue, shoe polish, or toluene (cleaning fluid).

hallucinations Sensory errors caused by a disturbance in the brain. They may be temporary and fleeting or may be recurrent and long-term. Hallucinations may be a side effect of legally administered drugs (such as some narcotics, particularly MORPHINE that is administered for severe pain). They may also be caused by illegal medications, such as hallucinogenic drugs. In addition, they may also be induced by AMPHETAMINE, COCAINE, CRACK COCAINE, METHAMPHETAMINE, and high doses of DEXTROMETHORPHAN.

Individuals who are severely alcoholic and who are undergoing DELIRIUM TREMENS, an outcome that may occur with withdrawal from alcoholism, may suffer from terrifying hallucinations. Such individuals should be treated in a hospital, where they can receive medication to mitigate the physical and psychological effects of alcohol withdrawal.

Hallucinations may also be caused by psychosis, such as the psychosis in SCHIZOPHRENIA and sometimes in BIPOLAR DISORDER or severe DEPRESSION. In some acute cases, it may be difficult for doctors to determine the cause of hallucinations until drug testing and other further evaluation of the patient have occurred.

People who have schizophrenia or other psychotic disorders who are untreated may suffer from both hallucinations and delusions. With treatment, these problems may be decreased or even eliminated altogether. However, the underlying disease is still present, and if the person who has schizophrenia stops taking effective medication, eventually the psychotic symptoms recur.

Types of Hallucinations

Hallucinations may be visual, auditory, or tactile. People who are hallucinating may experience one or more of these types of hallucinations. With visual hallucinations, the person thinks that he or she sees someone or something that is not present. With auditory hallucinations, the person thinks that he or she hears voices or sounds that are not present. Tactile hallucinations occur when the person feels as if someone or something is touching him or her, when there is no one touching the person. All hallucinations may be frightening (although some are benign). One of the most terrifying forms of a tactile hallucination is FORMICATION, when the individual feels insects (which are not actually present) on or *under* the skin.

Hallucinations may be accompanied by delusions, or false beliefs, such as the paranoid delusion that someone is plotting against the individual.

See also DELUSIONS; PSYCHIATRIC DISORDERS; PSYCHOSIS; SCHIZOPHRENIA.

hallucinogenic drugs Drugs that have a major psychiatric effect on the user, and may cause them to experience HALLUCINATIONS as well as major mood shifts, including swings from euphoria to profound sadness, extreme terror, and so forth. The term *hallucinogens* is actually a misnomer since these drugs *may* produce hallucinations, but they do not always cause these sensory misperceptions.

Hallucinogenic drugs have been romanticized by some individuals in the past, for example, those who stated that these drugs could be used to expand an individual's mental horizons, such as Dr. Timothy Leary. He later became disenchanted with hallucinogens. Others point out the serious physical and mental health risks that are associated with the use of hallucinogens.

Hallucinogenic drugs were popular in the 1960s and 1970s, but they are no longer the drugs of choice among most drug abusers, largely because

154

their effects are highly unpredictable and are often unpleasant. A person could take a hallucinogenic drug on one occasion and have a pleasurable experience and then take the same drug in the same dose on another occasion and experience terrifying hallucinations. According to the National Survey on Drug Use and Health, in 2004, 929,000 people used hallucinogens, or less than 1 percent of all illicit drug users.

Most hallucinogenic drugs are Schedule I illegal drugs under the CONTROLLED SUBSTANCES ACT, such as LYSERGIC ACID DIETHYLAMIDE (LSD), METHYLENEDIOXYMETHAMPHETAMINE (MDMA/Ecstasy), MESCALINE, and other drugs. LSD is the most potent hallucinogen known in the United States, but it is used by few people in comparison to other drugs; for example, about 23 million people in the United States have tried LSD in their lifetimes, but there were only 141,000 current users of the drug in 2004.

The effects of hallucinogenic drugs may be as follows:

- elevated blood pressure
- increased heart rate
- dilated pupils
- sensory distortions
- thought disorders

Individuals may also experience long-term effects, such as *flashbacks* to the hallucinatory experiences the individual had while under the influence of the drug, yet these flashbacks may occur months or even years later, and when the individual has not taken the drug. These flashbacks can be very distressing.

At very high dosages, some over-the-counter drugs may create hallucinogenic effects, for example, high dosages of DEXTROMETHORPHAN.

In some cases, hallucinogenic drugs may trigger psychotic symptoms that may continue long after the drug is no longer in the body.

See also CANADA; COLLEGE STUDENTS; MESCALINE; PHENCYCLIDINE (PCP).

hashish/hashish oil An illegal and very potent drug that is derived from the Indian hemp plant,

Cannabis sativa, the same plant from which MARIJUANA is derived. Hashish and hashish oil are derived from the resinous secretions of the flowering parts of the hemp plant, in contrast to marijuana, which is derived from the leaves, flowers, stems, and seeds of the plant.

As with marijuana, it is the delta-9-tetrahydrocannabinol (THC) substance in hashish that is believed to cause both the intoxication and the psychological effects of cannabis products. The THC content of hashish may range from 5 to 12 percent; however, hashish oil has a much higher THC content of from 20 to 80 percent. According to the World Health Organization in their 2006 report, the primary sources of hashish worldwide are Morocco, Afghanistan, and Pakistan.

Hashish is a Schedule I drug under the CONTROLLED SUBSTANCES ACT with no lawful medical use in the United States.

Hashish is compressed into balls or cake and then pieces are broken off and the drug is smoked in pipes. Some people mix hashish with cigarette or pipe tobacco, and it may also be smoked using a water pipe.

Hashish oil is made by using a solvent to extract the cannabinoids from the plant to create a viscous liquid. One or two drops of this liquid is equivalent to one marijuana cigarette. This concoction ranges in color from light to very dark brown.

The frequent use of hashish can lead to a psychotic intoxication for two or more days. Some people become addicted to hashish.

See also SCHEDULED DRUGS.

United Nations Office on Drugs and Crime. *World Drug Report 2006*. Vol. 1. *Analysis*. United Nations, June 2006. Available online. URL: http://www.unodc.org/pdf/WDR_2006/wdr2006_volume1.pdf. Downloaded July 28, 2006.

hepatitis Inflammation of the liver, often caused by a viral infection, that is commonly known as hepatitis. Hepatitis is a risk for individuals who share needles to inject illegal drugs. Toxic hepatitis is caused by dangerous contaminants in manufactured drugs; some street drugs such as Ecstasy can have direct toxic effects on the liver.

Alcoholic hepatitis, however, may be caused by the chronic consumption of alcohol, which has severely damaged the liver. In some cases, patients have *both* viral hepatitis and alcoholic hepatitis, a very dangerous combination. Patients may become so ill with hepatitis that the only cure is liver transplantation. Without transplantation, they will die because life cannot be sustained without liver function.

Types of Hepatitis

Alcoholic Hepatitis In contrast with most early cases of viral hepatitis, in which there may be few or no symptoms, alcoholic hepatitis does present distinct symptoms, such as abdominal pain, nausea and vomiting, weakness, and fever. Because of their already damaged immune system, patients who have alcoholic hepatitis are at risk for contracting other infections as well, further weakening their bodies.

Patients who have alcoholic hepatitis must stop drinking immediately, and many require DETOXIFICATION treatment. The patient's recovery depends on the severity of the illness when the patient stops drinking and the extent of damage that has already occurred to the liver; however, regardless of how severely damaged the liver is, it is always advisable to stop drinking in order to prolong life. Only a physician can determine the status of the liver.

Toxic Hepatitis Some substances have direct toxic effects on the liver and should be avoided. Contaminants from the manufacture of METHAMPHETAMINE can include high levels of substances harmful to the liver. In addition, individuals who seek to use hallucinogenic mushrooms can accidentally ingest poisonous mushrooms that cause abrupt and life-threatening liver toxicity. Some common over-the-counter medications, such as acetaminophen (Tylenol), if overused, can cause liver toxicity by causing the death of liver cells, especially in overdose situations. Individuals who have been diagnosed with hepatitis should avoid acetaminophen altogether.

Viral Hepatitis There are three primary forms of contagious hepatitis, including hepatitis A, B, and C. Hepatitis A is very common, and usually individuals who have this form of the disease have no symptoms. Treatment is not recommended if the illness is identified, usually inadvertently during routine testing.

Other forms of hepatitis are less common, such as hepatitis B and C. Individuals who have ALCOHOLISM are the most likely to contract hepatitis B and C, as are drug users who inject their drugs. Hepatitis B and/or C can become very serious and even life-threatening. In some cases, patients need liver transplantation.

Symptoms and Diagnostic Path

When symptoms occur with hepatitis A, they may include abdominal pain, fatigue, headache, light-colored stools, darkened urine, and jaundice. Routine liver enzyme tests such as for serum alanine aminotransferase (ALT) show elevated levels in patients who have hepatitis A.

With hepatitis B and C, patients often also have no symptoms. When there are symptoms, they may include jaundice, fatigue, darkened urine, abdominal pain, loss of appetite, and nausea.

Doctors check for hepatitis with routine liver enzyme tests, which show elevated levels if the condition is present. Occasionally, special blood tests can used to detect the virus, especially with hepatitis C; however, there are some false negative results, as a result of which despite negative findings for the virus, patients really are infected. The symptoms may be better evidence of the disease than laboratory tests provide.

Treatment Options and Outlook

There is no known cure for any form of hepatitis as of this writing other than liver transplantation, although some patients, especially those infected with hepatitis A, recover with no therapy. With all other forms of hepatitis, patients should avoid alcohol to prevent further damage to the liver.

With hepatitis B, treatment may include injected interferon and other antiviral medications. For patients who have hepatitis C, ribavarin or lamivudine may be given along with interferon.

The liver enzyme levels among patients diagnosed with hepatitis B or C should be checked periodically by the physician. Hepatitis B and C patients also have an increased risk for developing liver cancer (hepatocellular carcinoma). With hepatitis C, about 70 percent of infected individuals eventually have chronic liver disease, according to the Centers for Disease Control and Prevention (CDC), although this degenerative process may take many years before it becomes evident or troublesome.

Risk Factors and Preventive Measures

Individuals who are at risk for contracting hepatitis A may live with a person who already has the disease or may eat in a restaurant staffed by an infected worker. Contact with blood or body fluids can allow hepatitis A to be transmitted; however, type A is readily transmitted by contact with feces of an infected individual (thus, the need for hand washing prior to food handling). Most people in the United States should not worry about contracting hepatitis A; however, hepatitis A is widespread in Africa and Southeast Asia and can be contracted by travelers to these areas.

Hepatitis B is primarily transmitted through blood or contact with body fluid. Sexual partners may contract type B or C from a partner. Blood transfusion may also allow the virus to be transmitted to the recipient. With hepatitis B or C, children who have been sexually abused or were born to infected mothers are at risk for both hepatitis B and C infection.

Preventive measures against hepatitis B and C include avoiding shared needles, avoiding contact with the blood or bodily fluids of an infected individual, and using the same safe sex measures as recommended in preventing infection with the HUMAN IMMUNODEFICIENCY VIRUS (HIV).

See also ALCOHOL ABUSE AND DEPENDENCE AND HEALTH PROBLEMS; DRUG ABUSE AND DEPENDENCE AND HEALTH PROBLEMS; HEROIN; INTRAVENOUS/INJECTING DRUG USE/IV DRUG USERS.

Adamec, Christine, and Laurie C. Miller, M.D. *The Encyclopedia of Adoption.* New York: Facts On File, 2006.

Minocha, Anil, M.D., and Christine Adamec. *The Encyclopedia of the Digestive System and Digestive Disorders.* New York: Facts On File, 2004.

heroin   An illegal and highly addictive drug that is processed from MORPHINE, which itself is derived from opium poppies. Heroin is actually more potent than morphine for complex chemical rea-

sons. AFGHANISTAN is the world's largest producer of heroin, although most of the heroin that is used by addicts in the United States is from South America and MEXICO. Heroin is usually sold as either a brown or a white powder, although sometimes it is sold as a sticky black substance that is known as "black tar heroin." Most heroin is combined with other drugs or with substances such as powdered milk, starch, sugar, or quinine. In some cases, the drug is laced with strychnine or other poisons.

According to the United Nations Office on Drugs and Crime, an estimated 9.2 million people worldwide abused heroin in 2003. In the United States, heroin was involved in nearly 8 percent of all drug-related emergency room visits in 2003.

Users of heroin experience a "rush," or a feeling of euphoria, which is the most pronounced reaction with the initial or early use of the drug. Once individuals are addicted to heroin, the drug is needed to prevent WITHDRAWAL symptoms. After the drug takes effect, the user generally feels drowsy and mental function is impaired. (This is sometimes referred to as nodding.) The heart rate slows, as does the breathing. In some cases, breathing slows so much that the individual dies. Another side effect of heroin abuse for new users is copious vomiting. This produces such an aversive reaction in some people that they never try heroin again.

According to the National Institute on Drug Abuse (and although it sounds ludicrous to most people), some addicted individuals withdraw from heroin solely so that they may take the drug again later and reexperience the initial euphoria that is induced by heroin. Of course, they also become readdicted to the drug.

Heroin can be injected, sniffed/snorted, or smoked. Snorting or smoking the drug is more appealing to some drug abusers, who fear contracting diseases such as HEPATITIS or the HUMAN IMMUNODEFICIENCY VIRUS (HIV), from shared needles. They may also mistakenly believe that they can only become addicted to heroin if they inject the drug. However, the use of heroin by any delivery system will lead to drug dependence.

An intravenous injection of the drug has the fastest action of all delivery methods, or seven or eight seconds. An intramuscular injection of the drug takes five to eight minutes before the effects are experienced. When heroin is either smoked or snorted, the effects are usually experienced within about 10 to 15 minutes.

Because heroin is an illegal drug in the United States, there is no "quality control" over either its purity or the actual contents of the drug that is sold to individuals as heroin. In some cases, the drug is adulterated. The *Journal of the American Medical Association* reported in 2005 on 26 cases of heroin addicts who became very ill from heroin that was adulterated with clenbuterol, a veterinary medication that is also used illicitly by some people as an alternative to ANABOLIC STEROIDS. In the mid-1990s, there were cases of widespread poisoning as a result of heroin that was adulterated with scopolamine.

The more pure that the heroin is, the greater its effect on the body. In most cases, heroin sold on the street has a purity of from 1 to 10 percent. However, in recent years, more incidents of much purer heroin have been reported, and the purity may reach 70 percent in some cases. When the purity level increases, so does the death rate from heroin overdose.

Historical Background

Heroin was first synthesized in the United States in 1874 but was not developed as a medication until 1898, when the Bayer Company in Germany introduced heroin as a painkiller, marketing it as a safe and effective drug. It was used as a cough suppressant, as well as a means to treat both tuberculosis and pneumonia. Heroin was also included in many liquid and other preparations and was freely available to most people. In about 1910, the addictive nature of heroin was acknowledged and the tide began to turn against the legal use of this drug.

Heroin was first controlled by the federal government under the Harrison Narcotic Act of 1914. Today heroin is a Schedule I drug under the CONTROLLED SUBSTANCES ACT of 1970; that means it is among the drugs that have the highest potential for abuse and dependence and have no valid medical use in the United States. As a result, heroin use is illegal in the United States.

In some parts of the world, such as in the United Kingdom, heroin is prescribed to treat pain among terminally ill patients, and in those locations, physicians may prescribe the drug to their patients; however, these countries continue to criminalize the selling of heroin by DRUG DEALERS or others.

Users of Heroin

In the United States, heroin is rarely used by adolescents, and the average age of those who try heroin for the first time is about 24 years. According to the Monitoring the Future survey, an annual survey of drug use among students in the eighth, 10th, and 12th grades, the lifetime use of heroin (having ever used the drug) was 1.6 percent among eighth graders, and 1.5 percent each among the 10th graders and 12th graders. Thus, it is not a common drug of abuse among adolescents.

According to the National Survey on Drug Use and Health, about 3.7 million people in the United States had used heroin at one point in their life, and 119,000 had used the drug within the past month before the survey in 2004. About 314,000 Americans abused or were addicted to heroin in 2003, and about 281,000 heroin users received drug treatment for their addiction.

Heroin Use in Selected Cities and States

According to their 2005 report, the Community Epidemiology Work Group, which reports on 21 areas in the United States on drug abuse patterns, heroin abuse continued to be high in Baltimore, Maryland, and Newark, New Jersey, and its use was relatively high in areas such as Boston, Chicago, New York, Philadelphia, San Francisco, Seattle, and Washington, D.C. However, there is a very wide disparity of heroin abuse from region to region. (See tables.) For example, in considering treatment for heroin as a percentage of all drug treatment (except for alcohol) the percentages ranged from a low of 3 percent in Hawaii in 2004 to a high of 81.8 percent in Newark, New Jersey, followed by 74.2 percent in Boston. (See Table I.)

Another aspect of drug use is the number of emergency room admissions that occur as a result of the side effects of drug abuse. As can be seen from Table II, however, heroin only represented a small number of emergency room admissions from illicit drugs in some regions, while it represented a large percentage in others. For example, in Atlanta, heroin admission represented 5.3 percent of all emergency department admissions, while in New-

TABLE I: PRIMARY HEROIN TREATMENT ADMISSIONS AS A PERCENTAGE OF ALL ADMISSIONS (EXCLUDING ALCOHOL), 2001–2004

Area/State	2001	2002	2003	2004
Atlanta	8.6	5.2	8.5	7.4
Baltimore	60.4	62.0	61.5	60.4
Boston	74.1	72.6	73.4	74.2
Chicago	NR	NR	NR	47.3
Denver	25.3	21.5	22.5	13.6
Detroit	46.9	42.7	43.1	46.0
Los Angeles	46.3	37.4	31.1	29.2
Broward County, Florida	NR	9.0	4.1	13.0
Minneapolis/St. Paul	6.4	7.1	6.7	6.5
New Orleans	18.3	14.6	13.4	13.6
New York	43.2	41.1	42.3	42.0
Newark	85.9	85.8	85.4	81.8
Philadelphia	33.9	29.6	31.4	33.5
St. Louis	15.0	13.7	11.7	14.6
San Diego	12.3	11.7	10.9	25.0[1]
San Francisco	54.4	47.4	35.8	42.8
Seattle	23.7	26.6	25.1	27.2
Washington, D.C.	47.0	46.9	51.2	NR
Arizona	15.4	14.0	11.7	19.6
Hawaii	5.1	4.7	3.6	3.0
Texas	16.4	15.9	13.6	14.0

[1] The 2004 data are from the state system, while prior data are from the county California Alcohol and Drug Data System (CADDS). The state's county data include more programs treating heroin abusers.
NR: not reported.
Source: National Institute of Drug Abuse. *Epidemiologic Trends in Drug Abuse.* Vol. 1, *Proceeding of the Community Epidemiology Work Group: Highlights and Executive Summary.* Bethesda, Md.: National Institutes of Health, June 2005, p. 13.

ark, New Jersey, nearly half (45.2 percent) of all drug admissions were of heroin abusers.

It should also be noted that the purity of heroin varies greatly from city to city. According to the *Epidemiologic Trends in Drug Abuse* report, the purity of heroin sold to addicts in 2003 ranged from 10 percent pure in Seattle to 61 percent pure in Newark.

Effects of Heroin Abuse

According to the National Institute on Drug Abuse, there are both short-term and long-term effects of heroin abuse. The short-term effects that many people who abuse heroin experience are

- a euphoric "rush"
- nausea and vomiting
- miscarriage (also known as "spontaneous abortion," which is an unplanned loss of the fetus)
- cloudy mental functioning

The long-term effects of heroin abuse are

- addiction
- contracting of other diseases, such as hepatic infections and HIV
- bacterial infections
- infection of the lining of the heart and the heart valves
- development of arthritis
- collapsed veins
- liver and kidney diseases
- lung complications (tuberculosis, pneumonia)

Withdrawal from Heroin

It is very difficult for most individuals to withdraw from heroin, once they are addicted to the drug, and DETOXIFICATION should occur only under the care of experienced medical professionals. Attempts to withdraw on one's own are very dangerous and can be fatal.

Withdrawal symptoms may occur within hours from the time of the last injection, and they may include muscle and bone pain, vomiting, insomnia, diarrhea, and uncontrollable leg movements. These symptoms peak within about 24–48 hours after the last heroin dosage was taken and usually subside in about a week; however, some individuals continue to have symptoms for months.

Treatment of Heroin Addiction

Many heroin addicts are maintained on METHADONE, an oral legal drug that is neither sedating nor intoxicating. It is used to suppress the CRAVING for heroin and is considered medically safe. It is also used for those not addicted to heroin but who need relief from chronic pain. However, use of methadone does not end addiction but replaces an addiction with heroin to an addiction to methadone.

TABLE II: NUMBER OF HEROIN EMERGENCY DEPARTMENT REPORTS BY AREA AND
TOTAL REPORTS FOR ALL ILLICIT DRUG REPORTS: 2004

Area	Total Number Illicit Drug Reports	Heroin Reports	Percentage of Heroin Reports of All Illicit Drug Reports
Atlanta	9,437	483	5.1
Baltimore	10,528	4,533	43.1
Boston	8,957	3,341	37.3
Chicago	12,909	4,163	32.2
Denver	3,882	609	15.7
Detroit	6,990	1,885	27.0
Houston	6,434	166	2.6
Los Angeles	5,675	712	12.5
Miami-Dade County, Florida	9,225	1,387	15.0
Minneapolis/St. Paul	7,782	779	10.0
New Orleans	3,248	490	15.1
New York	21,695	6,574	30.3
Newark	3,901	1,764	45.2
Philadelphia	7,413	1,935	26.1
Phoenix	5,783	755	13.1
St. Louis	4,092	601	14.7
San Diego	2,999	492	16.4
San Francisco	6,071	1,278	21.1
Seattle	7,445	2,171	29.2
Washington, D.C.	6,183	1,486	24.0

Source: Adapted from National Institute of Drug Abuse. *Epidemiologic Trends in Drug Abuse.* Vol. 1, *Proceeding of the Community Epidemiology Work Group: Highlights and Executive Summary.* Bethesda, Md.: National Institutes of Health, June 2005, p. 13.

Supporters of methadone maintenance say that this form of treatment is preferable to continuation on heroin, because methadone users are treated with clean needles and it is known what is present in the drug. When heroin users share dirty needles, they risk the transmission of many diseases, and do not know what substances may be adulterated with the heroin or how pure the drug may be.

Other addicts may be treated with BUPRENORPHINE. Some are treated with naloxone or NALTREXONE (ReVia), drugs that block the effects of heroin or MORPHINE, which may be effective at preventing RELAPSE. In some cases, METHADONE or BUPRENORPHINE may be combined with psychotherapy, such as with behavioral therapies.

Rather than being maintained on methadone, most heroin addicts are given DETOXIFICATION treatment, which helps them to avoid the most severe symptoms of withdrawal while under the care of a physician in an inpatient facility, such as a rehabilitation center or a hospital. The most effective forms of treatment for heroin addiction are residential programs lasting at least three months.

According to the Treatment Episode Data Set (TEDS), which provides information on substance abuse admissions nationwide in the United States, the percentage of total treatment admissions for heroin abuse increased from 12 percent in 1993 to 25 percent in 2003. This is a greater percentage than among those who were hospitalized for cocaine addiction. Most of the patients (68 percent) who were admitted were male and about half (47 percent) were non-Hispanic whites.

See also DRUG ABUSE AND DEPENDENCE AND HEALTH PROBLEMS; HEPATITIS; INTRAVENOUS/INJECTING DRUG USE/IV DRUG USERS; NARCOTICS; OPIATES; SCHEDULED DRUGS.

Centers for Disease Control and Prevention. "Atypical Reactions Associated with Heroin Use—Five States, January–April 2005." *Morbidity and Mortality Weekly Report* 54 (2005): 793–796.

Joseph, Donald E., ed. *Drugs of Abuse.* Washington, D.C.: U.S. Department of Justice, 2005.

National Institute of Drug Abuse. *Epidemiologic Trends in Drug Abuse.* Vol. 1. *Proceeding of the Community Epidemiology Work Group. Highlights and Executive Summary.* Bethesda, Md.: National Institutes of Health, June 2005.

homelessness Lack of a home. Individuals who are substance abusers or addicts have a higher risk of homelessness than others. In a study of incarcerated inmates reported by the Bureau of Justice Statistics in 2005, more than two-thirds (68 percent) of the inmates had either a substance abuse or dependence problem. Of those inmates who abused or were dependent on drugs, 16.5 percent reported being homeless in the past year, compared to 9.1 percent of the other inmates.

In a study on the prevalence of mental health and substance abuse disorders among both homeless and low-income housed mothers reported in 1998 in the *American Journal of Psychiatry,* the researchers studied 220 homeless mothers and 216 housed mothers on public assistance. They found that the groups had similar rates of substance abuse disorders and psychiatric disorders, although the homeless women had higher rates of substance abuse. In addition, both groups of women had high rates of POST-TRAUMATIC STRESS DISORDER (PTSD).

Among the homeless women, 41.1 percent had a lifetime prevalence of any alcohol or drug abuse or dependence, compared to 34.7 percent of the housed women. The homeless women had a past-month prevalence of 4.6 percent of any substance use disorder, compared to 3.7 percent of the housed women. The homeless women had a 3.6 percent rate of past-month alcohol or drug abuse or dependence, compared to the housed women, who had a rate of 1.9 percent.

In considering psychiatric disorders, in some cases, the housed women had higher rates; for example, the homeless women had a rate of 9.6 percent for a one-month prevalence of major depressive disorder, compared to the rate of 11.6 percent for the housed women. The homeless women had a rate of 12.7 percent for any anxiety disorder in the past month, compared to 15.3 percent for the housed women.

See also CRIMES AND CRIMINALS; JAIL INMATES.

Bassuk, Ellen, M.D., John C. Buckner, Jennifer N. Perloff, and Shari S. Bassuk. "Prevalence of Mental Health and Substance Use Disorders among Homeless and Low-Income Housed Mothers." *American Journal of Psychiatry* 155 (1998): 1,561–1,564.

homicide See DEATH.

human immunodeficiency virus (HIV) See ACQUIRED IMMUNE DEFICIENCY SYNDROME (AIDS)/ HUMAN IMMUNODEFICIENCY VIRUS (HIV).

hydrocodone A narcotic painkiller that has a significant risk for abuse as well as dependence (addiction), primarily among those who use it for nonmedical purposes or who have received it for legitimate pain but have a prior history of substance abuse. Some forms of hydrocodone are Schedule II drugs under the CONTROLLED SUBSTANCES ACT. Others, such as hydrocodone that is combined with acetaminophen or ibuprofen, are Schedule III drugs, including such drugs as Lorcet, Lortab, Vicodin, Vicoprofen, Tussionex, and Norco. Among those aware of prescription drug abuse, hydrocodone prompts concern.

As with other prescription medications for moderate to severe pain, most pain patients do not develop a dependency (addiction) on hydrocodone; however, among those individuals who use the drug illegally, it is highly addictive. (See PAIN MANAGEMENT AND NARCOTIC MEDICATIONS.)

Because some forms of hydrocodone are Schedule III drugs, a physician can usually phone in a prescription for hydrocodone to a pharmacy and offer refills of the medication to patients. In contrast, for Schedule II drugs physicians may only write a prescription for 30 days and a new prescription is required every 30 days. As a result, some physicians may be more likely to prescribe hydrocodone than OXYCODONE or other Schedule II drugs. Note that as of this writing, the Drug Enforcement Administration has expressed an interest in reclassifying hydrocodone as a Schedule II drug, but no action toward reclassification has been taken yet.

Hydrocodone, as well as all other scheduled narcotics, is often offered for sale on the Internet to virtually any person who presents a valid credit card; however, federal and state governments are seeking the means to overcome this problem. This is complicated by the fact that such Web sites open and close with rapidity, and some of the sites are located in other countries, where the sale of narcotics may not be illegal.

Forms and Uses of Hydrocodone

Hydrocodone is made in a generic form as well as under several brand names, such as Vicodin, Lorcet, or Percocet (all containing hydrocodone with acetaminophen—also known as Tylenol) as well as Percodan (hydrocodone combined with aspirin).

Hydrocodone is prescribed to patients who have moderate to severe pain, such as those who have cancer or extreme chronic pain from arthritis, back pain, and other painful conditions. The drug is also sold illegally on the street by DRUG DEALERS, who themselves buy it through drug traffickers. In some cases, they obtain the drug from people who have submitted legitimate prescriptions and subsequently sold their drugs illegally. Sometimes hydrocodone is stolen from pharmacies or from dentists or doctors.

The drug may also be stolen from the medicine cabinets of patients, although this is the least efficient way of obtaining the drug, since most people have only a limited supply of narcotics in their bathrooms. However, because of this abuse, all legally prescribed narcotics should be kept under lock and key. Another reason for locking up narcotics is that sometimes others, such as elderly individuals or those with poor sight, mistakenly take narcotics from the medicine cabinet, mistaking them for other drugs.

Hydrocodone is sometimes abused by pharmacists, physicians, and others, who have ready access to this drug. For example, some pharmacists divert the drug by filling prescriptions for hydrocodone and other scheduled drugs, with fewer doses than ordered. They then keep (skim) the rest of the prescription for themselves or for sale to drug traffickers.

Abuse and Abusers of Hydrocodone

According to some reports, such as an article in the *Journal of Pain* in 2005, hydrocodone is the second

TABLE I: NONMEDICAL USE OF HYDROCODONE PRODUCTS[1] IN THE UNITED STATES IN LIFETIME, BY AGE GROUP: PERCENTAGES, 2003 AND 2004

Total		Ages 12–17		Ages 18–25		Ages 26+	
2003	2004	2003	2004	2003	2004	2003	2004
7.1	7.4	5.0	5.6	16.3	17.4	5.7	5.9

[1] Vicodin, Lortab, and Lorcet.
Source: Substance Abuse and Mental Health Services Administration. *Results from the 2004 National Survey on Drug Use and Health: National Findings.* Rockville, Md.: Department of Health and Human Services, September 2005, p. 242.

most abused drug in the United States after OXY-CONTIN (a timed-release form of oxycodone). However, according to the National Survey on Drug Use and Health, there are greater numbers of lifetime abusers of hydrocodone products than of oxycodone products. It is unknown whether the greater number of abusers may be due to the fact that hydrocodone is easier to obtain than products containing oxycodone, such as OxyContin.

Individuals who are in the age bracket of 18 to 25 years are the most likely to abuse products containing hydrocodone, especially Vicodin, Lortab, Lorcet, and generic hydrocodone. (See Table I.) According to the *Results from the 2004 National Survey on Drug Use and Health,* the lifetime prevalence of the abuse of specific forms of hydrocodone rose significantly from 2003 to 2004, particularly among young adults ages 18 to 25 years. For example, among those ages 18–25, Vicodin, Lortab, and Lorcet had a lifetime prevalence (among individuals who ever used the drug) of 16.3 percent in 2003, which increased to 17.4 percent in 2004. The lifetime abuse of hydrocodone by individuals of all ages increased slightly from 7.1 percent in 2003 to 7.4 percent in 2004.

See also DIVERSION, DRUG; NARCOTICS; OPIATES; PAIN MANAGEMENT AND NARCOTIC MEDICATIONS; PRESCRIPTION DRUG ABUSE; SCHEDULED DRUGS.

Cicero, Theodore J., James A. Inciardi, and Alvaro Muñoz. "Trends in Abuse of OxyContin and Other Opioid Analgesics in the United States: 2002–2004." *Journal of Pain* 6, no. 10 (October 2005): 662–672.
Substance Abuse and Mental Health Services Administration. *Overview of Findings for the 2004 National Survey on Drug Use and Health.* Rockville, Md.: Department of Health and Human Services, September 2005.

impaired driving, involvement of alcohol and/or drugs A markedly substandard driving ability that is either induced or worsened by the abuse of alcohol and/or illicit drugs. (Lawfully prescribed drugs may sometimes impair driving, but this entry concentrates on drugs that were used unlawfully, as well as on excessive alcohol consumption that impairs concentration and driving ability.) Motor vehicle crashes are the number one cause of death in people ages one to 35, and they are often fueled by the abuse of alcohol and/or drugs.

Individuals who are impaired by alcohol and/or drugs often drive fast and recklessly, and their response times are slowed considerably. As a result, they cannot respond quickly to the same changes that an unimpaired driver could readily adjust to, such as seeing a small child suddenly step into a crosswalk and in response slowing or swerving away from the child.

Drivers under the influence of alcohol or drugs are also less likely to take safety precautions, such as wearing seat belts or using turn signals, and thus are more likely to be injured in car crashes caused by them or others.

According to the National Center for Statistics and Analysis, a division of the National Highway Transportation Safety Administration (NHTSA), alcohol was present in 42,636 car crash fatalities in 2004. Of these cases, 49 percent of the fatalities were drivers who had used alcohol, and 17 percent of those who died were passengers who were riding with the person using alcohol. Motorcycle riders who were using alcohol represented 8 percent of the alcohol-related fatalities.

Many adolescents and young adults who are impaired by alcohol and or drugs are at risk for car crashes and other injuries. According to the *National Survey on Drug Abuse and Health*, about 10 percent of youths in the United States ages 16–17 years old drove vehicles while under the influence of alcohol in 2004. This percentage doubled to 20 percent of young adults ages 18–20 years old and further increased to 28 percent for individuals in the age range of 21–25 years old.

The Effect of Drugs on Driving Vary

Many illicit drugs can impair driving. The NHTSA reported on the effects of particular drugs on driving ability in *Drugs and Human Performance Fact Sheets*, which was prepared by an international panel of experts on drug-impaired driving and was published in 2004. For example, in considering the effects of marijuana on driving, the report states:

> Epidemiology data from road traffic arrests and fatalities indicate that after alcohol, marijuana is the most frequently detected psychoactive substance among driving populations. Marijuana has been shown to impair performance on driving simulator tasks and on open and closed driving courses for up to approximately 3 hours. Decreased car handling performance, increased reaction times, impaired time and distance estimation, inability to maintain headway, lateral travel, subjective sleepiness, motor incoordination, and impaired sustained vigilance have all been reported. Some drivers may actually be able to improve performance for brief periods by overcompensating for self-perceived impairment. The greater the demands placed on the driver, however, the more critical the likely impairment. Marijuana may particularly impair monotonous and prolonged driving. Decision times to evaluate situations and determine appropriate responses increase. Mixing alcohol and marijuana may dramatically produce effects greater than either drug on its own.

With regard to cocaine and its effects on driving, the authors state:

> Observed signs of impairment in driving performance have included subjects speeding, losing control of their vehicle, causing collisions, turning in front of other vehicles, high-risk behavior, inattentive driving, and poor impulse control. As the effects of cocaine wear off subjects may suffer from fatigue, depression, sleepiness, and inattention. In epidemiology studies of driving under the influence cases, accidents, and fatally injured drivers, between 8–23% of subjects have had cocaine and/or metabolites detected in their blood. An examination of 253 fatally injured drivers in Wayne County, Michigan between 1996–1998, found that 10% of cases were positive for blood cocaine and/or metabolites. On review of accident and witness reports, aggressive driving (high speed and loss of vehicle control) was revealed as the most common finding.

See also INJURIES, CAUSED BY ALCOHOL AND/OR ILLICIT DRUGS.

National Center for Statistics and Analysis. "Alcohol-Related Fatalities in 2004." DOT HS 809 904. Washington, D.C.: National Highway Safety Transportation Administration, August 2005.

National Highway Traffic Safety Administration. *Drugs and Human Performance Fact Sheets.* Washington, D.C.: National Highway Traffic Safety Administration, 2004.

impulse control disorders One or more psychiatric problems chiefly characterized by an inability to cease performing harmful actions that the individual performs on the spur of the moment, accompanied by little or no thought. Compulsive gambling is one form of an impulse control disorder, as are kleptomania (compulsively stealing items), pyromania (compulsively fire setting), and trichotillomania (constantly pulling out head and/or body hair, sometimes to the point of baldness). Individuals who are obsessed with acting out their sexual ideas may also suffer from impulse control disorder.

Those who have an impulse control disorder are more likely than others to abuse alcohol and drugs or to become dependent on them. If they commit crimes, they are more likely to be caught than others, because their impulsive actions usually are not based on any type of plan and they do not make sufficient efforts to elude detection.

Some experts consider excessive and compulsive shopping another form of impulse control disorder. In a study of compulsive buyers, reported in the *American Journal of Psychiatry* in 1998, the compulsive buyers had about twice the risk for alcohol abuse or dependence (alcoholism) or drug abuse or dependence. Eighteen percent of the compulsive buyers either abused or depended on alcohol, compared to about 9 percent of a control group. In addition, about 12 percent of the compulsive buyers used or were dependent on drugs, compared to only about 5 percent of the control group subjects.

See also ANXIETY DISORDERS; ATTENTION DEFICIT HYPERACTIVITY DISORDER; BIPOLAR DISORDER; DEPRESSION; PSYCHIATRIC DISORDERS.

Black, Donald W., M.D., et al. "Family History and Psychiatric Comorbidity in Persons with Compulsive Buying: Preliminary Findings." *American Journal of Psychiatry* 155, no. 7 (July 1998): 960–963.

incarceration Being placed in a jail or prison, after either an arrest or a conviction for an infraction of the law. In general, most individuals in the United States who are arrested for drug offenses are incarcerated for selling drugs rather than for using them. However, in other countries, the possession of any illegal drugs for personal use, including MARIJUANA, may lead to a prison term of many years.

In addition to drug dealing, individuals who use drugs may be incarcerated for acts of aggression or violence; some drugs, such as ANABOLIC STEROIDS, COCAINE, and METHAMPHETAMINE, can markedly increase an individual's aggressive behavior. Methamphetamine can also lead to an abnormal hypersexuality, such that individuals may sexually assault others, including their own children, leading to an arrest for sexual abuse or rape and subsequent incarceration.

Some states have classified the use of drugs, particularly methamphetamine, in a home with children as a form of CHILD ABUSE, for which children may be removed from the home by child protective services.

At least half of all the individuals who are incarcerated in prisons in the United States have ANTISOCIAL PERSONALITY DISORDER (ASPD), a disorder in which these individuals behave in a lawless manner and cannot empathize with others. Others may have a diagnosis of CONDUCT DISORDER. Many people who have ASPD have substance abuse problems, as do those with conduct disorder.

According to the Bureau of Justice Statistics, about 17 percent of prisoners in state prisons and 18 percent of inmates in federal prisons reported that they committed their offense in order to get money to buy drugs. Of those who said that they had committed crimes to get drug money, most committed property crimes or drug-related crimes. (See Table I.)

Of those prisoners who were held for drug offenses in 2004 in state and federal prisons, the majority were convicted of drug trafficking, and in most cases, the drug involved in the offense was cocaine, followed by stimulants. The number of prisoners who were convicted of selling stimulants (such as METHAMPHETAMINE) nearly doubled from 1997 to 2004. (See Table II.) Among state and federal prisoners who used methamphetamine, white inmates were at least 20 times more likely than black inmates to report a recent use of methamphetamine.

TABLE I: PERCENT OF PRISON AND JAIL INMATES WHO COMMITTED OFFENSE TO GET MONEY FOR DRUGS

Offense	State prisoners 2004	Federal prisoners 2004
Total	16.6%	18.4%
Violent	9.8	14.8
Property	30.3	19.6
Drugs	26.4	25.3
Public-order	6.9	6.8

Source: Bureau of Justice Statistics. *Dependence Use and Dependence, State and Federal Prisoners, 2004.* Washington, D.C.: U.S. Department of Justice, October 2006, p. 6.

TABLE II: DRUG OFFENDERS IN STATE AND FEDERAL PRISONS AND THE DRUG INVOLVED IN THEIR OFFENSE

Type of drug involved in the offense	Percent of Drug Offenders			
	State		Federal	
	2004	1997	2004	1997
Marijuana/ hashish	12.7%	12.9%	12.4%	18.9%
Cocaine/crack	61.8	72.1	65.5	65.5
Heroin/other opiates	12.2	12.8	8.1	9.9
Depressants	2.2	1.2	1.4	0.6
Stimulants	18.6	9.9	18.7	11.0
Hallucinogens	1.7	1.1	2.3	1.7

Source: Bureau of Justice Statistics. *Dependence Use and Dependence, State and Federal Prisoners, 2004.* Washington, D.C.: U.S. Department of Justice, October 2006, p. 4.

In general, *prison* or the *penitionary* refers to permanent long-term (usually longer than one-year) incarceration for individuals who are convicted of felony crimes, such as multiple counts of drug abuse or for drug dealing, as well as for crimes such as burglaries and for violent crimes, such as assault, rape, CHILD ABUSE, and HOMICIDE. *Jail* usually refers to local facilities that incarcerate individuals, either for misdemeanors or, in the case of people who are accused of felonies, for holding in jail unless or until they are convicted. In addition, individuals may be incarcerated in jail for sentences of short duration.

It is important to note that countries outside the United States have their own drug enforcement laws, and in some countries, the penalties for violating these laws are very severe and may be as severe as life imprisonment for crimes that would seem minor in the United States, such as using and/ or selling MARIJUANA. The rights of the U.S. citizen do not extend past the borders of other countries, although assistance from the State Department may be solicited by individuals who are jailed for drug crimes in other countries. In some cases, tourists abuse drugs in other countries, mistakenly believing that the laws of those countries are comparable to or even far more lenient than the laws in the United States.

See also CRIME AND CRIMINALS; DRUG COURTS; DRUG DEALERS; GANGS; HOMICIDE; INTERNET DRUG TRAFFICKING/ILLEGAL PHARMACIES; JAIL INMATES; LAW ENFORCEMENT; ORGANIZED CRIME; TRAFFICKING OF DRUGS.

inhalants   Substances that are inhaled for the purpose of intoxication. This includes household products that are not produced to be inhaled. However, when they *are* inhaled for the purpose of drug abuse, they produce a mind-altering effect. Unfortunately the lifetime use (having ever used) of inhalants increased significantly among eighth graders, from 15.8 percent in 2003 to 17.3 percent in 2004. However, some improvements were noted from 2003 to 2004; for example, the number of 10th graders who disapproved of inhalants increased significantly. At the same time, however, the perceived risk of inhalants among students who were eighth graders declined; they apparently saw inhalants as less risky to health than in past years. (It is unknown why this perception of risk declined.) This probably accounts at least in part for the increased abuse rate among eighth graders. (See Table I.)

Categories of Inhalants

In general, there are four basic categories of inhalants: volatile solvents, aerosols, gases, and nitrates. Volatile solvents are liquids that vaporize at room temperature. Many common household products are volatile solvents, including dry cleaning fluids, paint thinners, glues, gasoline, correction fluid, and even felt-tip marker fluids. (See Table II for a list of the major types of substances that are abused as inhalants, the products in which they are found, and possible effects of the abuse.)

Aerosols are sprays with solvents and propellants, and they include many different common products, such as spray deodorants, hair spray, vegetable oil sprays for cooking, fabric protector sprays, and spray paints.

Gases used as inhalants include household and commercial products as well as medical anesthetics used abusively. Nitrous oxide is the most abused gas that is used as an inhalant, and it may be found in dispensers of whipped cream as well as butane lighters and products that boost the octane levels in race cars.

Nitrates, another category of inhalants, are used as sexual enhancing drugs. Whereas the other forms of inhalants act on the central nervous system, in contrast, nitrates relax the muscles and dilate the blood vessels. Examples of nitrates are isobutyl nitrate, isoamyl nitrate, and cyclohexyl nitrate. In past years, amyl nitrate ("poppers") was used to treat patients for heart pain, but the drug is no longer used for this purpose.

Abuse of Inhalants

Inhalant chemicals are inhaled in several different ways, such as by "snorting" (sniffing) the fumes directly from the container, spraying the aerosols into the mouth or nose, inhaling substances that were sprayed inside a paper or plastic bag, "huffing" (inhaling) an inhalant-soaked rag that is placed inside the mouth, or inhaling nitrous oxide from balloons.

The euphoric effects of inhalant abuse are very rapid (within seconds). It is believed that the dopamine in the brain is activated by inhalants. The effects on the body resemble those that are seen with alcohol, such as slurred speech and impaired

TABLE I: MONITORING THE FUTURE STUDY: TRENDS IN PREVALENCE OF INHALANT USE AMONG 8TH GRADERS, 10TH GRADERS, AND 12TH GRADERS

	8th Graders			10th Graders			12th Graders		
	2002	2003	2004	2002	2003	2004	2002	2003	2004
Lifetime Use	15.2	15.8	17.3	13.5	12.7	12.4	11.7	11.2	10.9
Annual Use	7.7	8.7	9.6	5.8	5.4	5.9	4.5	3.9	4.2
30-Day Use	3.8	4.1	4.5	2.4	2.2	2.4	1.5	1.5	1.5

Source: Adapted from National Institute on Drug Abuse. "High School and Youth Trends." *NIDA Info Facts,* December 2004, p. 4.

TABLE II: HAZARDS OF CHEMICALS FOUND IN COMMONLY ABUSED INHALANTS

Substance	Found in	Possible Effects
Amyl nitrate, butyl nitrate	"Poppers," video head cleaners	Sudden sniffing death syndrome, suppressed immunological function, injury to red blood cells (interfering with oxygen supply to vital tissues)
Benzene	Gasoline	Bone marrow injury, impaired immunologic function, increased risk of leukemia, reproductive system toxicity
Butane, propane	Lighter fluid, hair and paint sprays	Sudden sniffing death syndrome via cardiac effects, serious burn injuries (caused by flammability)
Freon	Refrigerants and aerosol propellants	Sudden sniffing death syndrome, respiratory obstruction and death (from sudden cooling, cold injury to airways), liver damage
Methyl chloride	Paint thinners and removers, degreasers	Reduction of oxygen-carrying capacity of blood, changes to the heart muscle and heartbeat
Nitrous oxide, hexane	Laughing gas	Death from lack of oxygen to the brain, altered perception and motor coordination, loss of sensation, limb spasms, blackouts caused by blood pressure changes, depression of heart muscle functioning
Toluene	Gasoline, paint thinners and removers, correction fluid	Brain damage (loss of brain tissue mass, impaired cognition, gait disturbance, loss of coordination, loss of equilibrium, limb spasms, hearing and vision loss), liver and kidney damage
Trichlorethylene	Spot removers, degreasers	Sudden sniffing death syndrome, cirrhosis of the liver, reproductive complications, hearing and vision damage

Source: Adapted from National Institute on Drug Abuse. "Inhalant Abuse." National Institute on Drug Abuse Research Report Series. Bethesda, Md.: National Institutes of Health, 2005.

coordination. Abusers may also experience HALLU-CINATIONS and DELUSIONS. Because the intoxication that is induced by an inhalant lasts only a few minutes, abusers may seek to prolong their euphoria by continuing to inhale the substance for hours. This is extremely dangerous and can even prove fatal.

Regular abuse of inhalants can cause headaches, and heavy and continued use may lead to unconsciousness and even death.

Inhalant Abusers

The abuse of inhalants falls sharply after about age 20. Drugs in the inhalant category are the only type of drugs that have their highest use among those in the eighth grade. It is also interesting to note that eighth-grade females are more likely to abuse inhalants than 8th-grade males; for example, in 2003, 4.7 percent of females had used inhalants compared to 3.4 percent of males. The percentage of male inhalant abusers was slightly higher among 10th-grade males (2.3 percent) than 10th-grade females (2.2 percent). Among seniors, males used inhalants at about twice the rate (2.0 percent) of female 12th graders (1.1 percent). The reason for the greater prevalence among female eighth graders is unknown.

Inhalant abusers may use the drug as a result of PEER PRESSURE. The effect of peer pressure fades with age, and although 21 percent of 18-year-olds had friends who also use inhalants in 2004, the percentage declined sharply to 4.5 percent of inhalant abusers ages 27–30 whose friends also abused inhalants. Some abusers may wish to treat an undiagnosed depression, although inhalants are obviously an ineffective way to resolve such a problem.

Among young adults in 2004, according to the Monitoring the Future study on college students and young adults, 11.6 percent of young adults ages 19–28 had ever used inhalants. The rate was lower for college students, or 8.5 percent.

Signs and Symptoms of Inhalant Abuse Indicators of possible inhalant abuse may include the following:

- drunk or disoriented appearance
- nausea or appetite loss
- paint or other unexplained stains on the face, hands, or clothes
- hidden solvent containers, empty spray paint cans, or chemical-soaked rags or clothing
- inattentiveness, lack of coordination, depression, and irritability
- slurred speech

Other effects may include impaired judgment, belligerence, muscle weakness, lethargy, and stupor. Confusion may occur, as may nausea and vomiting.

Serious Medical Consequences

According to the National Institute on Drug Abuse, prolonged sniffing of inhalants could lead to heart failure and death, all within a matter of minutes. Inhalants can damage the major organs of the body, including the heart, lungs, liver, and kidneys.

Some of the ways that abusers can die from the inhalants (whether one use or many uses), a phenomenon that is also called "sudden sniffing death," include the following:

- asphyxiation (from repeated sessions of inhalations, which cause the oxygen in the lungs to be displaced by inhaled fumes)
- choking (from inhalation or vomiting)
- convulsions or seizures
- fatal injury (from accidents that result from intoxication)
- suffocation (because air is blocked from entering the lungs, as when fumes are inhaled from a plastic bag placed over the head)

Treatment of Those Who Have Inhalant Abuse

Individuals discovered to be using inhalants should receive psychiatric treatment for possible anxiety disorders or depression. A medical evaluation for the toxic effects of inhalants is an essential response. Inhalant abusers should be urged to cease this abuse immediately, and minors should be monitored by their parents. Household products should be locked up until the problem is resolved. Unfortunately, it is relatively easy for minors to purchase household products that they can inhale. For this reason, spray paint is frequently locked up behind the counter in many stores.

See also ADOLESCENTS; GLUE; SCHEDULED DRUGS.

Johnston, Lloyd D., et al. *Monitoring the Future: National Survey Results on Drug Use, 1975–2004.* Vol. 2, *College Students and Adults Ages 19–45.* Bethesda, Md.: National Institute on Drug Abuse, National Institutes of Health, 2005.

Johnston, Lloyd D., et al. *Monitoring the Future: National Results on Adolescent Drug Use: Overview of Key Findings 2004.* Bethesda, Md.: National Institute of Drug Abuse, April 2005.

National Institute on Drug Abuse. "High School and Youth Trends." *NIDA Info Facts,* December 2004, 1–9.

National Institute on Drug Abuse. "Inhalant Abuse." National Institute on Drug Abuse Research Report Series. Bethesda, Md.: National Institutes of Health, 2005.

injection drug use See INTRAVENOUS/INJECTING DRUG USE/IV DRUG USERS.

injuries, caused by alcohol and/or illicit drugs Harm to the body, ranging from cuts and abrasions to burns or fractures as well as fatal injuries, all of which stem from the abuse of alcohol and/or illicit drugs. The harm may be experienced by the substance abuser and/or by others; for example, an individual driving while intoxicated may crash, injuring himself, his passengers, other drivers, or even pedestrians.

Injuries are common among those who manufacture METHAMPHETAMINE illegally in CLANDESTINE LABORATORIES because of the volatile nature of the chemicals used to make the drug. Individuals operating machinery or equipment while intoxicated may harm themselves or others.

Self-Harm

Substance abusers are more likely to suffer from injuries and death than others. They may suffer intoxication-related falls or injuries sustained in auto or motorcycle crashes due to driving under the influence of alcohol and/or drugs. About a third of those who die of accidents unrelated to car crashes have a blood alcohol concentration of 0.10 grams/100 milliliter (g/dL) or greater. (The legal level of intoxication while driving in all states is less than this level, or 0.08 g/dL.)

Individuals under the influence of alcohol and/or drugs are more likely to die from drowning, burns, hypothermia, SUICIDE, and HOMICIDE than those who are not under the influence of these substances.

Harm Inflicted upon Others

Individuals impaired by illicit drugs and/or alcohol are more likely than others to *cause* injuries to others, up to and including death. They may harm their children, their loved ones, or even total strangers. Drugs and/or alcohol may increase the aggression level of an individual, causing him or her to assault others.

Harm to children   Adults under the influence of alcohol and/or drugs are more likely to harm their loved ones, including small children, as a result of their greater likelihood of causing automobile accidents and of engaging in violent acts. For example, from 1997 to 2002, alcohol-related car accidents caused the deaths of 2,355 children. Of these, 68 percent of the children who died were riding with an intoxicated driver.

Alcohol and illicit drugs are strongly implicated in acts of CHILD ABUSE and neglect, and an estimated one-third to two-thirds of all the substantiated cases of child abuse in the United States involve substance abuse by parents or other caretakers.

Harm to other loved ones   Individuals under the influence of alcohol and/or drugs are more likely to harm and even kill loved ones, including adult partners or spouses as well as their own children.

Harm to unknown others   Sometimes the victims of alcohol and/or drug abuse are unknown to the abuser. They may be people who are killed or injured in car crashes caused by drunk drivers or individuals who the abuser feels are challenging him or her in some way. The abuser may be experiencing paranoid or aggressive symptoms, depending on the type of drug abused.

Drug and alcohol abusers may also be the victims of crime, including both violent and nonviolent crime. An estimated 40 percent of all crimes in the United States were committed when the perpetrator was under the influence of alcohol. In addition, about 40 percent of individuals convicted of rape or sexual assault reported that they were drinking at the time of their crime.

See also BINGE DRINKING.

Internet drug trafficking/illegal pharmacies   The selling of prescription drugs to individuals who order these drugs over the Internet on sites purporting to be "pharmacies" and usually with no requirement for a prescription from a physician. Some of these sites operate in the United States and Canada, but the great majority operate in other countries.

These sites sell many different types of drugs, including NARCOTICS and ANABOLIC STEROIDS as well as DIET DRUGS, drugs for erectile dysfunction, and medications for many different purposes. It is unknown how many such sites exist, because they constantly appear and disappear, in apparent attempts to elude law enforcement authorities. Some owners of illegal Internet pharmacies may own many different sites.

The person placing the drug order may be an adult but may also be a minor, often using a borrowed or stolen credit card. There have been a few cases of deaths of minors that were directly related to the abuse of illegal drugs that were purchased over the Internet, which purchases were unknown to their families. Adolescents are often impatient, and some may believe that the prescribed dose of a drug is insufficient and too slow-acting. As a result, they may take double, triple, or even greater levels of the drug than are recommended, believing that as a result the drug will work faster and more efficiently. They usually do not realize that by taking excessive doses of a medication, they can experience serious medical consequences, which can lead to ACCIDENTAL OVERDOSE DEATHS.

It is illegal for people in the United States to purchase prescribed drugs over the Internet without a valid prescription from a licensed medical doctor; however, despite these restrictions, it is believed that at least thousands of people do so.

Law Enforcement

A variety of federal, state, and local agencies are concerned about illegal purchases of drugs over the Internet, including the Food and Drug Administration (FDA) and the U.S. Customs and Border Protection (CBP). The CBP can seize controlled or noncontrolled prescription drugs that are mailed from foreign countries to individuals in the United States. The U.S. Postal Service is also active in the interdiction of illegal drugs that are sent through the mail.

The FDA has the right to take action against those who

- sell, distribute, or import adulterated or misbranded drugs
- sell, distribute, or import unapproved new drugs
- sell or dispense prescription drugs without a valid prescription
- sell counterfeit drugs

As reported by the FDA, in 2003, physician Mark Brown and pharmacist Luke Coukos pled guilty to indictments related to Internet drug sales. Dr. Brown surrendered his license to practice medicine in Ohio and Massachusetts as well as his Drug Enforcement Administration (DEA) registration (which had allowed him to prescribe SCHEDULED DRUGS). He admitted to authorizing 22,056 prescriptions for Schedule III and IV controlled diet drugs. The pharmacist, Coukos, admitted he had personally dispensed at least 43,066 controlled prescription drugs as well as 9,055 noncontrolled prescription drugs. He was sentenced to 60 months' incarceration and a $140,000 fine.

Possible Motivations of Drug Purchasers

Some individuals may purchase drugs over the Internet, failing to use a valid prescription from a doctor, because they do not wish to go to the doctor or they may not have a current physician. They may be adolescents, whose parents would disapprove of their drug use. Others may be addicted to substances for which they know a doctor would not give them a prescription.

Some people say that they wish to try a drug to which they are not yet addicted but that they (rightly) believe that their physician would not prescribe for them, since the use would be for recreational rather than medical purposes. Many drugs sold over the Internet are DIET DRUGS, and some individuals may believe that their physicians would disapprove of their taking such drugs.

In general, drugs sold over the Internet are much more expensive than if they were purchased legally; that is the key reason why such Web sites proliferate despite the efforts of law enforcement authorities: they are very profitable.

Many Internet Pharmacies Operate from Other Countries

Many companies that sell drugs over the Internet are located in countries outside the United States and Canada, where there is little or no quality control over medications; consequently, the drugs may be adulterated with other substances or may have *none* of the substance that was ordered by the consumer.

The General Accounting Office (GAO) in the United States made a study of Internet drug purchases (published in 2005) based on actual purchases of ANABOLIC STEROIDS through the Internet in order to determine how easy purchasing them was as well as whether the drug that was purchased was what was actually ordered. The researchers readily ordered and received 14 shipments of drugs, which were subsequently tested. In 10 of the shipments, the product contained no anabolic steroids.

In an earlier GAO study on Internet pharmacies published in 2004, the researchers obtained 68 samples of 11 different drugs from pharmacy Web sites in the United States, Canada, Argentina, Costa Rica, Fiji, India, Mexico, Pakistan, Philippines, Spain, Thailand, and Turkey. Six orders that were paid for were never received. The GAO purchased Accutane (an acne drug), Celebrex (a drug formerly prescribed for arthritis), Clozaril (for schizophrenia), Cobivir and Crixivan (for human immunodeficiency virus [HIV]), Epgoen (for anemia), Humulin N (for diabetes), Lipitor (for high cholesterol level), Viagra (for erectile dysfunction), Zoloft (for depression), and OXYCONTIN, Percocet, and Vicodin (for pain).

The researchers found that in the majority of the cases, either an online medical questionnaire was required to be completed by the consumer or there were no requirements at all for those ordering the drug—other than a valid credit card. However, some pharmacies in the United States and Canada *did* require a valid prescription from a physician.

The researchers also found that none of the 21 drugs that the researchers received from Internet pharmacies outside of the United States or Canada included labels that provided instructions for their use. In three cases, drugs that should have been shipped in a temperature-controlled environment arrived in noninsulated envelopes, and five samples included tablets that were enclosed in blister packs that had been punctured. In several cases, the drugs that were received were counterfeit versions of the drugs that were ordered, including counterfeit versions of Accutane, OxyContin, and Viagra.

The researchers also discovered that 21 percent of the pharmacies from which the researchers ordered drugs (14 of 68) were under investigation by regulatory agencies, such as the DEA or the FDA. Say the researchers:

> Consumers can readily obtain many prescription drugs over the Internet without providing a prescription—particularly from certain U.S. and foreign Internet pharmacies outside of Canada. Drugs available include those for which patients should be monitored for side effects or where the potential for abuse is high. For these types of drugs in particular, a prescription and physician supervision can help ensure patient safety. In addition to the lack of prescription requirements, some Internet pharmacies can pose other safety risks for consumers. Many foreign Internet pharmacies outside of Canada dispensed drugs without instructions for patient use, rarely provided warning information, and in four instances provided drugs that were not the authentic products we ordered. Consumers who purchase drugs from foreign Internet pharmacies that are outside of the U.S. regulatory framework may also receive drugs that are unapproved by FDA and manufactured in facilities that

the agency has not inspected. Other risks consumers may face were highlighted by the other foreign Internet pharmacies that fraudulently billed us, provided drugs we did not order, and provided false or questionable return addresses. It is notable that we identified these numerous problems despite the relatively small number of drugs we purchased, consistent with problems recently identified by state an federal regulatory agencies.

Little or No Oversight or Control over Narcotics and Other Drugs

One major concern that regulators have about illicit Internet pharmacies is that consumers may order dangerous drugs such as narcotics, without having a legitimate pain management problem, initiating or continuing a drug dependence problem. In addition, such drugs have many side effects of which consumers should be aware. They also should be told that narcotics (and many other drugs) can interact with alcohol.

A study by the GAO published in 2004 discussed their finding that it was possible to purchase HYDROCODONE easily over the Internet. Hydrocodone is a Schedule III narcotic, which is often abused. (See PRESCRIPTION DRUG ABUSE.) The researchers purchased 60 tablets of hydrocodone at an Internet site for $190 plus a $49 "consultation" fee. This price appeared to the researchers to be slightly lower than the street price for purchasing hydrocodone illegally. However, if a consumer has a legitimate prescription, these drugs normally cost about $26.

The GAO researchers also visited the physical location of one business, which had purported on its Web site to have a clinic on its premises. According to the report, "The site is a one-room storefront set up with several computers and telephones. The only individuals we saw going to or leaving the storefront appeared to be employees, and there was no sign on the premises indicating that the business was health related. When one of the employees was asked what kind of business is operated at the location, she responded that they do computer consultations.

Some Pharmacies on the Internet Are Legitimate

Some valid pharmacies will fill prescriptions for patients over the Internet; however, they require a valid written prescription that is received from a physician beforehand. Such pharmacies may provide an important service, because they will mail the drug to the consumer, who may be disabled, lack transportation, or otherwise find it difficult to go to a storefront pharmacy for another reason.

According to the FDA in a 2004 statement, one way to find out whether a pharmacy is legitimate is to note whether it is a member of the Verified Internet Pharmacy Practice Site (VIPPS), developed by the National Association of Boards of Pharmacy to denote lawful pharmacy sites that meet federal and state requirements. Legitimate pharmacies are not required to participate in this program, but it is one way for consumers to screen in legitimate pharmacy sites. As of 2006, there were 12 pharmacies listed as approved by the VIPPS system. The system can be accessed at http://www.vipps.info.com.

Some Indicators of Illegal Pharmacies

There are several indicators that may reveal that a purported pharmacy Web site is not legitimate. Some indicators are

- It is impossible to determine where the seller is physically located. There is no "Contact Us" icon, or if there is one, the only information that is provided is a toll-free number.
- It is impossible or difficult to determine what company or individual owns the site. A legitimate pharmacy openly uses their name on the site.
- There are many misspellings on the site and the wording and language seem somehow "off." This may indicate that the Web site is located in another country.
- The site owner has no requirement for a prescription from a physician.
- The price for the drug seems extremely high.
- A "consultation" fee is charged although no one asks any questions or takes any medical history.
- The seller seems to concentrate on only one category of drugs, such as a heavy concentration on anabolic steroids or diet drugs.

See also DIVERSION, DRUG; DRUG TESTING; LAW ENFORCEMENT; SCHEDULED DRUGS.

Cramer, Robert J. "Internet Pharmacies: Hydrocodone, an Addictive Narcotic Pain Medication, Is Available without a Prescription through the Internet." Washington, D.C.: General Accounting Office, June 17, 2004. Available online. URL: http://www.gao.gov/new.items/do4892t.pdf. Downloaded February 22, 2006.

General Accounting Office Report. "Anabolic Steroids Are Easily Purchased without a Prescription and Present Significant Challenges to Law Enforcement Officials." GAO-06-243R. Washington, D.C.: General Accounting Office, November 5, 2005.

General Accounting Office. "Internet Pharmacies: Some Pose Safety Risks for Consumers." GAO-04-820. Washington, D.C.: June 2004. Available online. URL: http://www.gao.gov/new.items/do4820.pdf. Downloaded February 23, 2006.

Hubbard, William K. "Statement of William K. Hubbard, Associate Commissioner for Policy and Planning, before the Committee on Government Reform, U.S. House of Representatives Hearing on Internet Drug Sales, March 18, 2004." Available online. URL http://www.fda.gov/ola/2004/internetdrugs0318.html. Downloaded January 15, 2006.

U.S. Customs and Border Protection. "Buying Prescription Medicine from Internet Foreign Pharmacies." News release, February 22, 2006. Available online. URL: http://www.cbp.gov/xp/cgov/newsroom/highlights/foreign_medication.xml. Downloaded February 23, 2006.

intervention   A planned meeting, usually under the supervision of a licensed and experienced mental health professional, in which family members and others confront a person who is an alcoholic or drug addict about the negative effects of the alcohol/drug use on the individual's life and on their own lives. The meeting usually occurs in a setting where the individual feels safe, such as his home. The goal of the meeting is to shock the addicted individual to the point where he or she will agree to enter into a rehabilitation facility immediately. The plan includes previous arrangements with a specific rehabilitation center the addicted individual may enter after the intervention.

The family members, friends, coworkers, and others who plan an intervention often believe that nothing else that they have tried has helped the individual to deal with his or her addiction. Often they report that the addicted individual does not even acknowledge that there *is* an addiction problem. Thus, they regard the intervention as a "last resort" solution. They hope it will compel the addicted person to realize or to accept that he or she is addicted and finally understand the negative consequences of that addictive behavior. These negative effects may include failing to meet family and work obligations, embarrassing family members or coworkers in public, not attending important events, or attending them in an impaired state.

Interventions can be effective and individuals do enter rehabilitative facilities after successful interventions. They may also fail, leaving the addicted person angry with those who participated in the intervention and still in denial about the addiction. For this reason, it is useful to have a trained professional assist in preparing the family and conducting the intervention. Licensed drug and alcohol counselors and other licensed mental health professionals who have special training (who are frequently recommended by the treatment facility) can be very helpful in this type of situation.

During the intervention, individuals in the group state what they will or will not do if the person fails to enter a rehabilitation facility. It is essential that they follow through on their promises in the event that the addict refuses therapy, to ensure that clear consequences result. Many people will find it difficult or impossible to fulfill these promises, such as refusing to help the individual or even to see him or her anymore. This is especially true if there is CODEPENDENCY between the addicted person and another person. However, unless the promised consequences occur, the probability of the individual's changing is decreased. Even with clear consequences, there is no guarantee that the alcoholic or drug addict will change.

See also FAMILY, EFFECT ON.

intravenous/injecting drug use/IV drug users Users of drugs that are injected into a vein, including such drugs as HEROIN, COCAINE, METHAMPHETAMINE, or MORPHINE. Other drugs can also be injected illegally by drug abusers or addicts, such as FLUNITRAZEPAM (ROHYPNOL), KETAMINE, PROPOXYPHENE, and OXYCONTIN. In most cases, intravenous (IV) drug users are already addicted to the drug that they inject or quickly become addicted to it.

These individuals risk many negative health consequences. In addition to the health risks from the abuse of the drug itself, they are vulnerable to the transmission of sexually transmitted diseases, including the HUMAN IMMUNODEFICIENCY VIRUS (HIV) or HEPATITIS through the use of shared dirty needles. They also risk harm to the skin and other injuries resulting from the errors that nonmedical drug users may make.

According to research by the National Survey on Drug Use and Health (NSDUH), reported in a 2005 *NSDUH Report,* there were an average of 354,000 individuals ages 12 and older in the United States who used needles to inject cocaine, heroin, methamphetamine, or other drugs in the past year in 2002 and 2003. Of these individuals, an estimated 168,000 injected heroin in the past year, and another 168,000 injected cocaine, while 119,000 injected methamphetamines, and 78,000 injected other stimulants. Males were twice as likely to inject drugs as females, although for both the percentage was less than 1 percent of the population.

Of those who injected drugs on the most recent occasion, 39.5 percent bought the needle they used from a pharmacy, while 20.5 percent said they were either given the needle or stole the needle from someone else. (See Table I.) It is estimated that about 64 percent of past-year injection drug users failed to clean the needle that they used with bleach before they injected drugs on the last occasion of injected drug use.

In a study of injecting drug users over the period 1980–2001 published in 2004 in *Archives of Internal Medicine,* the researchers found that of 667 patients, there were 153 deaths. Most of the deaths were among individuals ages 25–34 years old, and this finding confirms that intravenous drug abuse is a considerable risk for YOUNG ADULTS.

Most of the deaths were caused by overdoses in the early years of the study and then were caused by HIV and acquired immune deficiency syndrome (AIDS) in the later years. Say the researchers, "Injecting drug users have a very high risk of mortality. Infectious diseases from nonsterile injecting are the most obvious preventable cause of death."

TABLE I: ESTIMATED NUMBERS AND PERCENTAGES OF PAST-YEAR INJECTION DRUG USERS AGED 12 OR OLDER WHO REPORTED HOW THEY GOT THEIR NEEDLES THE LAST TIME THEY USED ONE TO INJECT DRUGS, 2002 AND 2003

How Needle Was Obtained	Estimated Number	Percentage
Bought from a pharmacy	140,000	39.5
Given by, stolen from a person	73,000	20.5
Needle exchange	59,000	16.7
Given by, stolen from a location	24,000	6.8
Other	56,000	15.7
Don't know/refused/no answer	3,000	0.8

Source: Office of Applied Studies. "Injection Drug Use Update: 2002 and 2003." *The NSDUH Report.* Rockville, Md.: Substance Abuse and Mental Health Services Administration, April 8, 2005, p. 2.

They also state: "The nature of drug misuse exposes misusers to health risks they would not normally incur. This risk behavior in drug users contributes to their causes of death being dissimilar to the general population, where cancer and circulatory disease predominate."

Childhood Sexual Abuse and Injection Drug Use

One study showed that individuals who were sexually abused as children or adolescents had an increased risk for an earlier onset of injection drug use. This research, which was published in 2005 in the *American Journal of Public Health*, analyzed the age at first injection among more than 2,000 injection drug users. The majority of the subjects were male (63 percent) and white (53 percent).

About 14 percent of the subjects reported being forced to engage in sexual intercourse in childhood or adolescence, although the researchers suspected that sexual abuse was underreported by the subjects. Most of those who report having been sexually abused (72 percent) experienced the abuse prior to their initiating injection drug use.

The researchers found that the younger the age when the individual was forced to engage in sex, the younger the age at which he or she would become an injection drug user as an adult; for example, of those who were sexually abused before age 13 years, the average age of initiating drug use was 17 years.

Of those who were sexually assaulted between the ages of 13 to 17 years, the average age of the first injection drug use was 18 years. Note that the average age of the first use of injection drug use among those subjects who were *not* sexually assaulted was 19 years. The researchers also noted that there was a link between physical abuse and the later abuse of drugs.

Say the researchers:

Although further investigation is needed to fully elucidate the association between sexual abuse and the initiation of substance use, we can conclude that childhood sexual abuse is strongly associated with early initiation of injection drug use and vulnerability to HIV infection among these young injection drug users. Furthermore, we observed, as have other researchers, that sexual abuse is associated with higher rates of trading sex for money or drugs. Whether or not the relation between sexual abuse and the initiation of injection drug use is causal, childhood sexual abuse can be considered a valuable marker of risk for behaviors that compromise the health of young adults.

The researchers also studied the age at first injection among those who were not sexually assaulted in terms of their race and ethnicity and found that this factor was significant. The average age of injection drug users was youngest among whites (17.5 years), followed by Hispanics (19.0 years) and African Americans (20 years).

See also DRUG ABUSE AND DEPENDENCE AND HEALTH PROBLEMS; HEROIN.

Copeland, Lorraine, et al. "Changing Patterns in Cause of Death in a Cohort of Injecting Drug Users, 1980–2001." *Archives of Internal Medicine* 165 (June 14, 2004): 1,214–1,220.

Office of Applied Studies. "Injection Drug Use Update: 2002 and 2003." *The NSDUH Report.* Rockville, Md.: Substance Abuse and Mental Health Services Administration, April 8, 2005.

Ompad, Danielle, et al. "Childhood Sexual Abuse and Age at Initiation of Injection Drug Use." *American Journal of Public Health* 95 (2005): 703–709.

jail inmates Individuals incarcerated for crimes. Jail inmates are more likely to have problems with substance abuse and dependence than individuals in the general population. According to the Office of Justice Programs, in 2002, 68 percent met the criteria for substance dependence or abuse. In contrast, in 2002, 9 percent of the population ages 12 and older were dependent on or abused drugs or alcohol. Of 610,296 inmates, 415,242 were either substance abusers or substance dependent. (See Table I.) About 80 percent of the jail inmates who met the criteria for substance dependence or abuse had a prior jail sentence or were on probation, compared to 60 percent of the other inmates.

One surprising finding was that in contrast to noninmates, female inmates were more likely to be dependent on or abuse alcohol or drugs than male inmates; 52 percent of female inmates were dependent versus 44 percent of male inmates. However, in the general population, about 6 percent of females were substance abusers, compared to nearly 13 percent of the male population.

Half of all convicted inmates in jail were under the influence of drugs or alcohol at the time when they committed their offenses. The researchers also found that jail inmates who met criteria for substance abuse or dependence were more likely than others to have a criminal record, or 70 percent for the substance abusers compared to 46 percent for the nonabusers. In addition, those who were dependent on or abused substances were almost twice as likely to have been homeless in the past year, or 16 percent of the substance abusers compared to 9 percent of the non-abusers.

In considering race and ethnicity, white inmates had the highest levels of substance abuse or dependence (78 percent), followed by African-American inmates (64 percent) and Hispanic inmates (59 percent). See Table II for further information.

Most of the inmates had a prior history of drug abuse in the month before they committed the offense (54.6 percent), with marijuana the most commonly abused drug, followed by cocaine or crack cocaine. (See Table III.)

TABLE I: PREVALENCE OF SUBSTANCE DEPENDENCE OR ABUSE AMONG JAIL INMATES BY PERCENT, 2002

Diagnosis	Estimated number of inmates	Percentage of Jail Inmates		
		Alcohol	Drugs	Alcohol or Drugs
Any dependence or abuse	415,242	46.6	53.5	68.0
Dependence and abuse	269,632	22.2	34.4	44.2
Dependence only	6,081	0.6	1.4	1.0
Abuse only	139,530	23.8	17.7	22.9
No dependence or abuse	195,054	53.4	46.5	32.0

Source: Karberg, Jennifer C., and Doris J. James. *Substance Dependence, Abuse, and Treatment of Jail Inmates, 2002.* Washington, D.C.: Bureau of Justice Statistics, July 2005, p. 3.

TABLE II: SUBSTANCE DEPENDENCE OR ABUSE AMONG JAIL INMATES, BY SELECTED CHARACTERISTICS, BY PERCENTAGE, 2002

Characteristic	Percentage of Jail Inmates		
	All	Dependence	Abuse only
All jail inmates	68.0	45.2	22.9
Gender			
Male	67.9	44.3	23.6
Female	69.2	51.8	17.4
Race/Hispanic origin			
White	77.7	55.4	22.3
Black	64.1	40.4	23.7
Hispanic	58.7	35.7	23.0
Other	66.0	45.4	20.7
Age			
24 or younger	66.1	40.3	25.8
25–34	70.5	48.1	22.4
35–44	71.4	50.4	21.0
45–54	61.9	41.7	20.3
55 or older	46.2	23.1	23.1
Most serious offense			
Violent	63.1	40.8	22.3
Property	71.7	50.6	21.1
Drug	72.1	49.6	22.4
Public-order	67.0	41.3	25.7

Source: Karberg, Jennifer C., and Doris J. James. *Substance Dependence, Abuse, and Treatment of Jail Inmates, 2002.* Washington, D.C.: Bureau of Justice Statistics, July 2005, p. 3.

More than a third of the inmates reported engaging in binge drinking in the past (39.9 percent) and 33.4 percent said that they had been drinking at the time that they committed the offense.

See also CRACK COCAINE; CRIME AND CRIMINALS; DRUG DEALERS; GANGS; INCARCERATION; LAW ENFORCEMENT; ORGANIZED CRIME.

Karberg, Jennifer C., and Doris J. James. *Substance Dependence, Abuse, and Treatment of Jail Inmates, 2002.* Washington, D.C.: Bureau of Justice Statistics, July 2005.

junkies See ADDICTION/DEPENDENCE.

TABLE III: PRIOR DRUG USE OF JAIL INMATES, BY TYPE OF DRUG, PERCENTAGE, 2002

	Percentage of Jail Inmates Who Used Drugs			
	All Inmates		Convicted Inmates	
	Ever	Regularly	In the Month before the Offense	At the Time of the Offense
Any drug	82.2	68.7	54.6	28.8
Marijuana or hashish	75.7	58.5	37.5	13.6
Cocaine or crack	48.1	30.9	20.7	10.6
Heroin/opiates	20.7	12.0	7.8	4.1
Depressants [1]	21.6	10.7	6.1	2.4
Stimulants [2]	27.8	17.1	11.4	5.2
Hallucinogens [3]	32.4	13.4	5.9	1.6
Inhalants	12.7	4.2	1.0	0.2

[1] Depressants include barbiturates, tranquilizers, and Quaaludes.
[2] Stimulants include amphetamines and methamphetamines.
[3] Hallucinogens include lysergic acid diethylamide (LSD), methylenedioxymethamphetamine (MDMA/Ecstasy), and phencyclidine (PCP).
Source: Karberg, Jennifer C., and Doris J. James. *Substance Dependence, Abuse, and Treatment of Jail Inmates, 2002.* Washington, D.C.: Bureau of Justice Statistics, July 2005, p. 5.

ketamine Created in 1963 as a substitute drug for PHENCYCLIDINE (PCP), ketamine is an odorless and tasteless drug that may be used as an anesthetic in the United States, primarily by veterinarians, under the brand names Ketaset and Ketalar. The drug may also be used in emergency surgery for humans. It is sometimes used illegally as a drug of abuse and referred to as "Special K," "Super K," or "cat Valium." Ketamine is a Schedule III drug under the CONTROLLED SUBSTANCES ACT. It is considered a CLUB DRUG because it is sometimes abused by young people at parties or night clubs. It is also sometimes used as a DATE RAPE DRUG.

Ketamine is a dissociative anesthetic that has some properties of all the following types of drugs: DEPRESSANTS, HALLUCINOGENIC DRUGS, STIMULANTS, and analgesics (painkillers). Most of the ketamine that is abused illegally in the United States is stolen from legitimate sources, such as from veterinary offices. It is also smuggled in from other countries, particularly MEXICO.

Ketamine is available in both liquid and powder forms. The drug is rapidly metabolized, and detection is difficult to impossible with toxicology tests after about 48 hours from ingestion. In its powdered form, ketamine can be smoked or snorted, while liquid ketamine is either injected or ingested after being placed into drinks. Some people sprinkle ketamine on marijuana or tobacco before they smoke the drug.

The fastest effects occur with intramuscular injection, and the onset of the effects of ketamine occurs within three to four minutes from the time of the injection. The effects last from about 45 to 90 minutes. If the subject takes the drug intranasally, the effects occur within five to 15 minutes, and the effects last from 10 to 30 minutes. When the drug is taken orally, effects occur within five to 20 minutes and may last up to 90 minutes.

Sometimes ketamine is used as a date rape drug, because it is sedating and dissociative (causing mental confusion). It can be slipped into the drink of an unknowing person; that is why it is unwise for anyone at a bar or a party either to leave a drink unattended or to consume a drink that was unattended. The Drug-Induced Rape Prevention Act of 1996 specifically names ketamine as a date rape drug, and anyone who is convicted of using ketamine to facilitate a rape and/or a violent crime may be imprisoned for up to 20 years.

Side Effects of Ketamine

Common side effects of ketamine ingestion are agitation, amnesia, delirium, memory loss, nausea, respiratory depression, temporary paralysis, and unconsciousness. These effects occur within several minutes of taking the drug. According to the Drug Enforcement Administration in *Drugs of Abuse,* low doses of ketamine can cause vertigo (dizziness), slurred speech, slowed reaction time, and euphoria. Intermediate doses of the drug may cause an altered body image, disorganized thinking, and vivid HALLUCINATIONS. High doses of the drug can lead to amnesia and coma. In some cases, ketamine may cause violent body spasms. Ketamine is generally associated with less violent and confused behavior than is PHENCYCLIDINE (PCP).

Some abusers of ketamine experience sensory detachment that can be terrifying and that has been described as a near-death experience. Such experiences, often called a "bad trip" when the drug of abuse is LYSERGIC ACID DIETHYLAMIDE (LSD), are referred to as the "K-hole" when the drug of abuse is ketamine.

TABLE I: ANNUAL PREVALENCE OF ABUSE OF KETAMINE AMONG HIGH SCHOOL STUDENTS, 2002 AND 2004 (PERCENTAGE)

	2002	2004
8th Graders	1.3	0.9
10th Graders	2.2	1.3
12th Graders	2.6	1.9

Source: Adapted from Johnston, Lloyd D., et al. *Monitoring the Future: National Survey Results on Drug Use, 1975–2004.* Vol. 2, *College Students & Adults Ages 19–45.* Bethesda, Md.: National Institute on Drug Abuse, National Institutes of Health, 2005, pp. 43, 93.

Ketamine Use Has Declined

The abuse of ketamine is low in the United States and appears to be on the decline. Among high school students, the annual prevalence of the use of ketamine in 2004 was 0.9 percent among 8th graders, 1.3 percent among 10th graders, and 1.9 percent among 12th graders. This is lower than the rate seen in 2002 among this population. (See Table I.)

In considering young adults, ages 19–30, who abused ketamine in 2004, less than 1 percent (0.6 percent) had abused the drug, with the greatest prevalence among those 19–20 and 21–22 years old who lived in the Northeast and the South. Individuals in large or very large cities were most at risk for ketamine abuse. As with most drugs, males were more likely to abuse ketamine than females. (See Table II.)

See also CLUB DRUGS; DATE RAPE DRUGS; MALICIOUS POISONING; SCHEDULED DRUGS; SEXUAL ASSAULTS.

Johnston, Lloyd D., et al. *Monitoring the Future: National Survey Results on Drug Use, 1975–2004.* Vol. 2, *College Students and Adults Ages 19–45.* Bethesda, Md.: National Institute on Drug Abuse, National Institutes of Health, 2005.

Joseph, Donald E., et al., eds. *Drugs of Abuse.* Washington, D.C.: U.S. Department of Justice, 2005.

khat   A stimulant drug that is chewed like tobacco. (Pronounced "cot.") Fresh khat continues cathinone, which is a Schedule I drug under the CONTROLLED SUBSTANCES ACT in the United States. Even when the leaves are no longer fresh (after about 48

TABLE II: ANNUAL PREVALENCE OF USE OF KETAMINE BY SUBGROUPS, 2004, AMONG AGES 19–30 YEARS (PERCENTAGES)

Total	0.6
Gender:	
Male	1.0
Female	0.3
Age:	
19–20	1.3
21–22	0.9
23–24	0.0
25–26	0.4
27–28	0.6
29–30	0.4
Region:	
Northeast	0.9
North Central	0.3
South	0.8
West	0.3
Population Density:[1]	
Farm/country	0.4
Small town	0.1
Medium city	1.1
Large city	0.7
Very large city	0.5

[1] A small town is defined as having less than 50,000 inhabitants; a medium city as 50,000–100,000; a large city as 100,000–500,000; and a very large city as having more than 500,000 residents.
Source: Adapted from Johnston, Lloyd D., et al. *Monitoring the Future: National Survey Results on Drug Use, 1975–2004.* Vol. 2, *College Students & Adults Ages 19–45.* Bethesda, Md.: National Institute on Drug Abuse, National Institutes of Health, 2005, p. 93.

hours) khat contains cathine, a Schedule IV substance. (Both cathinone and cathine are alkaloids of khat.)

Khat is derived from *Catha edulis,* a flowering evergreen shrub that is native to both East Africa and the Arabian peninsula. Fresh khat leaves are crimson-brown and glossy. The leaves, twigs, and shoots of khat are chewed by abusers. The drug can also be smoked, brewed in tea, or even sprinkled onto food.

The effects of the drug last from 90 minutes to three hours, but in some cases, effects may last as long as 24 hours.

It is believed that khat may be used by several million people worldwide, primarily by users in countries within Europe, East Africa, and the Arabian peninsula. According to the U.S. National Drug Intelligence Center, the abuse levels of khat in the United States are highest where there are many immigrants from Ethiopia, Somalia, and Yemen, such as in Boston, Columbus, Dallas, Detroit, Kansas City, Los Angeles, Minneapolis, Nashville, New York, and Washington, D.C. Also, some nonimmigrants in these areas have begun abusing khat as well.

Khat can cause such side effects as hypertension, insomnia, and rapid heartbeat (tachycardia). It can also cause HALLUCINATIONS, DELUSIONS, and manic behavior, and there have been some reports of khat-induced psychosis. Individuals may experience mild DEPRESSION with prolonged use. Damage to the circulatory, digestive, nervous, and respiratory systems also may occur.

See also STIMULANTS.

L

law enforcement Compelling compliance with federal, state, county, and city laws as well as the practice of arresting individuals who violate these laws. There are many laws surrounding the use of illegal drugs as well as the misuse of prescription drugs. For example, as a result of the CONTROLLED SUBSTANCES ACT in the United States, drugs are named and classified in terms of their addiction potential. Schedule I drugs are illegal and regarded as highly addictive, while Schedule II through V drugs have declining levels of addiction potential.

Individuals who are using Schedule I drugs can be arrested and incarcerated, as can individuals who abuse drugs in the other schedules. Law enforcement officers deal with those who engage in drug trafficking as well as those who possess illegal drugs. They arrest drug dealers as well as criminals who commit crimes in order to obtain money to pay for the drugs to which they are addicted.

Numerous types of public officials enforce the laws against the sale and use of illegal drugs and an array of federal, state, county, and city government law-enforcement agencies back them up. According to the Office of National Drug Control Policy, there were about 1.8 million arrests for drug offenses in the United States in 2005.

The Drug Enforcement Administration (DEA) is a major agency enforcing the laws against the illegal use of narcotics and other prohibited drugs. The U.S. Coast Guard patrols specific coastal areas where drugs may be in transit. U.S. Customs and Border Protection (CBP), under the jurisdiction of the Department of Homeland Security, monitors the borders of the United States for drugs. The Immigration and Customs Enforcement (ICE) agency is another organization monitoring international drug trafficking. These are only a few of the many organizations involved in law enforcement against illegal drugs in the United States.

Drug enforcement is a major part of the duties of police at many levels. For example, an estimated 90 percent of the staff of local police departments perform drug-enforcement functions, and an estimated 95 percent of arrests by local sheriffs involve drug enforcement.

According to the Federal Bureau of Investigation's Uniform Crime Report, there were 1,745,712 drug abuse violations in states and local areas in 2004. Drug abuse violations are defined as state and/or local offenses related to the unlawful possession, sale, use, growing, manufacture and making of narcotics, including opium, cocaine, marijuana, synthetic narcotics, and dangerous nonnarcotic combinations, such as BARBITURATES.

See also CRIME AND CRIMINALS; GANGS; HOMICIDE; INCARCERATION; JAIL INMATES; ORGANIZED CRIME.

lysergic acid diethylamide (LSD) A hallucinogenic drug that was first popular in the 1970s but is used relatively infrequently in the 21st century. The drug was first synthesized in 1938 from the ergot rye fungus by Dr. Albert Hofman, a Swiss research chemist working for Sandoz Pharmaceuticals. However, its effects were unknown until Dr. Hofman himself consumed LSD by accident in 1943 and subsequently experienced its hallucinatory effects. When he reported on his findings others became interested in the drug.

LSD is illegal to use in the United States and is a Schedule I drug under the CONTROLLED SUBSTANCES ACT. In general, a physical tolerance is not seen with LSD because repeated and frequent dosages are rare. Some research indicates a cross-tolerance between LSD and mescaline or psilocybin. If LSD is taken with lithium (used to treat bipolar disorder) or fluoxetine (Prozac), an antidepressant, it may induce seizures.

Initially, LSD was used in research on mental illness, and it was believed that LSD might provide a breakthrough treatment for severe psychiatric illnesses, such as SCHIZOPHRENIA. Later in the 1960s, users such as Dr. Timothy Leary, who had previously experimented with PSILOCYBIN, encouraged adolescents and young adults to "turn on, tune in, and drop out" with LSD. In 1963, Leary was dismissed from his professorial position at Harvard University. (Leary became disenchanted with the drug and became interested in computers in the latter part of the 20th century.)

Only a tiny dosage of LSD is needed to create effects. In general, doses of LSD range from 20 to 80 mcg, or one-millionth of a gram. It has many forms: tiny "microdot" tablets, thin gelatinous squares, impregnated sugar cubes, and occasionally a liquid. Effects from the drug occur within 30–60 minutes and the peak of the drug's effects occur within about 90 minutes from the time of ingestion. For most individuals, the drug's effects have completely ended within five to 12 hours.

Researchers have found that LSD stimulates a subtype of serotonin sensitive receptors that are known as S_2 receptors. This effect causes the hallucinogenic experience of the LSD user.

Current Users of LSD

According to the *National Survey on Drug Use and Health* for 2004, although an estimated 23.4 million people in the United States had tried LSD in their lifetime, there were only about 141,000 current users in 2004.

With regard to the use of LSD in the past year by percentage, less than 1 percent (0.2 percent) of people ages 12 and older used LSD in both 2003 and 2004. The percentage of people who used LSD in the past month before the survey was even lower, at 0.1 percent in both 2003 and 2004. Usage was slightly higher among young adults who were ages 18 to 25 years, as with the usage of nearly all illicit drugs (with the exception of inhal-

ants, which are primarily abused by adolescents). Among young adults, usage of LSD in the past year was 1.0 percent, and in the past month, it was much lower, or 0.3 percent. As a result, it can be concluded safely that LSD is not a major drug of abuse in the United States.

Physical and Psychological Reactions to LSD

Physical reactions to LSD may include

- lowered body temperature
- increased blood sugar level
- dilated pupils
- heavy perspiration
- increased heart rate

Psychological reactions to LSD may include

- HALLUCINATIONS
- impaired depth perception
- distorted perception of time
- distorted perceptions of the shape and size of objects
- distortion of the user's body image

One use of LSD can cause a lifelong impact on an individual user. For example, the drug induces hallucinations and delusions, and the individual may act on what he thinks he sees or what she believes to be true. A person who is convinced that he can fly may leap off the roof of a building, suffering severe injuries (such as broken limbs or a broken back) or even death.

In some cases, use of LSD can cause psychosis, inducing a state of psychotic DEPRESSION or SCHIZOPHRENIA.

Users of LSD may also suffer from "flashbacks," or the experience of feeling that they are reliving their former hallucinatory experiences months or sometimes even years later, although they have not reused the drug. Antidepressants may help to reduce the symptoms associated with flashbacks.

See also CANADA; COLLEGE STUDENTS; DELUSIONS; HALLUCINATIONS; HALLUCINOGENIC DRUGS.

Gwinnell, Esther, M.D., and Christine Adamec. *The Encyclopedia of Addictions and Addictive Behaviors*. New York: Facts On File, 2006.

Joseph, Donald E., ed. *Drugs of Abuse*. Washington, D.C.: U.S. Department of Justice, 2005.

Levinthal, Charles F. *Drugs, Society, and Criminal Justice*. New York: Pearson Education, 2006.

Substance Abuse and Mental Health Services Administration. *Overview of Findings for the 2004 National Survey on Drug Use and Health*. Rockville, Md.: Department of Health and Human Services, September 2005.

malicious poisoning The administration of alcohol and/or drugs to individuals without their knowledge or consent and for a malevolent purpose. According to the Drug Awareness Network (DAWN), data from hospital emergency rooms throughout the United States indicate that most individuals victimized in this manner are females. In most cases, the victims are white and ages 25–29 years old. (See Table I.)

DAWN includes the following types of cases in their definition of malicious poisoning:

- drug-facilitated assault
- drug-facilitated SEXUAL ASSAULT
- homicide when the weapon was a drug
- product tampering

There were an estimated 1,300 emergency room visits to hospitals in the United States in 2003 by patients who were administered substances without their knowledge or permission. Most patients (87 percent) were treated and released.

Alcohol in combination with other drugs represented 765 cases (59 percent). MARIJUANA represented 202 cases (16 percent), followed by stimulants such as AMPHETAMINES or METHAMPHETAMINE, for 194 cases (15 percent). Other substances such as opioids/opiate painkillers were administered in 183 cases (14 percent). PHENCYCLIDINE (PCP) was administered to 24 patients (2 percent) and METHYLENEDIOXYMETHAMPHETAMINE (MDMA/ECSTASY) was given to 23 patients. (See Table II.) Multiple drugs were involved in 63 percent of the cases. Interestingly, so-called DATE RAPE DRUGS such as FLUNITRAZEPAM (ROHYPNOL) represented negligible percentages that were not reported by DAWN.

TABLE I: ESTIMATED CASES OF MALICIOUS POISONING, BY PATIENT AND VISIT CHARACTERISTICS TO HOSPITAL EMERGENCY DEPARTMENT, 2003

Patient/Visit Characteristics	Estimated Visits
Total Drug-Related Emergency Department	1,300
Gender	
Male	311
Female	989
Age	
0–5 years	—
6–11 years	6
12–17 years	—
18–20 years	57
21–24 years	91
25–29 years	571
30–34 years	195
35–44 years	184
45–54 years	24
54+	—
Race/ethnicity	
White	1,089
Black	102
Hispanic	35
Unknown	72
Chief complaint(s)	
Intoxication	252
Altered mental status	454
Psychiatric condition	11
Chest pain	35
Respiratory problems	19
Digestive problems	77
Other	614

Source: Adapted from Office of Applied Studies, Substance Abuse and Mental Health Services Administration. *Drug Abuse Warning Network, 2003: Interim National Estimates of Drug-Related Emergency Department Visits.* DAWN Series D-26. Publication no. SMA 04-3972. Rockville, Md.: Department of Health and Human Services, 2004.

**TABLE II: ESTIMATED NATIONWIDE INCIDENTS OF
MALICIOUS POISONINGS BY DRUG, 2003**

Drug Category and Selected Drugs	Estimated Visits
Total Drug-Related Emergency Department Visits	1,300
Alcohol in combination with other drugs	765
Cocaine	—
Heroin	14
Marijuana	202
Stimulants	194
MDMA (Ecstasy)	23
Gamma-hydroxybutyrate (GHB)	—
Flunitrazepam (Rohypnol)	—
PCP	24
Opiates/opioid analgesics	183

Source: Adapted from Office of Applied Studies, Substance Abuse
and Mental Health Services Administration. *Drug Abuse Warning
Network, 2003: Interim National Estimates of Drug-Related Emergency
Department Visits.* DAWN Series D-26. Publication no. SMA 04-3972.
Rockville, Md.: Department of Health and Human Services, 2004.

The primary complaint of patients who were
maliciously poisoned was an altered mental state.
DAWN estimated that about 7 percent of the malicious poisoning cases had a diagnosis of assault, SEX-
UAL ASSAULT, or sexual abuse. The rates of malicious
poisoning nationwide were low; the average patient
was female, white, and ages 25–29 years old.

See also CRIME; DATE RAPE DRUGS; EMERGENCY
TREATMENT; INCARCERATION; SCHEDULED DRUGS.

Office of Applied Studies, Substance Abuse and Mental
Health Services Administration. *Drug Abuse Warning
Network, 2003: Interim National Estimates of Drug-Related
Emergency Department Visits.* DAWN Series D-26. Publi-
cation no. SMA 04-3972. Rockville, Md.: Department
of Health and Human Services, 2004.

marijuana   The most commonly used illegal drug
in the United States as well as in many other countries worldwide. Marijuana (sometimes spelled *mari-
huana*) is also often referred to as *cannabis.* According
to the United Nations Office on Drugs and Crime,
an estimated 146.2 million people around the globe
abused cannabis in 2003. In the United States, marijuana was involved in nearly 13 percent of all drug-

related emergency room visits in 2003, or 79,663
cases, according to the National Institute on Drug
Abuse. Some pregnant women abuse marijuana;
according to a study published in 2006 in *Maternal
and Child Health;* in a sample of 1,632 women, 6 percent used marijuana during their pregnancy. (See
PREGNANCY AND SUBSTANCE ABUSE.)

Sometimes abusers combine marijuana with
other drugs, such as HEROIN, KETAMINE, METHAM-
PHETAMINE, or CRACK COCAINE. Most marijuana
users also abuse alcohol.

Most of the marijuana that is abused by people
in the United States is illegally trafficked into the
country from MEXICO, but some of the drug enters
from CANADA and the Caribbean. Marijuana is usually transported for sale by criminal organizations
and independent smugglers.

Marijuana is a drug that is derived from the
dried seeds, stems, shredded leaves, and flowers of the hemp plant, *Cannabis sativa.* It is also a
Schedule I drug under the CONTROLLED SUBSTANCES
ACT classification for SCHEDULED DRUGS. Marijuana
use induces a state of euphoria by stimulating the
release of dopamine, a brain chemical. This is the
primary reason why the drug is abused.

Marijuana affects the central nervous system.
The active chemical in marijuana, which causes
the intoxicating effect of the drug, is delta-9-tet-
rahydrocannabinol (THC), which is also the active
ingredient in HASHISH. The amount of THC in marijuana has steadily increased since 1990 and remains
significantly higher than the level of THC in the
drug in the 1960s and 1970s. As a result, the drug
is more potent than that used by individuals in the
past, such as during the Vietnam War.

Marijuana also impairs brain function, and it is
the second most frequently found substance among
drivers who are involved in fatal car crashes. (Alcohol is the *most* frequently found substance in fatal
car accidents.)

According to the National Institutes of Health,
about 10 percent of the population in the United
States uses marijuana on a regular basis. DRUG TEST-
ING can detect marijuana in the urine for up to 30
days after use because METABOLITES of marijuana
are present for up to 30 days after the use of the
drug. Some individuals continue to show marijuana
metabolites in the urine for months after ceasing

use of the drug, because THC is absorbed into the body fat and then released into the bloodstream in response to weight loss, exercise, or other physical changes.

Most users smoke marijuana in rolled cigarettes ("joints") or hollowed-out cigars ("blunts"), although the drug can also be ingested in foods. The effects of marijuana are more immediate and shorter-lasting when the drug is smoked than when it is eaten; for example, marijuana rapidly enters the brain when it is smoked, and the effects of the drug may last one to three hours. If marijuana is eaten, the effects begin about 30 to 60 minutes after ingestion and may last for about four hours.

Individuals who are intoxicated by marijuana may exhibit some or all of the following symptoms and signs:

- euphoria
- increased auditory and visual perception
- increased appetite (the "munchies")
- difficulty concentrating
- impaired coordination
- altered sense of time
- irritability
- lethargy

Users of Marijuana

An estimated 94 million Americans (40 percent) age 12 and older have used marijuana at least once in their lifetimes. The use of the drug is the heaviest among adolescents and among YOUNG ADULTS who are ages 18–25 years old. According to the National Survey on Drug Use and Health, there were 14.6 million current users of marijuana in the United States in 2004. About 2.1 million people tried marijuana for the first time in 2004, or about 6,000 people per day. This was about the same level as the number of people who tried marijuana for the first time in 2003.

During the period 2002 to 2004, marijuana use declined among males ages 12 to 17 years old, from 9.1 percent in 2002 to 8.1 percent in 2004. However, over the same period, the rate remained about the same among female adolescents, or 7.2 percent in 2002 and 7.1 percent in 2004.

In considering the daily use of marijuana/hashish (marijuana was not broken out from hashish, a drug also derived from the cannabis plant) in the past 30 days, information derived from the Monitoring the Future study in 2004 indicates that the rates of usage were highest for 12th graders, college students, and young adults. See Table I.

Studies have shown that the majority of marijuana users (55 percent) in 2004 obtained the drug free from others they knew or shared marijuana with someone else. Of those who purchased the drug, about 53 percent purchased the drug within their apartment, home, or dormitory, according to the National Survey on Drug Use and Health. In addition, most of those who obtained the drug free (65 percent) received it in these home locations as well. As a result, users did not have to go to unfamiliar or dangerous neighborhoods to purchase the drug, as with drugs such as CRACK COCAINE or HEROIN.

Myths about Marijuana

There are many different myths about marijuana use and abuse, such as the myth that marijuana is a

TABLE I: TRENDS IN THIRTY-DAY PREVALENCE OF DAILY USE OF MARIJUANA FOR EIGHTH, TENTH, AND TWELFTH GRADERS, COLLEGE STUDENTS, AND YOUNG ADULTS (AGES 19–28)

	1994	1995	1996	1997	1998	1999	2000	2001	2002	2003	2004
8th Graders	0.7	0.8	1.5	1.1	1.1	1.4	1.3	1.3	1.2	1.0	0.8
10th Graders	2.2	2.8	3.5	3.7	3.6	3.8	3.8	4.5	3.9	3.6	3.2
12th Graders	3.6	4.6	4.9	5.8	5.6	6.0	6.0	5.8	6.0	6.0	5.6
College students	1.8	3.7	2.8	3.7	4.0	4.0	4.6	4.5	4.1	4.7	4.5
Young adults	2.8	3.3	3.3	3.8	3.7	4.4	4.2	5.0	4.5	5.3	5.0

Source: Adapted from Johnston, Lloyd D., et al. *Monitoring the Future: National Survey Results on Drug Use, 1975–2004*. Vol. 2, *College Students & Adults Ages 19–45*. Bethesda, Md..: National Institute on Drug Abuse, National Institutes of Health, 2005, p. 53.

harmless or even a beneficial drug. The key myths about marijuana were described by the Office of National Drug Policy in a 2004 booklet. According to this source, there are 10 primary myths about marijuana, which are each debunked.

Myth one: marijuana is harmless The first myth is that marijuana is a harmless drug with no ill effects. In fact, however, marijuana significantly impairs thinking and concentration and affects an individual's performance at school and at work. College students who have used marijuana regularly have experienced problems with impaired memory and learning for up to 24 hours after they used the drug. In one study, the researchers discovered that frequent users of marijuana (seven or more times a week) had mathematical and verbal deficits as well as memory problems.

Marijuana can increase the risk for the subsequent development of psychiatric problems, such as DEPRESSION, ANXIETY DISORDERS, and other mental health problems, especially among young people; for example, research has shown that adolescents 12–17 years old who smoked marijuana on a weekly basis had three times the risk of experiencing thoughts about committing SUICIDE compared to those who were not regular users of the drug. Other studies have shown that the use of marijuana increases the risk of the development of depression by about four times.

Marijuana also impairs driving ability. Research has shown that of trauma patients who were injured while driving a car or a motorcycle, 15 percent had been smoking marijuana and an additional 17 percent had traces of marijuana and alcohol in their bloodstream. Thus, nearly a third of trauma patients had abused marijuana. An estimated 36 million people ages 12 and older reportedly drive their vehicles while under the influence of marijuana, alcohol, and/or another illegal drug each year. In one study of reckless drivers in Tennessee who were *not* under the influence of alcohol, these individuals were tested for drugs, and one-third of them tested positive for marijuana use.

Risky behavior is also linked to marijuana use, such as an increased risk for having multiple sex partners, failing to use condoms, and initiating sex at an early age.

According to the Drug Enforcement Administration (DEA), marijuana contains carcinogens (cancer-causing agents) as well as known toxins, similar to those in cigarettes or other nicotine products.

Myth two: marijuana is not addictive Contrary to popular belief, some people do become addicted to marijuana, and heavy users experience WITHDRAWAL effects if they stop using the drug. According to the Office of National Drug Policy report on marijuana myths, "The desire for marijuana exerts a powerful pull on those who use it, and this desire, coupled with withdrawal symptoms, can make it hard for long-term smokers to stop using the drug. Users trying to quit often report irritability, anxiety, and difficulty sleeping. On psychological tests they also display increased aggression, which peaks approximately one week after they last used the drug."

Some individuals enter rehabilitation facilities with a primary diagnosis of marijuana dependence, and an estimated two-thirds of all adolescents receiving drug treatment are addicted to marijuana. The earlier in life that a person starts using marijuana, the more likely he or she is to become dependent on it. For example, among those who were admitted to treatment facilities for primary marijuana dependence, more than half (56 percent) had begun using the drug by age 14.

Myth three: marijuana is not as harmful to health as is tobacco Marijuana is *not* a more benign drug than tobacco, and the amount of tar that is inhaled as well as the level of absorbed carbon monoxide that is present are an estimated three to five times greater than those absorbed by individuals who smoke tobacco. Some studies have shown a linkage between respiratory problems and marijuana smoking in young people. About three to four joints of smoked marijuana cause damage that is roughly equivalent to that caused by smoking more than 20 tobacco cigarettes.

Myth four: marijuana makes you mellow Another myth is that marijuana is benevolent and inevitably makes the user feel relaxed and at ease. Although this may be true with infrequent usage, research has shown that adolescents and young people who use marijuana on a weekly basis have a four times greater risk than others of exhibiting violent behavior. Other studies have shown that incidents of physical attacks, stealing, and destruction of personal property directly increase with the number of days that marijuana is smoked. Marijuana use is also associated with a greater probability of committing weapons offenses. In addition, there is a link between marijuana abuse and an increased risk for serious crimes, such as attempted homicide and reckless endangerment.

Myth five: marijuana is useful in treating cancer and other diseases   Some individuals believe that smoking marijuana will alleviate the pain of chronic severe diseases or of terminal illnesses such as cancer. In fact, some states have passed laws approving the use of "medical marijuana" for ill individuals. The federal government actively disputes this use and considers smoking marijuana to be medically unproven and illegal.

However, it should be noted that DRONABINOL (MARINOL), a marijuanalike preparation, is used in the treatment of cancer-related nausea and appetite problems associated with ACQUIRED IMMUNE DEFICIENCY SYNDROME (AIDS). Marinol's active ingredient is delta-9-tetrahydrocannibinol (THC), which is also the chemical in marijuana that can cause intoxication. The drug can cause dizziness, clumsiness, sedation, a false sense of well-being, and difficulty in thinking.

Myth six: marijuana is less popular among teens than other drugs   Many individuals mistakenly believe that adolescent drug users primarily abuse drugs other than marijuana, such as METHYLENEDIOXYMETHAMPHETAMINE (MDMA/ECSTASY), COCAINE, or METHAMPHETAMINE. In fact, however, according to the Monitoring the Future study in 2003, a study of students in the eighth, 10th, and 12th grades, marijuana is not only the *most* popular drug of abuse among students, but has also been the most widely used illegal drug among high school seniors for the entire 29 years that the Monitoring the Future study has been performed each year.

In 2003, 46.1 percent of high school seniors had ever used either marijuana or hashish, in comparison to 14.4 percent who had used amphetamines, 8.3 percent who had used Ecstasy, and 10.6 percent who had ever used hallucinogens.

Marijuana was also the most popular drug among those in the eighth and 10th grades as well; in 2003, 17.5 percent of 8th graders had ever used marijuana/hashish, and 36.4 percent of 10th graders had ever used the drug.

Myth seven: purchasing marijuana does not hurt others   Marijuana may be depicted as a drug of peace and love by many supporters and users of the drug, but it is important to keep in mind that the use of marijuana is also part of a very large business of DRUG DEALERS and organized criminals in the United States, particularly in California, as well as in other countries, such as MEXICO. Illegal aliens are smuggled into the United States from Mexico to work in marijuana fields, and campers, hunters, and others have been threatened at gun point or fired upon when they accidentally arrived at these illegal sites.

However, it should also be noted that those who favor the legalization of marijuana believe that it is the criminalizing of the drug that has drawn in a criminal element, since it is only criminals who can make a profit at selling marijuana. Such individuals believe the drug could be sold under government control and taxed.

Myth eight: my children won't use marijuana   Many parents are convinced that their children will never try marijuana or, if they do try the drug, they will not continue to use it. As a result, these parents believe that there is little or no reason to mention the subject with their children. Yet studies have shown that more than half of adolescents ages 12–17 have reported that if they wanted marijuana, it would be easy for them to obtain the drug. As mentioned, most adolescents do not buy the drug from street drug dealers; rather, they purchase or receive it free from a friend, and nearly 9 percent of students have reported buying marijuana on the grounds of a school. Nor are children in suburban or rural areas safe from being offered marijuana. There is ready access to marijuana in most areas if children and adolescents wish to try the drug.

PEER PRESSURE is another strong factor influencing the use of marijuana. Adolescents like to imitate the behavior of their friends, and studies such as those by the National Household Survey on Drug Abuse have demonstrated that adolescents who have friends who have used marijuana are themselves 30 times more likely to use the drug than those whose friends did *not* abuse marijuana. Adults are also influential over their children (although often they do not realize the extent of their influence), and children and adolescents who know an adult who has used marijuana in the past month are nine times more likely to use the drug than children who have no adult role models who use marijuana.

As can be seen from Figure I, the frequency of past marijuana use has a clear correlation with thefts of $50 or more among adolescents ages 12 to 17 years. For example, only 2.9 percent of those who never abused marijuana had stolen items, whereas those who used marijuana from one to 11 days in the past year had a theft rate of 8.3 percent. The rate continues to rise with use, and adolescents who used marijuana for 300 or more days had a theft rate of 31.7 percent.

In addition, among adolescents who attacked someone with the intent to harm him or her, the rate of marijuana use was linked to the percentage of teenagers who exhibited this behavior, as shown in Figure II. For example, among those who had not abused marijuana in the past year, the rate of violence was 5.9 percent, nearly doubling to 11.4 percent for those who used marijuana from one to 11 days in the past year. The highest rate was seen among adolescents who used marijuana 300 or more days in the past year, or 32.9 percent, five times the rate of those who did not use marijuana.

The use of handguns by adolescents was also correlated with the number of days of marijuana use. Among those adolescents who did not abuse marijuana in the past year, 2.5 percent carried a handgun. That rate increased to 3.2 percent for those who used marijuana from one to 11 days. Among those who used marijuana for 300 or more days in the past year, the rate of carrying a handgun was 22.2 percent, or about seven times the rate of those who did *not* abuse marijuana. (See Figure III.)

FIGURE I

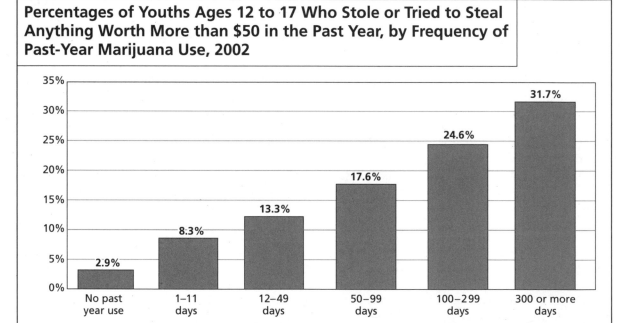

Percentages of Youths Ages 12 to 17 Who Stole or Tried to Steal Anything Worth More than $50 in the Past Year, by Frequency of Past-Year Marijuana Use, 2002

Source: Office of Applied Studies, "Marijuana Use and Delinquent Behaviors among Youths," *The NSDUH Report*, Substance Abuse and Mental Health Services Administration, January 9, 2004.

© Infobase Publishing

FIGURE II

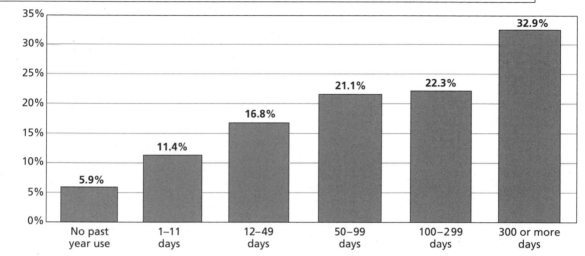

Percentage of Youths Ages 12 to 17 Who Attacked Someone with the Intent to Seriously Hurt Them in the Past Year, by Frequency of Past-Year Marijuana Use, 2002

Source: Office of Applied Studies, "Marijuana Use and Delinquent Behaviors among Youths," *The NSDUH Report*, Substance Abuse and Mental Health Services Administration, January 9, 2004.

© Infobase Publishing

Myth nine: parents can do little or nothing to stop their children from experimenting with marijuana Many parents assume that they are powerless to prevent their children from using marijuana, but studies have demonstrated that this belief is wrong. In fact, research has shown that parents exert a powerful influence over children, even when children are overtly rebellious and emotional.

Studies from the National Household Survey on Drug Use have shown that when adolescents believed their parents disapproved of marijuana use, they had a much lower use of the drug. In 2000, among those adolescents who believed their parents would disapprove of marijuana use, 4.9 percent of adolescents had used the drug in the past month. Among adolescents who believed that their parents did not strongly disapprove of the use of marijuana, 27 percent used the drug in the past month.

Some parents are reluctant to talk to their children about marijuana use, since they may have used marijuana themselves during their youth. They may feel that because they used marijuana then, they would be hypocrites to tell their children to avoid the drug. However, parents can caution children about avoiding mistakes that they may have made; for example, most parents who smoke cigarettes would not wish their children to start smoking. Parents may tell their children about the risks of marijuana use and (if true) state that they feel their own use was a mistake. If they do not believe their use was a mistake, they can instead emphasize the risks associated with marijuana use, such as arrest for possession of the drug or poor performance in school.

Myth 10: the government sends otherwise innocent people to prison for only casual marijuana use The reality is that it is extremely rare for peo-

FIGURE III

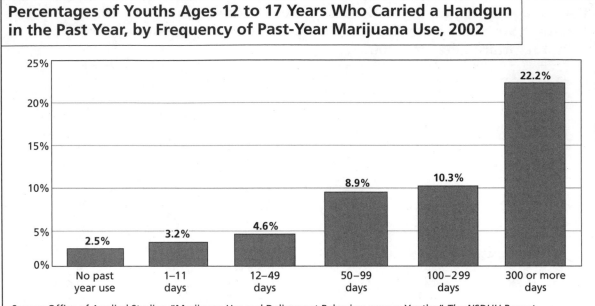

Percentages of Youths Ages 12 to 17 Years Who Carried a Handgun in the Past Year, by Frequency of Past-Year Marijuana Use, 2002

Source: Office of Applied Studies, "Marijuana Use and Delinquent Behaviors among Youths," *The NSDUH Report*, Substance Abuse and Mental Health Services Administration, January 9, 2004.

© Infobase Publishing

ple who have small amounts of marijuana, especially among first-time users of the drug, to be sent to prison for the use of marijuana only. Most states have made marijuana possession a misdemeanor or even a lesser crime, rather than the more serious crime of a felony, as with drugs such as heroin or methamphetamine.

Simple statistics do not support the belief that prisons are packed with first-time marijuana offenders. For example, according to the Office of National Drug Policy, in 2002 there were 1.2 million people incarcerated in prisons for all types of crimes. About 3,600 of these individuals were incarcerated for a first offense. Thus, less than 1 percent of all criminals were imprisoned for their first marijuana offense, since many first offenders committed an array of other crimes.

Instead, federal and state law enforcement authorities primarily concentrate on drug traffickers, and thus, most prison inmates who are convicted of drug offenses are imprisoned for drug trafficking, including the sale of marijuana and other drugs.

Health Consequences of Marijuana Use

There are many possible serious health and psychiatric consequences that are associated with the consumption of marijuana, particularly when the drug is used on a frequent or chronic basis. Multiple studies have demonstrated that continued cannabis use can impair an individual's cognitive ability, at least over the short term, and may even trigger a serious mental illness, such as DEPRESSION or SCHIZOPHRENIA. In addition, as mentioned, some individuals who use marijuana will develop an abuse or dependence on the drug. (See MARIJUANA/CANNABIS USE DISORDERS.)

According to the National Institute of Drug Abuse, the following consequences may occur with marijuana use.

Acute signs (which are present during marijuana intoxication)

- impaired short-term memory
- impaired attention, judgment, and other cognitive functions
- impaired coordination and balance
- increased heart rate

A key persistent sign (lasting longer than intoxication, but the effects may not be permanent)

- impaired memory and learning skills

Long-term effects (cumulative, potentially permanent effects of chronic abuse)

- can lead to addiction
- increases risk of chronic cough, bronchitis, and emphysema
- increases risk of cancer of the head, neck, and lungs

The chronic use of marijuana may also lead to changes in personality or the development of personality disorders. Other psychiatric effects may include

- disorientation
- acute panic reactions
- psychosis
- depersonalization (the inability to distinguish oneself from others)
- paranoia
- changed body image
- lack of motivation (amotivational syndrome)

Studies have also shown that the use of marijuana is associated with increased absences from jobs, a greater number of accidents, and more worker compensation claims. Marijuana also affects memory and learning for days or weeks from the last use of the drug. One study of 129 COLLEGE STUDENTS found that of those students who had smoked the drug on at least 27 of the past 30 days, their memory and attention skills were significantly impaired, even when they had not used the drug for 24 hours or longer.

Some studies have also shown that among those who are ages 18 and older, those individuals who first used marijuana before age 12 were twice as likely (21.0 percent) to have had a serious mental illness, defined as a disorder that met the criteria for mental, behavioral, or emotional disorders in the *Diagnostic and Statistical Manual of Mental* Disorders (*DSM-IV*) in the past year, compared to those adults who first used marijuana at age 18 or older (10.5 percent).

Amotivational Syndrome The heavy abuse of marijuana over the long term may lead to the development of a condition that is known as *amotivational syndrome*. Signs of this syndrome may include both impaired judgment and memory, as well as apathy, poor concentration, and the loss of any interest in the achievement of personal goals. Another indicator of amotivational syndrome is poor personal hygiene.

Crime and Marijuana Use

The abuse of marijuana is common among individuals arrested for crimes throughout the United States, and nearly half (44 percent) of those arrested in major cities test positive for marijuana use. The arrestees in a study in 2003 were asked about their usage of marijuana in the past week, month, and year, and this information is displayed in Table III.

As can be seen from the table, more than half the male arrestees reported using marijuana in the past year and the median number of days on which marijuana was used by males was 10.5 days. Among female arrestees, the abuse rates of marijuana were higher than among the general population but lower than those of male arrestees.

TABLE III: MALE AND FEMALE ARRESTEES REPORTING USE AND ACQUISITION OF MARIJUANA IN THE PAST WEEK, MONTH, AND YEAR, 2003 (MEDIAN IN THE UNITED STATES)

Past Marijuana Use by Arrestees	Male	Female
Used in past 7 days	39.3%	30.0%
Used in past 30 days	44.9%	36.0%
Used in past year	51.9%	44.4%
Average number of days used in past 30 days	10.5 days	9.1 days

Source: National Institute of Justice *Drug and Alcohol Use and Related Matters among Arrestees, 2003.* 2004. Available online. URL: http://www.ncjrs.gove/nij/adam/ADM2003.pdf. Downloaded May 19, 2006.

Criminal Penalties   There are state and federal penalties for the possession of marijuana, although DRUG DEALERS are usually treated much more harshly than "recreational" (infrequent) users of marijuana. Users of small amounts of marijuana are often charged with a misdemeanor offense, while selling marijuana is a felony. See Table II for federal penalties for the trafficking (selling) of marijuana, which are increasingly severe after the first offense.

In 2003, the DEA made 5,679 arrests related to cannabis, or about 21 percent of all DEA arrests for the year.

Marijuana use is common among juveniles who are arrested for crimes, and in one study, about 57 percent of male juveniles and 32 percent of female juveniles who were arrested tested positive for marijuana use.

Treatment Programs

There are few treatment programs exclusively designed for marijuana abuse, and most treatment programs concentrate instead on alcohol abuse or alcoholism or the abuse of drugs such as cocaine or heroin. However, marijuana dependence is

TABLE II: FEDERAL TRAFFICKING PENALTIES FOR MARIJUANA, HASHISH, AND HASHISH OIL

	Quantity	First Offense	Second Offense
Marijuana	1,000 kg or more mixtures; or 1,000 or more plants	Not less than 10 years, not more than life.	Not less than 20 years, not more than life.
		If death or serious injury, not less than 20 years, not more than life.	If death or serious injury, then life.
		Fine not more than $4 million individual, $10 million other than individual	Fine not more than $8 million individual, $20 million other than individual.
Marijuana	100 kg to 999 kg mixture; or 100–999 plants.	Not less than 5 years, not more than 30 years.	Not less than 10 years, not more than life.
		If death or serious injury, not less than 20 years, not more than life.	If death or serious injury, then life.
		Fine not more than $2 million individual, $5 million other than individual	Fine not more than $4 million individual, $10 million other than individual.
Marijuana	50 to 99 kg mixture	Not more than 20 years.	Not more than 30 years.
	50 to 99 plants	If death or serious injury, not less than 20 years, not more than life.	If death or serious injury, then life.
Hashish	More than 10 kg		Fine $2 million individual, $10 million other than individual.
Hashish oil	More than 1 kg	Fine $1 million individual $5 million other than individual	
Marijuana	Less than 50 kg	Not more than 5 years. Fine not more than $250,000, $1 million other than individual	Not more than 10 years. Fine $500,000 individual, $2 million other than individual.
	1 to 49 plants		
Hashish	10 kg or less		
Hashish oil	1 kg or less		

Source: Joseph, Donald E., et al., eds. *Drugs of Abuse.* Washington, D.C.: U.S. Department of Justice, 2005, p. 11.

linked to many problems, such as an increased risk for crime, and thus treatment is important. In addition, psychiatric disorders, such as depression, anxiety and some personality disorders, have been linked to chronic marijuana abuse. Marijuana can also impair memory and learning. Students who use marijuana are less likely to graduate from high school. Workers who smoke marijuana are more likely to have problems at work, including increased lateness, absences, accidents, and job turnover. A study of postal workers who were tested for marijuana found that those who tested positive had 85 percent more injuries and 55 percent more industrial accidents than those who tested negative.

One study indicated that adult marijuana users benefited from 14 sessions of cognitive-behavior therapy (CBT) as well as two sessions of individual treatment. Most participants were men in their early 30s who had smoked marijuana daily for more than 10 years. The treatments helped the men become aware of what triggered their marijuana abuse and enabled them to create strategies to avoid these triggers.

Another study showed that giving patients vouchers redeemable for goods such as sports equipment, passes to movies, or vocational training, improved outcomes.

To date, there are no medications that are specifically designed to treat marijuana abuse and dependence.

See also ADOLESCENTS AND SUBSTANCE ABUSE; CRIME AND CRIMINALS; IMPAIRED DRIVING, INVOLVEMENT OF ALCOHOL AND/OR DRUGS; INJURIES; JAIL INMATES; LAW ENFORCEMENT; YOUNG ADULTS.

Arria, Amelia M., et al. "Methamphetamine and Other Substance Use during Pregnancy: Preliminary Estimates from the Infant Development, Environment, and Lifestyle (IDEAL) Study." *Maternal and Child Health* 10, no. 3 (2006): 293–302.

Arseneault, Louise. "Cannabis Use in Adolescence and Risk for Adult Psychosis: Longitudinal Prospective Study." *British Medical Journal* 325 (November 23, 2002): 1,212–1,213.

Gwinnell, Esther, M.D., and Christine Adamec. *The Encyclopedia of Addictions and Addictive Behaviors.* New York: Facts On File, 2005.

Johnston, Lloyd D., et al. *Monitoring the Future: National Survey Results on Drug Use, 1975–2004.* Vol. 2, *College Students & Adults Ages 19–45.* Bethesda, Md.: National Institute on Drug Abuse, National Institutes of Health, 2005.

Joseph, Donald E., ed. *Drugs of Abuse.* Washington, D.C.: U.S. Department of Justice, 2005.

Matochik, John A., et al. "Altered Brain Tissue Composition in Heavy Marijuana Users." *Drug and Alcohol Dependence* 77 (2005): 23–30.

National Institute of Justice. *Drug and Alcohol Use and Related Matters among Arrestees, 2003.* 2004. Available online. URL: http:www.ncjrs.gove/nij/adam/ADM2003.pdf. Downloaded May 19, 2006.

National Institute on Drug Abuse. "Marijuana Abuse." National Institute on Drug Abuse Research Report Series, Washington, D.C., National Institutes of Health, 2005. available online. URL: http://www.drugabuse.gov/ResearchReports/marijuana/default.html. Downloaded February 26, 2006.

Office of Applied Studies, Substance Abuse and Mental Health Services Administration. *Overview of Findings from the 2004 National Survey on Drug Use and Health.* Publication no. SMA 05-4061. Rockville, Md.: Department of Health and Human Services, September 2005.

Office of Applied Studies. "Age at First Use of Marijuana and Past Year Serious Mental Illness." *The NSDUH Report,* 3 May 2005: 1–3.

Office of National Drug Control Policy. *Marijuana Myths and Facts: The Truth behind 10 Popular Misperceptions.* Available online. URL: http://www.whitehousedrugpolicy.gov/publications/marijuana_myths_facts/marijuana_myths_f acts.pdf. Downloaded on January 16, 2006.

Rey, Joseph M., and Christopher C. Tennant. "Cannabis and Mental Health." *British Medical Journal* 325 (November 23, 2002): 1,183–1,184.

Substance Abuse and Mental Health Services Administration. *Overview of Findings from the 2004 National Survey on Drug Use and Health.* Washington, D.C.: Department of Health and Human Services, September 2005.

marijuana/cannabis use disorders   The abuse of or dependence on (addiction) marijuana, as opposed to occasional experimentation or recreational use of the drug, just as those who use alcohol once or occasionally but not to the point of abuse or dependence are not regarded as alcohol abusers or alcoholics. Of course, marijuana is a Schedule I drug under the CONTROLLED SUBSTANCES ACT, and as a result, any user is subject to state and federal penalties. In general, it is the sale of marijuana that is punished more harshly than the use of the drug in the United States. In some other countries, possession of cannabis alone is grounds for lengthy periods of INCARCERATION.

Marijuana abuse and dependence are common problems among juvenile detainees and adult jail and prison inmates. Abuse or dependence on marijuana is also associated with psychiatric problems, particularly ANXIETY DISORDERS and DEPRESSION. In addition, some studies have demonstrated a link between marijuana abuse and the later development of psychotic disorders, such as SCHIZOPHRENIA.

Cannabis Abuse

According to the *Diagnostic and Statistical Manual–IV-TR (DSM-IV-TR)*, published by the American Psychiatric Association, cannabis (marijuana) abuse is defined as abuse that "can interfere with performance at work or school and may be physically hazardous in situations such as driving a car. Legal problems may occur as a consequence of arrests for cannabis possession. There may be arguments with spouse or parents over the possession of cannabis in the home or its use in the presence of children." If physical or psychological problems are also present, the *DSM* advises that a diagnosis of cannabis dependence should be considered by the physician.

Cannabis Dependence

According to the *DSM*, those who are dependent on cannabis are chronic users who have developed a PHYSICAL TOLERANCE to the drug.

Says the *DSM*,

Individuals with Cannabis Dependence may use very potent cannabis throughout the day over a period of months or years, and they may spend several hours a day acquiring and using the substance. This often interferes with family, school, work, or recreational activities. Individuals with Cannabis Dependence may also persist in their use despite knowledge of physical problems (e.g.,

chronic cough related to smoking) or psychological problems (e.g., excessive sedation and a decrease in goal-oriented activities resulting from repeated use of high doses).

Abuse and Dependence Prevalence Has Increased Significantly

According to Wilson M. Compton, M.D., and colleagues in their study on marijuana, reported in the *Journal of the American Medical Association* in 2004, the use of marijuana in 2001–2 was at about the same level as in 1991–92; however, despite this similarity in use, the rate of marijuana use disorders was significantly higher than in earlier years.

The researchers found that the rate of marijuana abuse or dependence increased slightly from 1.2 percent in 1991–92 to a rate of 1.5 percent in 2001–2. Although on the surface, this may not seem to be a major increase, it actually translated into 2.2 to 3 million more individuals who abused or were dependent on marijuana. The study also found sharp increases among African Americans and Hispanics. It is unknown why this increase occurred, but the researchers speculated that it might have been related to increased potency of marijuana in the 21st century.

Treatment of Marijuana Abuse and Dependency

Many treatment centers concentrate primarily or solely on the rehabilitation of individuals who abuse or are addicted to drugs such as COCAINE or HEROIN, rather than marijuana. Other centers specialize in treating patients who are alcoholics. However, many individuals who are heavy users of marijuana also abuse other drugs and/or alcohol, and as a result, their multiple addictions often need to be addressed in a rehabilitative facility.

Because many heavy users of marijuana have taken the drug for years, often daily or several times a week, inpatient facilities concentrate on teaching them how to change their thinking about the drug through such therapies as cognitive-behavioral therapy. This therapy teaches the individual to challenge basic beliefs and replace them with more logical and healthful ones. For example, the belief that the individual cannot change is replaced with the thought that change is possible and good. The idea that the individual is worthless is substituted with the idea that the person has talents and abilities and needs to develop them. The marijuana user must also stop denying that marijuana use is not a problem for them and that it must be avoided entirely.

Because the individual will be returning home after leaving an inpatient facility, former marijuana users are trained to reject others who offer them marijuana. It is best if they do not return to living with other drug users because doing so makes it easier for them to fall back into the trap of drug abuse. Avoidance of marijuana after years of use is not easy, but it is possible.

See also PSYCHIATRIC PROBLEMS.

American Psychiatric Association. *Diagnostic and Statistical Manual of Mental Disorders*. 4th ed. Washington, D.C.: American Psychiatric Association, 2000.

Compton, Wilson M., M.D. "Prevalence of Marijuana Use Disorders in the United States 1991–1992 and 2001–2002." *Journal of the American Medical Association* 291, no. 17 (May 5, 2004): 2,114–2,121.

medication contract   See TREATMENT CONTRACT.

meperidine (Demerol)   A strong narcotic painkiller that is used by physicians for both cancerous and severe noncancerous pain.

Meperidine was first introduced as a painkilling drug in the 1930s, and its use continues. It is a Schedule II drug under the CONTROLLED SUBSTANCES ACT. Meperidine is used prior to anesthesia and is also used as a drug to relieve moderate to severe pain, as occurs among women delivering babies. It is also used as a postoperative drug to control pain. Meperidine is used heavily by many emergency room doctors in order to control severe pain. Because this practice is widely known, sometimes individuals addicted to NARCOTICS go to emergency rooms, lying that they are suffering from severe pain, for the sole purpose of obtaining an injection of meperidine.

Meperidine is similar to MORPHINE, but it is not as long-lasting a drug. Meperidine is currently available in tablets, syrups, and in an injectable form. There are generic forms of meperidine as well as the brand names of Demerol, Mepergan, and other options.

Some individuals have illegally produced analogues to meperidine in CLANDESTINE LABORATORIES. During the synthesis of the analogue, a neurotoxic by-product, 1-methyl-4 phenyl-hz,s,b-tetrahydopyridine (MPTP), is produced. As a result, some people who have consumed these illegal analogues developed an irreversible Parkinsonian-like syndrome. According to the Drug Enforcement Administration, MPTP destroys the same neurons that are damaged in those individuals who develop Parkinson's disease, a severe degenerative neurologic disorder.

See NARCOTICS; OPIATES; PAIN MANAGEMENT; PRESCRIPTION DRUG ABUSE; SCHEDULED DRUGS.

Joseph, Donald E., ed. *Drugs of Abuse*. Washington, D.C.: U.S. Department of Justice, 2005.

mescaline   A HALLUCINOGENIC DRUG that is derived from the peyote cactus plant, *Lophophora williamsii*. It has sometimes been used in Native American tribal religious rituals. Mescaline can be produced synthetically in CLANDESTINE LABORATORIES; however, most clandestine laboratories in the United States concentrate on the manufacture of METHAMPHETAMINE.

Mescaline is an illegal drug in the United States and a Schedule I drug under the CONTROLLED SUBSTANCES ACT. It is not a common drug of abuse among people in the United States who abuse drugs.

Doses of mescaline used by abusers may range from 0.3 to 0.5 gram, according to the Drug Enforcement Administration, and its effects may last for up to 12 hours. According to a 2004 study by the Substance Abuse and Mental Health Services Administration, of recent hallucinogen initiates ages 12 and older, only about 2.5 percent had used mescaline.

Anthropologists have found that, based on radiocarbon dating, mescaline was used as far back as 5,700 years ago in what is now Shumla Cave number five on the Rio Grande in Texas. According to an article in *Lancet*, "From a cultural point of view, our identification of mescaline strengthens the evidence that Native Americans already recognized and valued the psychotropic properties of peyote as long as 5700 years ago."

In the 1960s some physicians believed that mescaline was a cure for SCHIZOPHRENIA, and they tested the drug on their patients with the condition. The patients did not improve.

Mescaline is not a popular drug of abuse among those ages 12 and older who use hallucinogens. According to the Substance Abuse and Mental Health Administration, about 2.5 percent of those ages 12 and older who had used hallucinogens had used mescaline in the past year in 2004 and 2005. Other hallucinogens were far more popular; for example, 61 percent of males and 41 percent of females who had used hallucinogens had used PSILOCYBIN. ECSTASY was the next most popular drug among hallucinogen users, and was used by 38 percent of male hallucinogen users and 50 percent of female users.

According to the National Institute of Drug Abuse (NIDA), the abuse of mescaline can cause an altered state of perception, flashbacks, as well as an increased body temperature, blood pressure, and heart rate. It can also cause a loss of appetite, sleeplessness, numbness, weakness, and tremors.

See CANADA; COLLEGE STUDENTS; HALLUCINATIONS; HALLUCINOGENIC DRUGS; LYSERGIC ACID DIETHYLAMIDE (LSD); SCHEDULED DRUGS.

Bruhn, Jan G., et al., "Mescaline Use for 5700 Years," *The Lancet* 359 (May 5, 2002): 1,866.

Joseph, Donald E., ed. *Drugs of Abuse.* Washington, D.C.: U.S. Department of Justice, 2005.

Office of Applied Studies, "Patterns of Hallucinogen Use and Initiation: 2004 and 2005," *The NSDUH Report,* July 5, 2007, pp. 1–4.

methadone   A long-acting (up to 24 hours or sometimes 36 hours) synthetic narcotic, which has been available in the United States since 1947. It is also known as an *agonist blocker.* Methadone acts within about 30 minutes. Individuals taking methadone do not experience the euphoria produced by heroin or other opiates that are abused; unfortunately, sometimes individuals seeking this euphoria take very high doses of methadone to attain a "high," but this strategy does not work, is very dangerous, and can lead to an overdose. Methadone also blocks the CRAVING for heroin, and it is not sedating when the dosage is right for the patient. (Dosages must be individualized.)

Several studies have shown that methadone reduces the death rate of heroin addicts. It also decreases the rate of infectious disease; for example, patients taking methadone maintenance are significantly less likely to contract the HUMAN IMMUNODEFICIENCY VIRUS (HIV) or infectious diseases such as HEPATITIS.

Methadone is a Schedule II drug under the CONTROLLED SUBSTANCES ACT. In addition to its use for heroin addicts, methadone is prescribed as a narcotic analgesic for the relief of moderate to severe pain. (See PAIN MANAGEMENT AND NARCOTIC MEDICATIONS.)

The drug is available in tablets and injectable solutions. It also has intramuscular and subcutaneous forms. When tested in the urine, methadone remains in the system for two to four days. Only physicians who are certified by the Substance Abuse and Mental Health Services Administration may prescribe or dispense methadone to patients being treated for opiate addiction; however, any physician may prescribe the drug to treat chronic pain.

Methadone was originally developed as a substitute drug for MORPHINE during World War II in Germany, when morphine was in short supply. In 1947, methadone was approved as a painkilling drug (Dolophine) in the United States. In the 1960s, physicians began recommending methadone as a treatment for heroin addicts. The New York Academy of Sciences first recommended the establishment of methadone maintenance clinics in 1963.

In 1965, the first methadone maintenance treatment center opened in New York City, launched by Dr. Vincent Dole and Dr. Marie Nyswander. They pioneered methadone maintenance, and many clinics were opened nationwide after their initial success.

The 1974 Narcotic Treatment Act established guidelines for the treatment of addicts with methadone. In 1997, a National Institutes of Health consensus conference supported methadone treatment for heroin addicts.

Side Effects and Medication Interactions

According to Krantz and Mehler in their article on treating opioid dependence in 2004 in *Archives of Internal Medicine,* common side effects of methadone use are constipation, sweating, diminished libido, and mild nausea. Less common effects are facial flushing, itching, insomnia, urinary retention, and euphoria. Some patients experience weight gain with this drug.

Some medications may reduce the efficacy of methadone, such as BARBITURATES, while other medications, such as erythromycin or the antidepressant fluvoxamine (Luvox), increase the levels.

Methadone Maintenance

An estimated 240,961 heroin addicts in the United States were treated with methadone in 2004 (22 percent of all patients receiving treatment for substance dependence), up from the 145,610 patients treated in 1998. According to the World Health Organization, methadone maintenance is the dominant method of treatment for opioid addiction worldwide.

Patients go to the clinic daily for their methadone dosage, which is slowly titrated up to a higher dose over four to six weeks. The clinic may refuse to administer a higher dosage to patients who are found not to be drug-free through urinalysis.

Some patients are treated for about six months, but most are treated on a long-term and indefinite basis.

In general, those patients who do best receive methadone maintenance and both individual and group counseling.

Krantz and Mehler state that they favor methadone maintenance as a treatment: "Methadone is the most inexpensive and well-validated agent for opioid maintenance, which leads to 1-year treatment retention rates of 80% with concomitant reductions in illicit opioid use."

Methadone maintenance facilities According to the *National Survey of Substance Abuse Treatment Services*, most methadone patients in 2004 were treated in private for-profit and nonprofit facilities. Clients received methadone at any of three types of care: outpatient, nonhospital residential, and hospital inpatient.

Pros and cons of methadone maintenance programs Individuals who are on methadone maintenance programs develop a PHYSICAL TOLERANCE to methadone and need higher doses of the drug to achieve the same effect; however, advocates say that it is important to keep in mind that methadone is manufactured legally (in contrast to heroin), and thus it is not adulterated, as heroin and other illegal drugs often are. As a result, there is a significantly lesser risk of harm to the individual. In addition, the person who is dependent on methadone need not resort to criminal activities, such as stealing or PROSTITUTION, to obtain the money that is needed to purchase drugs. Some studies have shown that methadone maintenance has decreased criminal activities by 50 percent.

On the other hand, dissenters argue that those on methadone maintenance have exchanged one drug for another, rather than altogether overcoming their drug dependence. In addition, they may be stigmatized by the need to go to a clinic daily to obtain their dosage of methadone.

Methadone as a Pain Medication

Some patients are prescribed methadone for severe chronic pain, as with cancer or terminal diseases as well as severe back pain. However, some patients may be resistant to taking methadone because they may fear that others may think that they are taking the drug because they are heroin addicts. They may also fear developing an addiction to the drug and fear potentially severe side effects. Patients should be counseled that addiction is rare among patients treated for pain, unless they have a past history of drug abuse or addiction.

Diversion of Methadone

It is estimated that about 900,000 people abuse methadone nonmedically each year, whether they obtain the drug from someone on methadone maintenance or through other means. Of those who do use methadone nonmedically, the greatest percentage of abusers are YOUNG ADULTS ages 18–25 years. In addition, about 1 percent of high school seniors have abused methadone at least once.

Federal law allows opiate treatment programs to give patients a single take-home dose on those days that the clinic is closed. In addition, treatment providers may also give up to a one-month supply of methadone to long-term methadone patients. Some of these take-home doses are illegally traded for other drugs or are sold.

Methadone is also sometimes diverted from patients receiving the drug for chronic pain. According to the National Drug Intelligence Center, the most common methods of diversion of methadone for pain are fraudulent prescriptions, the actions of unscrupulous physicians and pharmacists, and theft of the drug.

Illegal use of methadone creates a risk of overdose. Methadone overdoses may cause decreases in the heart rate and blood pressure, severe respiratory depression, coma, and death.

See also BUPRENORPHINE; NARCOTICS; PAIN MANAGEMENT; PRESCRIPTION DRUG ABUSE; SCHEDULED DRUGS.

Krantz, Mori J., M.D., and Philip S. Mehler, M.D. "Treating Opioid Dependence: Growing Implications for Primary Care." *Archives of Internal Medicine* 164 (February 9, 2004): 277–288.

National Drug Intelligence Center. "Methadone Fast Facts." Washington, D.C.: Department of Justice. Available online. URL: http://www.usdoj.gov/ndic/pubs6/6096/6096p.pdf. Downloaded June 23, 2006.

Office of Applied Studies. *National Survey of Substance Abuse Treatment Services (N-SSATS): 2004: Data on Substance Abuse Treatment Facilities.* Rockville, Md.: Substance Abuse and Mental Health Services Administration, August 2005.

Substance Abuse and Mental Health Services Administration. *Results from the 2004 National Survey on Drug Use and Health: National Findings.* Rockville, Md.: Department of Health and Human Services, September 2005.

Vocci, Frank, Jane Acri, and Ahmed Elkasef. "Medication Development for Addictive Disorders: The State of the Science." *American Journal of Psychiatry* 162, no. 8 (August 2005): 1,432–1,440.

methamphetamine A highly addictive drug that is often illegally manufactured. According to the Substance Abuse and Mental Health Services Administration, although the prevalence of illicit methamphetamine use was about the same in 2002, 2003, and 2004, the number of past-month methamphetamine users who met the criteria for abuse or dependence more than doubled, from 27.5 percent of methamphetamine users in 2002 to 59.3 percent in 2004.

It should be noted that a legal form of methamphetamine, Desoxyn, is infrequently used to treat patients who have ATTENTION DEFICIT HYPERACTIVITY DISORDER, as well as those who have narcolepsy. It is a Schedule II drug under the CONTROLLED SUBSTANCES ACT. Desoxyn is also occasionally used as an antiobesity medication, under the guidance of a physician. However, most methamphetamine is illegally manufactured in CLANDESTINE LABORATORIES and is subsequently illegally sold and consumed by drug abusers. The powdered form of the drug in its illegal form can be swallowed, injected, or snorted. It is extremely dangerous and addictive, as is crystal methamphetamine, which is a more concentrated and often much more pure form of the drug.

Methamphetamine is a form of AMPHETAMINE and the most commonly abused form. The drug acts as a central nervous system stimulant on the body. When tested for in the urine, methamphetamine can be detected from two to four days after the drug is used; however, detection may occur up to a week later in cases of heavy abuse. The effects of the drug may last as briefly as 20 minutes and as long as 12 hours, depending on the individual, the drug dosage, and other factors.

According to a 2006 report from the Executive Office of the President, most of the methamphetamine (75–85 percent) that is abused in the United States is made by using chemical precursors that were diverted from international commerce. The balance is made from precursors that are purchased at the wholesale or retail level. However, state laws controlling retail access to precursors have had the effect of limiting the production of methamphetamine in clandestine laboratories in the United States.

According to this report, the federal government has three primary aspects to their plan of tightening the international market for pseudoephedrine and related precursors: obtaining better information about the international trade of these chemicals, implementating the Combat Methamphetamine Epidemic Act of 2005 (Combat Meth Act), and performing law enforcement and border control activities as well as a continued partnership with Mexico.

The Combat Meth Act requires retailers to keep chemicals that can be used as precursors (a drug or chemical, usually a lawful one that is used with other drugs to create an illegal drug) behind store counters or in a locked cabinet that is inaccessible to customers. For example, individuals who operate CLANDESTINE LABORATORIES in the United States and other countries use ephedrine and pseudoephedrine as precursors to create METHAMPHETAMINE. In addition, retailers must maintain a written or electronic list of transactions of these products. The retailer may not sell more than 3.6 grams of the products in a day or 7.5 grams in 30 days to the same customer. As of April 8, 2006, no liquids (capsules, tablets, and gel capsules) of ephedrine, pseudoephedrine, and phenylpropanolamine may be sold in bottles but must be sold instead in blister packs. There are other requirements as well. For example, the seller must keep a logbook to record all sales of products containing ephedrine, pseudoephedrine, and phenylpropanolamine. The seller must record in the logbook the product and quantity sold. In addition, the customer must enter his or her name, address, date, and time of the sale and sign the logbook. The customer must also show a photo identification to the seller. One exception to the photo ID requirement is if the customer buys one package with not more than 60 milligrams of pseudoephedrine, such as one 60 mg tablet or two 30 mg tablets; however, the exception does not apply to ephedrine or phenylpropanolamine.

CRYSTAL METHAMPHETAMINE (*crystal meth*, also called *ice*) is a crystallized form of methamphetamine that can be smoked; it is similar to crack cocaine. The drug is usually smoked in glass pipes. Crystal methamphetamine may also be injected.

It is less frequently abused than powder methamphetamine, but crystal methamphetamine is a drug of concern. According to the Monitoring the Future study, about 1.7 percent of U.S. males and 1.1 percent of females used crystal methamphetamine in 2004. As with methamphetamine itself, crystal methamphetamine is more popular among young adults than adolescents. About 2 percent of college students have used crystal methamphetamine, compared to about 8 percent of their same-age peers.

Note that some researchers and writers use the term *crystal meth* to denote *any* form of methamphetamine.

Users of Methamphetamine

According to the annual Monitoring the Future survey, which surveyed the extent of drug use among students in the eighth, 10th, and 12th grades, in 2004, 6.2 percent of high school seniors had ever used methamphetamine, as had 5.3 percent of 10th graders. Usage was low among eighth graders.

According to the 2004 National Survey on Drug Use and Health, about 11.7 million Americans ages 12 and older have ever tried methamphetamine. About 1.4 million used methamphetamine in the past year and more than a half-million (583,000) had used it in the past month.

The average age of the first use of methamphetamine by new users increased, from 18.9 years in 2002 to 22.1 years in 2004. According to the *NSDUH Report,* young adults 18–25 years old represented the largest group of illicit users of methamphetamine (1.6 percent). However, methamphetamine abuse also declines with age. An estimated 4 percent of young adults ages 19 and 20 use the drug annually, but this percentage declines to about 1 percent by the ages of 29 to 30 years.

The highest rate of usage was found among some races and ethnicities; for example, among Native Hawaiians or other Pacific Islanders, the usage rate was 2.2 percent. Among persons reporting two or more races, the rate was 1.9 percent. Although the usage rate was less than 1 percent among whites, Hispanics, Asians, and African Americans, the past-year use of methamphetamine was highest among whites (0.7 percent), followed by Hispanics (0.5 percent), and then African Americans (0.1 percent), and Asians (0.2 percent).

According to the National Survey on Drug Use and Health, 1.4 million people in the United States used methamphetamine in 2004 and 600,000 had used the drug in the past month. About 21,000 individuals who were addicted to methamphetamine received treatment in drug treatment centers in 1993, and that number increased by more than five times to 117,000 receiving treatment by 2003.

As can be seen from Table I, 5.2 percent of college students had ever used methamphetamine in 2004, as did 8.9 percent of young adults not in college. Less than 1 percent of both groups had abused the drug in the past month.

TABLE I: PERCENTAGE OF COLLEGE STUDENTS/YOUNG ADULTS USING METHAMPHETAMINE, 2003–2004

	College Students		Young Adults	
	2003 Others	2004 Others	2003	2004
Past month	0.6%	0.2%	0.7%	0.6%
Past year	2.6%	2.9%	2.7%	2.8%
Lifetime (ever used)	5.8%	5.2%	8.9%	9.0%

Source: Johnston, Lloyd D., et al. *Monitoring the Future: National Survey Results on Drug Use, 1975–2004.* Vol. 2, *College Students and Adults Ages 19–45.* Bethesda, Md.: National Institute on Drug Abuse, National Institutes of Health, 2005, p. 230.

The use by students in the eighth, 10th, and 12th grades is shown in Table II; as shown, 2.9 percent of 10th and 12th graders used methamphetamine in the past year in 2004, as did 1.8 percent of students in the eighth grade.

Arrestees and methamphetamine abuse   When individuals are arrested, they are usually tested for illegal drugs. Information from the *Drug and Alcohol Use and Related Matters among Arrestees, 2003,* released in 2004, indicates that MARIJUANA is the most common substance found in arrestees, followed by cocaine, crack cocaine, HEROIN, and methamphetamine, in that order of prevalence. However, note that at least a third of the individuals who are arrested abuse more than one drug.

Male individuals arrested in the West were most likely to test positive for methamphetamine, and the highest percentages of male methamphetamine users were found in the following locations: Honolulu, Hawaii (40 percent); Sacramento, California (38 percent); Phoenix, Arizona (38 percent); San Diego, California (36 percent); San Jose, California (37 percent); Spokane, Washington (32 percent).

Among female arrestees who tested positive for methamphetamine, a similar pattern was seen, with the highest abuse rates in Honolulu, Hawaii (57 percent); San Diego, California (47 percent); Salt Lake City, Utah (46 percent); San Jose, California (45 percent); and Portland, Oregon (30 percent).

In considering methamphetamine use among arrestees and their use in the past week, month, and year, females had a higher rate of abuse than males, whereas in nonprison populations, males dominate. For example, of arrestees in 2003, 4 percent of males and 9 percent of females had used the drug in the past seven days. In addition, the female arrestees used the drug on 8.4 days in the past month, compared to 7.1 days for the males. (See Table III.)

Because methamphetamine can induce irrational and violent behavior in individuals of both sexes, it may be that those women who are arrested for crimes are more violent than other women and that in some part, this violence stems from the use of drugs such as methamphetamine.

Individuals who have bipolar disorder   There are some indications that BIPOLAR DISORDER patients are more likely to abuse methamphetamine than others, probably in the manic phase of the illness. Since patients who have bipolar disorder often abuse alcohol as well, the diagnosis and treatment of the substance use disorder as well as the mental illness can be complicated. (See PSYCHIATRIC DISORDERS.)

Pregnant women and methamphetamine   Methamphetamine is sometimes abused by women who are pregnant. In one study of 1,632 pregnant women, reported in 2006 in *Maternal and Child Health,* 5.2 percent of the women said that they had abused methamphetamine during their pregnan-

TABLE II: PERCENTAGE OF STUDENTS REPORTING METHAMPHETAMINE USE, 2004–2005

	8th grade		10th grade		12th grade	
	2004	2005	2004	2005	2004	2005
Past month	0.6%	0.7%	1.3%	1.1%	1.4%	0.9%
Past year	1.5	1.8	3.0	2.9	3.4	2.9
Lifetime (ever used)	2.5	3.1	5.3	4.1	6.2	4.5

Source: National Institute on Drug Abuse and University of Michigan. *Monitoring the Future 2005: Data from In-School Surveys of 8th, 10th, and 12th Grade Students.* Bethesda, Md.: National Institutes of Health. December 2005.

TABLE III: REPORTED METHAMPHETAMINE USE AND ACQUISITION BY ARRESTEES, 2003, BY PERCENTAGE

Past Methamphetamine Use by Arrestees	Male	Female
Used in past 7 days	4.0%	9.0%
Used in past 30 days	4.7%	11.3%
Used in past year	7.7%	15.3%
Average number of days used in past 30 days	7.1 days	8.4 days

Source: National Institute of Justice. *Drug and Alcohol Use and Related Matters among Arrestees, 2003.* 2004. Available online. URL: http:www.ncjrs.gove/nij/adam/ADM2003.pdf. Downloaded May 19, 2006.

cies. Methamphetamine was the third most abused drug among these pregnant women. The most commonly abused substance was alcohol (22.8 percent), followed by marijuana (6.0 percent), and then methamphetamine. Less than 1 percent of the women used HEROIN, BENZODIAZEPINES, and HALLUCINOGENIC DRUGS during their pregnancy.

The researchers stated that they will follow up on the effects of prenatal exposure to methamphetamine in future studies.

Children of methamphetamine users Some states classify an individual's methamphetamine use and/or the production of methamphetamine as a form of CHILD ABUSE in their state laws. In addition, it should be noted that the use of methamphetamine by addicted mothers during pregnancy causes their babies to undergo painful WITHDRAWAL symptoms at birth. The presence of methamphetamine (or other addicting drugs) in a child at birth is cause for removing an infant from the family in many states and may also be grounds for the termination of parental rights.

Methamphetamine use behavior and male/female differences In a study of 350 clients of a treatment system for methamphetamine abuse patients, published in 2004 in *Addictive Behaviors,* researcher Mary-Lynn Brecht and her colleagues in an array of findings about these individuals found common factors among methamphetamine abusers as well as some differences between male and female users.

In their sample, more than half the subjects (56 percent) were male and nearly half (46 percent) were non-Hispanic white, followed by Hispanics (29 percent), African Americans (16 percent), and other races. The median income of the subjects was $14,000. The average age of the subjects when they began using methamphetamine was 19 years.

Most of the subjects obtained the drug for the first time from a friend (59 percent), and their initial primary motivations to use the drug were that they wanted to get high and have fun and that their friends had used the drug, they wanted increased energy, and they wanted to experiment. All of the subjects used alcohol and nearly all (99 percent) also used marijuana. Many of the subjects used other drugs, such as cocaine (87 percent), HALLUCINOGENIC DRUGS (75 percent), crack cocaine (71 percent), INHALANTS (56 percent), and PHENCYCLIDINE (PCP) (55 percent). About half of the subjects had ever injected drugs (47 percent) and more than a third had ever shared needles (36 percent). Most of the subjects became regular users of methamphetamine within about two years of their first use of the drug.

The methamphetamine users reported many types of problems. The majority experienced side effects such as weight loss (84 percent), sleeplessness (78 percent), financial problems (73 percent), paranoia (67 percent), legal problems (63 percent), HALLUCINATIONS (61 percent), work problems (60 percent), violent behavior (57 percent), and dental problems (55 percent). More than half (56 percent) reported having ever sold methamphetamine to others.

In the study, males who abused methamphetamine were more likely to have work problems than female abusers (70 percent males to 48 percent females) and to suffer from hypertension (31 percent males, compared to 16 percent females). Females reported more skin problems than males (47 percent of females to 27 percent of males). There were no differences between males and females with regard to violent behavior.

The researchers also found that a significant number of the methamphetamine users had experienced physical or sexual abuse in childhood; for example, 44 percent of the females and 24 percent of the males reported childhood sexual abuse. About a third of both males and females reported childhood physical abuse.

More than a fourth of all the subjects (27 percent) reported having ever attempted SUICIDE.

The subjects reported a very high rate of criminal behavior: 94 percent had been arrested at least once, and more than half (51 percent) had been arrested more than five times. Males had a three times greater rate of five or more arrests compared to females.

The researchers found that there was an average of nine years from the first use of methamphetamine to admission to treatment, for both males and females. The average initiation treatment was about three months, and after the first treatment, more than half (58 percent) of the subjects relapsed and began using methamphetamine again within six months of their discharge from the treatment center.

Paraphernalia used by methamphetamine users The presence of all or most of the following items may indicate possible methamphetamine abuse:

- syringes
- burned spoons
- short straws
- surgical tubing

Effects of Methamphetamine on the Body

Users of methamphetamine experience a rush of euphoria and energy, which is the key reason why the drug is abused and why it is so addictive. Even one use of the drug can lead to addiction.

Methamphetamine affects key brain chemicals Methamphetamine (and crystal methamphetamine) boosts the supply of dopamine, a brain chemical, as well as, to a lesser extent, boosting the level of serotonin, another neurochemical. However, methamphetamine also causes a *depletion* of these brain chemicals, which accounts for the *crash*, or the feelings of depression and anxiety that occur when the effects of the drug wear off. These effects are not always transient. Some studies of methamphetamine abusers have shown that, even three years after the use of the drug, their dopamine neurons were still damaged. In addition, studies of animals that were administered methamphetamine have shown that their serotonin neurons were damaged by the drug. It is unknown whether this damage was permanent.

Physical side effects The following physical side effects may be present in a person using methamphetamine:

- hyperthermia (elevated temperature/fever) or hypothermia (very low body temperature)
- excessive sweating
- dilated pupils
- convulsions
- extreme itching
- tachycardia (rapid heartbeat)
- insomnia

Psychiatric effects that may occur include the following:

- PSYCHOTIC BEHAVIOR (hallucinations and/or paranoia)
- delusions, such as FORMICATION (feeling as if insects or parasites are crawling underneath the skin)
- confusion
- paranoia
- aggressiveness
- euphoria

The long-term use of methamphetamine can lead to the following damaging effects on the body:

- heart attack
- kidney failure
- stroke, caused by permanent damage to blood vessels in the brain that triggers brain bleeding
- seizures
- lung damage
- infections of the heart lining and valves
- contracting HIV, hepatitis B, and C, and other bloodborne viruses
- contracting tuberculosis
- liver disease
- extreme anorexia

- permanent psychosis
- death

Behavioral indicators of possible methamphetamine use include the following:

- periods of excessive sleep or sleeplessness (24–48 hours)
- diminished appetite
- constant talking
- change in friends (to individuals of whom family members may disapprove)
- repetitious behavior (taking apart and reassembling items repeatedly; pulling out hair; picking at skin)
- withdrawal from friends and family
- excessively high levels of self-confidence
- loss of interest in personal appearance and hygiene
- secretiveness

Methamphetamine may also induce aggressive behavior and also may heighten sexuality to an extreme. Some users become hypersexual to the extent that they engage in sexual activities for very long periods. Some users may abuse children because of their excessive arousal.

Methamphetamine and Car Crashes According to the National Highway Safety Transportation Administration (NHSTA) in a 2004 report on the effects of drugs on human performance, methamphetamine is associated with car crashes, high speed, failure to stop, impatience, and inattentive driving. In a review of 101 cases of driving under the influence in which methamphetamine was the only drug that was implicated, the NHTSA reported the following:

> Driving and driver behaviors included speeding, lane travel, erratic driving, accidents, nervousness, rapid and non-stop speech, unintelligible speech, disorientation, agitation, staggering and awkward movements, irrational or violent behavior, and unconsciousness. Impairment was attributed to distraction, disorientation, motor excitation, hyperactive reflexes, general cognitive impairment, or withdrawal, fatigue and hypersomnolence [excessive sleepiness].

Admissions to Substance Abuse Treatment

Along with the increased number of those who abuse methamphetamine there is an increased need for the treatment of those who have become addicted to the drug. The number of admissions to substance abuse treatment centers that were caused by methamphetamine/amphetamine have quadrupled since 1993; for example, in 1993, there were 13 treatment admissions per 100,000 people ages 12 and older in the United States. This rate increased to 56 admissions per 100,000 in 2003. States with the highest admission rates were Oregon (251 admissions per 100,000 people), Hawaii (241 per 100,000), and Iowa (213 per 100,000). This increase is primarily due to methamphetamine rather than amphetamine abuse. (See Table IV.)

Some states have experienced a marked jump in admissions to treatment centers from 1993 to 2003; for example, South Dakota's rate increased from five per 100,000 people in 1993 to 90 per 100,000 in 2003. Iowa's rate increased even further, from 13 per 100,000 in 1993 to 213 per 100,000 in 2003. The admission rate in Wyoming rose from 15 per 100,000 in 1993 to 209 per 100,000 in 2003.

Legislative Action to Limit Methamphetamine

Many clandestine laboratories that produce methamphetamine illegally for consumption by people in the United States are actually located in other countries, particularly MEXICO. However, because doing so can be highly profitable, some clandestine laboratories operate within the United States.

The Methamphetamine Anti-Proliferation Act (MAPA) was passed in 2000 in the United States and took effect in 2001. This law controls the use of over-the-counter (OTC) drugs that are illegally used, often in clandestine laboratories, to produce methamphetamine. Drugs directly affected included pseudoephedrine and phenylpropanolamine. Many decongestants and cold medications contain these two drugs, and when used as instructed, they are not harmful. However, illicit drug manufacturers

**TABLE IV: PRIMARY METHAMPHETAMINE/
AMPHETAMINE EMERGENCY DEPARTMENT ADMISSION
RATES PER 100,000 POPULATION AGED 12 OR OLDER,
BY STATE: 1993 AND 2003**

	1993	2003
United States	13	56
Northeast		
Connecticut	1	4
Maine	2	5
Massachusetts	<1	2
New Hampshire	<1	2
New Jersey	3	2
New York	2	4
Pennsylvania	3	2
Rhode Island	2	2
Vermont	5	4
South		
Alabama	1	45
Arkansas	13	130
Delaware	2	2
District of Columbia	—	2
Florida	2	7
Georgia	3	39
Kentucky	—	20
Louisiana	4	21
Maryland	1	3
Mississippi	—	23
North Carolina	<1	4
Oklahoma	19	117
South Carolina	1	9
Tennessee	—	6
Texas	7	17
Virginia	1	4
West Virginia	<1	—
Midwest		
Illinois	1	19
Indiana	3	28
Iowa	13	213
Kansas	15	65
Michigan	2	7
Minnesota	8	100
Missouri	7	84
Nebraska	8	117
North Dakota	3	44
Ohio	3	3
South Dakota	5	90
Wisconsin	<1	5
West		
Alaska	4	13
Arizona	—	36
California	66	212
Colorado	18	86
Hawaii	52	241
Idaho	20	72
Montana	30	133
Nevada	9	176
New Mexico	7	10
Oregon	98	251
Utah	16	185
Washington	18	143
Wyoming	15	209

Note: The primary substance of abuse is the main substance reported at the time of admission. Arkansas, Oregon, and Texas do not distinguish between amphetamine and methamphetamine. However, it is logical to conclude that the large portion of the increase in admissions in these states is due to methamphetamine abuse.
Source: Office of Applied Studies. "Trends in Methamphetamine/Amphetamine Admissions to Treatment: 1993–2003." The DASIS Report 9. Rockville, Md.: Substance Abuse and Mental Health Services Administration, 2006, p. 3.

buy large quantities of these drugs to aid them in producing methamphetamine.

MAPA limited the number of tablets or capsules containing these drugs; for example, the purchase of 30 tablets containing more than three grams of the pseudoephedrine hydrochloride is not a regulated transaction; however, a purchase of 31 tablets of this drug *is* a regulated transaction. Purchases are still allowed when regulated, but the pharmacy or other medication distributor would be required to answer questions about the intended use of the drug.

More recently, in 2005 the Combat Methamphetamine Act, a law that requires pharmacies to place all over-the-counter medications that contain pseudoephredrine behind the store counters, so that consumers must request the product if they wish to purchase it, was passed. In addition, the law limits the amount of products containing pseudoephedrine that a customer may buy. Individuals who purchase these medications must also show photo identification and sign a log book.

According to the Drug Enforcement Administration in their 2005 publication *Drugs of Abuse,* some chemicals used to manufacture methamphetamine are acetone, acetic anhydride, benzyl chloride, ephedrine, gamma-butyrolactone (GBL), hydriotic acid, hydrochloric acid, iodine, isosafrole, methylamine, phosphorus (red, white, and yellow), pro-prionic anhydride, and sulfuric acid.

Individuals who violate the laboratory supply part of the law may receive a civil fine of up to $25,000, and businesses that violate this provision of the law may receive a fine of up to $250,000. Some experts believe that this law is insufficiently enforced.

See also ADOLESCENTS; CHILD ABUSE; DRUG TEST-ING; PEER PRESSURE; SCHEDULED DRUGS; STIMULANTS; YOUNG ADULTS.

Arria, Amelia M., et al. "Methamphetamine and Other Substance Use during Pregnancy: Preliminary Estimates from the Infant Development, Environment, and Lifestyle (IDEAL) Study." *Maternal and Child Health* 10, no. 3 (2006): 293–302.

Brecht, Mary Lynn, et al. "Methamphetamine Use Behaviors and Gender Differences." *Addictive Behaviors* 29 (2004): 89–106.

Executive Office of the President. *Synthetic Drug Control Strategy: A Focus on Methamphetamine and Prescription Drug Abuse.* Washington, D.C.: Office of National Drug Control Policy, 2006.

Johnston, Lloyd D., et al. *Monitoring the Future: National Survey Results on Drug Use, 1975–2004.* Vol. 2, *College Students and Adults Ages 19–45.* Bethesda, Md.: National Institute on Drug Abuse, National Institutes of Health, 2005.

Joseph, Donald E., ed. *Drugs of Abuse.* Washington, D.C.: U.S. Department of Justice, 2005.

Kyle, Angelo D., and Bill Hansell. *The Meth Epidemic in America: Two Surveys of U.S. Counties: The Criminal Effect of Meth on Communities: The Impact of Meth on Children.* National Association of Counties. Washington, D.C., July 2005.

National Institute of Justice. *Drug and Alcohol Use and Related Matters among Arrestees, 2003.* Available online. URL: http:www.ncjrs.gove/nij/adam/ADM2003.pdf. Downloaded May 19, 2006.

National Highway Traffic Safety Administration. *Drugs and Human Performance Fact Sheets.* Washington, D.C.: U.S. Department of Transportation, April 2004.

National Survey on Drug Use and Health. "Methamphetamine Use, Abuse, and Dependence: 2002, 2003, and 2004." *The NSDUH Report,* 16 September 2005. Available online. URL: http://www.oas.samhsa.gov/2k5/meth/meth.htm. Downloaded March 11, 2006.

Office of Applied Studies. "Methamphetamine Use, Abuse, and Dependence: 2002, 2003, and 2004." *The NSDUH Report.* National Survey on Drug Use and Health. Rockville, Md.: Substance Abuse and Mental Health Administration, pp. 1–3.

Office of Applied Studies. *Treatment Episode Data Set (TEDS) Highlights—2003: National Admissions to Substance Abuse Treatment Services.* Drug and Alcohol Services Information System Series: S-27. Rockville, Md.: Substance Abuse and Mental Health Services Administration, June 2005.

Substance Abuse and Mental Health Services Administration. *Results from the 2004 National Survey on Drug Use and Health: National Findings.* Rockville, Md.: Department of Health and Human Services, September 2005.

methylenedioxymethamphetamine (MDMA/Ecstasy)

A drug of abuse that is also classified as a form of AMPHETAMINE. MDMA is primarily abused for its euphoria-inducing qualities. It is an illegal Schedule I drug under the CONTROLLED SUBSTANCES ACT. The drug is a central nervous system stimulant. In the 1990s, MDMA was a popular drug at dance parties known as raves, which largely fell out of favor in the 21st century, when alarmed parents and law enforcement authorities became vigilant about the heavy drug abuse occurring at these parties.

MDMA may cause many physical and psychological side effects, such as a reduction in an individual's mental abilities (such as memory), irritability, muscle cramps, and sweating. It should also be noted that many users of MDMA simultaneously consume other drugs, such as COCAINE, MARIJUANA, METHAMPHETAMINE, and alcohol. Thus, in many cases, it can be difficult to determine the specific effects of the MDMA.

MDMA causes the brain to increase the output of serotonin, a brain chemical; however, this rapid surge of serotonin subsequently causes a depletion of serotonin for up to days after the drug is taken.

Some users of MDMA will "stack" the drug, taking consecutive doses as the effects wane. This type of dangerous drug bingeing occurs most frequently on weekends. Some individuals develop a PHYSICAL TOLERANCE to MDMA, but the extent of this tolerance among users is unknown.

Once the drug is consumed, MDMA METABOLITES (other chemicals that are formed as a direct result of using MDMA) delay or interfere with the body's ability to break down the drug, and consequently, if an additional dose of MDMA is taken in the same period, the high blood levels of the drug escalate the risk for cardiovascular effects, such as a heart attack. MDMA continues to affect an individual one week (or longer) after it has been taken.

The drug is usually taken orally in tablets or capsules in doses of 50–200 mg; however, the dosages vary greatly since the drug is often formulated in CLANDESTINE LABORATORIES. The effects of MDMA are experienced in 30–45 minutes, peaking in about 60–90 minutes. These effects continue for three to six hours.

In about 80 percent of the cases, drugs that are sold as MDMA by DRUG DEALERS or others actually do contain MDMA, and the remaining 20 percent contain no MDMA. In some cases when no MDMA is present, the drug actually contains methamphetamine, amphetamine, or both of these drugs, according to the Drug Enforcement Administration (DEA).

In some cases, individuals are given MDMA without their permission or knowledge. (See MALICIOUS POISONING.)

MDMA was first synthesized in 1912, according to the DEA, and it was initially patented as an appetite suppressant. (MDMA may no longer be used as a DIET DRUG.) MDMA did not become popular as a drug of abuse until the 1980s. The DEA banned MDMA in 1985.

In the 1970s, some psychiatrists used MDMA as a psychotherapeutic drug, although no research had confirmed its validity at that time; nor had the Food and Drug Administration (FDA) approved the drug's use for humans. Some therapists during that time referred to MDMA as "penicillin for the soul," because they believed that the drug would be effective at enhancing the insights of patients into their personal problems. However, it was not until 2000 that the first clinical study was approved to test whether, under carefully monitored conditions and with ongoing psychotherapy, MDMA might help in the treatment of patients diagnosed with POST-TRAUMATIC STRESS DISORDER (PTSD). (Results have not been released on this study, as of this writing.)

Users of MDMA

According to the United Nations Office on Drugs and Crime, an estimated 8.3 million people worldwide abused Ecstasy in 2003. The average age of users of MDMA in the United States in 2004 was 19.5 years. According to the National Survey on Drug Use and Health, more than 11 million people ages 12 and older have reported using MDMA at least once in their life. About 450,000 people were current users, who had used MDMA in the past month in 2004. Hospital emergency rooms treat patients whose primary drug of abuse is MDMA, and most of these patients are ages 18–20 years old.

Most users of MDMA are adolescents and YOUNG ADULTS. For example, among young adults between the ages of 18 to 25 years, about 15 percent had ever tried the drug in 2003, compared to 14 percent in 2004. However, the past-year usage remained the same from 2003 to 2004, or 2.1 percent each year. In addition, the past-month usage remained at less than 1 percent, or 0.4 percent each year. In contrast, among adolescents ages 12 to 17 years, the lifetime usage (having ever tried) of MDMA was slightly up, from 10.7 percent in 2003 to 11 percent in 2004.

In considering student drug abusers in the eighth, 10th, and 12th grades, the Monitoring the Future study indicates that from 1996 to 2004 the annual prevalence of MDMA peaked in the years 2000–2001. As can be seen from Table I, abuse levels have declined since that time. (See Table I.)

MDMA is primarily a drug of abuse for white youths and young adults; however, it is increasingly also a drug of abuse for African-American young adults. Some research also indicates that the drug is popular among urban gay and bisexual males.

Effects of MDMA

Users of MDMA may experience the following psychological side effects:

- increased impulsivity
- euphoria
- aggression
- sadness
- restlessness
- irritability

TABLE I: TRENDS IN ANNUAL PREVALENCE OF USE OF MDMA (ECSTASY) FOR STUDENTS IN 8TH, 10TH, AND 12TH GRADES, 1996–2004

	1996	1997	1998	1999	2000	2001	2002	2003	2004
8th Grade	2.3	2.3	1.8	1.7	3.1	3.5	2.9	2.1	1.7
10th Grade	4.6	3.9	3.3	4.4	5.4	6.2	4.9	3.0	2.4
12th Grade	4.6	4.0	3.6	5.6	8.2	9.2	7.4	4.5	4.0

Source: Johnston, Lloyd D. et al. *Monitoring the Future: National Results on Adolescent Drug Use: Overview of Key Findings 2004*. Bethesda, Md.: National Institute of Drug Abuse, April 2005, p. 48.

- reduction of interest in sex
- psychiatric illnesses
- lasting cognitive impairments

They may also experience the following physical side effects:

- nausea
- hyperthermia (elevated body temperature, which may be severe enough to cause organ failure and death)
- blurred version
- increased muscle tension
- tremors
- sleep disturbances
- dehydration
- high blood pressure
- heart failure
- kidney failure
- muscle cramps
- involuntary teeth clenching and teeth grinding

Symptoms of an MDMA overdose may include the following:

- high blood pressure
- faintness
- panic attacks
- loss of consciousness
- seizures

According to the National Institute on Drug Abuse, research on adolescent and young adult users of MDMA has indicated that nearly half

(43 percent) met the diagnostic criteria for drug dependence, in terms of continuing to use the drug although knowing it was causing physical or psychological harm, experiencing WITHDRAWAL effects when the drug was not used, and having a PHYSICAL TOLERANCE to the drug.

Treatment for Abuse of MDMA

If patients who have abused MDMA are treated in the emergency room, the symptoms are treated, such as lowering a high fever and managing psychiatric symptoms, or irritability. Treatment is sometimes complicated because the patient has combined MDMA with other drugs, such as ALCOHOL, MARIJUANA, and COCAINE.

There is no specific treatment protocol for users of MDMA, although cognitive-behavioral psychotherapy, in which individuals are trained to detect the flaws in their distorted thinking and thus to change their behavior, is effective in some patients. MDMA users may also benefit from patient support groups.

As of this writing, there are no medications specifically used to treat individuals who abuse or are dependent on MDMA.

See also EMERGENCY TREATMENT; HALLUCINOGENIC DRUGS; SCHEDULED DRUGS.

Johnston, Lloyd D., et al. *Monitoring the Future: National Results on Adolescent Drug Use: Overview of Key Findings 2004*. Bethesda, Md.: National Institute of Drug Abuse, April 2005.

Joseph, Donald E., ed. *Drugs of Abuse*. Washington, D.C.: U.S. Department of Justice, 2005.

National Institute on Drug Abuse. *MDMA (Ecstasy) Abuse*. Research Report, Washington, D.C., 2006. Available online. URL: http://wwwdrugabuse.gov/PDF/RRmdma.pdf. Downloaded April 6, 2006.

Substance Abuse and Mental Health Services Administration. *Results from the 2004 National Survey on Drug Use and Health: National Findings.* Rockville, Md.: Department of Health and Human Services, September 2005.

methylphenidate (Ritalin/Concerta/Focalin, etc.)

A central nervous system stimulant drug that is sometimes used to treat patients for ATTENTION DEFICIT HYPERACTIVITY DISORDER (ADHD). Methylphenidate is a Schedule II drug under the CONTROLLED SUBSTANCES ACT that has proved very effective in treating the symptoms of impulsivity, hyperactivity, and distractibility among many ADHD patients.

In 2006, the Food and Drug Administration (FDA) decided to place a "black box" warning on drugs with methylphenidate, cautioning that patients who have preexisting heart disease should not take the drug.

Brand names of methylphenidate include Ritalin, Concerta, Metadate CD, and Focalin. There is also a generic form of methylphenidate. In addition, Daytrana, a transdermal skin patch of methylphenidate, was approved by the FDA in 2006 for use by children in the United States. (The drug is not specifically approved for use by adults, but it can be prescribed as an off-label drug by physicians.)

There are both short-acting and long-acting forms of methylphenidate. The short-acting forms such as Ritalin and generic methylphenidate, act within about 30–60 minutes, and their effects last about two to five hours. Focalin is a short-acting form of methylphenidate whose effects last about four hours.

Long-acting forms of the drug, such as Ritalin SR or Ritalin LA, require about an hour to take effect; effects may last seven to 12 hours, depending on the product. Note that long-acting methylphenidate is also available in a generic form.

Concerta, another form of methylphenidate, is a long-acting extended-release tablet. The drug effect peaks in about one or two hours after it is taken and lasts about 12 hours. Another drug, Metadate CD, includes both an immediate and an extended-release form of methylphenidate. About 30 percent of the dosage is immediately released when the drug is taken, and then the rest of the methylphenidate is continuously released over time, lasting about 12 hours altogether.

Abuse of Methylphenidate

Methylphenidate is sometimes a drug of abuse, used to decrease appetite, induce euphoria, or improve concentration; some adolescents try the drug to see how it affects them.

In some cases, the drug is diverted from patients who have legitimate prescriptions. Sometimes adolescent patients willingly give away or sell the drug to their peers, or, others forcibly take the drug from them. Some college students give their prescribed methylphenidate to friends or roommates who want to improve their focus or concentration in their studies. These individuals may later visit physicians, convinced that they have ADHD. However, improved concentration with methylphenidate alone does not indicate that a person has attention deficit hyperactivity disorder.

The annual Monitoring the Future survey data on secondary school students in the United States revealed that 2.5 percent of the eighth-grade students had abused Ritalin in 2004, as had 3.4 percent of 10th graders and 5.1 percent of 12th graders. As with most abused drugs, the largest proportion of abusers are young adults ages 18–25. According to the *National Survey on Drug Use and Health,* in 2004, the lifetime prevalence of methylphenidate abuse was 5.4 percent among young adults, followed by 1.8 percent among youths ages 12–17 years old.

Some drug abusers combine methylphenidate with alcohol or other drugs: a very dangerous combination. Even more dangerous is injection of the drug after it has been dissolved in water, because this formulation includes some nonsoluble ingredients. As a result, these ingredients can block the small blood vessels and may produce severe damage to the lungs and the retina of the eye. Toxic dosages of methylphenidate can lead to dangerous side effects; for example, HALLUCINATIONS and/or aggression may develop. Some patients have psychotic symptoms. A patient who has abused methylphenidate may become violently aggressive.

Side Effects of Methylphenidate

Side effects of the normal use of methylphenidate prescribed by a physician may include nervousness and insomnia. Patients may also experience decreased appetite, although this effect usually abates over time. Other side effects may include headache, dizziness, and increased blood pressure and heart rate. Some patients experience a rash.

Overdosage Signs of an overdosage of methylphenidate may include the following:

- vomiting
- convulsions
- delirium
- cardiac arrythmias
- sweating
- hallucinations

If an overdosage has occurred or may have occurred, emergency medical services should be sought.

See also DIVERSION, DRUG; SCHEDULED DRUGS; STIMULANTS.

Joseph, Donald E., ed. *Drugs of Abuse.* Washington, D.C.: U.S. Department of Justice, 2005.

Morton, A. Alexander, and Gwendolyn G. Stockton. "Methylphenidate Abuse and Psychiatric Side Effects." *Journal of Clinical Psychiatry 2*, no. 5 (2000): 159–164.

Rosack, Jim. "Methylphenidate Skin Patch Approved for ADHD." *Psychiatric News* 41, no. 1 (January 6, 2006): 1, 37.

Substance Abuse and Mental Health Services Administration. *Results from the 2004 National Survey on Drug Use and Health: National Findings.* Rockville, Md.: Department of Health and Human Services, September 2005.

Mexico A Latin American country that is the source for many illegal drugs that are sold in the United States and Canada, such as COCAINE, HEROIN, and MARIJUANA. In addition, CLANDESTINE LABORATORIES in Mexico create large supplies of METHAMPHETAMINE that is illegally transported into the United States. In 2005, the homeland security adviser directed that a strategy be developed to deal with the drug threat from Mexico.

The Mexican government has worked to destroy and seize illegal drugs. In 2005, about 30 metric tons of cocaine and 887 kilograms of methamphetamine were seized by the government of Mexico, along with 14.5 metric tons of marijuana. Many means of transporting illegal drugs were also seized, such as 1,643 vehicles, 60 maritime vessels, and eight aircraft.

Mexico also extradited 41 drug fugitives to the United States, up from 34 fugitives in 2004. Those individuals were accused of trafficking in narcotics as well as of money laundering and other crimes. In 2005, the Mexican Supreme Court ruled that life sentences in prison without the possibility of parole did not violate the Mexican Constitution's prohibition on cruel punishments. This was considered in the United States to be a key breakthrough, which will help facilitate the extradition of fugitives from Mexico who face life imprisonment in the United States for their violent crimes and drug trafficking.

The Mexican government has also ordered the destruction of illegal drugs; for example, in 2005, the Mexican government estimated that about 30,882 hectares of marijuana were destroyed, as were 20,464 hectares of opium poppy crops. (A hectare is a metric measurement that is roughly equivalent to 2.5 acres.)

According to the International Narcotics Control Strategy Report on Mexico, released by the Bureau for International Narcotics and Law Enforcement Affairs in March 2006, Mexico is the primary transit country for the entry of cocaine into the United States, and 70–90 percent of the cocaine sent to the United States passes through Mexico, after being smuggled into Mexico from COLOMBIA. In addition, Mexico is a major supplier of heroin to consumers in the United States, and about 30 percent of the heroin consumed in the United States is shipped from Mexico.

Within Mexico, the National Council against Addictions estimated that about 911,000 Mexican people ages 12 to 65 years old used illegal drugs in 2005, which was about the same incidence as in 1998. The highest rates of abuse occurred in two cities bordering the United States, Tijuana and Ciudad Juarez, as well as in Mexico City and Guadalajara.

See also AFGHANISTAN.

Bureau for International Narcotics and Law Enforcement Affairs. "Canada, Mexico, and Central America." International Narcotics Control Strategy Report, Department of State. Available online. URL: http://www.state.gov/p/inl/rls/nrcrpt/2006/vol1/html/62107.htm. Downloaded May 3, 2006.

mood stabilizers Medications that are given to control the rapid mood swings from elation to depression (and back again) that are characteristic among individuals who have BIPOLAR DISORDER. Lithium and valproate (Depakote, Depakene) are the most commonly used medications for the treatment of bipolar disorder. Lithium is a naturally occurring element, while valproate is an antiseizure drug.

Mood-stabilizing drugs are not themselves drugs of abuse, but their potential effects on patients who have already-existing substance abuse disorders should be considered, particularly since individuals who have bipolar disorder have a greater risk than other individuals of abusing alcohol and/or drugs.

Some studies indicate that lithium may not work as well for patients who have both bipolar disorder and a substance use disorder and that an antiseizure drug such as valproate is better tolerated among this population. In addition, medication compliance (taking the medication at the right dose and the right frequency) among patients is more likely to occur when patients are prescribed valproate rather than lithium, possibly because valproate has fewer side effects than lithium. For example, lithium has a greater tendency to lead to a considerable weight gain than valproate, a side effect that can decrease compliance among bipolar disorder patients.

Other drugs that are sometimes used as mood stabilizers to treat bipolar disorder include the antiseizure drugs carbamazapine (Tegretol) and oxcarbazepine (Trileptal). In some cases, physicians have treated bipolar patients both with and without substance abuse problems with antipsychotic drugs, such as olanzapine (Zyprexa) or aripiprazole (Abilify).

See also ANTIDEPRESSANTS; ANXIETY DISORDERS; BENZODIAZEPINES; PSYCHIATRIC DISORDERS.

morphine A narcotic painkiller that has been used effectively for centuries in surgical procedures and the treatment of severe pain that is caused by cancer and other illnesses. It is also used to treat the pain of myocardial infarction (heart attack) as well as for acute pulmonary edema. According to Miles Weatherall in *The Cambridge Illustrated History of Medicine*, morphine was first isolated from opium in 1806 by Frederick Sertürner, an apothecary's assistant in Germany, who nearly died from an accidental overdose of the drug.

Morphine is derived from the seed pod of the poppy plant, *Papavar somniferum*. It is a Schedule II drug under the CONTROLLED SUBSTANCES ACT. In the United States, morphine is marketed as a generic drug and is also sold under a variety of brand names, such as Astramorph, Duramorph, Infumorph, Kadian, Morphine Sulfate, MS-Contin, MSIR, Oramorph SR, Roxanol, and RMS.

Morphine can be given to patients either orally, intravenously, intramuscularly, or rectally. In addition, morphine may be delivered to chronic severe pain patients in a pump system that is implanted. These pumps are preprogrammed such that only a dosage up to a specific amount of the drug may be released, precluding excessive intake by patients.

According to the Drug Enforcement Administration, about 15 percent of the morphine that is used in the United States is used in its original state and the rest is converted to either CODEINE or other derivatives.

In the United States, morphine was first manufactured as both an anesthetic and a painkiller in 1832. Morphine was also the primary narcotic painkiller that was used to treat the wounded soldiers during the Civil War in the United States. According to Charles F. Levinthal in his book on drugs of abuse, "Following the war, morphine dependence among Civil War veterans was so common that it was called the 'soldier's disease' or the 'army disease.'"

During the Victorian era of the late 19th century, morphine was used or was included in other remedies to treat headaches, menstrual cramps, colic, diarrhea, and many other illnesses. At that time, morphine was an easily attainable drug. According to Levinthal, women who were dependent on morphine represented about half the cases of drug dependence in the 1890s.

Morphine is still used for acute pain management in the 21st century, although there is an extensive array of other effective narcotic analgesics from which doctors may choose to treat pain.

As with other narcotics, morphine may induce a pronounced state of sedation as well as severe constipation. Some patients develop HALLUCINATIONS from the drug, which abate as its effects wear off.

Abuse of Morphine

Morphine is also a drug of abuse. It is used illegally by some who have become addicted to the drug; however, most people in the United States who are addicted to controlled drugs are addicted to other substances, such as HEROIN, OXYCODONE, and/or COCAINE.

Withdrawal from morphine causes distinct symptoms that are noticeable to others. In the early stages of withdrawal, the person's eyes water, the nose runs, and he or she experiences increased perspiration. As the withdrawal from morphine progresses, the individual experiences a loss of appetite, tremors, irritability, nausea, restlessness, and drug craving. Many addicted individuals undergoing withdrawal become severely depressed, and vomiting is also common. The blood pressure and heart rate increase. Flu-like symptoms such as chills may occur, as do pains in the bones and muscle spasms. If either morphine or a drug that blocks the effects of morphine (such as naloxone, NALTREXONE or BUPRENORPHINE) is administered, withdrawal symptoms will quickly stop. If no drug is given, most of the obvious physical symptoms will end within about seven to 10 days. However, the PSYCHOLOGICAL DEPENDENCE on morphine will still be present.

Long after the body no longer requires the drug and exhibits withdrawal symptoms, the formerly addicted individual continues to think about morphine and may feel very frightened and overwhelmed without it. If no drug treatment is begun, most individuals will relapse into morphine addiction as soon as they possibly can.

Treatment of Morphine Dependence

Individuals who are addicted to morphine may undergo DETOXIFICATION in a treatment facility that is managed by trained and experienced physicians who are also experts in addiction medicine.

Some morphine addicts are maintained on a program pioneered by Dr. Vincent Dole and Dr. Marie Nyswander. The first methadone clinic opened in New York City in 1965 and was later followed by others nationwide. However, most morphine addicts are treated with such medications as buprenorphine and naltrexone. In addition, drugs in the benzodiazepine class may be used to treat individuals going through withdrawal from morphine.

There are also self-help groups on the order of Alcoholics Anonymous for individuals addicted to morphine and other narcotics, for example, Narcotics Anonymous.

See also HEROIN; METHADONE; NARCOTICS; SCHEDULED DRUGS.

Joseph, Donald E., et al., eds. *Drugs of Abuse*. Washington, D.C.: U.S. Department of Justice, 2005.

Levinthal, Charles F. *Drugs, Society, and Criminal Justice*. New York: Pearson Education, 2006.

Weatherall, Miles. "Drug Treatment and the Rise of Pharmacology." In the *Cambridge Illustrated History of Medicine,* edited by Ray Porter, 246–278. Cambridge: Cambridge University Press, 2001.

naltrexone (ReVia) A long-acting drug that is approved by the Food and Drug Administration (FDA) to treat ALCOHOLISM (alcohol dependence) and is often effective in blocking the CRAVING for alcohol and thus preventing RELAPSE. Some studies indicate that the drug may be more effective for individuals who have a family history of alcoholism. Several studies indicate that naltrexone combined with cognitive-behavioral therapy is an effective treatment for alcohol dependence. However, some studies, such as that by Krystal and colleagues, did not find naltrexone to be effective in treating men for chronic and severe alcoholism.

Other drugs that are also used to treat alcohol dependence are DISULFIRAM (ANTABUSE) and ACAMPROSATE (CAMPRAL). According to the Substance Abuse and Mental Health Services Administration, an estimated 12 percent of treatment facilities in the United States used naltrexone in 2003. More facilities (17 percent) used disulfiram and 5 percent used buprenorphine.

Naltrexone is also sometimes used in the treatment of opioid dependence and was originally developed to treat opiate addiction. It was later discovered to be effective in treating alcoholism. In general, naltrexone works best for highly motivated individuals, such as addicted physicians and medical personnel. Patients must have undergone DETOXIFICATION and be opiate-free before starting the naltrexone to aid them in staying off drugs. If patients continue to use opioids when they use naltrexone, the drug can cause severe WITHDRAWAL symptoms.

Some BIPOLAR DISORDER patients are also treated with naltrexone, which is a drug that does not cause the weight gain that is commonly associated with other treatments for bipolar disorder (such as lithium or various antipsychotic medications),

although other side effects may be experienced. In addition, some researchers have found that naltrexone is helpful in treating patients who have a pathological gambling disorder.

Patients who have liver disease or kidney impairment should avoid naltrexone, as should those who have a history of SUICIDE attempts. Naltrexone has been shown to be effective in treating alcoholism in a variety of studies, such as those by Garbutt and associates in 2005 and Anton and colleagues in 2006.

In the Anton study, published in the *Journal of the American Medical Association* in 2006, the subjects were divided into nine different groups. Four groups received medical management and no combined behavioral intervention (CBI), a form of therapy. Of the four groups in this set, one group received the placebo drug, another group received naltrexone, a third group received acamprosate (a drug approved by the FDA for the treatment of alcoholism), and a fourth group received a combination of naltrexone and acamprosate. Another set of four groups received a combination of CBI and medical management. In this second set of groups, one group received the placebo drug; the second group received naltrexone; the third group received acamprosate; and the fourth group received a combination of naltrexone and acamprosate. Last, a ninth group received CBI only and no drugs.

The researchers found that all groups showed a significant decrease in drinking; however, the patients who improved most were those who received either naltrexone or CBI, both with medical management.

In a study reported in *Archives of Internal Medicine* in 2003, the researchers studied 197 alcoholic subjects; one group received naltrexone and primary care management (PCM) while the other group received naltrexone and cognitive-behavioral therapy (CBT). Several other subgroups of the original group were subsequently studied. The researchers found that naltrexone over 10 weeks of treatment was effective when combined with PCM or CBT.

Say the researchers:

For 6 months after initial treatment, maintenance of improvement was enhanced by continued naltrexone treatment in responders to PCM, but the effect was not statistically significant in responders to CBT. Thus, when naltrexone is used, a primary care alternative to specialty alcohol dependence treatment may yield a similar result if naltrexone use is maintained after the treatment initiation phase in conjunction with monthly follow-up appointments. The major benefit of this may be to increase access to effective treatment for alcohol dependence by enlisting primary care providers into the treatment system.

See also ACAMPROSATE; BUPRENORPHINE; DELIRIUM TREMENS; DETOXIFICATION; DISULFIRAM; LEVO-ALPHA-ACETYLMETHADOL (LAAM); METHADONE.

Anton, Raymond F., M.D., et al. "Combined Pharmacotherapies and Behavioral Interventions for Alcohol Dependence: The COMBINE Study: A Randomized Controlled Trial." *Journal of the American Medical Association* 293, no. 17 (May 3, 2006): 2,003–2,017.

Collins, Eric D., M.D., et al. "Anesthesia-Assisted vs. Buprenorphine- or Clonidine-Assisted Heroin Detoxification and Naltrexone Induction: A Randomized Trial." *Journal of the American Medical Association* 294, no 8 (August 24/31, 2005): 903–913.

Garbutt, James C., M.D., et al. "Efficacy and Tolerability of Long-Acting Injectable Naltrexone for Alcohol Dependence: A Randomized Controlled Trial." *Journal of the American Medical Association* 293, no. 13 (April 6, 2005): 1,617–1,625.

Krystal, John H., M.D., et al. "Naltrexone in the Treatment of Alcohol Dependence." *New England Journal of Medicine* 345, no. 24 (December 13, 2001): 1,734–1,739.

National Institute on Alcohol Abuse and Alcoholism. *Helping Patients Who Drink Too Much: A Clinician's Guide.* Rockville, Md.: National Institutes of Health, 2005.

O'Brien, Charles P., M.D. "Anticraving Medications for Relapse Prevention: A Possible New Class of Psychoactive Medications." *American Journal of Psychiatry* 162, no. 8 (August 2005): 1,423–1,431.

O'Malley, Stephanie S., et al. "Initial and Maintenance Naltrexone Treatment for Alcohol Dependence Using Primary Care vs. Specialty Care." *Archives of Internal Medicine* 163 (July 28, 2003): 1,695–1,704.

narcotics Generally refers to drugs that are derived from opium, opium derivatives, and synthetic substitutes; however, some experts refer to all drugs that are scheduled by the CONTROLLED SUBSTANCES ACT and controlled by the Drug Enforcement Administration (DEA) as narcotics. According to the United Nations Office on Drugs and Crime, an estimated 6 million people worldwide abuse opiates and an additional 9.2 million people worldwide abuse HEROIN.

The word *narcotic* was derived from the Greek word for stupor because of the lethargy that opium-based drugs induce. Narcotics can be addicting, although when they are used over the short term, the risk for drug dependence is low, particularly when the drug is used to control moderate to severe pain of cancer and acute and chronic painful diseases, such as broken bones, severe back pain, or arthritis. Narcotics are also used as anesthetics.

Depending on the particular drug, narcotics may be taken orally, by injection, intranasally, or through a transdermal skin patch. Some individuals in severe chronic pain receive narcotics through an implanted pump, such as a morphine pump. This is a device that releases periodic doses of morphine directly into the bloodstream with no need for regular injections into the skin. The morphine pump is refilled by the physician or a staff member on a periodic basis and the amount of drug that can be released within a given period is regulated by the pump. Individuals who use a morphine pump may not increase the amount or the frequency of their dosage.

Narcotics are also available as suppositories or in a form that can be sucked like a lollipop. When narcotics are abused, they are usually sniffed, injected, or smoked rather than taken orally as a tablet. The reason for this is that the oral form is the slowest-acting form of a narcotic.

Effects of Narcotics

In general, narcotics are sedating and may cause the following side effects, which are more pronounced if the drug is used to excess, as with abuse:

- drowsiness
- inability to concentrate
- apathy
- constipation
- nausea and vomiting
- respiratory depression

When used illegally, narcotics can cause other complications, because often these drugs are adulterated with other substances that may be harmful. In addition, many injection drug users share contaminated needles. As a result, illegal users of narcotics risk very serious complications, such as endocarditis (an inflammation of the lining of the heart) and abscesses of the brain and the lung. They are also at risk for contracting diseases such as HEPATITIS or the HUMAN IMMUNODEFICIENCY VIRUS (HIV).

Sometimes individuals willingly or unknowingly take an excessive dose of narcotics. Signs of a narcotic overdose include the following:

- cold and clammy skin
- convulsions
- mental confusion
- trouble with breathing (the cause of most deaths from a narcotic overdose, according to the Drug Enforcement Administration)
- pinpoint pupils of the eyes
- extreme drowsiness

Tolerance and Dependence with Narcotics

Once individuals begin taking narcotics for any reason for more than a short period of a week or two, they will develop a TOLERANCE to the drug, needing greater doses to achieve the same effect. For example, if the narcotic is taken lawfully for pain control, eventually higher doses will be needed to achieve the same level of pain relief. If the drug is taken illegally, tolerance is likely to occur faster because the street user is likely to take higher doses of narcotics much more frequently than the patient in pain who is under the supervision of a physician.

Some people become addicted to narcotics, particularly illegal drug users. Addiction, also known as dependence, includes not only an increased tolerance to the drug but also a physical and psychological need for it. In addition, the individual's work and family life are affected. Essentially, the person addicted to narcotics centers his or her life on getting and using narcotics, and little else (or nothing else) is important because of the powerful hold of the addiction.

Withdrawal/Detoxification and Treatment

If the person who is dependent on a narcotic cannot or does not wish to use the narcotic anymore, then he or she will go through WITHDRAWAL, which can be extremely unpleasant and even life-threatening. As a result, withdrawal, which is also called DETOXIFICATION when it occurs in a drug facility, should occur only under the supervision of an experienced physician. According to the Drug Enforcement Administration, shorter-acting narcotics usually cause a shorter and more intense form of withdrawal, while longer-acting narcotics generally cause a longer period of withdrawal symptoms that are less severe.

The early physical symptoms of withdrawal from narcotics may include nausea, loss of appetite, tremors, irritability, and drug CRAVING. As the withdrawal progresses, patients may experience vomiting and depression. Other physical symptoms may include chills alternating with sweats and elevated heart rate and blood pressure. Individuals may also suffer from bone pain, muscle pain, and muscle spasms. In general, the symptoms of narcotic withdrawal abate in seven to 10 days. However, the PSYCHOLOGICAL DEPENDENCE usually lingers and may lead to resumption of drug abuse.

Individuals may be treated for narcotic dependence through detoxification. Some individuals who are addicted to narcotics, particularly HEROIN, are maintained on other narcotics, primarily METHADONE. However, use of newer medications, such as BUPRENORPHINE, is increasing.

It is important to remember that even when the body has undergone detoxification and there are no further physical effects of the drug, often psychological dependence continues, and it is this problem that often leads to relapse. As a result, the psychological elements surrounding the addiction must also be addressed if there is any hope for a sustained recovery. Some self-help groups, such as Narcotics Anonymous or Cocaine Anonymous, may be useful to individuals because they involve working with others who have overcome their addiction and who understand firsthand how difficult it is to resist the drug.

See also DIVERSION, DRUG; HYDROCODONE; OPIATES; OXYCODONE; OxyContin; PRESCRIPTION DRUG ABUSE; SCHEDULED DRUGS.

Joseph, Donald E., et al., ed. *Drugs of Abuse.* Washington, D.C.: U.S. Department of Justice, 2005.

Substance Abuse and Mental Health Services Administration. *Results from the 2004 National Survey on Drug Use and Health: National Findings.* Rockville, Md.: Department of Health and Human Services, September 2005.

obsessive compulsive disorder (OCD) A psychiatric disorder and a form of an ANXIETY DISORDER that is characterized by compulsive and repetitive behavior, such as constantly counting or frequently washing hands. The individual who has OCD is fully aware that these actions are irrational and unnecessary, and yet he or she cannot refrain from performing them. Individuals who have OCD have a slightly greater risk for substance abuse than those who do not have it. According to the National Institute of Mental Health (NIMH), individuals who have obsessive compulsive disorder have a 3.3 percent increased risk of substance abuse compared to those who do not have OCD.

Individuals who have OCD may use drugs and/or alcohol to attempt to cope with the anxiety caused by their obsessive and compulsive actions. They may also use alcohol or drugs to try to dampen their compulsions.

Many people who have OCD have other concurrent psychiatric problems, such as DEPRESSION, other anxiety disorders, ATTENTION DEFICIT HYPERACTIVITY DISORDER, and EATING DISORDERS.

According to NIMH, about 3.3 million adults in the United States have OCD, or about 2 percent of the population age 18 and older. (OCD can also occur in individuals younger than 18 years.) The disorder affects men and women at equal rates and typically first appears in childhood or adolescence.

Symptoms and Diagnostic Path

Say Brian Martis, M.D., and his colleagues in their chapter on obsessive compulsive disorder in the *Clinical Manual of Anxiety Disorders.* "Obsessive-compulsive disorder (OCD) is characterized by obsessions and compulsions that intrude into a person's psychological and daily life by creating distress, taking inordinate periods of time, and increasing the risk of comorbidity, such as major depression. Obsessions are intrusive, disturbing, and incessant thoughts, ideas, images, or urges. Compulsions are repetitive mental or motor activities that mostly occur in response to obsessions and serve to neutralize anxiety."

Common obsessions are a concern about contamination, pathologic doubt (such as a fear that the individual has harmed someone in a car crash when there was no car crash), or somatic symptoms, such as fatigue or hypochondria. The person who has OCD may be obsessed with creating order and symmetry, as manifested in ritualistic arranging and rearranging of items.

Common compulsions are checking items (and rechecking, over and over), as with frequently taking inventory of items, washing to excess, and counting items. Some individuals who have OCD have religious obsessions and feel they must pray for hours or even all day. Obsessive fears are manifested in constantly checking to see that doors are locked, stoves are turned off, and so forth, not once but repeatedly and despite knowing that previous checks revealed no problem. Some people who have OCD hoard objects, collecting massive amounts of material that they are unwilling to throw out or to allow anyone else to throw out.

The individual who may have OCD should be treated by a psychiatrist, who is best qualified to diagnose and treat this disorder. Thorough questioning of the individual is needed because patients may be resistant and/or embarrassed to reveal some or all of their obsessive behavior.

Psychiatrists question individuals who may have OCD about their current and past medical and psychiatric history. They also seek to determine whether the behavior is causing the patient problems at work and at home.

Treatment Options and Outlook

OCD is often treated with medication and psychotherapy. In general, that combination produces the best outcome for most patients. If the person who has OCD also has a substance use disorder, both problems should be addressed.

In a study of 60 substance abusers admitted to a drug-free therapeutic community, reported in 1992 in the *Journal of Substance Abuse Treatment*, the researchers placed the subjects in three groups. In one group, the subjects received treatment that addressed both their OCD and their substance abuse. In another group, the subjects were treated only for substance abuse. In a third group, the subjects received treatment for their substance abuse and were trained in progressive muscle relaxation.

The researchers found that the subjects who were treated for both their substance abuse *and* their OCD remained in treatment longer than the subjects in the other groups. They also had a greater reduction in their OCD symptoms and, at 12-month follow-up, had significantly greater abstinence rates than the subjects in the other groups. The findings indicate that ignoring either their OCD or substance abuse is not helpful for the patient who has both of these disorders.

Medications and OCD　The mainstay treatment for most OCD patients are antidepressants. Clomipramine (Anafranil) is approved by the Food and Drug Administration (FDA) for the treatment of OCD. Antidepressants such as fluoxetine (Prozac), fluvoxamine (Luvox), paroxetine (Paxil), citalopram (Celexa), and sertraline (Zoloft) have proved effective as well. Some studies indicate that velafaxine (Effexor) is also helpful.

Some experts, such as Michael A. Jenike, M.D., a professor of psychiatry at Harvard Medical School, believe that high dosages of antidepressants are necessary to treat OCD, although, paradoxically, some patients have responded to lower dosages than considered therapeutic.

In general, clomipramine should be avoided by the elderly, since it can cause confusion in this population. The medications should be taken on a regular basis and not only on days when the patient feels distressed by symptoms. It may be 10–12 weeks before patients notice significant improvements in their symptoms.

Some OCD patients respond to monoamine oxidase (MAO) inhibitors, such as penelzine (Nardil) or tranylcypromine (Parnate). Patients who take these drugs must be very careful with their diet because some foods and medications cannot be taken together with MAOs. Rarely, antipsychotic medications may be prescribed to patients who have severe OCD, in addition to an antidepressant.

Psychotherapy treatment　Psychotherapy is also often effective for OCD patients. Cognitive-behavioral therapy, in which the patient is taught to challenge irrational thoughts, may be helpful. Some therapists use exposure therapy, in which the patient is exposed to distressing circumstances, such as when the patient who is obsessed with cleanliness is exposed to dirt and is not allowed to wash her hands. Instead, the patient is trained to deal with the anxiety and avoid the compulsive rituals that surround it.

Family therapy may be needed because often extreme OCD behavior affects the entire family. Family members may be angry or embarrassed by their relative's actions.

Risk Factors and Preventive Measures

Studies indicate that there may be a genetic link to OCD, particularly among first-degree relatives (siblings and parents), and especially when the relatives were age 19 or younger at the age of onset. Some experts believe that OCD is caused by an abnormality in brain functioning, particularly in the striatum of the brain. OCD is not triggered by excessively clean parents (although their excessive cleanliness may reflect a genetic tendency toward OCD) or by those who are otherwise ineffective or poor parents.

There are no measures to prevent OCD. If it does occur, then treatment should be sought.

See also ANTISOCIAL PERSONALITY DISORDER; BIPOLAR DISORDER; DEPRESSION; DUAL DIAGNOSIS; PSYCHIATRIC DISORDERS.

Fals-Stewart, W., and J. Schafer. "The Treatment of Substance Abusers Diagnosed with Obsessive-Compulsive Disorder: An Outcome Study." *Journal of Substance Abuse Treatment* 9, no. 4 (Fall 1992): 365–370.

Jenike, Michael, M.D. "OCD Medication: Adults." Available online. URL: http://www.ocfoundation.org/ocd-medication-adults.html. Downloaded March 12, 2006.

Khouzam, Hani Raoul, M.D. "Obsessive-Compulsive Disorder: What to Do If You Recognize Baffling Behavior." *Postgraduate Medicine* 106, no. 7 (December 1999). Available online. URL: http://www.postgradmed.com/issues/1999/12_99/khouzam.htm. Downloaded March 12, 2006.

Martis, Brian, M.D., et al. "Obsessive-Compulsive Disorder." In *Clinical Manual of Anxiety Disorders.* Washington, D.C.: American Psychiatric Press, 2004.

National Institute of Mental Health, Obsessive-Compulsive Disorder. Available online. URL: http:www.nim.nih.gov/medlineplus/obsessivecompulsivedisorder.html. Downloaded March 12, 2006.

Stahl, Stephen M. *Essential Psychopharmacology: The Prescriber's Guide.* Cambridge: Cambridge University Press, 2005.

open air markets, drug dealing in   The selling and buying of drugs in specific public places, such as public streets and neighborhoods, and at specific times, although some open air markets operate around the clock, particularly for users of HEROIN or CRACK COCAINE. Most open air drug markets are located within the inner city or urban areas. They are often in economically depressed neighborhoods and are more likely to operate in areas with a high rate of rental properties or public housing not occupied by the owners.

Many individuals actively seek out drugs from strangers in such places despite the high risk of arrest, primarily because of their addiction to these substances. The most common types of drugs sold in open air markets are COCAINE, crack cocaine, heroin, and MARIJUANA.

For buyers and sellers, the primary advantages of the open market are that they know where and when to buy drugs and they can weigh the quality of the drug with the price. The primary disadvantage is that LAW ENFORCEMENT officials are also aware of open air markets and can, at any time, decide to arrest buyers and sellers. Another disadvantage is that the buyer can be cheated or robbed. In addition, violence is common in heavily used open air markets.

Those who operate in open markets may change their practices to a *closed market,* in which they only sell drugs to people they know or for whom someone else will vouch. They may rely heavily on cell phones and pagers to manage their drug selling.

Open air markets are a problem for law enforcement officials. If they arrest one or two drug dealers, others will usually take their place. However, police have devised tactics to combat this. One tactic is high-visibility policing. In New York, for example, police officers on foot have patrolled areas known to be open-air markets, and their high visibility has resulted in reduced drug trafficking. Another tactic is to arrest drug buyers. This is most effective against occasional or new users. This is called a *reverse sting* because buyers rather than drug dealers are arrested, whereas usually law enforcement officials concentrate on arresting drug dealers. Generally, the penalties for drug buying are not severe, but the process of being arrested, going to jail, going to court, and risking the possibility of having their car impounded, has served as a deterrent to some drug buyers. In Miami, Florida, of 1,725 people arrested in 18 reverse sting operations, only seven people were repeat offenders.

Say authors Alex Harocopos and Mike Hough in their article on drug dealing in open air markets for the Office of Community Oriented Policing Services, "The continued use of this type of operation led to two significant changes: the first was a lower arrest rate. The second was that those getting arrested were predominantly problem users implying that the number of the casual and novice users had decreased."

In another tactic, police in Fort Lauderdale, Florida, monitored vehicles in the open air market, traced their owners, and sent them postcards that their car had been seen in a high-crime area. This tactic decreased the number of drug-related arrests as well as the traffic volume in the area. There are many other tactics that police can employ to discourage open-air drug markets, such as working with the community and encouraging landlords to take a more active role.

See also ADDICTION/DEPENDENCE; CRIME AND CRIMINALS; DRUG DEALERS; HEROIN; METHAMPHETAMINE.

Harocopos, Alex, and Mike Hough. *Drug Dealing in Open-Air Markets.* Washington, D.C.: Office of Community Oriented Policing Services, U.S. Department of Justice, January 11, 2005.

opiates/opium   Opiates include narcotic drugs that are directly or indirectly derived from the opium poppy as well as drugs that are synthetically similar to natural opium. HEROIN and MORPHINE are naturally derived opiates. Heroin is illegal in the United States, while examples of synthetically derived opiates such as OXYCONTIN and products containing HYDROCODONE and OXYCODONE are lawful when prescribed by physicians for PAIN MANAGEMENT.

Historical Background

Opium, a drug derived from the opium poppy, is an ancient drug that has been used and abused for more than 5,000 years. The first known depiction of the opium poppy was found in the language of ancient Sumeria in southern Iraq in 3100 B.C.E. The Ebers Papyrus of 1500 B.C.E. includes prescriptions detailing the use of the berry of the poppy. In the *Odyssey,* by the Greek poet Homer, opium is described as the drug that quiets all pains and quarrels. The returning crusaders came back to Europe with opium they obtained in Arab countries.

In more modern times before 1800, opium was readily available in multidrug prescriptions that anyone could buy. (There was no Food and Drug Administration.) Many people did not know, however, that the concoctions they purchased contained opium, nor did they know it was an addicting drug.

In the 19th century, doctors used opium to treat severe pain, menstrual problems, diabetes, sexually transmitted diseases, and many other ailments. It was available in powdered or gum forms, although most people drank laudanum (a mixture of opium and other ingredients). At that time, it was socially unacceptable for women to drink alcohol, and women consumed opium products at about three times the rate of men. Males were more likely to drink alcohol. Ironically, many products including opium also had high levels of alcohol. (There were no required labels that listed the ingredients of products at that time.)

Professionals in the latter part of the 19th century realized that opium was addictive; however, their solutions were not always effective. For example, the famous psychiatrist Sigmund Freud prescribed cocaine as a cure for opium addiction, and he did not realize for years that cocaine itself is an addictive drug.

Positive benefits have also accrued from opium; for example, morphine was isolated from opium by Frederick Sertürner in 1806; however, morphine did not become widely used until during and following the Civil War in the United States. Morphine is still used today as a powerful painkiller.

In the present, many legal and illegal drugs are derived from opium poppies, although there are also many drugs that are synthetically derived.

According to the United Nations Office on Drugs and Crime, 15.2 million people abused opiates worldwide in 2003, and of this number, 9.2 million individuals abused heroin.

Opium is sometimes used in the drug paregoric to treat diarrhea, but it is rarely used in its pure form in the United States and most Western countries. Instead, most opium is broken down into its constituents, particularly into drugs in the chemical classes of phenanthrenes. The primary phenanthrenes are CODEINE and MORPHINE.

If opiates are taken on a regular basis, such as by patients who have chronic pain, these patients will eventually develop a TOLERANCE to opiates and therefore will need a greater dose to achieve the same effect. This tolerance is *not* the same as an ADDICTION/DEPENDENCE, which also involves a CRAVING for the drug and the act of centering one's life around both acquiring and using the drug, to the detriment of the individual's personal, family, and work life.

Some patients develop a PSEUDOADDICTION to opiates, or an apparent addiction, because they are undertreated for their pain, and as a result, they may actively seek pain medications from other physicians. Such patients, if given adequate pain control, do not meet the criteria for addiction.

Patients who are addicted to opiates may be treated with METHADONE on a maintenance basis or may be given other drugs to help them withdraw from opiates, such as BUPRENORPHINE or NALTREXONE. DETOXIFICATION from opiates is often provided in a hospital or a rehabilitative setting. Patients receiving methadone maintenance are treated on an outpatient basis and they go to the clinic to receive their injection of methadone.

Wide Disparity among Cities

The level of abuse of opiates varies from region to region of the United States. According to *Epidemiologic Trends in Drug Abuse* in 2005, there was a wide variation among the number of emergency room reports of abuse for various opiates in 2004, ranging from few reports in Los Angeles, to many reports in some cities, such as New York. (See Table I.)

See also NARCOTICS; SCHEDULED DRUGS.

Evans, Christopher, J. "Secrets of the Opium Poppy Revealed." *Neuropharmacology* 47 Supplement (2004): 293–299.

TABLE I: NUMBERS OF EMERGENCY DEPARTMENT REPORTS FOR OPIATES BY DRUG AND AREA: 2004

Area	Total Opiate Reports
Atlanta	815
Baltimore	1,006
Boston	1,332
Chicago	1,041
Dallas	786
Denver	583
Detroit	1,102
Houston	1,013
Los Angeles	32
Miami	252
Minneapolis/St. Paul	903
New Orleans	1,070
New York	2,057
Newark	420
Philadelphia	871
Phoenix	1,071
St. Louis	657
San Diego	577
San Francisco	533
Seattle	1,277
Washington, D.C.	671

Source: National Institute of Drug Abuse. *Epidemiologic Trends in Drug Abuse.* Vol. 1, *Proceeding of the Community Epidemiology Work Group: Highlights and Executive Summary.* Bethesda, Md.: National Institutes of Health, June 2005, p. 19.

National Institute of Drug Abuse. *Epidemiologic Trends in Drug Abuse.* Vol. 1, *Proceeding of the Community Epidemiology Work Group: Highlights and Executive Summary.* Bethesda, Md.: National Institutes of Health, June 2005.

organized crime   Crime that is under the control of large organizations, which are often associated with teenage GANGS, as opposed to crimes committed by individuals. Because there is a great deal of profit to be made through the trafficking of illegal drugs, organized crime groups operating within the United States and other countries are actively involved in this highly lucrative (albeit, dangerous) activity. Drug trafficking is a multibillion-dollar business worldwide, and thus, traffickers actively resist attempts to curtail their activities and resort to violence to continue them.

TABLE: DRUG TRAFFICKING ORGANIZATIONS OR CRIMINAL GROUPS OPERATING IN REGIONS OF THE UNITED STATES, BY TYPE OF DRUG AND ETHNICITY OF THE CRIMINAL GROUPS

Region	Cocaine	Methamphetamine	Heroin	Marijuana	MDMA (Ecstasy)
Great Lakes	Mexican Colombian African-American	Mexican Asian	Mexican Colombian Nigerian African-American	Mexican Asian Middle Eastern Caucasian	African-American Asian Caucasian
Florida/Caribbean	Colombian Mexican Dominican Caribbean-based Venezuelan Haitian Puerto Rican Jamaican Bahamian Cuban Honduran Panamanian Nicaraguan Salvadoran Guatemalan Caucasian African-American European	Caucasian Mexican	Colombian Dominican Caucasian Venezuelan Cuban Honduran Panamanian Nicaraguan Salvadoran Guatemalan Puerto Rican African-American	Mexican Jamaican Colombian African-American Caucasian Cuban Haitian Honduran Panamanian Nicaraguan Salvadoran	African-American Asian Caucasian
Mid-Atlantic	African-American Caucasian Colombian Dominican Mexican Puerto Rican	Caucasian Hispanic Mexican	African-American Asian Caucasian Colombian Dominican Mexican Puerto Rican West African	African-American Asian Caucasian Cuban Colombian Dominican Mexican Puerto Rican	Israeli Caucasian Colombian Dominican African-American Cuban
New England	African-American Caucasian Colombian Dominican Haitian Honduran Panamanian Nicaraguan Salvadoran Guatemalan Jamaican Mexican Puerto Rican	Cambodian Chinese Laotian Vietnamese Caucasian Mexican Puerto Rican	Cambodian Chinese Laotian Vietnamese Caucasian Colombian Dominican Haitian Honduran Panamanian Nicaraguan Salvadoran Guatemalan Mexican Puerto Rican	African-American Cambodian Chinese Laotian Vietnamese Caucasian Colombian Dominican Haitian Honduran Panamanian Nicaraguan Salvadoran Guatemalan Jamaican Mexican Puerto Rican	Cambodian Chinese Laotian Vietnamese Caucasian

(table continues)

TABLE (continued)

Region	Cocaine	Methamphetamine	Heroin	Marijuana	MDMA (Ecstasy)
New York/ New Jersey	African- American Caucasian Colombian Dominican Jamaican Mexican Puerto Rican	Caucasian Filipino Mexican	African- American Asian Caucasian Colombian Dominican Mexican Pakistani Puerto Rican West African Nigerian	African- American Asian Caucasian Colombian Dominican Jamaican Mexican	Caucasian Colombian Dominican Jamaican Mexican Vietnamese
Pacific	Mexican Caucasian Vietnamese Samoan Tongan African- American	Mexican Caucasian African-American	Mexican Caucasian African- American	Caucasian Mexican Vietnamese Indonesian Malaysian African- American	Vietnamese Caucasian Indonesian Malaysian African- American Mexican
Southeast	Mexican African- American	Mexican Caucasian African-American Hispanic Asian	African- American Mexican Caucasian	Mexican African- American Caucasian Asian	Vietnamese Mexican
Southwest	Mexican Colombian African- American	Mexican Asian	Mexican Colombian	Mexican Jamaican Asian Caucasian	Asian
West Central	Caucasian Hispanic Mexican	Caucasian Hispanic Mexican Native American	Asian Caucasian Hispanic Mexican	African- American Caucasian Hispanic Mexican Vietnamese	Asian Caucasian Vietnamese

Source: National Drug Intelligence Center. *National Drug Threat Assessment 2007.* Washington, D.C.: U.S. Department of Justice, pp. 29–30.

Organized crime is also associated with human trafficking (illegal buying and selling of people for forced labor and/or PROSTITUTION). Both children and adults are frequently trafficked for criminal purposes. Crime bosses may use drugs to addict individuals so that they are easier to control and to entice or compel them more readily to commit criminal acts. Some crime groups use individuals to transport the drugs inside their bodies, such as cocaine bags that are swallowed and later excreted. These bags are very dangerous because they can burst within the digestive system and kill the person acting as a drug mule.

According to the 2007 annual report of the National Drug Intelligence Center of the Justice

Department, trafficking organizations and criminal groups range "from small, loosely knit groups that distribute one or more drugs at the retail level to complex, international organizations with highly defined command and control structure that produce transport, and distribute large quantities of one or more illicit drugs. Among these groups, Mexican organizations are the most widespread and influential traffickers of illicit drugs in the country." Colombian groups are still powerful with regard to the smuggling of heroin and cocaine into the United States, but they have a diminished role because of the expanded power of Mexican groups.

There are a variety of criminal groups and drug-trafficking organizations in the United States and their race and ethnicity, as well as the drugs they specialize in selling, vary in different regions of the country. For example, according to the National Drug Intelligence Center in its 2007 report, methamphetamine is primarily sold by Mexicans and Asians in the Great Lakes region, while in New England, methamphetamine drug dealers are of many different ethnicities, including Cambodian, Chinese, Laotian, Vietnamese, Caucasian, Mexican, and Puerto Rican. (See table) Motorcycle gangs also sell methamphetamine in New England.

In 2007 the National Drug Intelligence Center reported that Mexican and Asian criminal groups were increasingly important in the distribution of drugs in the United States. In addition, as the domestic production of methamphetamine decreased, Mexican drug-trafficking organizations began supplementing local dealers. According to the report from the National Drug Intelligence Center, "These stronger more organized, and insulated distribution groups have proven to be much more difficult for local law enforcement to detect and disrupt than the local dealers they have replaced."

Criminal groups have also become more active in distributing marijuana, and the potency of this drug has sharply increased, more than doubling from 2000 to 2005 owing to higher cultivation methods. The major trafficking of marijuana is from Asian drug trafficking groups. In addition, Mexican drug traffickers have begun producing high-potency marijuana.

Trafficking of MDMA has sharply increased since 2004, primarily due to Asian traffickers based in Canada.

See COLOMBIA; CRIME AND CRIMINALS; DRUG DEALERS; INCARCERATION; JAIL INMATES; LAW ENFORCEMENT; MEXICO; OPEN AIR MARKETS, DRUG DEALING IN.

oxycodone   A narcotic medication and a controlled substance that is the active ingredient in more than 20 prescription drugs, such as OXYCONTIN, Percocet, and Percodan. Oxycodone is also combined with ibuprofen (5 mg of oxycodone and 400 mg of ibuprofen) and marketed as Combunox, an oral combination tablet for moderate to severe pain. This drug has been proved effective for the short-term management of acute, moderate, to severe pain, according to Oldfield and Perry in *Drugs* in 2005.

Drugs that contain oxycodone are Schedule II drugs under the CONTROLLED SUBSTANCES ACT. Oxycodone has been used since 1917 to treat postoperative pain and continues to be commonly prescribed for moderate to severe pain.

Medications containing oxycodone may be legally prescribed for patients who have moderate to severe pain, but they have abuse potential when used by patients who have a history of substance abuse. As a result, drugs with oxycodone are closely monitored by organizations such as the Drug Enforcement Administration (DEA). Patients taking these drugs should also be closely monitored by their physicians. Periodic drug testing of these patients may be useful, since legally prescribed oxycodone is sometimes diverted illegally to others. Studies have shown that physicians do not always judge accurately which patients are most likely to give or sell their drugs to others. A drug screen can reveal that the patient is *not* taking the drug. Patients who fail to take their prescribed narcotics should not be given additional prescriptions in most cases. In addition, drug testing can check for other drugs, such as COCAINE and MARIJUANA, that the patient should not be using.

Physicians who prescribe drugs that contain oxycodone or other narcotics have a specific DEA number that allows them to prescribe them. This license can be withdrawn if physicians are known to overprescribe or otherwise misuse narcotics.

Abusers of Oxycodone

Individuals who are ages 18 to 25 are the most likely people to ever abuse products containing oxycodone, particularly Percocet, Percodan, Tylox, and Oxy-Contin. (See Table I.) Of concern is that the abuse of oxycodone products increased from 8.9 percent of the population ages 18 to 25 years old in 2003 to 10.1 percent in 2004. Abuse increased among adolescents ages 12–17 years old, from 2.4 percent in 2003 to 2.7 percent in 2004. However, among those ages 26 or older, abuse slightly dropped, from 4.5 percent in 2003 to 4.4 percent in 2004.

Deaths from Oxycodone Products

Some researchers have looked at deaths in which drugs such as oxycodone, the active ingredient in the timed-release OxyContin, were suspected or known to be a factor in the death. This issue was researched and reported in the *Journal of Forensic Science* in 2005.

The researchers performed a retrospective review of cases that were investigated by the Palm Beach Country Medical Examiner's Office in Florida, studying 172 cases. In 18 cases, the deaths were attributed to oxycodone.

The rest of the 172 deaths included 117 deaths that were caused by combined drug abuse (multiple toxicity), 23 deaths caused by trauma, nine attributed to natural causes, and five caused by drugs other than oxycodone.

The researchers discovered that when oxycodone was present in the deceased person, in most cases other drugs were also present. The most common drug type found were BENZODIAZEPINES, and the most common drug combined with oxycodone was ALPRAZOLAM/ALPRAZOLAM XR (XANAX/XANAX XR). This was a new finding in 2005.

Note that drug users do not always die solely of the drug that they abused. They may die of multiple drug use or may die of another health problem altogether. There may also be a combination of reasons that contribute to the person's death.

In another study, published in 2004 in the *American Journal of Therapeutics,* the researchers studied the risk factors of dependence on hydrocodone and oxycodone among 534 patients who were admitted and then discharged in 2000 from an addiction detoxification unit. They found that 27 percent of the patients were dependent on prescription narcotics. Of these, most users were addicted to Vicodin (hydrocodone), or 53 percent, followed by OxyContin (19 percent).

They also found predictors of prescription narcotic abuse, such as other drug dependence diagnoses and medical complaints. Clearly before physicians prescribe any narcotics for pain, they should do a thorough check for a history of substance abuse.

See also ADDICTION/DEPENDENCE; DIVERSION, DRUGS; HYDROCODONE; METHADONE; NARCOTICS; OPIATES; OxyContin; PAIN MANAGEMENT; PRESCRIPION DRUG ABUSE; PRESCRIPTION DRUG MONITORING PROGRAMS, STATES WITH; SCHEDULED DRUGS.

TABLE I. NONMEDICAL USE OF OXYCODONE PRODUCTS IN LIFETIME, BY AGE GROUP IN THE UNITED STATES, 2003 AND 2004, IN PERCENTAGES

Total		12–17		18–25		26 or Older	
2003	2004	2003	2004	2003	2004	2003	2004
4.9	5.0	2.4	2.7	8.9	10.1	4.5	4.4

Source: Substance Abuse and Mental Health Services Administration. *Results from the 2004 National Survey on Drug Use and Health: National Findings.* Rockville, Md.: Department of Health and Human Services, September 2005, p. 242.

Kalso, E. "Oxycodone." *Journal of Pain Symptom Management* 29, Suppl. 5 (May 2005): S47–S56.

Miller, Norman S., and Andrea Greenfield. "Patient Characteristics and Risks Factors for Development of Dependence on Hydrocodone and Oxycodone." *American Journal of Therapeutics* 11, no. 1 (January/February 2004): 26–32.

Oldfield, V., and C. M. Perry. "Oxycodone/Ibuprofen Combination Tablet: A Review of Its Use in the Management of Acute Pain." *Drugs* 65, no. 16 (2005): 2,337–2,354.

Substance Abuse and Mental Health Services Administration. *Results from the 2004 National Survey on Drug Use and Health: National Findings.* Rockville, Md.: Department of Health and Human Services, September 2005.

Wolf, B. C., et al. "One Hundred Seventy Two Deaths Involving the Use of Oxycodone in Palm Beach County." *Journal of Forensic Science* 50, no. 1 (January 2005): 192–195.

OxyContin A narcotic medication that is a 12-hour timed-release form of OXYCODONE. OxyContin is a Schedule II analgesic drug that was created and continues to be manufactured by Purdue Pharma in Stamford, Connecticut. OxyContin was first approved for sale in the United States by the Food and Drug Administration (FDA) in 1995. It was aggressively advertised and became a very popular drug to treat chronic and acute pain. In 2007 Purdue Pharma, the manufacturer of OxyContin, and three company executives, including its president, chief attorney, and former medical director, pleaded guilty to over-marketing OxyContin and understating its addiction risk. As a consequence, the company agreed to pay fines of $634 million, the largest penalty ever assessed on any pharmaceutical company.

Starting in about 2000, however, some magazines and newspapers had begun to question the likelihood of addiction to OxyContin, and one publication discussed how to abuse the drug by smashing it and ingesting the entire 12-hour dose at once, either orally or by injecting the drug. There has been speculation that abuse of the drug escalated after that information was provided to the general public.

Among all abusers of illicit drugs among individuals ages 12 years and older in the United States in 2004, less than 1 percent (0.5 percent) were abusers of OxyContin, according to the Substance Abuse and Mental Health Services Administration in their *Overview of Findings for the 2004 National Survey on Drug Use and Health.*

OxyContin is legally prescribed to patients for moderate to severe pain, such as the pain of cancer, as well as severe noncancerous chronic pain stemming from back problems, arthritis, and sickle cell anemia. When abused, the drug is highly addictive, although patients who have legitimate pain and no prior history of substance abuse usually do not develop an addiction. As a result of the abuse of the drug, OxyContin carries a "black box" warning label describing its abuse potential. This is the only commonly prescribed opioid analgesic that carries such a warning.

In many cases of the abuse of OxyContin by new users, the abusers have a past history of substance abuse, and they are much more likely to have abused alcohol, cocaine, and other drugs, even than those who abuse other prescription painkillers. (See PRESCRIPTION DRUG ABUSE.)

Abusers of OxyContin

The Researched Abuse, Diversion and Addiction-Related Surveillance (RADARS) system, sponsored by Purdue Pharma, was developed to identify information on the abuse and diversion of OxyContin and other Schedule II and III drugs, according to Cicero and colleagues in their 2005 article on the abuse of prescribed analgesics in the *Journal of Pain.* The drugs that the researchers investigated included BUPRENORPHINE, FENTANYL, HYDROCODONE, MORPHINE, OxyContin, other oxycodone products, and METHADONE.

The researchers in the RADARS system identified several key characteristics of OxyContin abusers, based on 978 cases. They found that the average age of the abuser was 34.0 years, and men were much more likely (greater than 65 percent) to abuse OxyContin than women. Most of the abusers reported themselves as white (91 percent); African Americans (less than 5 percent) and Hispanics (less than 3 percent) were also included. Most of the abusers (91 percent) had a past and current history of multiple drug abuse. In addition, most of the abusers (70 percent) had obtained the OxyContin with a doctor's prescription.

The researchers also found different drug patterns in the locations of OxyContin abusers and abusers of other drugs. They say, "The results of these studies indicate that prescription drug abuse had become prevalent in the United States, and, unlike the pattern of abuse observed with illicit drugs such as heroin, which is heavily localized to the inner cities of very large metropolitan areas, it [OxyContin abuse] is most prevalent in rural, suburban, and small- to medium-sized urban areas."

In another report on OxyContin abuse, the researchers looked at patterns among those who abused the drug, reporting on their findings in the *Journal of Pain and Palliative Care Pharmacotherapy* in 2005. These researchers compared individuals who abused other prescription painkillers to those who specifically used OxyContin in a nonmedical (abusive) manner. Users of nonmedical OxyContin were more likely to have used needles to inject the OxyContin, and they were also more likely to have abused multiple drugs. In addition, the OxyContin abusers had higher rates of dependence than individuals who abused other prescription analgesics.

About 83 percent of those who misused OxyContin had abused other illegal or prescription drugs before ever using OxyContin nonmedically. The authors say that this information indicated that the initial nonmedical use of OxyContin is rarely the first time that individuals have ever abused drugs.

Thus, OxyContin apparently does not drive individuals to use other drugs, but the use of other drugs may lead to the abuse of OxyContin.

According to the National Survey on Drug Use and Health, the lifetime abuse (having ever used) of OxyContin is highest among those ages 18–25 years, and this abuse increased from 3.6 percent of YOUNG ADULTS in 2003 to 4.3 percent in 2004. In considering *all* oxycodone products that were abused, however, the abuse rate increased from 8.9 percent in 2003 to 10.1 percent in 2004 among young adults. However, this level was nearly doubled by those who abused HYDROCODONE products, or 16.3 percent in 2003, a percentage that increased to 17.4 percent in 2004.

Adolescent Abuse of OxyContin   In a 2004 article in the *Journal of the American Academy of Child & Adolescent Psychiatry,* Deborah Katz and Lon Hays discussed several cases of adolescents who became addicted to OxyContin. In one case, a 16-year-old girl who had no past history of substance abuse tried OxyContin for the first time when she was age 14, at the urging of a DRUG DEALER, who then compelled her into sexual activity. The girl also began abusing Percocet, a drug containing oxycodone. She became addicted and was treated in a rehabilitative facility. She was also hospitalized for two SUICIDE attempts.

The girl later began stealing needles from her pediatrician so she could inject OxyContin intravenously. She finally achieved success in abstinence from the drug through a long-term residential treatment and a "wilderness" program for adolescents. However, she reportedly continues to crave drugs. In addition, her mother's use of narcotics for severe chronic pain allegedly complicates the issue for the teenager.

In another case, a 17-year-old boy began using marijuana at age 12 and cocaine at age 16. He started abusing OxyContin at age 17. He stole the drug from his mother and began snorting it, rapidly escalating his drug use. He received DETOXIFICATION about a month after he began abusing OxyContin.

Say the authors, "Child and adolescent psychiatrists and other professionals who work with children need to be aware of risk factors, early symptoms of abuse, and methods of treatment for OxyContin abuse." They add, "A complete substance abuse history should include inquiry about OxyContin use as well as parents' or other family members' use of pain medications and their attitudes toward them. In many of the patients we have seen, parental dependence on opioids was a significant risk factor for adolescent abuse."

The authors conclude, "Because of the high relapse rate, these adolescents need close psychiatric follow-up with attention to depression, anxiety, and self-injurious behavior, family and school involvement in treatment, including evaluation of parental opioid use and availability of OxyContin within the home, and regular drug testing to ensure abstinence."

The RADARS System and the Abuse and Diversion of OxyContin

According to the authors of the article in the *Journal of Pain,* RADARS used three different methods to identify drug abuse: surveys of drug abuse experts (pain management specialists, experts in adult or adolescent treatment programs, methadone specialists, hospitals, and so forth), surveys of police agencies, and the monitoring of poison control centers for calls related to the abuse or intentional misuse of prescription medications.

The researchers in the RADARS system found that OxyContin and hydrocodone were the most prevalently and widespread abused narcotic drugs, followed by (in descending order) other oxycodone products, methadone, morphine, hyydromorphone, fentanyl, and buprenorphine. The authors indicated that although OxyContin abuse was considerable, it seemed to be part of a pattern of abuse of prescription drugs in general. They conclude, "We hypothesize that OxyContin may simply be the current drug of choice among recreational drug users and street addicts and that this preference will dissipate over time."

Misreporting on OxyContin

Some newspaper and magazine accounts have attempted to link deaths to OxyContin abuse alone, contending that the risk of death is higher among abusers of OxyContin than among those who abuse other narcotic analgesics. A common error among some reporters is to group other forms of oxycodone carelessly with OxyContin and mistakenly assume that *all* deaths were caused by OxyContin.

However, medical examiners are not able to isolate which form of oxycodone is a factor in the person's death or which caused the individual's death. In many cases, the abuse of multiple drugs, one of which may have been oxycodone, led to the individual's death. This type of factual error was made by an *Orlando Sentinel* reporter who wrote a five-part series on OxyContin abuse in 2003.

Among other errors, the *Orlando Sentinel* reporter alleged that two healthy men who had never abused drugs were prescribed OxyContin for their pain problems, and they subsequently became addicted to the drug. The point that the reporter sought to make was that normal and healthy men could become addicted when given OxyContin for pain.

Further investigation by others uncovered the fact that both men who were depicted as sterling characters who later succumbed to OxyContin addiction actually had a history of prior substance abuse. One of the men was previously convicted in a cocaine abuse case. The other was a long-term substance abuser who was previously hospitalized for an overdose of drugs other than OxyContin.

The newspaper issued a front-page retraction and the reporter resigned. However, the erroneous "facts" in the series continue to be reported in other published articles, as of this writing.

See also DIVERSION, DRUG; NARCOTICS; OPIATES; OXYCODONE; PAIN MANAGEMENT AND NARCOTIC MEDICATIONS; PRESCRIPTION DRUG ABUSE; SCHEDULED DRUGS; YOUNG ADULTS.

Cicero, Theodore J., James A. Inciardi, and Alvaro Muñoz. "Trends in Abuse of OxyContin and Other Opioid Analgesics in the United States: 2002–2004." *Journal of Pain* 6, no. 10 (October 2005): 662–672.

Katz, Debra A., M.D., and Lon R. Hays, M.D. "Adolescent OxyContin." *Journal of the American Academy of Child & Adolescent Psychiatry* 43, no. 2 (February 2004): 231–234.

Libby, Ronald T. "Treating Doctors as Drug Dealers: The DEA's War on Prescription Painkillers." *Policy Analysis* 545 (June 16, 2005). Available online. URL: http://www.cato.org/pubs/pas/pa545pdf. Downloaded November 16, 2005.

Miller, Normal S., and Andrea Greenfield. "Patient Characteristics and Risks Factors for Development of Dependence on Hydrocodone and Oxycodone." *American Journal of Therapeutics* 11, no. 1 (January/February 2004): 26–32.

Sees, K. L, et al. "Non-Medical Use of OxyContin Tablets in the United States." *Journal of Pain and Palliative Care Pharmacotherapy,* 19, no. 2 (2005): 13–23.

Substance Abuse and Mental Health Services Administration. *Overview of Findings for the 2004 National Survey on Drug Use and Health*. Rockville, Md.: Department of Health and Human Services, September 2005.

pain management and narcotic medications

Moderate to severe discomfort that is often treated by medications such as NARCOTICS as well as other therapies (physical therapy, special exercises, acupuncture, and so forth). In addition, patients who have existing substance abuse problems have been found in numerous studies to be at a greater risk for addiction to other substances than are those who have no past or current drug abuse history.

Some physicians specialize in pain management, such as treating the pain that stems from cancer or from noncancerous but chronic severe diseases, such as extreme back pain, arthritis, sickle-cell anemia, or stroke. Patients who have constant and unremitting pain may be treated with narcotics, including such drugs as FENTANYL, OXYCODONE, OxyCONTIN, METHADONE, and HYDROCODONE. These are SCHEDULED DRUGS that are carefully controlled by the federal government and by each state. They may also prescribe acetaminophen with codeine (Tylenol 3), PROPOXYPHENE (Darvon, Darvocet), and other controlled drugs.

Other physicians, such as family practitioners or general internists, treat their patients for many different medical problems, and they infrequently prescribe narcotics. Emergency department (ED) doctors often prescribe narcotic pain medications to emergency room patients for a day or two, but they do not usually follow up these patients. Instead, they advise ED patients to see their own physicians for a later evaluation and any further needed pain management.

Undertreatment and Overtreatment of Pain

Some experts believe it's more likely that patients in pain are undertreated than overtreated with narcotics, and past studies on cancer patients have supported this view. In some cases, patients who are undertreated for severe pain develop a PSEUDOADDICTION; they may seek out two or more doctors to alleviate their pain, because the dosage of the medication they have received is inadequate. However, they appear like drug abusers to others, by virtue of their drug-seeking behavior.

In contrast, few patients are overtreated, or prescribed excessively high dosages of narcotics, for pain. The task force for the College on Problems of Drug Dependence made a position statement on this issue in *Drug Dependence* in 2003: "Pain is still undertreated in this country and to reduce availability of opioids in an attempt to stem diversion to illicit sources would further exacerbate a problem already affecting many pain patients—inadequate pain relief."

Abuse of Drugs by Pain Management Patients

Although it is believed that the majority of patients who receive medications for pain do not abuse the drugs that they are prescribed, at the same time, it is clear that some *do* misuse or abuse their medications.

According to Jane Ballantyne and Jianren Mao in their 2003 article in the *New England Journal of Medicine*, behavior that should concern physicians who prescribe narcotics includes the following:

- patients who report that they have lost their prescriptions on two or more occasions
- patients who frequently go to the emergency room, seeking pain medications
- patients who often miss their follow-up appointments with the physician who prescribed the narcotic
- patients who unreasonably ask for increases in their dosages of narcotics

Some doctors use their own screening process of asking questions and seeking information on the patient's past or current doctors so they can determine whether the patient is seeking drugs for pain or for abuse. Doctors can find information on whether a patient has a past history of abusing prescription drugs in states with PRESCRIPTION DRUG MONITORING PROGRAMS.

Many doctors who specialize in pain management rely on DRUG TESTING (or the implied threat of drug testing) as a means to screen out individuals who may be using illegal drugs or other prescription drugs, although it is generally unknown how effective such methods are. Most doctors test only patients of whom they are suspicious. However, it may be better to test all patients randomly.

In one study reported in *Pain Physician* in 2003, the researchers studied patients who were being treated in an interventional pain management environment, to determine whether they were abusing other drugs. The researchers studied 100 patients who were receiving pain management treatment and were receiving controlled substances as part of their treatment. The researchers selected only patients who their physicians believed were at a low risk of abusing illicit substances or prescription drugs.

The subjects all had drug testing, and the researchers concentrated on whether the subjects tested positive for MARIJUANA, COCAINE, METHAMPHETAMINE, and AMPHETAMINE. The results were unanticipated: The researchers found that 13 percent of the patients tested positive for MARIJUANA use, and 3 percent tested positive for cocaine. One of the patients who tested positive for marijuana also tested positive for cocaine. As a result, 16 percent of the subjects were using illicit substances. (It is unknown whether the 16 percent of the patients who abused illegal drugs in the *Pain Physician* study had a history of past substance abuse. If they did, it was apparently unknown to their physicians.)

It should also be noted that the broad majority of the patients in this study, or 84 percent, did *not* test positively for illicit drug use; thus, in most cases, the physicians' evaluations of patients at low risk for drug abuse were accurate.

This study seems to bear out the need for random DRUG TESTING of all patients, since the combination of marijuana and/or cocaine with medications such as oxycodone, hydrocodone, or other narcotics can be a dangerous one.

Fear of Narcotics Prescriptions among Doctors and Patients

Because of the oversight from the Drug Enforcement Administration (DEA), some doctors fear that prescribing scheduled drugs to their patients in pain could lead to being labeled as overprescribers of narcotics—even when they are very careful to avoid prescribing inappropriate doses to their pain patients. There is evidence that both supports and refutes this concern.

Evidence refuting that excessive punitive actions are taken against doctors who prescribe narcotics. In a study reported in the *Journal of Pain and Symptom Management* in 2005, the researchers sought to determine how many physicians are actually charged with misconduct because of their prescribing patterns. Say the researchers, "Surveys of Wisconsin physicians, oncologists, and primary care physicians all find fear of disciplinary action a barrier to their prescribing the analgesic regimen that they would otherwise prescribe for patients in pain."

The researchers decided to determine whether there was any validity to physicians' fears about prescribing narcotics. They followed two parallel courses of investigation. In one course, they studied records of punitive actions taken against physicians by the New York State Board for Professional Medical Misconduct over the course of three years. The researchers also studied punitive actions against doctors for all medical boards in the United States over a nine-month period.

The researchers found that most physicians who had been disciplined had multiple violations. "Not a single physician, for whom information was available, was disciplined solely for overprescribing opioids. The actual risk of an American physician being disciplined by a state medical board for treating a real patient with opioids for a painful medical condition is virtually nonexistent."

They also discovered that, in the national sample, 43 percent of the doctors who had been disciplined had been prescribing for nonpatients or for themselves. In one case, a doctor had prescribed

MEPERIDINE (Demerol) for himself; in another case the doctor prescribed hydrocodone to his wife, who was addicted to the drug.

Twelve percent of the disciplined doctors had prescribed drugs to addicts without considering their known drug dependence problem. Nineteen percent had prescribed drugs when there was no indication for using narcotics.

Thirteen percent of the disciplined doctors were found incompetent; for example, the doctor had failed to take a patient history and/or give the patient a physical examination. Others failed to follow up on patients who were prescribed narcotic pain medication; for example, in one case a patient who had chronic herpes simplex was seen only once, but prescribed Vicodin (a form of hydrocodone) for five months in a row.

Eight percent of the disciplined doctors were engaged in sexual activity with individuals for whom they prescribed narcotics. In one case, the doctor had sex with a woman in his home, at motels, and in the office. This physician did not record these prescriptions; nor did he provide any medical reason for prescribing the drugs to the woman.

The authors advised that the patient's medical record should include documentation that supports the prescribing of narcotics as part of the treatment regimen. In addition, doctors should not prescribe narcotics to their friends or family members unless there is an existing doctor-patient relationship.

Evidence supporting punitive actions are taken against doctors who prescribe narcotics Not everyone agrees that doctors who are treating their pain patients in an organized and ethical manner need not fear repercussions from prescribing narcotics. Although state medical boards may not be heavy-handed with their physician investigations, the Drug Enforcement Agency may be very aggressive (although the agency has denied this allegation). In addition, some newspaper and magazine articles denouncing the use of narcotics, particularly OxyContin, have influenced public attitudes.

In his heavily documented article in *Policy Analysis*, Ronald T. Libby discusses many cases of physicians he says were punished by the DEA for prescribing narcotics. Says Libby, "The DEA's painkiller campaign has cast a chill over the doctor-patient candor necessary for successful treatment. It has resulted in the pursuit and prosecution of well-meaning doctors. It has also scared many doctors out of pain management altogether, and likely persuaded others not to enter it, thus worsening the already widespread problem of undertreated or untreated chronic pain."

Concludes Libby, "By demonizing physicians as drug dealers and exaggerating the health risk of pain management, the federal government has made physicians scapegoat for the failed drug war."

Patient Worries about Taking Narcotics

Some patients are extremely fearful of taking narcotics despite their severe pain or are resistant to the idea of allowing their children to use narcotics, as in the case of a terminally ill six-year-old in severe pain whose father refused to give permission for the child to receive pain-relieving narcotics. The reason: the father feared that the child would become an "addict." Yet the fear of addiction is rarely a valid problem among patients who take narcotics for pain. Studies have shown that very few patients who experience severe pain and who have no prior history of drug abuse will develop an addictive disorder.

They may develop a TOLERANCE to a narcotic and therefore need a higher dose to obtain the same pain relief. But they do not exhibit the same behavior as addicted individuals do, such as using a drug for nonmedical purposes, buying drugs from DRUG DEALERS, and ignoring family members, their job, and important aspects of their lives because they are entirely centered on obtaining and using drugs.

In contrast, patients who have severe pain who take narcotics under the careful guidance of physicians usually find that once their pain is under control, they are able to resume many aspects of their life that had formerly been neglected or ignored because of overwhelming pain.

Important Protections for Patients Who Use Narcotics

To protect patients as well as themselves, many doctors treat only those patients who have signed a TREATMENT CONTRACT, which is a written agreement that specifies what actions the doctor requires that patient to take or avoid. For example, the doctor may require the patient to agree to random drug testing.

The physician may also require that the patient agree to receive all SCHEDULED DRUGS only from the doctor, to prevent the problem of "doctor shopping," when patients go from doctor to doctor seeking to obtain prescriptions for narcotics. (An exception is made if the patient has suffered an emergency and urgently needs narcotics. However, in that case, the patient or family members should advise the emergency department staff that the patient already takes narcotics for pain.)

Other constraints may be set, such as that the patient understands that for most narcotics, refills cannot be provided on the prescription, and if the patient continues to need a Schedule II drug (such as a hydrocodone or oxycodone product), a new prescription will be required each month.

Patients should be advised in person (and sometimes in writing, as the doctor sees fit) that it is very important to strictly follow the instructions they are given for prescribed dosages. If they continue to have pain they should avoid taking higher dosages and call the doctor instead. Many patients think that if one pill does not work, two or three will be effective. This is a very dangerous attitude that may lead to an ADVERSE REACTION.

Patients should also inform their doctors of any other legal or illegal drugs that they are taking; doing so greatly reduces the risk of ACCIDENTAL OVERDOSE DEATHS if that drug is combined with the prescribed narcotic.

Patients should also be told that they should never give or sell their drugs to anyone (DRUG DIVERSION). It is against the law to do so. In addition, the person to whom they give the drug could experience a serous adverse reaction to the medication. Law enforcement authorities may hold the person who provided the drug liable in that case.

See also METHYLPHENIDATE; MORPHINE; NARCOTICS; OPIATES; PRESCRIPTION DRUG ABUSE; PROPOXYPHENE.

Ballantyne, Jane C., M.D., and Jianren Mao, M.D. "Opioid Therapy for Chronic Pain." *New England Journal of Medicine* 249, no. 20 (November 13, 2003): 1,943–1,953.

Gwinnell, Esther, M.D., and Christine Adamec. *The Encyclopedia of Addictions and Addictive Behaviors.* New York: Facts On File, 2006.

Libby, Ronald T. "Treating Doctors as Drug Dealers: The DEA's War on Prescription Painkillers." *Policy Analysis* 545 (June 16, 2005). Available online. URL: http://www.cato.org/pubs/pas/pa545pdf. Downloaded November 16, 2005.

Manchikanti, Laxmaih, M.D., et al. "Prevalence of Illicit Drug Use in Patients without Controlled Substance Abuse in Interventional Pain Management." *Pain Physician* 6 (2003): 173–178.

Richard, Jack, M.D., and Marcus M. Reidenberg, M.D. "The Risk of Disciplinary Action by State Medical Boards against Physicians Prescribing Opioids." *Journal of Pain and Symptom Management* 29, no. 2 (February 2005): 206–212.

Zacny, James, et al. "College on Problems of Drug Dependence Taskforce on Prescription Opioid Non-Medical Use and Abuse: Position Statement." *Drug and Alcohol Dependence* 69, no. 3 (2003): 215–232.

paranoia   The irrational belief that others are actively plotting to harm one. (In the event that others *are* actually plotting against a person, then the person is not paranoid.) Paranoia is a DELUSION, or false belief. Individuals who have psychotic disorders such as SCHIZOPHRENIA often experience paranoia, although medications can markedly increase the insight of the ill person. Sometimes individuals who have BIPOLAR DISORDER or DEPRESSION may exhibit PSYCHOTIC BEHAVIOR, such as paranoia.

Individuals who abuse some drugs, such as ANABOLIC STEROIDS, COCAINE, METHAMPHETAMINE, or PHENCYCLIDINE (PCP), may experience paranoia. MARIJUANA users may have paranoia, and HALLUCINOGENIC DRUGS may sometimes cause it. Drugs that are central nervous stimulants may induce paranoia, particularly when they are abused.

The danger of paranoia is that paranoid persons may behave in a violent or aggressive manner toward others, mistakenly believing that they are defending themselves or others about whom they care.

Because paranoid individuals are convinced that they are being persecuted, it is very difficult or impossible to reason with them or explain to them how and why they are wrong. At best, some doubt can be placed in their minds. Actively paranoid individuals can be very dangerous to themselves and others.

See also DELUSIONS; FORMICATION; HALLUCINA-TIONS; PSYCHIATRIC DISORDERS; PSYCHOSIS, DRUG-INDUCED.

peer pressure The influence of the people with whom an individual most strongly identifies. Peer pressure can affect people of any age but it is especially powerful among adolescents. Some adolescents engage in risky behavior, such as drug abuse or alcohol abuse, because they are actively encouraged to do so by their peers. Some studies have shown that girls are more susceptible to peer pressure than boys. Often drugs or alcohol are first used as a result of the urging of a friend, to which the adolescent succumbs. Studies have shown that the majority of people addicted to METHAMPHETAMINE were first given the drug by a person they considered a friend.

The consequences of the behavior may be severe. For example, an adolescent or young adult who engages in heavy drinking and then is urged by peers to drive very fast has a high risk of causing a car crash and suffering or causing severe injuries or even death. Alcohol and drug abuse is associated with an increased risk for physical and SEXUAL ASSAULTS, as well as sexually transmitted diseases and unplanned pregnancies.

One counter to peer pressure is for parents to talk to adolescents about the dangers of drug and alcohol use. Although many teenagers appear not to listen to their parents, the information is heard and processed by many adolescents, and as a result, a short talk by parents can change the mind of an adolescent who might otherwise drive under the influence of alcohol or drugs or a teenager who would get into the car of another adolescent who is using alcohol and/or drugs. Teachers can also help students learn how to resist peer pressure.

According to the National Institute of Drug Abuse, adolescents are particularly vulnerable to taking drugs because of the powerful influence of peer pressure. The institute's *Preventing Drug Use among Children and Adolescents: A Research-Based Guide for Parents, Educators, and Community Leaders* indicates that there are both risk factors in favor of and protective factors against drug abuse. These factors may change with age. For example, the report states, "risk factors within the family have greater impact on a younger child, while associating with drug-abusing peers may be a more significant risk factor for an adolescent." As a result, students in junior high and high school need assistance with social competence in their peer relationships and drug resistance skills as well as reinforcement of antidrug attitudes and strengthening of personal commitments against drug abuse.

According to the report, some risk factors that may lead to drug abuse are academic failure, early peer rejection, and a later association with deviant peers. (The deviant peers are the strongest risk factor for adolescents.) Said the report, "Studies have shown that children with poor academic performance and inappropriate social behavior at ages 7 to 9 are more likely to be involved with substance abuse by age 14 or 15."

Gender is also a factor, and boys are more frequently offered drugs than girls. However, girls are more susceptible to drinking alcohol in order to fit in than boys are. Studies have demonstrated that boys start drinking for other reasons and then seek out groups whose members also drink.

See also ADOLESCENTS AND SUBSTANCE ABUSE; YOUNG ADULTS.

National Institute of Drug Abuse. *Preventing Drug Use among Children and Adolescents: A Research-Based Guide for Parents, Educators, and Community Leaders.* 2nd ed. Bethesda, Md.: National Institutes of Health, 2003.

phencyclidine (PCP) A hallucinogenic drug that often causes a PSYCHOLOGICAL DEPENDENCE and CRAVING and can lead to compulsive drug-seeking behavior. PCP is a Schedule II drug under the CONTROLLED SUBSTANCES ACT. The drug is sometimes used in animal tests by laboratory and clinical researchers, primarily with mice, rats, and monkeys, and often in studies of SCHIZOPHRENIA that was induced by PCP. Most urine drug tests can detect the presence of PCP.

PCP was originally developed as a depressant drug in 1963, with the brand name of Sernyl. It was marketed as an anesthetic that would not depress the respiration or blood pressure. However, it was withdrawn from the market in 1965 after reports that as many as half of the patients who had been given phencyclidine exhibited HALLUCINATIONS, disorientation, and extreme anxiety. Nearly all PCP today in the United States is produced in CLANDESTINE LABORATORIES, often by GANGS.

Sometimes illicit purchasers of other drugs are given PCP rather than the drug they seek, such as METHYLENEDIOXYMETHAMPHETAMINE (MDMA/ECSTASY). Sometimes PCP is inserted into other drugs, such as MARIJUANA, without the user's knowledge or permission. Users may also purposely insert PCP into CRACK COCAINE or into food without the consumer's knowledge. (See MALICIOUS POISONING.)

Some individuals use the drug in a liquid form. PCP powder, also called "angel dust," can be inhaled ("snorted"). It is also available in pill form.

PCP is not a popular drug of abuse in the 21st century, and according to the *National Survey on Drug Use and Health* for 2004, less than 1 percent of the population (0.7 percent) in the United States used PCP in 2004. Less than 1 percent (0.2 percent) of all emergency room admissions were of patients who had used PCP and were suffering from the aftereffects. However, it is estimated that at least 6 million people in the United States ages 12 and older have used PCP at least once. The highest percentage of PCP users in 2004 were young adults ages 18–25 years, but even in this group, few used the drug; for example, 2.3 percent of adults in this age bracket had ever used PCP. Less than 1 percent of this group (0.3 percent) had used PCP in the past year.

The Effects of PCP

Phencyclidine may produce the following effects:

- loss of coordination despite an illusion of strength and invulnerability
- slurred speech
- involuntary eye movements
- sensory distortions
- auditory hallucinations (hearing sounds that were not made)
- amnesia
- severe mood disorders
- anxiety and a feeling of doom

- paranoia
- a psychosis that cannot be distinguished from schizophrenia

In addition, the PCP user often exhibits zombie-like behavior. According to *Drugs of Abuse*, published by the Drug Enforcement Administration, in discussing the effects of PCP abuse, "A blank stare, rapid and involuntary eye movements, and an exaggerated gait are among the more observable effects."

Long-term users of PCP can develop memory loss and difficulty with thinking and speaking, which can continue for about a year after use of the drug. Adolescent users of PCP may impair hormones that spur growth and as a result may experience a shorter stature than they would have attained without PCP abuse. The learning process may also be impaired in adolescent users of PCP.

If users of PCP abruptly discontinue the drug, they may develop DEPRESSION and a lack of energy.

In some rare cases, PCP can cause multiorgan failure. In 2005 in the *Israel Medical Association Journal,* the authors discussed a 42-year-old woman who entered the emergency room with confusion and a heart rate of 20 beats per minute. She had acute kidney and liver failure and extreme lethargy. Her urine toxin screen showed opiates and PCP. She went into cardiac arrest and despite the extreme efforts of the physicians, died three days later of multiorgan failure. The physicians speculated that the woman had experienced PCP-induced hyperthermia (very high fever), which led to liver failure and the ultimate shutdown of her other organ systems.

It is unknown whether the woman was aware that she had ingested PCP and the family refused to authorize an autopsy to determine the cause of death.

See also CANADA; HALLUCINATIONS; HALLUCINOGENIC DRUGS; KETAMINE; SCHEDULED DRUGS.

Joseph, Donald E., ed., et al. Drug Enforcement Administration. *Drugs of Abuse.* Washington, D.C.: U.S. Department of Justice, 2005.

Levinthal, Charles F. *Drugs, Society, and Criminal Justice.* New York: Pearson Education, 2006.

Stein, Gideon Y., M.D., et al. "Phencyclidine-Induced Multi-Organ Failure." *Israel Medical Association Journal* 7 (August 2005): 535–537.

Substance Abuse and Mental Health Services Administration. *Results from the 2004 National Survey on Drug Use and Health: National Findings.* Rockville, Md.: Department of Health and Human Services, September 2005.

physical dependence   See DEPENDENCE, PHYSICAL.

physical tolerance   See TOLERANCE, PHYSICAL.

polypharmacy   The illicit use of two or more drugs. Many individuals who abuse or are addicted to drugs use several types of drugs. For example, many individuals who use COCAINE on a regular basis also use MARIJUANA. Many drug abusers also use alcohol. Polypharmacy can be dangerous because there is no physician or pharmacist monitoring the use of these multiple drugs (since they are illegal), and thus, the risk of an ADVERSE REACTION increases.

Sometimes polypharmacy occurs inadvertently; for example, older individuals and even younger people who are taking many different medications may forget completely whether they took their medications or not, and as a result, may inadvertently receive a double dose of their drugs when they mistakenly assume that they have *not* taken their medications. (It is very risky to take high doses of drugs such as NARCOTICS and other sedating medications, especially among older people who may metabolize the medications at a significantly slower rate than younger people.) It is best for those who need to take regular medications and who are forgetful to use a weekly pill container to keep track of whether medications have been taken.

Sometimes people "share" their prescribed medications, which is illegal and also can be very dangerous. For example, they may believe that giving PROPOXYPHENE (Darvon, Darvocet) or OXYCODONE will help a friend who is in pain. However, that friend may experience a severe reaction to the drug because of other narcotics he or she already takes or other non-narcotics medications he or she receives. It is also very dangerous to combine two or more medications with alcohol, which can be fatal. Even a few tablets of the seemingly innocuous Tylenol (acetaminophen) is dangerous in combination with alcohol, and such use can lead to liver problems. Adolescents and adults can end up in hospital emergency rooms as a result of such "sharing" and this practice can even be fatal.

See also PRESCRIPTION DRUG ABUSE.

post-traumatic stress disorder (PTSD)   A form of ANXIETY DISORDER that is a delayed and long-lasting reaction to a traumatic event, such as a physical attack, a wartime experience, or severe circumstances, such as a flood or hurricane, when individuals feared that death or severe harm would occur to them or loved ones. At the same time the distressing event occurred, the individual experienced feelings of helplessness, fear, and horror. The severe emotions that occurred at the time of the incident may be triggered at a later date, even years later, by people, places, or items that remind the person of the trauma. The presence of PTSD increases the risk for the development of substance abuse as well as eating disorders.

According to the Substance Abuse and Mental Health Administration, of all the individuals who are exposed to a particular traumatic event, about 7 percent will exhibit symptoms of PTSD.

An estimated 5–6 percent of men and 10–14 percent of women have had PTSD at some point, typically due to violence or exposure to life-threatening events such as car crashes or natural disasters. It is likely that a large number of people who directly observed the September 11, 2001, destruction of the Twin Towers in New York City suffered from PTSD.

Individuals who have PTSD have a biological response in addition to the psychiatric response; for example, studies have shown that people who have chronic PTSD have elevated levels of norepinephrine and thyroid hormone and below-normal levels of cortisol. In addition, imaging studies such as positron-emission tomography and functional magnetic resonance imaging (fMRI) of individuals who have PTSD have shown that activity in the amygdala and anterior paralimbic region of the brain is increased, while activities in other parts of the brain, such as the anterior cingulate and the orbitofrontal areas, are decreased.

According to Rachel Yehuda in her article on PTSD in the *New England Journal of Medicine,* "Facts that contribute to the intensity of the response to a psychologically traumatic experience include the degree of controllability, predictability, and perceived threat; the relative success of attempts to minimize injury to oneself or others; and actual loss."

Yehuda says that incidents that involve violence are more likely to cause PTSD than other events such as car crashes or natural disasters; for example, one study reported that PTSD developed in 55 percent of those who were raped, compared to 7.5 percent of those who were in car crashes and 2 percent of those who learned about traumatic events. Another study indicated that 14 percent of individuals who learned of the sudden and unexpected death of a loved one experienced PTSD. This one type of event represented nearly a third of all PTSD cases, or 39 percent for men and 27 percent for women.

Many people who have PTSD actively avoid anything that reminds them of the feared event. Even without reminders, they may experience flashbacks, when they feel that they are reexperiencing the event and feeling the same emotions they experienced at the time when it occurred. People who have PTSD may develop other anxiety disorders, such as generalized anxiety disorder or panic disorder. They are also at an increased risk for DEPRESSION. Some individuals who have PTSD develop physical disorders, such as high blood pressure or asthma.

Individuals who have PTSD have an elevated risk for alcohol abuse and ALCOHOLISM and are at risk for addiction to drugs. It is likely that those who use alcohol and/or drugs are seeking to block out or blunt the emotional pain from the devastating experience that caused the PTSD.

Symptoms and Diagnostic Path

Individuals who have PTSD may exhibit some or all of the following behavior:

- easy and excessively exaggerated startle response
- difficulty in sleeping
- frequent nightmares

- active avoidance of people, places, or items that remind them of the trauma

Combat veterans Soldiers in wartime may experience PTSD because they face situations and dilemmas that they would normally never face in their lives, such as the need to kill or be killed, as well as respond to surprise attacks and constant stress. Letting down their guard could lead to death, and soldiers may become hypervigilant as a means of survival. When they return to a peacetime life, these habits and mindsets may become difficult or impossible to discard at will.

Adults abused as children Individuals who were severely abused as children may suffer from PTSD; for example, according to the Northwest Foster Care Alumni Study, based on 659 adults who were placed in foster care as maltreated children, 25 percent of these adults reported experiencing PTSD in the past 11 months. This rate is twice as high as reported by military war veterans, and it is more than six times greater than the rate reported in the general population.

Molested women and children According to the Substance Abuse and Mental Health Services Administration (SAMHSA), in their statistics source book published in 1998, women who were molested or raped as children had a greatly elevated risk of PTSD; among those who were molested, 33 percent had PTSD while among those who were raped, 64 percent suffered from PTSD.

Domestic violence PTSD is common among women who are victims of domestic violence. The SAMHSA researchers reported that women who were assaulted had a greatly elevated risk of suffering from PTSD (54 percent) compared to women who had not been assaulted (11 percent).

Treatment Options and Outlook

Therapy and medications may help the person who has PTSD. Antidepressants, sedatives, or sleep remedies may enable the individual to obtain a restful sleep. Selective serotonin reuptake inhibitor (SSRI) antidepressants are often used, and sertraline (Zoloft) and paroxetine (Paxil) have been specifically approved by the Food and Drug Administration (FDA) to treat PTSD. If patients do not respond to these medications, nefazone (Serzone) or venlafaxine (Effexor) may help them. Some patients improve with the addition of divalproex (Depakote)

Psychotherapy may help the individual to learn how to manage psychologically the stress that was initially induced by the disturbing event. Exposure therapy, in which the person is systematically desensitized to things that he or she relates to the traumatic event, may be effective, as may cognitive-behavioral therapy, in which the patient learns to challenge irrational thoughts and beliefs.

Says Yehuda:

No matter what the emotional response, the process of recovery requires acknowledgment of changes that have occurred as a result of the traumatic event. Although many traumatized persons attempt to avoid distressing emotions related to their experiences, being able to confront them will promote habituation, so that over time, their thoughts about and emotional responses to the event will become less distressing.

Risk Factors and Preventive Measures

Individuals who have been in environments that were extremely stressful are at risk for PTSD. There are no preventive measures against PTSD.

See also ANXIETY DISORDERS; BIPOLAR DISORDER; DEPRESSION; PSYCHIATRIC DISORDERS; SEXUAL ASSAULTS; VIOLENCE.

Campbell, Jacquelyn C. "Health Consequences of Intimate Partner Violence." *Lancet* 359 (April 13, 2002): 1,331–1,336.

Pecora, Peter J., et al. *Improving Family Foster Care: Findings from the Northwest Foster Care Alumni Study.* Seattle: Casey Family Services, 2005.

Rouse, Beatrice A., ed. Web Mounted Version prepared by Rick Albright, *Substance Abuse and Mental Health Services Administration (SAMHSA) Statistics Source Book, 1998.*

Stein, Murray B., M.D., Neal A. Kline, M.D., and Jeffrey L. Matloff. "Adjunctive Olanzapine for SSRI-Resistant Combat-Related PTSD: A Double-Blind, Placebo-Controlled Study." *American Journal of Psychiatry* 159, no. 10 (October 2002): 1,777–1,779.

Yehuda, Rachel. "Post-Traumatic Stress Disorder." *New England Journal of Medicine* 346, no. 2 (January 10, 2002): 108–114.

precursor See METHAMPHETAMINE.

pregnancy and substance abuse Use of alcohol or illegal drugs and/or the illegal use of prescribed drugs during pregnancy. Substance abuse during pregnancy can lead to serious health problems in the children who are later born, such as FETAL ALCOHOL SYNDROME, low birth weight, and long-term developmental disabilities. Newborn babies of mothers who are addicted to drugs will themselves be born addicted and will usually undergo distressing WITHDRAWAL symptoms after the birth.

Some drugs present special problems for pregnant women; for example, studies of COCAINE use, such as that reported in the *New England Journal of Medicine* in 1999, have demonstrated that cocaine use can increase the risk of miscarriage. Some experts say that the use of MARIJUANA in the first month of pregnancy can impede muscle movement in the newborn infant.

It should also be noted that many substances may be dangerous for pregnant women and their offspring; for example, excessive CAFFEINE consumption may be dangerous. In a study of 562 women in Sweden who miscarried in the first trimester of pregnancy, significantly more pregnancy losses occurred in women who ingested at least 100 mg of caffeine per day than in women who consumed lower amounts. Use of nicotine can lead to a severe decrease in birth weight. This is due to the shrinking of blood vessel size in the placenta, leading to poor fetal nutrition.

Some women abuse methamphetamine during their pregnancies; however, the effects of prenatal exposure are yet largely unknown. In one study reported in 2006 in *Maternal and Child Health,* 5.2 percent of 1,632 women had abused methamphetamine during their pregnancies. (See METHAMPHETAMINE.)

Types of Substances Abused by Women in Treatment Facilities

As can be seen from Figure I, as indicated in studies of both pregnant woman and control subjects who were admitted to treatment facilities for drug or alcohol treatment in 1999, the pregnant women who abused substances were more likely to use COCAINE (27 percent) than nonpregnant substance-

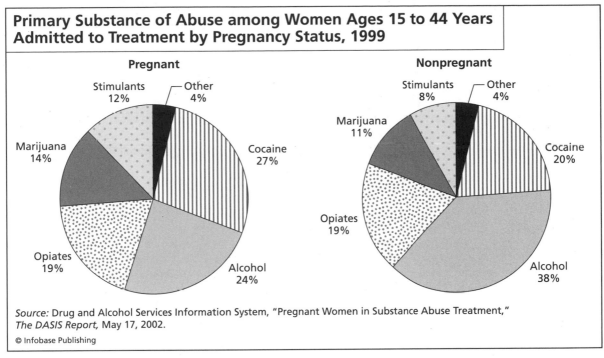

Primary Substance of Abuse among Women Ages 15 to 44 Years Admitted to Treatment by Pregnancy Status, 1999

Pregnant

Stimulants 12% — Other 4%
Marijuana 14%
Cocaine 27%
Opiates 19%
Alcohol 24%

Nonpregnant

Stimulants 8% — Other 4%
Marijuana 11%
Cocaine 20%
Opiates 19%
Alcohol 38%

Source: Drug and Alcohol Services Information System, "Pregnant Women in Substance Abuse Treatment," *The DASIS Report,* May 17, 2002.

© Infobase Publishing

Source: Drug and Alcohol Services Information System. "Pregnant Women in Substance Abuse Treatment," *The DASIS Report,* May 17, 2002.

abusing women (20 percent). However, pregnant women admitted to treatment were significantly *less* likely to be alcohol abusers (24 percent) than the nonpregnant women (38 percent).

Statistical Information

In 1989, the U.S. federal government mandated the public labeling of alcohol products to provide warnings to pregnant women that alcohol consumption is not recommended for pregnant women. Yet the Centers for Disease Control and Prevention (CDC) estimates that about 13 percent of pregnant women in the United States continue to drink during pregnancy,

Most women avoid illegal drugs during their pregnancy; however, some continue to abuse drugs throughout their pregnancy, despite warnings from their physicians, family members, friends, coworkers, and others. In 2003, according to the National Survey on Drug Use and Health, an estimated 4.3 percent of pregnant women used illegal drugs during the past month. However, younger pregnant

women, ages 15 to 25 years, were much more likely to use illegal drugs (8 percent) than older pregnant women ages 26 to 44 years old (1.6 percent.)

Some of the pregnant women were binge drinkers; an estimated 4 percent of pregnant women were binge drinkers of alcohol, consuming five or more drinks at the same time or within a couple of hours of each other. Younger pregnant women, ages 15 to 25 years old, were more likely to binge drink (5.0 percent) than those ages 26 to 44 years (3.3 percent). However, these rates were much lower than the rate of binge alcohol use among nonpregnant women of all ages, which was 23.2 percent.

Problems with Seeking Help

It is often very difficult for pregnant women who are substance abusers to obtain rehabilitative services, because most TREATMENT FACILITIES will not accept them as patients. In addition, some pregnant women who have drug and/or alcohol problems are afraid to seek out help because they fear that the children they already have could be removed from their home by child protective services workers. They also fear that when their new baby is born, state agencies could take the newborn away from them.

This fear has some validity because some states can take babies away from their mothers if there is evidence of drug or alcohol abuse in the newborn child; however, most states allow the mother time to undergo rehabilitative treatment before she risks losing her parental rights. (See Appendix XVI for information on state laws on child abuse that relate to drug abuse, which also includes such crimes as manufacturing drugs such as methamphetamine in the home as well as bearing children addicted to drugs or alcohol.) Some states have laws that require the testing of pregnant women who seek emergency services of any kind; such laws lead to early detection of substance abuse but create additional problems for women who forgo emergency treatment in order to avoid this kind of testing.

In one study of 244 pregnant women who had substance abuse problems in North Carolina, reported in the *American Journal of Drug and Alcohol Abuse* in 2001, 236 (97 percent) were referred for outpatient treatment, and 61 percent complied with the referral. The researchers found that those women who complied with their referrals to outpatient treatment were significantly more likely to have received substance abuse treatment in the past. (Forty-five percent of the women who complied had undergone prior substance abuse treatment versus 28 percent of the women who failed to comply with outpatient treatment.)

Possibly in these women, their substance abuse was no longer secret, and women who have undergone treatment in the past may think that they have more to gain and less to lose by having treatment.

Say the authors:

Women who have never been in substance abuse treatment might be afraid that seeking help would cause them to be labeled as a drug user and then shunned by friends and/or family members, causing them to leave treatment early or to forgo it. Women who have experienced treatment, however, may realize that it might be necessary to forge new drug-free relationships that could only be achieved through successful completion of a treatment program.

In addition, women who have previously been through treatment and experienced RELAPSE may have a greater chance of losing their parental rights than those who are referred for treatment for the first time.

See also DUAL DIAGNOSIS; SCHEDULED DRUGS.

Clark, Kathryn Anderson, et al. "Treatment Compliance among Prenatal Care Patients with Substance Abuse Problems." *American Journal of Drug and Alcohol Abuse* 27, no. 1 (2001): 121–136.

Cnattingius, Sven, M.D., et al. "Caffeine Intake and the Risk of First-Trimester Spontaneous Abortion." *New England Journal of Medicine* 343, no. 25 (December 21, 2000): 1,839–1,945.

Drug and Alcohol Services Information System. "Pregnant Women in Substance Abuse Treatment." *The DASIS Report.* (May 17, 2002). Available online. URL: http://www.oas.samhsa.gov/2k2/pregTX/pregTX1htm. Downloaded on August 17, 2007.

National Survey on Drug Use and Health. "Substance Use during Pregnancy: 2002 and 2003." *The NSDUH Report,* Office of Applied Studies, Substance Abuse and Mental Health Services Administration, June 2, 2005.

Ness, Roberta B., M.D., et al. "Cocaine and Tobacco Use and the Risk of Spontaneous Abortion." *New England Journal of Medicine* 340, no. 5 (February 4, 1999): 333–339.

Substance Abuse and Mental Health Services Administration. *Results from the 2004 National Survey on Drug Use and Health: National Findings.* Rockville, Md.: Department of Health and Human Services, September 2005.

prescription drug abuse   The misuse or abuse of legally prescribed drugs, particularly of substances that are classified as SCHEDULED DRUGS under the CONTROLLED SUBSTANCES ACT, such as narcotic painkillers, such as OXYCODONE, HYDROCODONE, OXYCONTIN, as well as many other narcotics. BARBITURATES and BENZODIAZEPINES, both central nervous system DEPRESSANTS, are also sometimes drugs of abuse. In addition, some stimulants, such as METHYLPHENIDATE (RITALIN/CONCERTA/FOCALIN, ETC.) and AMPHET-

AMINES, which are prescribed to individuals who have ATTENTION DEFICIT HYPERACTIVITY DISORDER (ADHD), are sometimes abused. Prescription drug abuse can destroy lives and lead to prison sentences.

Prescription drug abuse is a major and growing problem in the United States. Some people who would never consider using such illegal drugs as HEROIN, METHAMPHETAMINE, COCAINE, or CRACK COCAINE actively abuse other drugs, such as methylphenidate (Ritalin), ALPRAZOLAM (XANAX), PROPOXYPHENE (Darvon/Darvocet), and narcotic painkillers. Sometimes METHADONE, a drug used to treat heroin addicts, is also abused.

According to a 2006 report from the Executive Office of the President, the administration set a new goal of reducing prescription drug abuse by 15 percent by the end of 2008. Efforts will be made to determine how and why prescription drugs are abused and to clamp down on these various means, without preventing access to these drugs by consumers who need them for medical problems.

Abuse of Various Types of Drugs

The primary types of prescription drugs that are abused are narcotic painkillers, stimulants, and depressants (such as barbiturates or benzodiazepines).

Many people who will abuse one prescription drug will also abuse other prescription drugs. In addition, they often abuse alcohol as well. The combination of prescribed drugs and alcohol can be very dangerous and even fatal, particularly since the dosage of the prescribed drug that is used by the abuser is usually much higher than recommended by physicians. Some individuals purposely combine prescription drugs with alcohol in order to commit SUICIDE, although some of these deaths are accidental. Adolescents and young adults are particularly likely to combine alcohol with the abuse of prescription drugs. (See ACCIDENTAL OVERDOSE DEATHS.)

Abuse of narcotic painkillers Prescribed painkillers are commonly abused; of course, their legitimate use is often perceived as a godsend for individuals suffering from severe chronic pain caused by cancer, back problems, and other painful conditions.

Young adults ages 18 to 25 years old have the highest abuse rates of prescription drugs, and in 2005, 2 million people in this age group (6.1 percent) abused prescription drugs in the past month and 4.8 million (14.8 percent) abused them in the past year. (See Table I.)

In considering the lifetime prevalence (ever having abused) of narcotics, young adults had a rate of 24.3 percent in 2004, as reported by the National Survey on Drug Use and Health.

According to the National Survey on Drug Use and Health, among new abusers of prescription painkillers in 2004, the most commonly abused drugs were VICODIN, Lortab, or Lorcet, which are all forms of hydrocodone. Of those with a lifetime

TABLE I: CONTROLLED SUBSTANCE PRESCRIPTION DRUG ABUSE BY CATEGORY AND AGE GROUP, 2004

Drug Category	Age 12 or Older Number (in millions)	Percentage	Age 12 to 17 Number (in millions)	Percentage	Age 18 to 25 Number (in millions)	Percentage	Age 26 to Older Number (in millions)	Percentage
Prescription Drugs								
Past Month	6.0	2.5	0.914	3.6	2.0	6.1	3.1	1.7
Past Year	14.6	6.1	2.2	8.8	4.8	14.8	7.7	4.2
Pain Relievers								
Past Month	4.4	1.8	0.751	3.0	1.5	4.7	2.1	1.2
Past Year	11.3	4.7	1.9	7.4	3.8	11.9	5.6	3.0
Tranquilizers								
Past Month	1.6	0.7	0.161	0.6	0.566	1.8	0.889	0.5
Past Year	5.1	2.1	0.532	2.1	1.7	5.2	2.9	1.6

Source: Executive Office of the President. *Synthetic Drug Control Strategy: A Focus on Methamphetamine and Prescription Drug Abuse.* Washington, D.C.: Office of National Drug Control Policy, 2006, p. 31.

abuse of prescription painkillers, nearly half (48 percent) abused one of these drugs. The next most frequently abused drugs were either forms of PRO-POXYPHENE (Darvocet or Darvot) or Tylenol with codeine, and 34.3 percent of those who abused pain relievers misused these drugs. Third in terms of abuse were forms of oxycodone, including Per-cocet, Percodan, or Tylox, and 20 percent of those who initiated prescription painkiller abuse used these drugs.

Among new abusers who initiated the use of OxyContin, more than half (55.1 percent) were male and the average age at the time of the first prescription abuse was 25 years. Nearly 90 percent of recent initiates of OxyContin abuse in 2004 were non-Hispanic whites.

Among adolescents ages 12–17 years in 2004, 11.4 percent had ever abused prescription pain relievers and 5.1 percent abused these drugs in the past year.

Abuse of stimulants   Increasing numbers of adolescents and adults are diagnosed with ADHD and they are often treated with stimulants, such as methylphenidate or amphetamine. Among ado-lescents ages 12–17 years in 2004, 3.2 percent had ever abused stimulants.

Abusers of prescribed stimulants are usually ADOLESCENTS, COLLEGE STUDENTS, or YOUNG ADULTS. Physicians should warn patients, especially adoles-cents, that others may seek to use their medication, but such use is not only illegal, but very danger-ous.

In one study of students treated with psycho-stimulant drugs for ADHD in grades six through 11, reported in *Substance Use & Misuse,* 23 percent of the students were approached by others who wanted them to give, sell, or trade their stimulant medica-tions, a finding that prompts concern.

Abuse of depressants   Drugs that depress the central nervous system continue to be abused by some individuals. Barbiturate medications are com-monly abused; for example, among high school seniors, about 9.9 percent had ever abused barbi-turates in 2004, according to the Monitoring the Future reports. This usage was up 1 percent from 2003.

Among college students and their same-age peers in 2004, there was a lifetime barbiturate abuse prevalence of 7.2 percent for college students and 12.2 percent for their same-age peers.

Benzodiazepines, also known as tranquiliz-ers, are central nervous system depressants that are sometimes abused. According to the National Survey on Drug Use and Health, in 2004, 11.2 percent of young adults ages 18–25 abused benzo-diazepines, and the most commonly abused ben-zodiazepine was DIAZEPAM (Valium): 6.1 percent of individuals of all ages had ever abused Valium in 2004. Alprazalam (Xanax) was also a drug of abuse. Among college students, 10.6 percent had abused benzodiazepines, compared to the significantly greater 16.6 percent of their noncollege peers.

Among adolescents, ages 12–17 years, 3.2 per-cent had ever abused benzodiazepines.

Increase in the Abuse of Some Prescription Drugs

According to the National Survey on Drug Use and Health, 6 million people abused prescription drugs nonmedically in the United States in 2004, includ-ing 4.4 million who had abused analgesic (painkill-ing) drugs, 1.6 million who abused tranquilizers (benzodiazepines), 1.2 million who abused stimu-lants, and less than a million (0.3 million) who had abused sedatives (barbiturates).

This abuse level corresponds to the levels that were also seen in 2003; however, there were sig-nificant increases in the rates of the lifetime preva-lence of abuse (having ever abused) among those who abused some drugs, such as HYDROCODONE (Vicodin, Lortab, or Lorcet). The abuse of hydroco-done products increased from 15.0 percent in 2003 to 16.5 percent in 2004. In addition, OXYCODONE (Percocet, Percodan, or Tylox) abuse increased from 7.8 percent in 2003 to 8.7 percent in 2004. The lifetime abuse of OxyContin, a timed-release form of oxycodone, rose from 3.6 percent in 2003 to 4.3 percent in 2004.

In considering demographic information on those who abuse prescription drugs, the majority are white (74.7 percent) and have a family income of less than $50,000. (See Table II.)

Most people who abuse OxyContin have abused other legal and illegal drugs in the past; for exam-ple, 97 percent of OxyContin abusers have abused marijuana and/or other prescription pain relievers prior to the abuse of OxyContin. (See Table III.) As

TABLE II: DEMOGRAPHIC CHARACTERISTICS OF RECENT NONMEDICAL PAIN RELIEVER USE INITIATES, AGES 12 AND OLDER, 2004

Demographics	Number (Thousands)	Percentage
Total	2,422	100.0
Gender		
Male	1,093	45.1
Female	1,329	54.9
Race/Ethnicity		
White, non-Hispanic	1,809	74.7
Black, non-Hispanic	198	8.2
American Indian or Alaska Native, non-Hispanic	11	0.5
Asian, non-Hispanic	58	2.4
Hispanic 280		11.6
Family Income		
Less than $20,000	570	23.5
$20,000–$49,000	795	32.8
$50,000–$74,999	383	15.8
$75,000 or More	674	27.8

Source: Adapted from Substance Abuse and Mental Health Services Administration. "Nonmedical Users of Pain Relievers: Characteristics of Recent Initiates." *The NSDUH Report* 22 (2006), p. 3. Available online. URL: http://oas.samhsa.gov/2k6/pain/pain.pdf. Downloaded June 19, 2006.

can be seen from the table, there were significant differences between those who began abusing pain relievers that were not OxyContin and those who abused OxyContin. For example, 73.6 percent of those who abused other pain relievers were smokers, compared to 95.5 percent of those who abused OxyContin.

Although most of those who abused other pain relievers had abused alcohol (86.9 percent), the alcohol abuse rate was much higher among those who abused OxyContin, or 99.4 percent. The OxyContin abusers were also far more likely than the abusers of other pain relievers to have abused crack cocaine, heroin, HALLUCINOGENIC DRUGS, and every other category of drug.

Abusers of Prescription Drugs

In considering the abuse of prescription drugs in general, among adolescents, teenage females are significantly more likely to abuse prescription drugs than adolescent males. In 2004, 14.4 percent of teenage girls had ever abused prescription drugs in the United States, compared to 12.5 percent of teenage boys. In considering adolescents who had

TABLE III: PERCENTAGES OF SUBSTANCES USED PRIOR TO INITIATION OF NONMEDICAL PAIN RELIEVER USE OR OXYCONTIN USE IN THE PAST YEAR, AMONG RESPONDENTS AGES 12 OR OLDER IN 2004

Substance Use Categories	Pain Reliever Initiates Percentage	OxyContin Alone Initiates Percentage
Cigarettes	73.6	95.5
Alcohol	86.9	99.4
Marijuana	66.2	97.1
Cocaine/crack	13.0	63.8
Heroin	0.7	8.2
Hallucinogens	24.9	71.1
Inhalants	21.3	49.9
Nonmedical use of tranquilizers	12.2	59.8
Nonmedical use of stimulants	12.4	46.1
Nonmedical use of any other pain reliever (not OxyContin)	—	97.4
Use of marijuana, cocaine/crack, heroin, hallucinogens, inhalants, or the nonmedical use of tranquilizers, stimulants, or sedatives	73.8	99.1
Use of marijuana, cocaine/crack, heroin, hallucinogens, inhalants or the nonmedical use of tranquilizers, stimulants, or any other pain reliever (not OxyContin)	—	99.8

Source: Adapted from Substance Abuse and Mental Health Services Administration. "Nonmedical Users of Pain Relievers: Characteristics of Recent Initiates." *The NSDUH Report* 22 (2006), p. 3. Available online. URL: http://oas.samhsa.gov/2k6/pain/pain.pdf. Downloaded June 19, 2006

abused prescription drugs in the past month, an estimated 4.1 percent of adolescent girls were abusers, compared to 3.2 percent of adolescent boys.

In contrast to the pattern seen with many other drugs of abuse, females represented more than half (54.9 percent) of those who initiated the nonmedical use of prescription pain relievers in 2004.

In a 2005 study of more than 9,000 college students, discussed in *Drug and Alcohol Dependence,* the researchers found that illicit use of prescription painkiller drugs in the past year was a greater problem among students who had received prior prescription for pain medication. For example, only 4.4 percent of women with no previous prescribed use of painkillers used pain medications illicitly in the past year. More than double (9.4 percent) of those who had been previously prescribed painkillers in college were illicit users of drugs.

Prescription drug abuse rates of painkillers were higher for male college students than for their non-college peers; for example, 6.3 percent of male college students who had not previously used prescription painkillers abused these drugs compared to 15.4 percent of male college students who had been previously prescribed a painkiller in college and who then subsequently abused this type of drug.

Possible Reasons for the Popularity of Nonmedical Use of Prescribed Drugs

There are many reasons why the abuse of prescribed drugs may have increased. One is that some prescribed drugs can induce the same or similar mood states that illegal drugs induce, and if they are willing to do so illegally, many individuals would rather abuse a prescribed drug than an illegal drug. Prescription drug abuse may also seem to be more of a "white-collar crime," and thus, individuals may mistakenly believe that they are less likely to be prosecuted than if they were abusing cocaine or heroin. (Individuals who misuse prescription drugs, especially SCHEDULED DRUGS such as narcotics, are often prosecuted.)

Drugs that are used illegally, such as COCAINE, and METHAMPHETAMINE, do not have uniform dosages, and their level of purity depends on the manufacturer. In many cases, illegal drugs include adulterants, such as other drugs, talcum powder, and all sorts of other items that can cause severe

illness and even death upon ingestion. In contrast, many people are aware that prescription drugs are manufactured under strict control, and are not adulterated with other drugs.

As a result, individuals may perceive these drugs as safe. However, when individuals take prescribed drugs that were meant for others and with the sole aim of abusing these drugs, and/or they abuse their own prescribed medications, taking very high dosages, then these drugs are *not* safe.

Another reason why prescription drug abuse may be a growing problem is that most people do not wish to interact with DRUG DEALERS, because they fear being arrested and they may fear traveling to unsafe neighborhoods, where they risk being robbed and beaten, to purchase the drug. These individuals may be willing to make illegal purchases of prescribed drugs over the Internet or to buy prescribed drugs from friends in high school, college, or elsewhere, where they perceive the risk of physical harm is significantly lower than in interacting with drug dealers directly.

People who abuse prescription drugs may mistakenly believe that these drugs have a lower risk (or no risk) of addiction than illicit drugs such as crack cocaine, heroin, methamphetamine, and other illegal drugs. What most people who abuse scheduled prescription drugs do not realize is that some prescribed SCHEDULED DRUGS can be highly addictive, and that WITHDRAWAL from them can be as difficult as or even more difficult than withdrawal from illegal drugs.

Means of Obtaining Illegal Prescriptions or Drugs

Some people who abuse prescription drugs do so by altering valid prescriptions that they have received from a doctor, for example, changing a prescription for 10 pills to one for 90 pills. Or they may take a valid prescription and add another drug to the same prescription. If the prescription looks suspicious, most pharmacists will call the doctor for confirmation of the drug and the number of pills.

Some people engage in *doctor shopping,* in which they go to several or many different physicians, often complaining of severe pain solely for the purpose of obtaining prescriptions for prescribed painkillers (such as hydrocodone or oxycodone), which they then fill at different pharmacies. This is done for the purpose of abusing the drug or sometimes for selling the drug to others who will abuse it.

Some people call in their own prescriptions to pharmacies, pretending to be the doctor or a member of the doctor's staff, usually on a day when the doctor's office is closed and the pharmacist cannot double check. These individuals may be patients or employees of the physician.

Stealing prescription pads from the doctor is another way that individuals obtain drugs for the purpose of abuse. They then write prescriptions for themselves or others, usually fictitious people.

Other individuals steal prescribed drugs from the homes and medicine cabinets of family members, friends, and relatives, either for their own use or for sale to others. (See DIVERSION, DRUG.)

Many people illegally obtain prescription drugs online through Internet pharmacies that require no prescription, a serious problem in the United States and other countries. These pharmacies may be located in other countries, such as MEXICO or Thailand. Some minors have used parental credit cards or other means to order prescription painkillers and ANDROGENIC STEROIDS illegally. Deaths have been reported. (See INTERNET DRUG TRAFFICKING/ ILLEGAL PHARMACIES.)

Another way that individuals sometimes obtain drugs illegally is through well-meaning friends; for example, a person may receive a prescription for a narcotic painkiller from a physician or dentist and not need to use all the tablets that were prescribed. He or she may keep the remaining pills and, if a friend or relative complains of severe pain, give the drug to that person. This is not lawful and is very dangerous for the person who is given the drug, since he or she could suffer from a drug interaction or could experience serious side effects to the medication.

Treatment for Abuse of Prescription Drugs

Many abusers of prescription drugs may receive treatment in an outpatient rehabilitative program while others may need assistance in an inpatient program. They may need DETOXIFICATION from their drug of abuse and, once the addiction ends, usually need continued counseling. Often the CRAVING for the drug remains and can lead to RELAPSE if this problem is not addressed with counseling. Self-help groups may also be very helpful to individuals overcoming prescription drug abuse.

See also ALPRAZOLAM/ALPRAZOLAM XR (XANAX/ XANAX XR); AMPHETAMINE; BARBITURATES; BENZO- DIAZEPINES; CODEINE; CONTROLLED SUBSTANCES ACT; DIAZEPAM (VALIUM); HYDROCODONE; METHADONE; METHYLPHENIDATE (RITALIN/CONCERTA/FOCALIN, ETC.); MOOD STABILIZERS; MORPHINE; OXYCODONE; OXYCON- TIN; PAIN MANAGEMENT AND NARCOTIC MEDICATION; PRESCRIPTION DRUG MONITORING PROGRAMS, STATES WITH; PROPOXYPHENE; SCHEDULED DRUGS.

Executive Office of the President. *Synthetic Drug Control Strategy: A Focus on Methamphetamine and Prescription Drug Abuse.* Washington, D.C.: Office of National Drug Control Policy, 2006.

Friedman, Richard A., M.D. "The Changing Face of Teenage Drug Abuse—The Trend toward Prescription Drugs." *New England Journal of Medicine* 354, no. 14 (April 6, 2006): 1,448–1,450.

Johnston, Lloyd D., et al. *Monitoring the Future: National Survey Results on Drug Use, 1975–2004.* Vol. 2, *College Students and Adults Ages 19–45.* Bethesda, Md.: National Institute on Drug Abuse, National Institutes of Health, 2005.

Joseph, Donald E., et al., eds. *Drugs of Abuse.* Washington, D.C.: U.S. Department of Justice, 2005.

McCabe, S. E., C. J. Teter, and C. J. Boyd. "Illicit Use of Prescription Pain Medication among College Students." *Drug and Alcohol Dependence* 77 (2005): 37–47.

McCabe, S. E., C. J. Teter, and C. J. Boyd. "The Use, Misuse and Diversion of Prescription Stimulants among Middle and High School Students." *Substance Use and Misuse* 39, no. 7 (2004): 1,095–1,116.

Ness, Roberta B., M.D., et al. "Cocaine and Tobacco Use and the Risk of Spontaneous Abortion." *New England Journal of Medicine* 340, no. 5 (February 4, 1999): 333– 339.

Office of National Drug Control Policy. *Girls and Drugs: A New Analysis: Recent Trends, Risk Factors and Consequences.* Washington, D.C.: Executive Office of the President, February 9, 2006.

Substance Abuse and Mental Health Services Administration. "Nonmedical Users of Pain Relievers: Characteristics of Recent Initiates." *The NSDUH Report* 22 (2006): p. 3. Available online. URL: http://oas.samhsa. gov/2k6/pain/pain.pdf. Downloaded June 19, 2006.

prescription drug monitoring programs, states with

Programs within some states in the United States that monitor scheduled drug use in order to help prevent DRUG DIVERSION of narcotics. The first prescription drug monitoring program was established in 1940 in California.

In 2005, according to the National Alliance for Model State Drug Laws, 20 states were operating prescription drug monitoring programs, including California, Hawaii, Idaho, Illinois, Indiana, Kentucky, Maine, Massachusetts, Michigan, Mississippi, Nevada, New York, Oklahoma, Pennsylvania, Rhode Island, Texas, Utah, Washington, West Virginia, and Wyoming. Several states anticipated implementing programs as of 2005, including Alabama, New Mexico, and Tennessee.

In 2005, President George W. Bush signed the National All Schedules Prescription Electronic Reporting Act of 2005, enacting this new program as an incentive to create or enhance the electronic monitoring of scheduled prescription drugs in all 50 states. The law offers grants from the Department of Health and Human Services to states for establishing an electronic database monitoring program or improving their existing programs that monitor scheduled prescription drugs. The law authorized expenditures of $60 million through fiscal year 2010. It should be noted that at least a year passes before most new programs are implemented.

Costs for Programs

In 2002, the General Accounting Office (GAO) evaluated the start-up costs and annual operating costs for prescription drug monitoring programs in three states: Kentucky, Nevada, and Utah. (See Table I.)

Some states manage the program within state agencies, while others use private contractors to collect the data. In some cases, federal funds from grants may be used to finance part of the cost of the programs. For example, in 2005, the Office of Justice Programs under the Department of Justice announced awards of $6.3 million. The Harold Rogers Prescription Drug Monitoring Program within the Department of Justice also provided assistance to states in starting up a prescription drug monitoring program or enhancing an already-existing program. This program provides technical assistance

TABLE I: COSTS ASSOCIATED WITH THREE PRESCRIPTION DRUG MONITORING PROGRAMS

State	Year Implemented	Start-up Costs	Annual Operating Costs
Kentucky	1999	$415,000	$500,000
Nevada	1996	$134,000	$112,000
Utah	1996	$50,000	$93,000

Source: Adapted from U.S. General Accounting Office. *Prescription Drugs: State Monitoring Programs Provide Useful Tool to Reduce Diversion.* Washington, D.C.: Government Printing Office, May 2002.

to states and assistance to states that seek to share drug information with neighboring states.

Collection of Data

Prescription drug monitoring programs involve either the use of triplicate state-issued prescription pads or electronic transmission of data. With the multiple-copy prescription pads (used only for scheduled drugs), the doctor writes a prescription, keeps one copy, then gives the prescription to the patient. When it is filled, the pharmacist keeps a copy of the prescription and sends a copy to the state regulating agency. However, nearly all states use electronic prescription monitoring systems, in which the pharmacist sends prescription information electronically to the state agency. Some states rely primarily on electronic transmission but also keep a paper copy of the prescription.

Note that in those states that do *not* have prescription drug monitoring programs, some physicians who prescribe narcotics to patients for severe pain photocopy the prescription for their own records before it is given to the patient. This is done to protect the doctor, for example, if the patient should illegally try to change the prescription that the doctor wrote, such as by increasing the number of pills that the doctor has ordered. (In contrast, if the patient changes the number of refills, such as changing 0 to 1 or more, the pharmacy usually catches this error because Schedule II drugs cannot be refilled and doctors and pharmacists know this, although some patients do not.)

Pros and Cons of Prescription Monitoring Programs

Supporters of state prescription drug monitoring programs say that they can eliminate or at least reduce the number of prescription forgeries by patients as well as monitor questionable or illegal practices of doctors, such as among the few doctors who overprescribe narcotics. In addition, these programs can help to decrease "doctor shopping," the practice of some patients of going to multiple physicians and pharmacies to obtain the same narcotics, for the purpose of abusing them. They also point out that states that do not have drug monitoring programs usually must rely on tips from law enforcement authorities, physicians, and patients to discover cases of PRESCRIPTION DRUG ABUSE.

One study by the General Accounting Office revealed that the average investigation time of a doctor shopper was reduced from 156 days to 16 days in Kentucky because of the prescription drug monitoring program. In addition, the investigation time in Nevada for doctor shopping was reduced from 120 days to 20 days with the implementation of a drug monitoring program.

In some states, physicians may obtain information on individual patients and their use of narcotics. For example, according to a 2004 General Accounting Office report, in Kentucky, a doctor can ask for a drug history report on the same day as a patient's appointment and may receive the results within four hours of submitting the request. This information will keep the doctor informed of which narcotics, if any, have recently been prescribed to the patient. This information will also help the doctor to make better prescribing decisions. For example, if a patient was prescribed a form of OXYCODONE in the past month or two by another physician, the new doctor may wish to prescribe only a mild analgesic or choose to prescribe no medication at all.

The system in Kentucky is actively used, and in 2002, the program received about 400 physician requests daily.

There are some key areas of concern with prescription monitoring programs. Some people worry that patient confidentiality can be compromised with such a monitoring system; however, supporters say that only law enforcement agencies and the state agency receiving the information (and sometimes physicians) may see the information. However, in some states, the monitoring is contracted out to outside agencies, and as a result, some fear that the information could be compromised or leaked to others. This may be especially true in the case of celebrities or politicians, because that sort of negative information is often fascinating to the media and to the general public.

Another concern is that such a system may deter doctors from writing narcotic prescriptions for their patients who are in severe pain and who truly need them. The Drug Enforcement Administration counters this argument by saying that from 1990 to 1998, the production of Schedule II and III narcotics increased rather than decreased in the United States.

One area of increasing concern is that prescription monitoring programs do not capture the data when illegal drugs are ordered over Internet Web sites. (See INTERNET DRUG TRAFFICKING/ILLEGAL PHARMACIES.)

See also PRESCRIPTION DRUGS; SCHEDULED DRUGS.

Crosse, Marcia, Director. Health Care—Public Health and Military Health Care Issues. *Testimony before the Subcommittee on Health, Committee on Energy and Commerce, House of Representatives, Prescription Drugs: State Monitoring Programs May Help to Reduce Illegal Diversion.* Washington, D.C.: General Accounting Office, March 4, 2004.

General Accounting Office. Report to the Subcommittee on Oversight and Investigations, Committee on Energy and Commerce, House of Representatives. *Prescription Drugs: State Monitoring Programs Provide Useful Tool to Reduce Diversion.* Washington, D.C., May 2002.

Kraman, Pilar. *Prescription Drug Diversion.* Lexington, Ky.: The Council of State Governments, April 2004.

propoxyphene A central nervous system depressant medication that is used as a painkiller for mild to moderate pain. Propoxyphene is a Schedule IV drug under the CONTROLLED SUBSTANCES ACT because it has some addictive potential. (There are five categories of SCHEDULED DRUGS.) When it is combined with aspirin, the brand name of propoxyphene is Darvon. When combined with acetaminophen instead of aspirin, the brand name is Darvocet. The drug can be taken orally as a liquid, tablet, or capsule, or it may be injected.

There is a low rate of PRESCRIPTION DRUG ABUSE of propoxyphene in the United States. According to the *National Survey on Drug Use and Health* in 2004, the lifetime nonmedical use of propoxyphene among all ages in 2003 (the most recent data as of this writing) was significantly less than 1 percent (0.1 percent). The incidence of abuse increased slightly to 0.2 percent in 2004.

Patients should tell their doctors if they are taking any other prescribed or over-the-counter medications, particularly medications in the categories of pain relievers, anticoagulants (blood thinners), antidepressants, antihistamines, cough medications, muscle relaxants, sedatives, seizure medications, sleeping pills, tranquilizers, or vitamins. Knowing what other medications the patient takes, the physician can determine whether there could be any interactions with these drugs and propoxyphene. For example, propoxyphene can interact with antidepressants such as amitriptyline (Elavil) or with antihistamines such as Benadryl. Blood thinners such as coumadin (Warfarin) combined with propoxyphene can cause a dangerous thinning of the blood.

In addition, the patient should inform the doctor if he or she has any history of kidney or liver disease or ALCOHOLISM, since propoxyphene affects the liver and the kidneys. Patients should not drive a car or operate any heavy equipment or machinery until they know whether the drug causes them to become drowsy.

When taken as directed, propoxyphene may cause some side effects, including upset stomach, constipation, skin rash, headache, dizziness, light-headedness, and mood changes.

Abuse or Overdose of Propoxyphene

When abused, high doses of propoxyphene can cause serious medical problems, including coma, seizures, and even accidental death. Some symptoms of propoxyphene overdose are muscle spasticity, slow or labored breathing and/or breathing difficulties, pupils so dilated that they are pinpoints, blue fingernails or lips (cyanosis), nausea and vomiting, abdominal cramps, low blood pressure, and drowsiness.

Propoxyphene when combined with alcohol produces effects more severe than those produced by either substance alone; the effect is commonly described as a synergistic interaction to differentiate it from an addictive interaction. Although the most frequently seen synergistic interaction is that of benzodiazepines and alcohol, propoxyphene with alcohol can be a much more dangerous combination.

The long-term use of propoxyphene, even when used legitimately rather than as a drug of abuse, can cause gastrointestinal damage, such as stomach bleeding and ulcers. (These effects may be primarily caused by propoxyphene that is combined with aspirin.) Kidney and liver damage may also occur with long-term use. Serious medication interactions may also occur with some drugs, such as blood thinners like Coumadin (warfarin). This combination can cause internal bleeding and even death. Clearly, when the drug is not used therapeutically and excessive dosages of propoxyphene are abused, the risks for developing these serious medical problems are further increased.

See also ADVERSE REACTION; DRUG ABUSE AND DEPENDENCE AND HEALTH PROBLEMS; PRESCRIPTION DRUG ABUSE; SCHEDULED DRUGS.

Joseph, Donald E., et al., eds. *Drugs of Abuse.* Washington, D.C.: U.S. Department of Justice, 2005.

Substance Abuse and Mental Health Services Administration. *Results from the 2004 National Survey on Drug Use and Health: National Findings.* Rockville, Md.: Department of Health and Human Services, September 2005.

prostitution   Providing sexual favors in exchange for money or other items of value. Prostitution is illegal in all states of the United States, except in some parts of Nevada. Many prostitutes abuse alcohol and drugs, and often they also become addicted to drugs such as COCAINE or HEROIN. Some addicted individuals resort to prostitution to obtain money for drugs, while other individuals have not used drugs in the past but become users after their entry into prostitution.

Gang members may encourage or compel females to engage in prostitution to support the gang and some gangs operate prostitution rings.

Susan McClanahan and her colleagues studied 1,142 female detainees and found that about a third of the women had ever engaged in prostitution. About half of the women met the criteria for moderate or severe cocaine or opiate abuse or dependence.

The two primary factors that led women into prostitution were running away from home and childhood sexual victimization. The subjects who practiced moderate or severe cocaine or opiate abuse or dependence had a higher likelihood of engaging in prostitution than those who did not: 53.2 percent versus 13.9 percent for the women not on drugs.

The researchers also sought to determine whether drug use primarily occurred before or after prostitution, and they found that among women who prostituted themselves one or more times per week and who also had a diagnosis of moderate or severe cocaine or heroin abuse or dependence, 67.4 percent began using drugs before they began routinely prostituting themselves. Of the other women who were drug abusers or addicts, 22.3 percent said that their substance abuse occurred after they began prostituting themselves. (The remaining women were not sure whether the drug problem started before or after the prostitution.)

Say the researchers:

Addict-prostitutes tend to be heavy users and report that narcotic use increases with further involvement in prostitution. Although entrance into prostitution before addiction may be due to effects of sexual abuse, entering prostitution after developing an addiction may be an economic necessity. Addiction complicates women's efforts to leave prostitution, and drug treatment needs to begin early in their prostitution careers. Prostitutes who use drugs are also at a significantly higher risk for HIV infection.

See also CRIME AND CRIMINALS; JAIL INMATES.

McClanahan, Susan F., Gary M. McClelland, Karen M. Abram, and Linda A. Teplin. "Pathways into Prostitution among Female Jail Detainees and Their Implications for Mental Health Services." *Psychiatric Services* 50, no. 12 (December 1999): 1,606–1,613.

pseudoaddiction An apparent addiction of a patient whose moderate to severe pain is under-controlled by the medications that are currently prescribed to him or her. The physician may refuse to increase the dosage or frequency of the patient's narcotics, and the patient, still in debilitating pain, may react by seeking narcotics from other physicians, in an attempt to obtain adequate pain treatment. This behavior, which may be mislabeled "doctor shopping," may also be mistakenly identified as drug addiction; however, the individual is not a drug addict in this case, because if his or her pain were adequately controlled, the patient would not have sought pain medications from other physicians. In addition, the patient is not a doctor shopping in the classic sense of seeking drugs to satisfy an addiction.

See ADDICTION/DEPENDENCE.

psilocybin A hallucinogenic drug that is derived from mushrooms, sometimes referred to as magic mushrooms, which are native to regions of MEXICO and South America. Psilocybin is chemically known as O-phosphoryl-4-hydroxy-N,N-dimethyl-tryptamine. Some sellers coat the psilocybin mushrooms in chocolate in order to disguise the bad taste, primarily transporting the drug through the mail to individuals throughout the United States. The mushroom is also cultivated in some parts of the United States, such as in Arkansas, California, North Dakota, Oregon, Rhode Island, South Dakota, and Wisconsin.

Most drug distributors of psilocybin are white males between the ages of 18 and 21 years, according to the National Drug Intelligence Center in the United States. These individuals are usually local DRUG DEALERS. According to the Substance Abuse and Mental Health Services Administration, of those ages 12 and older using a hallucinogen for the first time, 61 percent of males and 41 percent of females used psilocybin.

Psilocybin is an illegal Schedule I substance under the CONTROLLED SUBSTANCES ACT. It is not a commonly used drug of abuse in the United States. The lifetime use of psilocybin among adults ages 18 to 25 years was 13.4 percent in 2002, compared to 2.3 percent among adolescents ages 12 to 17 years.

At doses of 10 to 20 mg, the use of psilocybin may produce one or more of the following effects in those who abuse the drug:

- dilated pupils
- muscle relaxation
- visual and auditory hallucinations
- emotional distress

The drug is derived from dried or brewed mushrooms, and its effects are highly variable, based on the mushrooms that were used, as well as on the preservation and age of the extracted drug. Many species of "magic" mushrooms contain psilocybin as well as other, unknown chemicals. The hallucinogenic effect and the level of toxicity from ingesting this drug usually cannot be determined in advance, which is another reason why consumption of this drug is very dangerous. Psilocyn (4-hydroxy-N,N-dimethyltrptamine) is a similar drug to psilocybin and is also obtained from mushrooms.

Research on the effects of psilocybin was published in 2006 in *Psychopharmacology* based on a study performed at Johns Hopkins Medical School. In this study, subjects who had previously used hallucinogens were screened out, as were subjects with a serious mental disorder, such as bipolar disorder or SCHIZOPHRENIA. This was the first study on psilocybin performed in about 40 years. The study subjects received either psilocybin or methylphenidate (Ritalin). About half the subjects reported regular participation in religious activities, and all subjects had at least an intermittent interest in religion.

The researchers found that the psilocybin induced powerful spiritual experiences and positive changes in both attitude and behavior among some participants, while the methylphenidate had no such effect. (Keep in mind that the dosage of the drug was carefully controlled by researchers, in contrast to the psilocybin that is illegally purchased by users.) Some participants said it was the most powerful experience of their lives, akin to the birth of a child.

In contrast, some subjects said that the drug (which they did not know was psilocybin) caused them to be anxious, paranoid, and fearful, and several said they felt as if they had been in a war. Several participants who took psilocybin said they would never wish to repeat the experience. The researchers stated that in a less controlled environment, such reactions could cause panic and endanger users.

Cautioned the study authors, "It is important that the risks of hallucinogen use not be underestimated. Even in the present study in which the conditions of volunteer preparation and psilocybin administration were carefully designed to minimize adverse effects, with a high dose of psilocybin, 31% of the group of carefully screened volunteers experienced significant fear and 17% had transient ideas of reference/paranoia. Under unmonitored conditions, it is not difficult to imagine such effects escalating to panic and dangerous behavior. Also, the role of hallucinogens in precipitating or exacerbating enduring psychiatric conditions and long-lasting visual perceptual disturbances should remain a topic of research." Further research is likely to occur as a result of this study.

See also HALLUCINOGENIC DRUGS.

Griffiths, R. R., W. A. Richards, U. McCann, and R. Jesse. "Psilocybin Can Occasion Mystical-Type Experiences Having Substantial and Sustained Personal Meaning and Spiritual Significance," *Psychopharmacology* 187, no. 3 (August 2006): 268–283.

Joseph, Donald E., et al., eds. *Drugs of Abuse.* Washington, D.C.: U.S. Department of Justice, 2005.

psychiatric disorders   Mental health problems, which may range from those that are transient and responsive to treatment to chronic long-term disorders that can be very difficult to treat. Many substance abusers or those who are dependent on alcohol or drugs also have serious psychiatric problems, such as DEPRESSION and/or ANXIETY DISORDERS in addition to their drug and/or alcohol abuse or dependence. (This is sometimes called a DUAL DIAGNOSIS.)

In addition, patients who have some psychiatric disorders such as BIPOLAR DISORDER, CONDUCT DISORDER, or ANTISOCIAL PERSONALITY DISORDER are often drug and/or alcohol abusers. As well, individuals who have ATTENTION DEFICIT HYPERACTIVITY DISORDER, particularly those who are untreated for the disorder, have an increased risk for substance-induced disorders. Patients who are diagnosed with SCHIZOPHRENIA have a five-fold greater risk of developing drug or alcohol problems compared to the general population.

In some cases, psychiatric disorders are predictive for outcome; for example, in a study reported in the *American Journal of Psychiatry* in 2003, researchers analyzed 425 subjects who were dependent on at least one substance. They found that antisocial personality disorder was predictive for the use of a greater number of substances than among those without this disorder, and they also found that generalized anxiety disorder was predictive for alcohol and/or drug dependence diagnoses. They also found that outcomes among men were more closely associated with their psychiatric status than the outcomes among women. Among women, the researchers found that drug-dependent women who had psychiatric disorders had better outcomes than or similar outcomes to drug-dependent women who had no psychiatric disorder.

In addition, they found that phobias among women predicted a *better* outcome than among treated individuals who did not have phobias. They speculated that phobic women might have higher harm avoidance levels, although more research needs to be done to determine possible causes for this finding.

Alcohol Abuse and Dependence and Psychiatric Problems

Those who abuse alcohol or who are alcoholics have a high rate of psychiatric disorders. For example, data from *Alcohol Research & Health* in 2002 indicated that 11.3 percent of those who abused alcohol had major depressive disorder (depression). In addition, among those who were alcoholics, the

rate of depressive disorder was more than double the rate of alcohol abusers, or 29.2 percent.

The rate of anxiety disorders was very high among substance abusers: 29.1 percent among those who were alcohol abusers and more than a third (36.9 percent) of those dependent on alcohol. (See Table I.)

Substance Abuse and Psychiatric Disorders

Many individuals who abuse or who are dependent on illicit substances have psychiatric disorders; for example, according to the National Institute of Mental Health (NIMH), individuals who have antisocial personality disorder have a 15.5 percent greater risk than those who do not have psychiatric disorders for having a substance abuse problem. In addition, individuals who have BIPOLAR DISORDER who are in a manic state have a 14.5 percent increased risk of abusing drugs. Those who have panic disorder, a form of anxiety disorder, have a 4.3 times greater risk of having a substance abuse disorder and those who have OBSESSIVE COMPULSIVE DISORDER have a 3.4 times greater risk of substance abuse.

In some cases, the use of a particular drug has a risk of inducing psychiatric disorders, as with the abuse of AMPHETAMINE, ANABOLIC STEROIDS, COCAINE, METHYL-ENEDIOXYMETHAMPHETAMINE (MDMA/ECSTASY), KET-AMINE, and METHAMPHETAMINE.

Treatment for Psychiatric Disorders Has Somewhat Increased

Ronald Kessler and his colleagues studied the prevalence of mental disorders in the United States

TABLE I: PREVALENCE OF PSYCHIATRIC DISORDERS IN PEOPLE WHO HAVE ALCOHOL ABUSE AND ALCOHOL DEPENDENCE, ONE-YEAR RATE[1]

	Alcohol Abuse	Alcohol Dependence
Mood disorders	12.3 percent	29.2 percent
Major depressive disorder	11.3 percent	27.9 percent
Bipolar disorder	0.3 percent	1.9 percent
Anxiety disorders	29.1 percent	36.9 percent
Generalized anxiety disorder (GAD)	1.4 percent	11.6 percent
Panic disorder	1.3 percent	3.9 percent
Post-traumatic stress disorder	5.6 percent	7.7 percent

[1] The one-year rate is the percentage of people who met the criteria for the disorder during the year prior to the survey.
Source: Petrakis, Ismene L., M.D., et al. "Comorbidity of Alcoholism and Psychiatric Disorders." *Alcohol Research & Health* 26, no. 2 (2002): p. 82.

from 1990 to 2003. Although they found that the prevalence of psychiatric disorders had not changed in that period, they also discovered that the rate of treatment for these disorders had increased; for example, about 20 percent of patients who had a psychiatric disorder diagnosis received treatment over the period 1990–1992, while 33 percent of patients who had psychiatric disorders received treatment in 2001–3. However, it should also be noted that it is still true that *most* people who had psychiatric disorders still did not receive any treatment.

Treatment for individuals who have both psychiatric disorders and a substance abuse or dependence problem can be very complex.

See also ANTISOCIAL PERSONALITY DISORDER; ANXIETY DISORDERS; ATTENTION DEFICIT HYPERACTIVITY DISORDER; BINGE DRINKING; BIPOLAR DISORDER; CHILD ABUSE; CONDUCT DISORDER; DEPRESSION; DUAL DIAGNOSES; EATING DISORDERS; HOMELESSNESS; IMPULSE CONTROL; PSYCHIATRISTS; SCHIZOPHRENIA; SUICIDE.

Compton III, Wilson M., M.D., et al. "The Role of Psychiatric Disorders in Predicting Drug Dependence Treatment Outcomes." *American Journal of Psychiatry* 160, no. 5 (May 2003): 890–895.

Kessler, Ronald C., et al. "Prevalence and Treatment of Mental Disorders, 1990 to 2003." *New England Journal of Medicine* 352, no. 24 (June 16, 2005): 2,515–2,523.

Petrakis, Ismene, L., M.D., et al. "Comorbidity of Alcoholism and Psychiatric Disorders." *Alcohol Research & Health* 26, no. 2 (2002): 81–89.

psychiatrists Medical doctors trained in diagnosing and treating individuals who have severe psychiatric problems, such as ANXIETY DISORDERS, ATTENTION DEFICIT HYPERACTIVITY DISORDER, BIPOLAR DISORDER, DEPRESSION, and substance-induced disorders. Many patients who have psychiatric problems also have concurrent substance abuse problems, although it is often unclear or impossible to determine which factor is the driving force for the other problem: the psychiatric problem or the substance abuse.

Psychiatrists may treat the individual with medication and/or with therapy, although many psychiatrists refer patients who need psychotherapy to psychologists. Psychiatrists may manage rehabilitation facilities for individuals seeking to overcome their problems with drugs and/or alcohol.

See also ANTISOCIAL PERSONALITY DISORDER; DUAL DIAGNOSIS; EATING DISORDERS; PSYCHIATRIC DISORDERS; PSYCHOSIS, DRUG-INDUCED; PSYCHOTIC BEHAVIOR; SCHIZOPHRENIA.

psychological dependence A feeling and a compulsion that a person must have and use a substance of abuse, which persists well after addicted individuals have undergone rehabilitation and/or DETOXIFICATION for drugs and/or alcohol. When the recovered individual feels sad, depressed, or confused or experiences other intense emotions, he or she may feel drawn to use the substance that formerly provided relief by masking their psychological pain, either in a sedating or a stimulating manner. Recovered individuals may also associate with others who frequently use alcohol and/or drugs and who encourage them to resume their destructive behavior. Should they do so, they have relapsed and are often easily readdicted to the substance.

The psychological dependence that an individual has toward a substance can be an intense one, and it is usually the primary cause of RELAPSE in individuals who have successfully undergone rehabilitation but who then use the substance again. With recovery, they had overcome the body's physical need for the drug or alcohol, but the person's mind continues to be drawn to the substance. Some organizations, such as Alcoholics Anonymous or Narcotics Anonymous, seek to help individuals to master their psychological dependence on alcohol or drugs.

Psychological dependence is also experienced by individuals who have not become physically dependent on a particular drug or substance. The experience of needing a drug or fearing being without the drug can lead some individuals to stockpile medication or to seek additional prescriptions to prevent running out of them. Some individuals must carry a supply of a particular medication with them at all times, since being without the drug can lead to anxiety and/or panic.

The legal and illegal drugs that are the riskiest in terms of psychological dependence are also the ones with the quickest onset of action. Some examples of such drugs are ALPRAZOLAM (Xanax), DIAZEPAM (Valium), HYDROCODONE (Lortab, Lorcet), as well as COCAINE, CRACK COCAINE and nicotine.

All of these drugs have a rapid onset and a very short duration of action on the body. In addition, any drug that is either smoked or injected has a greater likelihood of causing a psychological dependence than do oral drugs because the smoked or injected drugs have a much more immediate effect on the body.

Most narcotic painkillers also have a risk for psychological dependence when they are abused, although the risk is much lower when the drug is used short-term to treat pain and under the supervision of a physician.

According to the Drug Enforcement Administration in *Drugs of Abuse.*

"The psychological dependence associated with narcotic addiction is complex and protracted. Long after the physical need for the drug has passed, the addict may continue to think and talk about the use of drugs and feel strange or overwhelmed coping with daily activities without being under the influence of drugs. There is a high probability that relapse will occur after narcotic withdrawal when neither the physical environment, nor the behavioral motivators that contributed to the abuse have been altered."

See also ADDICTION/DEPENDENCE; CRAVING; DENIAL.

psychosis, drug-induced   A mental disorder in which the individual is unable to distinguish reality from unreality as a direct result of drug abuse. Often such individuals are a threat to themselves and others, since they act on DELUSIONS (false beliefs, such as believing others are persecuting them) and HALLUCINATIONS (false sensory experiences, such as seeing or hearing people who are not there or having tactile experiences when no one and nothing is touching them). Some individuals who have become psychotic under particular drugs, such as AMPHETAMINE, COCAINE, or METHAMPHETAMINE, are very aggressive, violent, and difficult to control.

Hallucinogenic drugs such as PHENCYCLIDINE (PCP), lysergic acid diethylamide (LSD), or METHYLENEDIOXYMETHAMPHETAMINE (MDMA/ECSTASY),

may also trigger a psychotic break. Some individuals recover from a drug-induced psychosis, while others remain psychotic.

Alcoholic individuals who are undergoing WITHDRAWAL from alcohol may experience DELIRIUM TREMENS, a form of induced psychosis from which the individual usually recovers within days or weeks. (It is best for this individual to receive medical treatment because there is a risk of death with untreated delirium tremens.)

Some researchers believe that a drug-induced psychosis may be induced by cannabis (MARIJUANA), while others dispute this claim and say that, at most, marijuana may trigger a psychosis in individuals who are genetically prone to SCHIZOPHRENIA. In one study of 2,437 subjects ages 14 to 24 years old in Munich, Germany, reported in 2005 in the *British Medical Journal,* the researchers found that cannabis moderately increased the risk for psychosis; however, the risk was higher among subjects who had some evidence of a predisposition toward psychosis.

Say the researchers, "Frequent use of cannabis was associated with higher levels of risk in a dose-response fashion. Associations were independent of other variables known to increase the risk for psychosis. Also, the effect of cannabis remained significant after we corrected for baseline use of other drugs, tobacco, and alcohol."

Note that it should not be assumed that a person who is psychotic must have abused drugs. In some individuals, a psychosis may be genetically linked and also may be triggered by an unknown event.

See also PSYCHIATRIC DISORDERS; PSYCHIATRISTS.

Hénquet, Cecile, et al. "Prospective Cohort Study of Cannabis Use, Predisposition for Psychosis, and Psychotic Symptoms in Young People." *British Medical Journal* 330 (2005): 11–15.

psychotic behavior   The actions of a person who is unable to distinguish reality from the DELUSIONS and/or HALLUCINATIONS he or she experiences. The range of psychotic behavior is great. A person may shrink in fear from others who are no threat, because the individual is paranoid and sees them as a threat. Others may exhibit violent behavior because of auditory hallucinations telling them to attack people. Some may try to brush imaginary insects off the body, because they have a sensation of crawling insects on or under the skin. (See FORMICATION.)

In some cases, psychotic behavior is triggered by illicit drugs, such as AMPHETAMINES, COCAINE, and METHAMPHETAMINE, as well as hallucinogens such as LYSERGIC ACID DIETHYLAMIDE (LSD), PHENCYCLIDINE (PCP), or METHYLENEDIOXYMETHAMPHETAMINE (MDMA/ECSTASY). (See PSYCHOSIS, DRUG-INDUCED.)

In the case of amphetamines, constant use for a week or longer may induce a severe form of psychosis known as amphetamine psychosis. The symptoms of amphetamine psychosis may be difficult or even impossible to distinguish from those of SCHIZOPHRENIA. Many people recover from amphetamine psychosis, but an estimated 5 to 15 percent do *not* recover.

According to a study of mostly male prisoners (78 percent), 10 percent of the prisoners were psychotic as a result of abuse of amphetamine or cocaine abuse. The study was reported in a 2002 issue of *British Journal of Psychiatry*. The prisoners had a rate of psychosis that was 20 times greater than found in the general population.

The researchers also found that early use of drugs was a potential trigger for psychosis. The researchers conclude, "Early use of cocaine and amphetamines almost triples the risk of psychosis in addition to the effect exerted by drug dependence."

Individuals who are psychotic are unable to care for themselves or for others, such as their children. They may neglect or even abuse their children because of their break from reality. (See CHILD ABUSE.)

Psychotic behavior can often be treated with drugs, such as antipsychotic medications. However, some cases of drug-induced psychosis are less responsive to antipsychotic drugs than they are in the cases of mentally ill individuals who have not abused illegal drugs.

See also BIPOLAR DISORDER; DUAL DIAGNOSIS; FORMICATION; PSYCHIATRIC DISORDERS; PSYCHIATRISTS; PSYCHOTIC DISORDERS, DRUG-INDUCED; SCHIZOPHRENIA.

Farrell, M., et al. "Psychosis and Drug Dependence: Results for a National Survey of Prisoners." *British Journal of Psychiatry* 181, no. 5 (2002): 393–398.

PTSD   See POST-TRAUMATIC STRESS DISORDER.

racial/ethnic differences and drug and alcohol abuse In considering race or ethnicity alone in relation to drug and/or alcohol abuse or dependence, some racial and ethnic groups have a significantly higher rate of substance abuse than others. In many cases, whites (Caucasians) lead all other racial and ethnic groups in terms of the percentage of those who have drug and alcohol abuse problems. However, some groups, such as American Indians or Alaska Natives, have a high rate of drug abuse and dependence compared to that of other races and ethnicities. In general, Asians have a low rate of alcohol or drug abuse and dependence.

Definition of Racial/Ethnic Groups

In the United States, the following definitions are used for racial or ethnic groups. *American Indian* or *Alaska Native* is used to denote a person who has origins in any of the original peoples of North and South America (including Central America) and who maintains a cultural identification, either through tribal affiliations or community recognition.

The *Asian* or *Pacific Islander* is an individual who has origins in any of the original peoples of the Far East, Southeast Asia, the Indian subcontinent, or the Pacific Islands, including such areas as China, India, Japan, Korea, the Philippine Islands, Hawaii, and Samoa.

The *black* or *African American* is a person having origins in any of the black racial groups of Africa.

The *Hispanic* is a person of Mexican, Puerto Rican, Cuban, Central or South American, or other Spanish culture or origin, regardless of race.

The *white* is a person having origins in any of the original peoples of Europe, North Africa, or the Middle East.

It should also be noted that some individuals are members of more than one racial or ethnic group.

Drug Abuse and Race/Ethnicity

According to the National Institute on Drug Abuse, in general, whites have a higher rate of illegal drug abuse than blacks, although the rates of abuse differ according to the drug. In contrast, American Indian/Alaska Natives have a significantly higher rate of drug abuse. (This group also has a high rate of alcohol abuse and ALCOHOLISM.) For example, in considering the current abuse of illicit drugs among individuals age 12 to 17 years old in 2004, 9.3 percent of blacks and 11.1 percent of whites had abused drugs. However, among American Indians or Alaska Natives, 26.0 percent currently abused illicit drugs, nearly three times the rate for blacks. *Current drug abuse* was defined as the use of an illicit drug during the month before the National Survey on Drug Use and Health had occurred.

Hispanics had a drug abuse rate between the percentages of whites and blacks in terms of current illicit drug use, or 10.2 percent. (See Table I.)

Among some Hispanic subgroups, such as Puerto Ricans, drug abuse is higher than for all other groups except American Indians/Alaska Natives. For other subgroups of Hispanics, the rates are either at or below the rates of drug abuse for blacks and whites.

In considering Asian subgroups, Koreans in the United States have about the same level of illegal drug abuse as blacks or whites; however, all other subgroups of Asians have a lower rate of abuse.

Alcohol Use

In considering the use of alcohol among differing races and ethnicities, whites had the heaviest consumption in the United States in 2004. Among whites, 32.6 percent used alcohol in the past month, compared to 26.6 percent among Hispanics, 26.4 percent among those reporting two or more races,

TABLE I: RATE OF CURRENT ILLICIT DRUG USE AMONG YOUTHS AGES 12–17, BY RACE AND PERCENTAGE, 2004

American Indians or Alaska Natives	26.0
Two or more races	12.2
Whites	11.1
Hispanics	10.2
African Americans	9.3
Asians	6.0
All youths	10.6

Source: Adapted from Substance Abuse and Mental Health Services Administration. *Overview of Findings for the 2004 National Survey on Drug Use and Health.* Rockville, Md.: Department of Health and Human Services, September 2005, p. 18.

24.3 percent among American Indians or Alaska Natives, 19.1 percent among blacks, and 16.4 percent among Asians. Note that alcohol use does not always denote alcohol abuse or alcoholism.

Heavy Alcohol Use and Binge Drinking There are also racial differences when considering heavy alcohol use and BINGE DRINKING; for example, among adolescents ages 12–17 years in 2004, 4.7 percent of American Indians or Alaska Natives were heavy alcohol abusers, compared to 3.3 per of blacks and 2.7 percent of both whites and Hispanics. When considering binge drinking again American Indians/Alaska Natives had the highest percentage of binge drinkers, 15.1 percent of this group, followed by whites at 12.6 percent.

In contrast, blacks had a much lower rate, or 4.9 percent, who were binge drinkers, and Asians also had a low rate (5 percent). (See Table II.)

The rates of heavy alcohol use and binge drinking were much higher among young adults ages 18–25 years than among adolescents; for example, among whites, nearly half (47.7 percent) of young adults had engaged in binge drinking, followed by young adults who were American Indians or Alaska Natives (42.3 percent). (See Table III.)

Specific Drugs and Ethnic/Racial Groups
Some data sources that provide substance abuse information on a specific type of drug limit their data to black, white, and Hispanic groups, and when such information is provided, often it is Hispanics who lead in drug abuse, followed by whites and then blacks. For example, in *Drug Use among Racial/Ethnic Minorities,* published by the National Institute on Drug Abuse in 2003, among youths who abused drugs within the past 30 days, by percentage among high school seniors, the rate was highest among Hispanics (24.6 percent), followed by whites (22.7 percent) and then blacks (19.0 percent).

This pattern was also seen with INHALANTS, HALLUCINOGENIC DRUGS, LYSERGIC ACID DETHYLAMIDE (LSD), and powdered COCAINE. The one exception was with CRACK COCAINE, in which Hispanics led in the percentage of abuse, followed by blacks and then whites. (See Table IV.)

National Institute on Drug Abuse. *Drug Use among Racial/Ethnic Minorities,* Bethesda, Md.: National Institutes of Health, 2003.

TABLE II: ALCOHOL USE, BINGE ALCOHOL USE, AND HEAVY ALCOHOL USE BY RACE AND ETHNICITY, AMONG PERSONS AGES 12–17 YEARS, BY PERCENTAGE, 2004

	Alcohol Use	Binge Alcohol Use	Heavy Alcohol Use
Not Hispanic or Latino	17.5	10.8	2.7
White	19.9	12.6	3.3
Black or African American	9.8	4.9	0.6
American Indian or Alaska Native	18.5	15.1	4.2
Asian	9.4	5.0	0.5
Two or more Races	18.2	11.8	3.3
Hispanic or Latino	18.0	12.3	2.7

Note: Binge alcohol use is defined as drinking five or more drinks on the same occasion (such as at the same time or within a couple of hours of each other) on at least one day in the past 30 days. *Heavy alcohol use* is defined as drinking five or more drinks on the same occasion on each of five or more days in the past 30 days.
Source: Adapted from Substance Abuse and Mental Health Services Administration. *Overview of Findings for the 2004 National Survey on Drug Use and Health.* Rockville, Md.: Department of Health and Human Services, September 2005, p. 253.

TABLE III: ALCOHOL USE, BINGE ALCOHOL USE, AND HEAVY ALCOHOL USE AMONG PERSONS AGES 18 TO 25 YEARS, BY PERCENTAGE 2004

	Alcohol Use	Binge Alcohol Use	Heavy Alcohol Use
Not Hispanic or Latino	63.1	42.6	16.4
White	67.7	47.7	19.4
Black or African American	48.5	25.7	5.9
American Indian or Alaska Native	55.8	42.3	13.1
Asian	46.6	23.1	6.9
Two or More Races	68.6	47.2	17.7
Hispanic or Latino	48.2	35.0	9.0

Note: Binge alcohol use is defined as drinking five or more drinks on the same occasion (such as at the same time or within a couple of hours of each other) on at least one day in the past 30 days. *Heavy alcohol use* is defined as drinking five or more drinks on the same occasion on each of five or more days in the past 30 days.
Source: Adapted from Substance Abuse and Mental Health Services Administration. *Overview of Findings for the 2004 National Survey on Drug Use and Health.* Rockville, Md.: Department of Health and Human Services, September 2005, p. 254.

TABLE IV: ESTIMATED PREVALENCE OF LIFETIME, ANNUAL, 30-DAY, AND DAILY USE OF SELECTED DRUGS, BY RACE/ETHNICITY FOR STUDENTS IN THE UNITED STATES IN GRADES 8, 10, AND 12, BY PERCENTAGE, IN 2000

Estimated Prevalence	Marijuana			Inhalants			Hallucinogens			LSD			Cocaine			Crack cocaine		
	8th	10th	12th	8th	10th	12th	8th	10th	12th	8th	10th	12th	8th	10th	12th	8th	10th	12th
Lifetime																		
White, non-Hispanic	19.0	40.1	49.4	19.9	18.5	16.7	4.9	10.5	14.9	4.2	9.1	13.2	4.2	7.4	9.9	2.8	3.7	4.4
Black, non-Hispanic	23.8	39.5	45.7	10.5	6.6	4.6	1.3	1.4	2.1	0.9	1.2	1.7	1.4	1.2	1.9	0.9	0.9	0.8
Hispanic	27.1	46.0	55.0	23.1	17.6	15.4	6.8	8.6	15.3	5.8	7.6	13.1	8.9	12.4	13.3	5.6	6.8	6.3
Annual																		
White, non-Hispanic	14.9	32.6	38.2	10.9	8.4	6.4	3.1	7.6	9.9	2.6	6.5	8.3	2.5	4.7	6.2	1.7	2.2	2.5
Black, non-Hispanic	16.1	27.6	30.0	4.3	2.0	1.9	0.7	1.0	1.6	0.5	0.9	1.3	0.8	0.6	1.0	0.4	0.5	0.5
Hispanic	20.1	34.8	40.5	12.2	6.3	6.3	4.0	5.2	9.6	3.5	4.6	7.6	4.7	8.0	7.6	2.9	4.0	3.4
30-day																		
White, non-Hispanic	8.4	20.2	22.7	5.2	2.9	2.1	1.2	2.9	3.2	1.0	2.2	2.3	1.1	1.8	2.5	0.8	0.8	1.0
Black, non-Hispanic	9.3	15.8	19.0	2.3	1.1	1.3	0.5	0.5	0.9	0.3	0.5	0.8	0.4	0.3	0.8	0.2	0.3	0.4
Hispanic	12.7	20.5	24.6	5.6	2.3	3.1	2.0	2.0	3.8	1.7	1.6	2.4	2.7	3.0	3.6	1.5	1.4	2.1

Source: National Institute on Drug Abuse. *Drug Use among Racial/Ethnic Minorities.* Bethesda, Md.: National Institutes of Health, 2003, pp. 72–73.

Substance Abuse and Mental Health Services Administration. *Overview of Findings for the 2004 National Survey on Drug Use and Health.* Rockville, Md.: Department of Health and Human Services, September 2005.

relapse The recurrence of the abuse of alcohol and/or drugs after a period during which the substance of abuse is not used. Many individuals who experience a relapse mistakenly believe that relapse indicates that they cannot ever overcome their problem with ALCOHOLISM or drug dependence; however, relapses are common and even expected by most substance abuse counselors. Even when treatment has been successful, often the basic CRAVING for alcohol or drugs remains.

Some factors may increase the odds of a relapse, such as associating with friends who continue to use the substance that the individual is actively trying to avoid, whether it is ALCOHOL, MARIJUANA, or another drug. In addition, increased levels of STRESS escalate the likelihood of a relapse, as the individual struggles to deal with whatever the problem is. If the individual has learned healthier ways to cope with increased stress, the likelihood of relapse is decreased. Some individuals seek to prevent relapse by joining a twelve-step group, such as Alcoholics Anonymous or Cocaine Anonymous.

See ADDICTION/DEPENDENCE; ALCOHOLISM; DRUG TREATMENT; TREATMENT FACILITIES.

Rohypnol   See FLUNITRAZEPAM/ROHYPNOL.

runaway/throwaway youths   Children ages seven to 17 who either run away from home or are purposely sent away from their homes by their parents or other caretakers. According to the National Center for Juvenile Justice in their 2006 report on juvenile offenders and victims, there were an estimated 1.7 million youths who left home because they ran away or their caretakers ordered them to leave in 1999. Most of these youths were whites (57 percent) and most were ages 15–17 years old (68 percent). There were equal numbers of males and females. Most of the youths who ran away or were ordered away were gone for less than a week (77 percent), and the largest proportion of the displacements occurred in the summer (39 percent). Some of the youths (21 percent) had left home or were ordered from home in relation to CHILD ABUSE (physical or sexual abuse), and these youths feared they would be abused again upon their return home.

Drugs were involved in many of these cases, according to researchers; for example, 19 percent of the youths were dependent (addicted) to substances and 18 percent were in the company of someone who was known to abuse drugs. Less than 1 percent of the youths said that they had exchanged sex for drugs, money, food, or shelter, and 2 percent said that they were with a sexually exploitive person.

See also ADOLESCENTS; CHILD ABUSE; FOSTER CARE; SEXUAL ASSAULTS.

Snyder, Howard N., and Melissa Sickmund. *Juvenile Offenders and Victims: 2006 National Report.* Washington, D.C.: National Center for Juvenile Justice, March 2006.

scheduled drugs Legal and illegal drugs that are classified under the CONTROLLED SUBSTANCES ACT and are under the control of the Drug Enforcement Administration (DEA). In addition to federal control, these drugs are under state control. Scheduled drugs are considered to have a potential for abuse and dependence. There are five drug schedules. Schedule I includes only illegal drugs with a high potential for abuse. Schedules II–V are drugs that are lawful if they are used under the direction of a physician but also have varying levels of abuse and dependence potential. Schedule I drugs have the greatest abuse potential among the five schedules and Schedule V drugs have the least abuse potential. (See Appendix XIV for a listing of scheduled drugs.)

According to the DEA in their 2005 book *Drugs of Abuse,* several key factors are considered in determining under which schedule a drug should be placed. For example, the criteria for placing a drug under Schedule I are as follows:

- The drug or other substance has a high potential for abuse.
- The drug or other substance has no currently accepted medical use in treatment in the United States.
- There is a lack of accepted safety for use of the drug or other substance under medical supervision.

Examples of drugs that are Schedule I drugs are HEROIN, LYSERGIC ACID DIETHYAMIDE (LSD), and MARIJUANA. Note that the federal government does not recognize any medical use of marijuana as of this writing, despite the fact that some states have passed laws "legalizing" marijuana. Only Congress has the authority to change existing federal laws on marijuana, a move that is actively opposed by organizations such as the DEA.

In classifying Schedule II drugs, the following criteria are used:

- The drug or other substance has a high potential for abuse.
- The drug or other substance has a currently accepted medical use in treatment in the United States or a currently accepted medical use with severe restrictions.
- Abuse of the drug or other substance may lead to severe psychological or physical dependence.

Examples of Schedule II drugs are COCAINE, METHADONE, METHAMPHETAMINE, MORPHINE, and PHENCYLIDINE (PCP).

The criteria for Schedule III drugs are as follows:

- The drug or other substance has less potential for abuse than the drugs or other substances in Schedules I and II.
- The drug or other substance has a currently accepted medical use in treatment in the United States.
- Abuse of the drug or other substance may lead to moderate or low physical dependence or high psychological dependence.

Examples of Schedule III drugs are ANABOLIC STEROIDS, CODEINE, HYDROCODONE with aspirin or acetaminophen, and some BARBITURATES.

The criteria for Schedule IV drugs are as follows:

- The drug or other substance has a low potential for abuse relative to the drugs or other substances in Schedule III.
- The drug or other substance has a currently accepted medical use in treatment in the United States.

- Abuse of the drug or other substance may lead to limited physical dependence or psychological dependence relative to the drugs or other substances in Schedule III.

Examples of drugs that are in Schedule IV are PRO- POXYPHENE (Darvon, Darvocet), DIAZEPAM (Valium), and ALPRAZOLAM (Xanax).

The criteria for Schedule V drugs are as follows:

- The drug or other substance has a low potential for abuse relative to the drugs or other substances in Schedule IV.
- The drug or other substance has a currently accepted medical use in treatment in the United States.
- Abuse of the drug or other substances may lead to limited physical dependence or psychological dependence relative to the drugs or other substances in Schedule IV.

Cough medicines with codeine are an example of a Schedule V drug.

See also CRIME AND CRIMINALS; HYDROCODONE; LAW ENFORCEMENT; METHADONE; NARCOTICS; ORGA- NIZED CRIME; OXYCODONE; OxyContin; PRESCRIPTION DRUG ABUSE.

Joseph, Donald E., ed., et al. *Drugs of Abuse*. Washington, D.C.: U.S. Department of Justice, 2005.

schizophrenia   A severe psychiatric thought dis- order that is characterized by psychosis and the inability of the individual to distinguish reality from fantasy. It is also characterized by auditory and/or visual HALLUCINATIONS and DELUSIONS. Auditory hallucinations are generally more common than visual or tactile hallucinations. In some cases, drugs may induce a state that is difficult or impossible to distinguish from schizophrenia, particularly in the case of the excessive use and abuse of ANABOLIC STEROIDS, COCAINE, AMPHETAMINE, and METHAM- PHETAMINE. Hallucinogenic drugs may also trigger PSYCHOTIC BEHAVIOR that resembles the behavior of a person who has schizophrenia.

According to the National Institute of Mental Health, men and women are affected by schizo- phrenia at the same frequency, and an estimated 2.4 million adults ages 18 and older in the United States have schizophrenia (about 1.1 percent of the adult population). Among men, the illness usually appears in the late teens or early twenties. Among women, the onset may occur in the twenties or early thirties. However, schizophrenia can also occur in childhood or adolescence.

Many people diagnosed with schizophrenia are substance abusers. For example, the Epidemiologic Catchment Area study determined that about 34 percent of people diagnosed with schizophrenia or schizophreniform disorder (a disorder related to schizophrenia) together had met the criteria for alcohol use disorder at some point in their lives, and about 28 percent met the criteria for a drug misuse disorder (with the exception of nicotine dependence). In addition, schizophrenia patients have a five-fold risk of developing drug or alcohol problems compared to the general population.

In one study of patients who had schizophrenia and schizoaffective disorder (a psychotic disorder that is a combination of schizophrenia and a mood disorder, such as either DEPRESSION or BIPOLAR DIS- ORDER) reported by Alain Dervaux and colleagues in the *American Journal of Psychiatry* in 2001, the researchers studied 100 hospitalized patients, of whom 91 individuals were diagnosed with schizo- phrenia and nine with schizoaffective disorder. Of these patients, 41 were substance abusers.

The researchers sought to determine whether there were factors contributing to the substance dis- order, and they found that significantly high levels of impulsivity and sensation seeking were present among the psychotic patients who were substance abusers. The researchers disputed that the patients were seeking to self-medicate their symptoms, as has often been hypothesized by others when there is drug abuse. They state: "Our results indicate that schizophrenic patients with a lifetime comorbidity of substance abuse or dependence are more impul- sive and seek more intense sensations than schizo- phrenic patients without abuse or impulsivity."

In another study, reported in *Psychiatric Bulletin*, on the patterns of substance misuse in schizophre- nia patients and conducted in Dublin, Ireland, the researchers Rita M. Condren, John O'Connor, and Roy Browne found that the patterns of illicit drug use and alcohol abuse were similar in the schizophrenia patients and the control group. For example, 45 percent of the schizophrenia patients abused illicit drugs, compared to 43 percent of the control groups. However, the patients who had schizophrenia had a significantly higher use of alcohol (33 percent) than the controls (25 percent).

The most commonly abused drug among the schizophrenia patients was MARIJUANA (42 percent), compared to a 40 percent abuse rate among the control group. The patients who had schizophrenia had a lower rate of consuming some substances such as METHYLENEDIOXYMETHAMPHETAMINE (MDMA/ECSTASY) (4 percent), versus the 20 percent rate among the control subjects, as well as METHADONE (2 percent), versus the 5 percent among the controls. The schizophrenia patients had a higher rate of abusing multiple substances (18 percent) than the controls (11 percent).

Another study of 262 patients who had schizophrenia or schizoaffective disorder was reported in the *American Journal of Drug and Alcohol Abuse* in 2000. Most of the patients (80 percent) were African American and most (56 percent) were male. Among these patients, 23 percent were currently using alcohol and 16 percent were currently using illicit drugs.

The researchers found that the substance-abusing patients had a higher rate of missing their psychiatric appointments than those who did not abuse alcohol or drugs, and that they also had a higher number of psychiatric hospitalizations over the past two years. The research also revealed that drug abuse was correlated with both negative and positive symptoms, while alcohol abuse was correlated only with negative symptoms when the patient received alcohol treatment. (Note that the term *positive symptoms* in schizophrenia refers to acting out and aggression, while *negative symptoms* refers to withdrawal and depressive symptoms.)

The author states that her data "underline the importance of the relation of substance use to outcome in schizophrenia and the need for further research into the nature and treatment of these patients with DUAL DIAGNOSES and their poor outcome. The reason for this poor outcome most likely involves a number of factors. Substance abuse has been associated with poor treatment adherence, which in turn can be associated with poor outcome. Also, there is much conjecture about substance-abuse causing neuronal damage and diminished cognitive performance over time."

Symptoms and Diagnostic Path
The symptoms of schizophrenia usually appear in late adolescence or early adulthood and they are seen in both males and females. Individuals who have schizophrenia exhibit unusual behavior that is often noticeable to the average person because it is unusual and obvious. However, a trained mental health professional must diagnose schizophrenia and differentiate it from BIPOLAR DISORDER, DEPRESSION with psychotic features, or other psychotic disorders that may be present. In addition, people who have schizophrenia are at risk for other psychiatric disorders, such as depression and ANXIETY DISORDERS.

Individuals who have schizophrenia may exhibit some or all of the following:

- hallucinations
- delusional thinking, such as PARANOIA
- very poor personal hygiene
- confused thinking
- flat affect (a lack of detectable emotion) or florid (agitated) affect

Treatment Options and Outlook
In the recent past, there was little hope for individuals who had schizophrenia, who usually remained ill for much of their lives. Many were homeless and unmedicated, and often they died well before others of their generation. However, medication breakthroughs have enabled some schizophrenia patients to lead productive lives. Medications such as aripiprazole (Abilify) or clozapine (Clozaril) help patients to maintain clearer thinking than medications used in the past, which caused heavy sedation, extreme weight gain, and chronic tics associated with TARDIVE DYSKINESIA.

Many patients who have severe psychiatric illnesses such as schizophrenia and also who abuse substances have not been treated in the past, in part because of a lack of facilities but also in part because of a sense of hopelessness about such patients among some practitioners and among members of society at large. This is tragic because many patients can benefit from treatment for both schizophrenia and substance-induced disorders.

Robert Drake and Kim Mueser in their article in *Alcohol Research & Health,* state, "These positive findings have fueled attempts to develop more effective interventions for AUD [alcohol use disorder] among schizophrenia patients." They point out that treatment is very important in this population, because individuals who have both mental illness and substance use disorders are often homeless or incarcerated.

Drake and Mueser recommend the following steps for patients who have schizophrenia and alcohol use disorder:

1. engagement, which involves building a trusting treatment relationship
2. persuasion, which entails developing motivation to manage both illnesses and pursue recovery
3. active treatment, which encompasses development of the skills and supports needed for illness management and recovery
4. relapse prevention, which involves strategies to avoid and minimize the effects of relapses

Risk Factors and Preventive Measures

Schizophrenia appears to have a genetic risk, although it may be triggered by unknown environmental agents in vulnerable individuals. It is unknown how to prevent the disease, since there are no warnings, and once it is present, it is already a problem that must be treated. However, it should also be noted that sometimes the abuse of drugs can trigger a schizophrenic episode in a vulnerable person; thus, the avoidance of drug abuse may limit the risks for those for whom schizophrenia is a family health problem.

Some studies indicate that schizophrenia can be triggered by heavy and chronic abuse of marijuana in individuals, particularly adolescents who are susceptible to the development of schizophrenia. These studies indicate that the marijuana was not used to self-treat any already existing symptoms of psychosis. Authors Degenhardt and Hall reviewed the results of six longitudinal studies on marijuana use and schizophrenia for their 2006 article for the *Canadian Journal of Psychiatry.* Concluded these authors, "It is most plausible that cannabis use precipitates schizophrenia in individuals who are vulnerable because of a personal or family history of schizophrenia."

According to Sunjiv Kumra, M.D., in an article in *Minnesota Medicine* in 2007, repeated abuse of marijuana (also known as cannabis) may affect the development of frontal white matter in the brain based on research at the University of Minnesota.

Researchers at the University of Minnesota studied white matter development in adolescents with schizophrenia and also in adolescents who were healthy. In addition, the researchers observed age-related changes. According to Dr. Kumra, the frontal lobe is involved in auditory hallucinations (hearing voices) and working memory.

The researchers discovered that white matter abnormalities were more dramatic among adolescents with schizophrenia and the use of marijuana. Some researchers have previously postulated that individuals may develop schizophrenia first and then begin to use drugs in order to cope with their symptoms; however, some current researchers now believe that the drug use precedes and may cause the psychotic symptoms of schizophrenia.

See also ANTISOCIAL PERSONALITY DISORDER; BIPOLAR DISORDER; DEPRESSION; DUAL DIAGNOSIS; PSYCHIATRIC DISORDERS; PSYCHOSIS, DRUG-INDUCED.

Condren, Rita M., John O'Connor, and Roy Browne. "Prevalence and Patterns of Substance Misuse in Schizophrenia." *Psychiatric Bulletin* 25 (2001): 17–20.

Degenhardt, L., and W. Hall, "Is Cannabis Use a Contributory Cause of Psychosis," *Canadian Journal of Psychiatry* 51, no. 9 (August 2006): 556–565.

Dervaux, Alain, M.D., et al. "Is Substance Abuse in Schizophrenia Related to Impulsivity, Sensation Seeking, or Anhedonia?" *American Journal of Psychiatry* 158, no. 3 (March 2001): 492–494.

Drake, Robert E., M.D., and Kim T. Mueser, "Co-Occurring Alcohol Use Disorder and Schizophrenia." *Alcohol Research & Health* 26, no. 2 (2002): 99–102.

Kumra, Sanjiv, M.D, "Schizophrenia and Cannabis Use," Minnesota Medicine 90 (January 2007). Available online at URL: http://ww.mmaonline.net/Publications/MNMed2007/January/clinical-Kumra.cfm. Downloaded September 20, 2007.

National Institute of Mental Health. "The Numbers Count: Mental Disorders in America." Rockville, Md.: National Institutes of Health, 2006. Available online. URL: http://www.nimh.nih.gov/publicat/numbers.cfm#readNow. Downloaded April 22, 2006.

Swofford, Cheryl D. "Double Jeopardy: Schizophrenia and Substance Use." *American Journal of Drug and Alcohol Abuse* (August 2000). Available online. URL: http://www.findarticles.com/p/articles/mi_m0978/is_3_26-ai_65803039.print. Downloaded January 10, 2006.

schools and school policies Elementary, middle, and high schools and the rules that they impose on students, such as that a student who takes any non-authorized drug, whether legal or illegal, to school may be suspended or expelled. Such policies, when followed to extremes, have sometimes caused problems for students who have taken minor analgesics to school, such as acetaminophen or aspirin. In some cases, students taking insulin for their diabetes have also had problems with restrictive school policies. However, in general, they are meant to serve as a deterrent to students who might otherwise take illegal drugs such as MARIJUANA or METH-AMPHETAMINE to school.

Some students abuse drugs or have access to drugs, by their own admission, and sometimes this drug abuse takes place on school grounds. According to the 2005 report from the National Center for Education Statistics on indicators of school crime and safety, nearly half (45 percent) of students in grades 9–12 said that they had consumed at least one drink of alcohol in the past 30 days and 5 percent said they had consumed at least one drink on school property within the past 30 days.

About 12 percent of the schools said that they experienced the distribution of illegal drugs in their schools, or 85,000 incidents. About half the schools reported drug incidents to the police. Researchers also found that 22 percent of students reported using marijuana anywhere in the past 30 days, and 6 percent said that they had used marijuana on school property in the past 30 days.

Nearly a third of students say that drugs are accessible to them in school. About 29 percent of students in grades 9–12 nationwide in 2003 said that drugs had been made available to them on

TABLE I: PERCENTAGE OF STUDENTS IN GRADES 9–12 WHO REPORTED THAT DRUGS WERE MADE AVAILABLE TO THEM ON SCHOOL PROPERTY DURING THE PREVIOUS 12 MONTHS, BY SELECTED STUDENTS AND SCHOOL CHARACTERISTICS: SELECTED YEARS, 1999–2003

Student or School Characteristic	1999	2001	2003
Total	30.2	28.5	28.7
Sex			
Male	34.7	34.6	31.9
Female	25.7	22.7	25.0
Race/ethnicity			
White	25.8	28.3	27.5
Black	25.3	21.9	23.1
Hispanic	36.9	34.2	36.4
Asian	25.7	25.7	22.5
American Indian	30.6	34.5	31.3
Pacific Islander	46.9	50.2	34.7
More than one race	36.0	34.5	36.6
Grade			
9th	27.6	29.0	29.5
10th	32.1	29.0	29.2
11th	31.1	28.7	29.9
12th	39.5	26.9	24.9
Urbanicity			
Urban	30.3	32.0	31.1
Suburban	29.7	26.6	28.4
Rural	32.1	28.2	26.2

Source: Adapted from: DeVoe, Jill F., et al. *Indicators of School Crime and Safety: 2005.* Washington, D.C.: U.S. Department of Education and U.S. Department of Justice, October 2005. p. 89.

school property. (See Table I.) Males were more likely to report that drugs were available to them at school (31.9 percent) than females (25 percent). Students of more than one race, Hispanics, and Pacific Islanders were most likely to say that drugs were made available to them at school, and urban students were the most likely of urban, suburban, and rural students to say that drugs were available.

In 2003, 21 percent of the students said that street GANGS had been present in their schools in the past six months.

Some schools took action with regard to the use of drugs or alcohol; for example, 10 percent of public schools took one or more serious disciplinary actions for the distribution of illegal drugs and 20 percent acted in the cases of the possession or use of illegal drugs or alcohol. A serious disciplinary action included suspensions for five days or more, which represented 83 percent of all disciplinary actions. Other serious disciplinary actions included expulsions or transfers. Eleven percent of the students who were punished were expelled and about 7 percent were transferred to specialized schools.

Many schools also have general security policies; for example, 75 percent locked or monitored doors and 34 percent controlled access to the school grounds by using locked or monitored gates. Nearly all schools (97 percent) required visitors to sign in or check in when entering the school.

Middle schools and high schools had higher security measures than elementary schools; for example, about 13 percent of high schools required students to wear picture IDs, as did 6 percent of middle schools and 2 percent of elementary schools. About 4 percent of elementary schools performed random metal detector checks on students, as did 15 percent of secondary schools.

See also ADOLESCENTS; ATTENTION DEFICIT HYPER-ACTIVITY DISORDER; DIVERSION, DRUG; METHYLPHENI-DATE (RITALIN/CONCERTA/FOCALIN, ETC.).

DeVoe, Jill F., et al. *Indicators of School Crime and Safety: 2005.* Washington, D.C.: U.S. Department of Education and U.S. Department of Justice, October 2005.

self-help groups   Organizations that are designed to help individuals to help themselves with a particular problem that the group members all share. The most famous self-help group in the United States and the world is Alcoholics Anonymous, a group that was originally formed by Bill H. in 1935. Bill H. was a man who had ALCOHOLISM who had developed the theory that alcoholism was a disease, which he believed could be controlled by working with others who had experienced the same problem.

Today there are numerous self-help groups nationwide as well as in other countries, designed to assist individuals with a broad array of addictive behavior, such as Narcotics Anonymous and Cocaine Anonymous, many of which have modeled their organizations on the basic principles of Alcoholics Anonymous.

In many cases, people who attend self-help support groups benefit by meeting and exchanging information with others who intimately understand the problems that they face and who may give them the courage and the information that they need to realize they can overcome their addiction.

In some cases, the court may order that individuals attend specific self-help group meetings, as a condition for regaining the legal custody of their children or avoiding incarceration.

sexual assaults   Rape or other forms of sexual attacks, which vary depending on state laws. BINGE DRINKING, alcohol abuse, and drug abuse are all associated with an increased risk for sexual assaults by the perpetrator. In addition, substance abuse of the victim also increases the risk for sexual assault. For victims, substance abuse may decrease the ability to make a conscious decision to consent or decline to have sex. It also decreases the inhibitions of predators, who perpetrate sexual assaults that they probably would not have made without the presence of drugs and/or alcohol.

Among inmates in jail for sexual assaults, about half said that they had used alcohol or drugs when they committed the crime.

Some research has looked at drug use among sexual assault victims. According to a study of 144 women who identified themselves as sexual assault victims, commissioned by the National Criminal Justice Reference Service, nearly 62 percent of the subjects tested positive for drugs in toxicology studies of their hair and urine, and 4 percent of the sexual assault victims were given DATE RAPE DRUGS without their knowledge or permission. (Other studies have estimated that about 40 percent of sexual assault victims used drugs and/or alcohol at the time of the assault.) The victims in this study ranged from 18 to 56 years, with an average age of 27 years.

There are many long-term consequences of sexual assaults. Many women who have been sexually assaulted suffer from POST-TRAUMATIC STRESS DISORDER (PTSD), anxiety, and DEPRESSION, and often they subsequently turn to the abuse of alcohol and/or drugs as a means to relieve their anxiety and depression. Sexual assault victims also have an increased risk for SUICIDE.

See also CHILD ABUSE; CRIME AND CRIMINALS; VIOLENCE.

Negrusz, Adam, Matthew Juhascik, and R. E. Gaensslen. "Estimate of the Incidence of Drug-Facilitated Sexual Assault in the United States." Washington, D.C.: U.S. Department of Justice. November 2005. Available online. URL: http://www.ncjrs.gov/pdffiles1/nij/grants/21200.pdf. Downloaded June 19, 2006.

sleep remedies, addictive Prescribed medications that are given to individuals who are severely and/or chronically unable to sleep. Most individuals under severe STRESS may need such drugs for a brief period, such as a few weeks, but some individuals continue to use the medications for a longer period. Many sleep remedies are Schedule IV drugs under the CONTROLLED SUBSTANCES ACT, because they entail some risk for addiction, particularly if they are abused.

Examples of prescribed sleep remedies are eszoplicone (Lunesta), zaleplon (Sonata), and zoldipem (Ambien, Ambien CR). Another sleep remedy, that is *not* a scheduled drug, is ramelton (Rozarem). If the drug is effective, it usually works in about an hour, causing the individual to fall asleep and decreasing the number of times during the night when the person awakens. In some cases, such as among individuals who are suicidal, sleep remedies may increase the risk for suicidal ideation; as a result, DEPRESSION patients usually should not be treated with sleep remedies alone. In general, prescribed sleep remedies work best when they are not taken with food.

Some individuals who use prescribed sleep remedies experience rebound insomnia for one or two nights after stopping a prescribed sleep remedy. Physicians may choose to taper medications down from sleep remedies rather than stopping them suddenly, to prevent such rebound insomnia.

Not all sleep remedies are prescribed. Some insomnia patients take mild over-the-counter sedatives or herbal remedies, such as melatonin.

stimulants Drugs that affect the central nervous system and reverse the effects of fatigue on mental and physical tasks. Stimulants are sometimes called "uppers." Some stimulants are legally used, such as CAFFEINE. Nicotine is also a legal stimulant when it is used by adults—nicotine is *not* legally used by minors in the United States.

Prescribed stimulants are Schedule II drugs under the CONTROLLED SUBSTANCES ACT, and they include medications given to treat individuals for ATTENTION DEFICIT HYPERACTIVITY DISORDER, such as METHYLPHENIDATE (RITALIN, CONCERTA, FOCALIN, ETC.), and AMPHETAMINES (Dexedrine and Adderall, Adderall XR). COCAINE and CRACK COCAINE are stimulants, as are some drugs are prescribed to treat obesity, such as phentermine (Adipex, Fastin, and Lonamin).

Stimulants generally have both legal and illegal uses. Cocaine (powder) may be used legally by physicians to treat diseases of the eyes or nose; however, it may not be used lawfully by individuals on their own.

Stimulants can be taken orally or injected or smoked. Individuals who abuse stimulants may develop a PSYCHOLOGICAL DEPENDENCE on the drugs as well as a physical TOLERANCE, needing higher doses to achieve the same effect of high energy and euphoria.

High doses of stimulants can cause insomnia, headache, dizziness, chest pain, abdominal cramps, and vomiting. High doses or chronic use may also induce aggression, panic, and psychotic symptoms, such as HALLUCINATIONS and PARANOIA. An overdose of stimulants can lead to hyperthermia (high body temperature), seizures, and even death.

See also DEPRESSANTS; SCHEDULED DRUGS.

stress Often refers to an emotional and physiological reaction to a problem and sometimes used to describe the stressor itself. When individuals are under extreme or moderate stress, they may react in unhealthy ways, such as drinking alcohol to excess, using illegal drugs, or abusing prescription drugs. In addition, if they have had past problems with substance abuse, overstressed individuals may find themselves relapsing into excessive drinking or drug use as well as overeating and/or smoking.

Examples of common stressors are

- a death in the family
- a severe illness of an individual or a loved one

- the breakup of an important relationship
- a move to another home
- the loss of a job

It is not possible to remove all stress from life; however, most individuals can learn coping skills and improve their responses to stressful situations. Stress management may include psychotherapy or membership in a twelve-step group, such as Alcoholics Anonymous. It may also include the substitution of healthy habits for bad habits, such as exercising and using other options in replacement for the abuse of substances.

When the individual who has had a substance abuse problem feels that a RELAPSE may be likely to occur, he or she may increase the frequency of learned coping strategies, such as seeing a therapist weekly instead of monthly, attending more twelve-step meetings, and exercising daily instead of weekly and/or for a longer period during each session. Some individuals may need to add antidepressant medications in order to help them to get through a particularly difficult time in their lives.

Some individuals have suffered from extremely stressful events, such as a natural disaster, a physical or sexual assault, or a wartime experience, and such people often experience an anxiety disorder known as POST-TRAUMATIC STRESS DISORDER (PTSD). Individuals who have PTSD have an increased risk for substance abuse in the future, although treatment may mitigate the risk.

Brady, Kathleen T., M.D., and Susan C. Sonne. "The Role of Stress in Alcohol Use, Alcoholism Treatment, and Relapse." *Alcohol Research & Health* 23, no. 4 (1999): 263–271.

suicide Voluntarily seeking to end one's life. Individuals who abuse or are dependent on alcohol and/or drugs have an increased risk of attempting (and sometimes succeeding at) suicide. In 2002, 31,655 people committed suicide in the United States, or about 11 per 100,000 individuals. According to the National Institute of Mental

Health, more than 90 percent of those who commit suicide have a diagnosable mental disorder, either a depressive disorder or a substance abuse disorder. The highest suicide rates in the United States are among white males older than age 85 years. Men are four times more likely to die from suicide than women, despite the fact that women attempt suicide two or three times more often than men.

Individuals who abuse alcohol and/or illicit drugs are more likely than others to have depression or anxiety disorders. They are also more likely to have other psychiatric problems. These problems may contribute to the decision to attempt suicide.

Data from the Drug Awareness Warning Network (DAWN) on Suicide

Many people attempt suicide by using drugs or alcohol, or drugs are found present in their system after a suicide attempt. According to the Drug Awareness Warning Network (DAWN), an annual survey of hospital emergency rooms that captures data on drug- and alcohol-related emergencies, 40,044 people who had attempted suicide were treated in 2003. In the largest proportion of cases, (22,348), central nervous system agents were present in these individuals, followed by psychotherapeutic agents (18,207 cases). (See Table I.)

As seen in Table I, alcohol and another drug in combination were the agents found among many people who attempted suicide. Alcohol alone was only used in 18 cases, while alcohol in combination with another drug was used in 10,429 cases.

When drugs alone were used in suicide victims, central nervous system agents were used most commonly (22,348 cases), followed by analgesics (18,029 cases).

When illicit drugs were used in conjunction with attempted suicide, COCAINE was used most frequently, or in 4,544 cases, followed by MARIJUANA (3,603 cases).

As indicated by DAWN data for 2003, most people who attempted suicide were females and were white. The largest single age range for those attempting suicide was 35–44 years. (See Table II.)

TABLE I: ESTIMATED NUMBERS OF DRUG-RELATED SUICIDE ATTEMPTS OF INDIVIDUALS TREATED IN HOSPITAL EMERGENCY DEPARTMENTS, 2003

Drug Category and Selected Drugs	Estimated Visits
Total Drug-Related Emergency Department Visits	40,044
Major substances of abuse	
Alcohol	10,447
Alcohol-in-combination	10,429
Alcohol alone	18
Cocaine	4,544
Heroin	495
Marijuana	3,603
Stimulants (amphetamines or methamphetamine)	1,141
Methylenedioxymethamphetamine (MDMA/Ecstasy)	35
Phencyclidine (PCP)	187
Inhalants	12
Other Substances	
Psychotherapeutic agents	18,207
Antidepressants	7,479
Benzodiazepines	9,143
Central nervous system agents	22,348
Analgesics	18,029
Opiates/opioids	8,047

Source: Adapted from Office of Applied Studies, Substance Abuse and Mental Health Services Administration. *Drug Abuse Warning Network, 2003: Interim National Estimates of Drug-Related Emergency Department Visits.* DAWN Series D-26. Publication no. SMA 04-3972. Rockville, Md.: Department of Health and Human Services, 2004.

See also DEPRESSION; EMERGENCY TREATMENT; PSY-CHIATRIC DISORDERS.

Office of Applied Studies, Substance Abuse and Mental Health Services Administration. *Drug Abuse Warning Network, 2003: Interim National Estimates of Drug-Related Emergency Department Visits.* DAWN Series D-26. Publication no. SMA 04-3972. Rockville, Md.: Department of Health and Human Services, 2004.

TABLE II: SUICIDE ATTEMPTS, BY PATIENT AND VISIT CHARACTERISTICS, OF DRUG-RELATED SUICIDE ATTEMPTS OF INDIVIDUALS TREATED IN HOSPITAL EMERGENCY DEPARTMENTS, 2003

Patient/Visit Characteristics	Estimated Visits
Total drug-related emergency department visits	40,044
Gender	
Male	13,089
Female	26,923
Age	
12–17 years	5,190
18–20 years	3,100
21–24 years	5,879
25–29 years	4,539
30–34 years	3,765
35–44 years	10,760
45–54 years	4,289
55–64 years	1,313
65 years and older	1,185
Unknown age	15
Race/ethnicity	
White	25,460
Black	3,859
Hispanic	3,947
Race/ethnicity not tabulated	853
Unknown	5,925
Chief complaint(s)	
Overdose	36,094
Intoxication	1,983
Seizures	36
Altered mental status	7,310
Psychiatric condition	11,342
Chest pain	277
Digestive problems	358
Other	2,265

Source: Adapted from Office of Applied Studies, Substance Abuse and Mental Health Services Administration. *Drug Abuse Warning Network, 2003: Interim National Estimates of Drug-Related Emergency Department Visits.* DAWN Series D-26. Publication no. SMA 04-3972. Rockville, Md.: Department of Health and Human Services, 2004.

tardive dyskinesia   A movement disorder that is caused by some older antipsychotic drugs prescribed to patients who had SCHIZOPHRENIA or other psychotic disorders. The disorder causes involuntary movements of the tongue, such as tongue thrusting, as well as writhing movements of the arms and legs. The individual may appear to be under the influence of illegal drugs to some people. These movements can be disturbing to others and cause embarrassment to the individual. Newer antipsychotic medications have a much lower risk of causing tardive dyskinesia than older antipsychotic drugs, such as haloperidol (Haldol).

thebaine   A constituent of opium that is a Schedule II drug, as classified by the CONTROLLED SUBSTANCES ACT. Thebaine is not used by physicians; it is converted by manufacturers into many other drugs, including BUPRENORPHINE, nalbuphine, naloxone, NALTREXONE, OXYCODONE, and oxymorphone. According to the Drug Enforcement Administration, the United States is the number one consumer of thebaine.

tolerance, physical   The need to take higher dosages of a drug in order to achieve the same effect. Drugs that have an addictive potential cause a physical tolerance. Physical tolerance develops among those who use NARCOTICS, whether the drug is used legally, as for pain management, or illegally and for the purposes of abuse. Individuals may develop a physical tolerance to other drugs, such as ANABOLIC STEROIDS, BENZODIAZEPINES, COCAINE, and MARIJUANA. However, when the drug is used illegally, very high doses may be taken in the early phase of usage and there may be a rapid escalation of the dosage.

When an opiate is administered legally by a physician for a pain problem, or a benzodiazepine is used for anxiety, the lowest dose of the drug that can control the symptom is used and dosages are increased slowly and carefully.

A person who has a physical tolerance to a drug is not addicted unless the other elements of addiction are also present, such as a CRAVING for the drug (or alcohol) and a psychological dependence on the drug or alcohol. In addition, the individual's life centers on either planning to obtain the drug or alcohol or consuming the substance. Other issues that are not related to either obtaining or consuming the drug are assigned tertiary importance (if that) by the addicted person.

See also PSEUDOADDICTION.

trafficking of drugs   The illegal sale of illicit drugs and/or the nonmedical use of prescription drugs. Some drugs are sold directly to individuals by DRUG DEALERS while other drugs, such as ANABOLIC STEROIDS and some NARCOTICS, are sold illegally through INTERNET DRUG TRAFFICKING/ILLEGAL PHARMACIES. In terms of large quantities of drugs, ORGANIZED CRIME and GANGS are usually involved in the transfer and sale of illegal drugs.

In some cases drug dealing in open air markets occurs in public areas, such as when drugs such as MARIJUANA and COCAINE are sold in poor and crime-ridden neighborhoods. (See OPEN AIR MARKETS, DRUG DEALING IN.) In addition, some drugs are received from people who have legitimate prescriptions but who give away or sell their drugs. (See DIVERSION, DRUG.) Adolescents and YOUNG ADULTS are the most likely to give away or sell scheduled medications or illicit substances. Many adolescents who are being treated for ATTENTION DEFICIT HYPER-

ACTIVITY DISORDER with STIMULANTS report that they have been approached by others who are seeking their drugs.

Some individuals manufacture their own drugs (particularly METHAMPHETAMINE) in illegal CLANDESTINE LABORATORIES and subsequently sell them.

In some cases, individuals from other countries trafficking drugs into the United States by swallowing packets of drugs, using their own bodies as a means of transportation. This is extremely dangerous because the packets can burst open in the digestive system, killing the individual.

Global Drug Trafficking

Despite a continuing "war on drugs," the global trafficking of drugs into the United States and other countries is a multi-billion dollar business, and drugs such as marijuana, cocaine and HEROIN are trafficked into other nations from AFGHANISTAN, MEXICO, COLOMBIA, and many other countries. In many cases, drug traffickers hire individuals to bring the drugs into the United States, sometimes having them swallow bags of cocaine and other drugs or inserting the bags rectally into the individual so that the drugs cannot be detected in a routine search. This is an extremely dangerous practice because the bags can break in the digestive system and cause harm and even death to the carrier.

The Drug Enforcement Administration sends agents into other countries to combat drug trafficking. However, the profits are so high despite the risks of INCARCERATION that many individuals continue their drug trafficking as long as possible. There is also a great deal of violence associated with the global trafficking of drugs, as rival groups vie for markets and profits. In addition, drug traffickers may also be involved in the forced prostitution of children and adults.

See also CRIME AND CRIMINALS; JAIL INMATES; ORGANIZED CRIME.

treatment The means by which the alcohol abuser, alcoholic, drug abuser, or drug addict ends reliance on a substance. Some patients receive rehabilitative treatment in an inpatient facility, but the majority of substance abusers who are treated receive some form of outpatient treatment, whether it is a standard program, an intensive program, a combination of day treatment and partial hospitalization, or maintenance on METHADONE. In some cases, hospitalized patients may be placed in an intensive DETOXIFICATION program.

A treatment contract is a signed agreement between a physician and a patient with regard to narcotic drugs to be prescribed. Such an agreement is used most frequently by physicians who specialize in PAIN MANAGEMENT.

There are a variety of issues that may be addressed in the treatment contract; for example, the doctor may wish the contract to stipulate that the patient will obtain his or her narcotic medications from only one physician and/or from only one pharmacy. Physicians wish to prevent patients from obtaining narcotic prescriptions from two or more doctors, because they will lose oversight about the amount of pain medication the patient is taking and some patients will use dangerous levels of the drug. Of course, patients who wish to abuse the drug may sign the contract anyway, but some patients may not realize the dangers of obtaining pain medications from more than one doctor, and this provision of the treatment contract will alert them to this danger.

Patients who sign the treatment contract may still obtain their nonnarcotic medications from other physicians, although they should be sure to tell the doctor who prescribes the narcotic about all other drugs they take, to prevent any adverse reactions.

The treatment contract may also explain the doctor's policy with regard to who may pick up the patient's prescription from the office, as well as what will happen if the patient reports that the prescription is misplaced. Doctors know that sometimes patients really do lose their prescriptions; however, they also know that some small number of patients will lie about having lost their prescription in order to obtain more drugs than the physician prescribes.

The doctor may include a statement in the treatment contract that the patient will not give or sell his or her narcotic medications to others. In addition, the doctor may wish the patient to stipulate that he or she will not use any illegal scheduled drugs, such as marijuana or cocaine.

The agreement may also stipulate that the patient must give the doctor a certain number of hours' or days' notice before calling for more medications.

The agreement may also stipulate that the patient is willing to have random drug tests, as requested by the physician.

With new or even established patients, it can be difficult sometimes to determine who is likely to misuse medications, although there are some patterns, such as strong requests for a particular drug or for higher than normal dosages of a narcotic. Yet such conditions do *not* invariably indicate that a patient is prone to abuse or addiction, since, with the advent of the Internet, many patients seek to self-educate about medications as well as illnesses. In addition, patients may know which pain medications have worked well for them in the past and request specific drugs for that reason.

The treatment contract may stipulate that if the patient fails to adhere to the terms of the agreement, then the physician may choose to stop treating the patient.

Rehabilitative, hospital, and other types of facilities provide outpatient or residential treatment programs for patients who have drug and/or alcohol dependence. There were 13,454 treatment facilities in the United States in 2004, with the largest number of facilities and *clients* (patients) in California. (See Table I.)

TABLE I: NUMBER OF TREATMENT FACILITIES AND NUMBER OF CLIENTS BY STATE OR JURISDICTION IN THE UNITED STATES, 2004

State	Total Facilities	Number of Clients
Total	13,454	1,072,251
Alabama	137	12,106
Alaska	69	2,503
Arizona	215	23,527
Arkansas	58	3,165
California	1,779	140,401
Colorado	425	30,501
Connecticut	227	21,363
Delaware	45	3,977
District of Columbia	51	5,365
Federation of Micronesia	1	—
Florida	569	45,215
Georgia	258	17,238
Guam	1	178
Hawaii	92	178
Idaho	73	3,618
Illinois	572	4,017
Indiana	416	42,709
Iowa	128	8,220
Kansas	214	9,796
Kentucky	308	18,261
Louisiana	164	12,313
Maine	184	7,109
Maryland	362	34,449
Massachusetts	330	35,998
Michigan	562	42,121
Minnesota	254	9,679
Mississippi	115	6,095
Missouri	224	17,566
Montana	48	2,715
Nebraska	105	4,976
Nevada	88	8,335
New Hampshire	60	3,517
New Jersey	331	29,687
New Mexico	120	11,517
New York	1,066	120,451
North Carolina	280	26,169
North Dakota	53	2,383
Ohio	460	36,133
Oklahoma	156	8,738
Oregon	222	18,735
Palau	1	42
Pennsylvania	449	38,796
Puerto Rico	182	10,974
Rhode Island	56	6,590
South Carolina	102	13,641
South Dakota	50	1,991
Tennessee	195	13,139
Texas	538	33,820
Utah	120	9,732
Vermont	37	2,668
Virginia	195	22,298
Virgin Islands	3	135
Washington	353	34,298
West Virginia	87	7,103
Wisconsin	309	17,354
Wyoming	50	2,887

Source: Office of Applied Studies. *National Survey of Substance Abuse Treatment Services (N-SSATS): 2004: Data on Substance Abuse Treatment Facilities.* Rockville, Md.: Substance Abuse and Mental Health Services Administration, August 2005, pp. 90–91.

Treatment facilities may be inpatient or outpatient facilities; those offering outpatient treatment are far more common. Most patients who received treatment for substance abuse in 2004 received outpatient treatment (89 percent), and 9.5 percent received treatment in a nonhospital residential facility. Only a tiny percentage, 1.5 percent of the patients, were treated in a hospital.

Numbers of Individuals Receiving Treatment in Treatment Facilities in the United States and Types of Treatment

In 2004, 1,066,351 individuals received treatment for a substance abuse problem. Of these, 493,552 abused both alcohol and drugs (nearly half of all patients receiving treatment), 210,696 abused alcohol only, and 362,103 abused drugs only. About two-thirds of substance abuse facilities (62 percent) focused primarily on substance abuse treatment, while about 26 percent of the facilities considered both substance abuse and mental health issues to be their paramount concerns.

As can be seen from Table III, treatment with methadone was increasingly popular; 14 percent received methadone maintenance in 1998, and by 2004, that percentage had increased to 22.5 percent.

Types of Patients

There are many different types of patients who are substance abusers and have unique needs, although not all facilities can accommodate every type of patient. (See Table II.) According to the National Survey of Substance Abuse Treatment Services (N-SSATS): 2004: Data on Substance Abuse Treatment Facilities, released in 2005, different populations were treated in treatment facilities; for example, 31 percent of the facilities offered programs or groups for adolescent substance abusers, and the greatest percentage of such facilities were run either by tribal or local governments.

About a third (35 percent) of the facilities offered programs or groups for patients who had both mental health and substance abuser disorders, and services for this population were most common in government-operated facilities.

Some facilities (27 percent) offered programs or groups for criminal justice clients who were not incarcerated and were not among those found

guilty of driving while intoxicated (DWI). About 31 percent of the treatment facilities offered programs for driving under the influence (DUI) or DWI offenders.

Eleven percent of the treatment facilities offered programs or groups for people who had ACQUIRED IMMUNE DEFICIENCY SYNDROME (AIDS)/HUMAN IMMUNODEFICIENCY VIRUS (HIV).

About 29 percent of all facilities offered programs or groups in sign language for the hearing impaired.

Some facilities (5 percent) offered special programs for gays and lesbians who had substance abuse disorders. About 7 percent of the facilities offered programs or groups for older adults. Some facilities (30 percent) offered special programs or groups for adult women, while 23 percent of the facilities offered specific programs or groups for adult men. About 14 percent of the facilities offered programs or groups for both pregnant and postpartum women. (See Table II.)

Medications Given for Treatment

In some cases, if detoxification is the goal, medications may be provided to help the patient withdraw from the drug, such as BUPRENORPHINE (Subutrex, Suboxone), BENZODIAZEPINES, or antidepressants. In some cases, alternative narcotics are given to treat patients as outpatients, as when HEROIN addicts are given METHADONE on a regular basis. In this case, the addicted individuals do not receive inpatient treatment within a facility but usually live at home and go to the facility to receive their methadone.

The numbers of patients who are receiving methadone to treat addiction, specifically to heroin, increased from 145,610 in 1998 (14 percent of all patients receiving substance abuse treatment) to 240,961 patients in 2004 (22 percent of all patients receiving treatment for substance abuse).

Those Needing Treatment for Illicit Drug Use

According to the National Survey on Drug Use and Health, 8.1 million people needed treatment for illicit drug use in 2004, up from 7.3 million who needed treatment in 2003. Of the 8.1 million people who needed treatment, 6.6 million did *not* receive any treatment. It should also be noted that only about 9 percent (598,000 people) of those

TABLE II: FACILITIES OFFERING PROGRAMS OR GROUPS FOR SPECIFIC CLIENT TYPES, BY FACILITY OPERATION AND PRIMARY FOCUS OF FACILITY, 2004, BY PERCENTAGE

Facility Operation and Primary Focus	No. of facilities	Any program or group	Adolescents	Clients with cooccurring disorders	Criminal justice clients	Persons with HIV or AIDS	Gays or lesbians	Seniors or older adults	Adult women	Pregnant/ postpartum women	Adult men	DUI/DWI offenders
Total	13,454	82.3	30.9	35.4	27.2	10.9	5.5	6.7	30.1	14.0	23.0	30.8
Facility operation												
Private nonprofit	8,053	82.6	31.2	35.5	26.9	11.9	5.4	6.0	31.3	14.3	24.0	24.9
Private for-profit	3,488	82.0	29.9	30.5	29.4	9.1	6.7	8.1	25.5	21.2	22.2	31.7
Local, county, or community government	956	84.4	36.4	44.1	31.3	8.6	3.2	5.2	36.8	21.2	22.2	31.7
State government	458	85.8	31.7	50.2	25.1	14.6	4.1	7.0	36.0	18.1	23.4	20.7
Federal government	327	65.1	5.5	41.0	5.5	7.6	2.8	10.4	18.0	4.0	15.9	21.4
Dept. of Veterans Affairs	185	68.1	—	53.5	4.9	10.3	2.2	14.1	18.4	3.8	14.6	16.2
Dept. of Defense	102	53.9	2.9	19.6	2.0	2.0	3.9	2.9	16.7	2.9	12.7	33.3
Indian Health Services	34	76.5	41.2	38.2	17.6	8.8	2.9	14.7	17.6	8.8	29.4	11.8
Other	6	100.0	16.7	33.3	16.7	16.7	—	—	33.3	—	33.3	33.3
Tribal government	172	84.9	55.8	29.1	22.7	7.0	7.6	15.1	37.8	18.0	28.5	41.3
Primary focus of facility												
Substance abuse treatment services	8,340	82.1			28.3	12.5	5.2	5.6	33.6	16.9	26.6	29.0
Mental health services	1,104	72.2			14.8	3.6	3.0	8.1	11.7	3.5	7.2	21.0
Mix of mental health and substance abuse treatment services	3,558	86.6			29.4	8.9	6.7	8.9	28.2	11.0	20.0	39.3
General health care	219	65.3			9.1	15.1	3.2	8.2	18.3	10.0	14.2	15.1
Other/unknown	233	x			27.9	15.5	9.0	7.3	33.0	12.4	26.6	26.6

Source: Office of Applied Studies. *National Survey of Substance Abuse Treatment Services (N-SSATS): 2004: Data on Substance Abuse Treatment Facilities.* Rockville, Md.: Substance Abuse and Mental Health Services Administration, August 2005, p. 55.

TABLE III: CLIENTS IN TREATMENT BY TYPE OF TREATMENT, 1998–2004, AND CLIENTS RECEIVING METHADONE BY TYPE OF CARE RECEIVED, NUMBER AND PERCENTAGE DISTRIBUTION

	Number of Clients					Percentage Distribution				
	1998	2000	2002	2003	2004	1998	2000	2002	2003	2004
Total	1,038,378	1,000,896	1,136,287	1,092,546	1,072,251	100.0	100.0	100.0	100.0	100.0
Type of care received										
Outpatient	915,798	891,547	1,020,214	968,719	954,551	88.2	89.1	89.8	88.7	89.0
Regular	686,730	739,794	616,957	587,975	564,300	66.1	73.9	54.3	53.8	52.6
Intensive	198,355	118,610	139,777	128,127	121,862	19.1	11.9	12.3	11.7	11.4
Detoxification	30,713	14,249	18,307	11,770	12,064	3.0	1.4	1.6	1.1	1.1
Day treatment/partial hospitalization	n/c	18,894	29,506	27,728	28,133	n/c	1.9	2.6	2.5	2.6
Methadone maintenance	n/c	n/c	215,667	213,119	228,192	n/c	n/c	19.0	19.5	21.3
Nonhospital residential	107,961	96,084	102,394	108,592	101,713	10.4	9.6	9.0	9.9	9.5
Detoxification	7,636	8,264	8,401	9,061	7,021	0.7	0.8	0.7	0.8	0.7
Rehabilitation	100,325	87,820	93,993	n/c	n/c	9.7	8.8	8.3	n/c	n/c
Short-term treatment (30 days or less)	n/c	n/c	n/c	22,926	21,758	n/c	n/c	n/c	2.1	2.0
Long-term treatment (more than 30 days)	n/c	n/c	n/c	76,605	72,934	n/c	n/c	n/c	7.0	6.8
Hospital inpatient	14,619	13,265	13,679	15,235	15,987	1.4	1.3	1.2	1.4	1.5
Detoxification	6,317	6,375	6,306	7,067	6,214	0.6	0.6	0.6	0.6	0.6
Treatment	8,302	6,890	7,373	8,168	9,773	0.8	0.7	0.6	0.7	0.9
Clients receiving methadone	145,610	172,502	225,500	227,003	240,961	14.0	17.2	19.8	20.8	22.5

Note: n/c Data not collected.
Source: Office of Applied Studies. *National Survey of Substance Abuse Treatment Services (N-SSATS): 2004: Data on Substance Abuse Treatment Facilities.* Rockville, Md.: Substance Abuse and Mental Health Services Administration, August 2005, p. 28.

who needed treatment but did not receive it actually believed that they needed treatment.

This failure to acknowledge their substance abuse problem is probably a key factor in those patients who fail to receive treatment. People who do not believe that they have a problem are unlikely to seek treatment unless they are compelled to do so by a court. This is not surprising, since many people are in denial about their drug dependence or alcoholism. Most people who felt they needed treatment but did not receive it (68 percent) said that they had made no effort to seek treatment, while the remainder said they did seek treatment but were unsuccessful.

Data from the National Survey of Substance Abuse Treatment Services

Each year the Substance Abuse and Mental Health Services Administration collects data on the location, characteristics, and use of alcoholism and drug abuse treatment facilities in the United States. They receive a very high response to their survey: in 2004, a 96 percent response rate. The researchers analyzed results from 13,454 facilities providing treatment to more than a million clients.

Services Offered by Treatment Facilities

Treatment facilities may offer a variety of different services; for example, most facilities offer comprehensive substance abuse assessment, and many offer a comprehensive mental health assessment as well. Many facilities offer substance abuse therapy and counseling in the forms of individual therapy, family therapy, aftercare counseling, and relapse prevention counseling.

Most facilities offer DRUG TESTING in the forms of blood and urine drug and/or alcohol screening or breathalyzer screening for alcohol, and many facilities also offer screening for HIV, other sexually transmitted diseases, and HEPATITIS B and C, as well as tuberculosis. Most offer case management services and many offer family or partner services for those who are victims of domestic violence. Some facilities provide transportation assistance to treatment facilities. Some offer employment counseling as part of their transitional services, as well as assistance in locating housing and obtaining social services.

The strategy developed to assist a person to overcome an addictive disorder or psychiatric problem, including whether the treatment is provided within a facility or in an outpatient setting, is known as a treatment plan. The treatment plan is developed by the physician or other person who is overseeing a patient's case. The treatment plan includes such factors as the estimated time that treatment will occur, whether treatment will occur in an inpatient (in a hospital or rehabilitative facility) or outpatient setting, and whether the plan is DETOXIFICATION (removal from drugs or alcohol) or another, such as METHADONE maintenance, often used to treat individuals who are addicted to HEROIN.

If detoxification is the plan, physicians must decide whether to use other medications to assist the individual with detoxification, such as BUPRENORPHINE or NALTREXONE.

treatment contract   See TREATMENT.

treatment facilities   See TREATMENT.

treatment plan   See TREATMENT.

Vicodin See HYDROCODONE; PRESCRIPTION DRUG ABUSE.

violence Acting in such a way as to inflict physical harm to another person, whether the person is known to the assailant or not. Some drugs are known to trigger aggression and rage in some individuals, including such drugs as ANABOLIC STEROIDS, AMPHETAMINE, COCAINE, and METHAMPHETAMINE. In some cases, HALLUCINOGENIC DRUGS may lead to violent behavior. Studies have shown that individuals who are using drugs and/or alcohol are more prone to violent behavior, such as assault and murder, than those who are not substance abusers.

In a study of 14,843 residents of New York City who were fatally injured from 1990 to 1992, the researcher Peter M. Marzuk and colleagues reported that cocaine use was determined to be present in 26.7 percent of the deaths. Many of these deaths were caused by violence.

Say the researchers, "Approximately one third of deaths after cocaine use were the result of drug intoxication, but two thirds involved traumatic injuries resulting from homicides, suicides, traffic accidents, and falls. If fatal injury after cocaine use was considered as a separate cause of death, it would rank among the five leading causes of death among those 15 to 44 years of age in New York City."

Adolescents and Violence

In a study of youth violence and illicit drug use, reported in 2006 in the *NSDUH Report*, based on statistics from 2002 to 2004, of those adolescents who did not use illicit drugs and were in school, 26.5 percent were violent. Of those in school who had used illegal drugs in the past year, nearly double, or 49.6 percent, had engaged in violent behavior. (See Table I.)

Adolescents who lived near the poverty level had a greater risk of violence than individuals in families with higher incomes, but if they were using illicit drugs, the risk was elevated further. For example, as can be seen from Table I, 33.4 percent of adolescents with no past year illicit drug use and whose family income was less than 125 percent of the federal poverty threshold had committed violent acts in the past year. However, in the case of adolescents in the same financial circumstances who had also used drugs, 57.3 percent exhibited violent behavior.

In every case in Table I, whether the factor considered was school status, poverty level, the region where the adolescent lived, or the type of county, the drug-abusing adolescent was more likely to be violent than the nonabusing adolescent. It also did not matter what race or gender the individual was—illegal drug use was predictive for violence in all cases.

In considering violent behavior and the drugs used by adolescents, those using methamphetamine had the highest percentage of violent behavior (69.3 percent), followed by adolescent users of cocaine (61.8 percent) and HALLUCINOGENIC DRUGS (61.4 percent). (See Table II.) Some people are surprised to learn that marijuana users are not inevitably passive, as in the general stereotype, and about half the adolescent marijuana users exhibited violent behavior. GANGS who distribute marijuana and other drugs often rely upon violence to achieve their ends.

TABLE I: PERCENTAGES OF YOUTHS AGES 12 TO 17 ENGAGING IN PAST YEAR VIOLENT BEHAVIOR, BY PAST YEAR ILLICIT DRUG USE AND SOCIODEMOGRAPHIC CHARACTERISTICS, 2002, 2003, AND 2004

	Past Year Illicit Drug Use (Percentage)	No Past Year Illicit Drug Use (Percentage)
School Status		
Currently enrolled/attending	49.6	26.5
Not currently enrolled/attending	54.0	27.4
Poverty Threshhold		
Less than 125 percent of federal poverty theshhold	57.3	33.4
125–199 percent of federal poverty threshhold	51.9	29.3
200–399 percent of federal poverty threshhold	48.0	25.1
400 percent or more of federal poverty threshhold	45.0	21.4
Region		
Northeast	52.3	28.1
Midwest	49.9	26.9
South	48.6	27.0
West	49.3	24.4
County Type		
Large metropolitan	50.3	26.7
Small metropolitan	49.1	26.6
Nonmetropolitan	49.5	25.9

Source: Office of Applied Studies. "Youth Violence and Illicit Drug Use," *The NSDUH Report.* Washington, D.C.: Substance Abuse and Mental Health Services Administration, 2006. Available online. URL: http://www.drugabusestatistics.samhsa.gov/2k6/youthViolence/youthViolence.pdf. Downloaded February 7, 2006, p. 2.

TABLE II: PERCENTAGES OF YOUTHS AGES 12 TO 17 ENGAGING IN PAST YEAR VIOLENT BEHAVIOR, BY TYPE OF ILLICIT DRUG USED IN PAST YEAR, 2002, 2003, AND 2004

Type of Illicit Drug	Past Year Violent Behavior (Percentage)
Methamphetamine	69.3
Cocaine	61.8
Hallucinogens	61.4
Inhalants	55.4
Nonmedical use of prescription pain relievers	53.6
Marijuana	49.7

Source: Adapted from Office of Applied Studies. "Youth Violence and Illicit Drug Use." *The NSDUH Report.* Washington, D.C.: Substance Abuse and Mental Health Services Administration, 2006. Available online. URL: http://www.drugabusestatistics.samhsa.gov/2k6/youthViolence/youthViolence.pdf. Downloaded February 7, 2006, p. 3.

The probability of violence also increased with the number of illegal drugs used; for example, 46 percent of the subjects who used one illicit drug reported past year violence, compared to 55 percent for those who used two illegal drugs and 62 percent for those who used three or more illicit substances.

See ADOLESCENTS; CHILD ABUSE; CRIME AND CRIMINALS; DOMESTIC VIOLENCE; GANGS; HOMICIDE; INCARCERATION; INJURIES, CAUSED BY ALCOHOL AND/ OR ILLICIT DRUGS; LAW ENFORCEMENT; ORGANIZED CRIME; RUNAWAY/THROWAWAY YOUTHS; SEXUAL ASSAULTS.

Grisso, Jeane Ann, M.D., et al. "Violent Injuries among Women in an Urban Area." *New England Journal of Medicine* 341, no. 25 (December 16, 1999): 1,899–1,905.

Kyriacou, Demetrios, M.D., et al. "Risk Factors for Injury to Women from Domestic Violence," *New England Journal of Medicine* 341, no. 25 (December 16, 1999): 1,892–1,898.

Marzuk, Peter M., M.D. "Fatal Injuries after Cocaine Use as Leading Cause of Death among Young Adults in New York City." *New England Journal of Medicine* 332, no. 26 (1995): 1,753–1,757.

Office of Applied Studies. "Youth Violence and Illicit Drug Use," *The NSDUH Report.* Washington, D.C.: Substance Abuse and Mental Health Services Administration, 2006. Available online. URL: http://www.drugabusestatistics.samhsa.gov/2k6/youthViolence/youthViolence.pdf. Downloaded February 7, 2006.

withdrawal What individuals experience when they are not receiving a substance, such as a drug or alcohol, to which they are addicted. The withdrawal may be voluntary, as when the person seeks DETOXIFICATION from a drug or alcohol, or it may be involuntary, as when the person does not have access to the addictive substance because of insufficient funds to purchase the drugs or for other reasons. Sometimes BENZODIAZEPINES are used to ease the process of withdrawal during detoxification.

Withdrawal from drugs or alcohol can be very physically and psychologically difficult, and it can also be extremely dangerous. If the withdrawal occurs suddenly and not under a physician's care, the patient may experience very severe consequences and even death, depending on the type of drug to which he or she is addicted and the degree of the addiction. Some individuals addicted to substances such as ALPRAZOLAM/ALPRAZOLAM XR (XANAX/XANAX XR) have died in jail from severe withdrawal symptoms. It is best for most addicted individuals to undergo detoxification under the control of an experienced physician.

See also DELIRIUM TREMENS; DETOXIFICATION.

Kosten, Thomas R., M.D., and Patrick G. O'Connor, M.D. "Management of Drug and Alcohol Withdrawal." *New England Journal of Medicine* 348, no. 18 (May 1, 2003): 1,786–1,795.

work Providing labor in exchange for pay and sometimes for benefits as well. Individuals who abuse alcohol and/or drugs often find it increasingly difficult to meet their work goals, and it is even more difficult for those who are dependent on alcohol or drugs to perform their necessary work duties. Individuals in some occupations, such as police officers, physicians, and airline pilots, have the potential to cause serious harm to many others if they are active substance abusers.

Some substance abusers have a spotty work history, moving from job to job. If an employed individual is identified as having a problem with drugs or alcohol, EMPLOYEE ASSISTANCE PROGRAMS may provide assistance to substance abusers, particularly in large corporations.

Unemployed drug users may find it very difficult to obtain jobs, because many employers require preliminary DRUG TESTING for major substances before an individual may be hired for a job. A failed test means that the individual will not be hired.

Unemployed adults have a greater risk of drug abuse than employed adults. According to the National Survey on Drug Use and Health, 19.2 percent of unemployed adults ages 18 and older were current illegal drug users, compared to 8.0 percent of those employed full-time and 10.3 percent of those employed part-time. However, some substance abusers are in the workforce, and of the 16.4 million users of illegal drugs in the United States, 12.3 million (75.2 percent) were employed either part- or full-time.

Substance Abuse and Mental Health Services Administration. *Overview of Findings for the 2004 National Survey on Drug Use and Health.* Rockville, Md.: Department of Health and Human Services, September 2005.

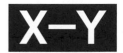

Xanax See ALPRAZOLAM/ALPRAZOLAM XR (XANAX/ XANAX XR).

young adults Individuals within the age group of about 18 to 25 years. (Some studies have an older age limit for young adults, such as age 18 to age 28 or 29 years.) Young adults have a higher likelihood of abusing alcohol and/or drugs, particularly MARIJUANA, than most other age groups. As can be seen in Table I, 57.4 percent of young adults had ever used marijuana. (See ADOLESCENTS AND SUBSTANCE ABUSE.)

Drug Abuse

Young adults ages 18–25 years old also represented the largest group of users of many drugs; for example, they were the largest illicit users of METHAMPHETAMINE (9.0 percent) in 2004 according to the National Survey on Drug Use and Health. In addition, the lifetime prevalence of powdered cocaine abuse was 15.2 percent among young adults, followed by 9.5 percent among college students.

The lifetime abuse of OXYCONTIN was the highest among young adults ages 18–25 years, and in fact, this abuse increased among young adults, from 3.6 percent in 2003 to 4.3 percent in 2004. In considering *all* OXYCODONE products that are abused (of which OxyContin is one), the abuse rate increased from 8.9 percent in 2003 to 10.1 percent in 2004 among young adults.

Individuals who are in the age bracket of 18 to 25 years are also the most likely to abuse HYDROCODONE products. According to the National Survey on Drug Use and Health, the lifetime prevalence of the abuse of Vicodin, Lortab, and Lorcet (brand names of hydrocodone products) increased among young adults from 16.3 percent in 2003 to 17.4 percent

in 2004. In contrast, the lifetime abuse of hydrocodone by individuals of all ages increased slightly, from 7.1 percent in 2003 to 7.4 percent in 2004.

HALLUCINOGENIC DRUGS, although not used to a great extent by young adults, were nonetheless abused most prominently by this age group compared to other ages; for example, the highest percentage of users of PHENCYCLIDINE (PCP) were young adults ages 18–25 years, though few of them used the drug; for example, 2.3 percent of those in this age bracket had ever used PCP.

According to the National Survey on Drug Use and Health, in 2004, 11.2 percent of adults ages 18–25 used BENZODIAZEPINES nonmedically. As indicated in Table I, BARBITURATES are also a major drug of abuse among young adults and college students; the rate rose from 3.2 percent of college students who ever used barbiturates in 1994 to 7.2 percent in 2004. Among young adults ages 19–28, the rate of abuse of barbiturates increased from 6.4 percent in 1994 to 9.7 percent in 2004. It is clear that the abuse of prescription drugs by young adults, as well as the abuse of illicit drugs, is a problem of concern.

Increases and decreases of drug abuse among young adults and college students As can be seen from Table I, the abuse of illicit drugs increased over the period of 1994–2004 among both young adults in general as well as the subpopulation of college students; for example, in 1994, 45.5 percent of college students and 57.5 percent of young adults had ever tried any illicit drug; however, by 2004, that percentage had further increased to 52.2 percent of college students and 60.5 percent of young adults who had ever tried an illicit substance.

The use of some drugs, however, has significantly decreased over time. For example, 12 percent of college students and 13.2 percent of young adults had ever tried inhalants in 1994. In contrast, in 2004, the percentage of college students who had ever tried inhalants was down to 8.5 per-cent and the percentage of young adults who had abused inhalants had dropped to 11.6 percent. In addition, the abuse of LYSERGIC ACID DIETHYLAMIDE

TABLE I: TRENDS IN LIFETIME PREVALENCE OF USE OF VARIOUS DRUGS BY COLLEGE STUDENTS AND YOUNG ADULTS (AGES 19–28)

	1994	1995	1996	1997	1998	1999	2000	2001	2002	2003	2004
Any Illicit Drug											
College Students	45.5	45.5	47.4	49.0	52.9	53.2	53.7	53.6	51.8	53.9	52.2
Young Adults	57.5	57.4	56.4	56.7	57.0	57.4	58.2	58.1	59.0	60.2	60.5
Marijuana/Hashish											
College Students	42.2	41.7	45.1	46.1	49.9	50.8	51.2	51.0	49.5	50.7	49.1
Young Adults	53.7	53.6	53.4	53.8	54.4	54.6	55.1	55.7	56.8	57.2	57.4
Inhalants											
College Students	12.0	13.8	11.4	12.4	12.8	12.4	12.9	9.6	7.7	9.7	8.5
Young Adults	13.2	14.5	14.1	14.1	14.2	14.2	14.3	12.8	12.4	12.2	11.6
Hallucinogens											
College Students	10.0	13.0	12.6	13.8	15.2	14.8	14.4	14.8	13.6	14.5	12.0
Young Adults	15.4	16.1	16.4	16.8	17.4	18.0	18.4	18.3	19.6	19.7	19.3
LSD											
College Students	9.2	11.5	10.8	11.7	13.1	12.7	11.8	12.2	8.6	8.7	5.6
Young Adults	13.8	14.5	15.0	15.0	15.7	16.2	16.4	16.0	15.1	14.6	13.4
Methylenedioxymethamphet-amine (MDMA/Ecstasy)											
College Students	2.1	3.1	4.3	4.7	6.8	8.4	13.1	14.7	12.7	12.9	10.2
Young Adults	3.8	4.5	5.2	5.1	7.2	7.1	11.6	13.0	14.6	15.3	16.0
Cocaine (powder)											
College Students	5.0	5.5	5.0	5.6	8.1	8.4	9.1	8.6	8.2	9.2	9.5
Young Adults	15.2	13.7	12.9	12.1	12.3	12.8	12.7	13.1	13.5	14.7	15.2
Crack Cocaine											
College Students	1.0	1.8	1.2	1.4	2.2	2.4	2.5	2.0	1.9	3.1	2.0
Young Adults	4.4	3.8	3.9	3.6	3.8	4.3	4.6	4.7	4.3	4.7	4.2
Heroin											
College Students	0.1	0.6	0.7	0.9	1.7	0.9	1.7	1.2	1.0	1.0	0.9
Young Adults	0.8	1.1	1.3	1.3	1.6	1.7	1.8	2.0	1.8	1.9	1.9
Amphetamines											
College Student	9.2	10.7	9.5	10.6	10.6	11.9	12.3	12.4	11.9	12.3	12.7
Young Adults	17.1	16.6	15.3	14.6	14.3	14.1	15.0	15.0	14.8	15.2	15.9
Methamphetamine											
College Students	—	—	—	—	—	7.1	5.1	5.3	5.0	5.8	5.2
Young Adults	—	—	—	—	—	8.8	9.3	9.0	9.1	8.9	9.0
Barbiturates											
College Students	3.2	4.0	4.6	5.2	5.7	6.7	6.9	6.0	5.9	5.7	7.2
Young Adults	6.4	6.7	6.6	6.5	6.9	7.4	8.1	7.8	8.0	8.7	9.7
Tranquilizers											
College Students	4.4	5.4	5.3	6.9	7.7	8.2	8.8	9.7	10.7	11.0	10.6
Young Adults	9.9	9.7	9.3	8.6	9.6	9.6	10.5	11.9	13.4	13.8	14.9

Source: Adapted from Johnston, Lloyd D., et al., *Monitoring the Future: National Survey Results on Drug Use, 1975–2004*. Vol. 2, *College Students and Adults Ages 19–45*. Bethesda, Md.: National Institute on Drug Abuse, National Institutes of Health, 2005, pp. 35–38.

(LSD) steadily decreased to the 2004 low of 5.6 percent of college students who had ever abused LSD and 13.4 percent of young adults who had abused this drug.

The use of some particular drugs, such as powdered cocaine, AMPHETAMINES, and, as mentioned earlier, barbiturates, has slightly increased, a matter that raises concern.

Alcohol Abuse

Young adults are at high risk for alcohol abuse and heavy drinking. For example, according to research provided by Chen and colleagues in 2004/2005 in *Alcohol Research & Health*, data from the 2001–2 National Epidemiologic Survey on Alcohol and Related Conditions (NESARC), indicated that the majority, or 70.8 percent, of men and women ages 18–24 years engaged in past-year drinking. The drinking rates were higher among men ages 18–24 years, and more than two-thirds (70.8 percent) of males drank compared to a lower rate for women (66.8 percent).

According to the researchers, the majority of men (52.3 percent) engaged in risk drinking or exceeding recommended daily limits, of more than four drinks per day. In considering race and ethnicity, the greatest percentage of drinkers in the

past year were whites (77.1 percent). A majority of college students, both full-time and part-time students, were past-year drinkers, and a majority of college students engaged in risky drinking. (See Table II.)

Drinking is also associated with behavior problems; for example, among young adults, in the past year, based on data from 2001–2, the average person drove after drinking three or more drinks on nearly five days. This rate rose to 6.2 days for college students. As can be seen from the table, the average man drinks on more days in a year (82.7 days for men versus 48.3 days per year for women), and he also drives under the influence of alcohol more frequently than the average woman. (See Table III.)

People of some races or ethnicities have significantly higher rates of drinking than others; for example, the data have shown that American Indians and Alaska Native young adults drank on average on 97.2 days per year, the highest level of drinking of all races. They were also intoxicated on more days; 39.8 days in a year. However, they had the lowest rate of driving under the influence of alcohol of all races; 1.8 days. In considering race, those who were the most likely to drive after drinking were Hispanic, followed by whites. In addition,

TABLE II: PREVALENCE OF DRINKING, EXCEEDING THE RECOMMENDED DAILY LIMIT, AND EXCEEDING THE WEEKLY LIMIT IN THE PAST YEAR, AMONG THE TOTAL POPULATION OF YOUNG ADULTS AGES 18–24 YEARS, ACCORDING TO SEX, RACE/ETHNICITY, AND COLLEGE ENROLLMENT STATUS, 2000–2002

Sex/Race/Ethnicity, College Enrollment Status	Past-Year Drinking	Exceeding Daily Drinking Limit[1]	Exceeding Weekly Drinking Limit[2]
Total	70.8%	45.9%	14.5%
Men	74.7%	52.3%	17.4%
Women	66.8%	39.4%	11.5%
White	77.1	52.5	17.3
Black	60.1	29.0	8.9
American Indian/Alaska Native	70.7	53.0	27.4
Asian/Native Hawaiian/Other Pacific Islander	59.1	36.5	10.5
College, full-time	60.4	37.3	17.9
College, part-time	76.3	45.9	14.6
Noncollege	68.3	43.3	12.9

[1] Consuming more than four drinks in a single day for men and more than three drinks in a single day for women.
[2] On average, consuming more than two drinks per day for men and more than one drink per day for women.
Source: Adapted from Chen, Chiung M., Mary C. Dufour, M.D., and Hsiao-ye Yi. "Alcohol Consumption among Young Adults Ages 18–24 in the United States: Results from the 2001–2002 NESARC Survey." *Alcohol Research & Health* 28, no. 4 (2004/2005): p. 272.

TABLE III: AVERAGE AGE OF DRINKING FREQUENCY, INTOXICATION, AND DRIVING AFTER DRINKING 3+ DRINKS IN THE PAST YEAR AMONG YOUNG ADULT DRINKERS AGES 18–24

Sex/Race/Ethnicity, College Enrollment Status	Drinking Frequency/ Days Per Year	Intoxication/ Days Per Year	Driving after Drinking 3+ Drinks, Days per Year
Total	66.4	18.0	4.8
Men	82.7	23.3	6.0
Women	48.3	11.9	3.5
White	69.7	18.9	5.1
Black	64.7	13.2	2.6
American Indian/Alaska Native	97.2	39.8	1.8
Asian/Native Hawaiian/Other Pacific Islander	54.4	22.3	4.0
Hispanic	53.0	13.4	5.8
College, full-time	71.8	21.1	6.2
College, part-time	55.8	15.7	2.5
Noncollege	65.3	16.7	4.5

Source: Adapted from Chen, Chiung M., Mary C. Dufour, M.D., and Hsiao-ye Yi. "Alcohol Consumption among Young Adults Ages 18–24 in the United States: Results from the 2001–2002 NESARC Survey." *Alcohol Research & Health* 28, no. 4 (2004/2005), p. 275.

full-time college students were more likely to drive while intoxicated than other groups of their own age. (See Table III.)

In another study, according to the National Survey on Drug Abuse and Health, 20.2 percent of young adults ages 18–20 years old drove while under the influence of alcohol in 2004, and this rate further increased to 28.2 percent for those individuals who were between the ages of 21 and 25 years old.

Types of alcohol consumed In considering the types of alcohol that are consumed by young adults ages 21–24 years who drank at home, the study by Chen and associates notes that the most popular alcoholic beverage was wine, which was consumed by 39 percent, followed by wine coolers (37.8 percent). There were also variations on the form of alcohol of choice depending on whether individuals were college students as well as on their race and ethnicity. However, if the alcohol was consumed in the homes of friends or relatives, the most popular types of alcohol were wine coolers, followed by wine. If the alcohol was consumed in a public place, the most popular type of alcohol was liquor, followed by beer. (See Table IV.)

There are many interesting variations in drinking patterns. For example, as indicated by the data in Table IV, only 19 percent of women drank beer with friends and relatives but nearly 51 percent drink beer when they were in public places. Perhaps women perceive that beer is a better beverage to drink in public, for whatever reason. The consumption of wine coolers by men at home or with friends and relatives is higher than their consumption in public. (Perhaps wine coolers are considered unmasculine by some men, who wish to convey a macho image in public.)

Even more strikingly, the consumption of liquor was only 20.5 percent at home and 22.4 percent with friends and relatives but rose to more than double, or 57.1 percent, of the type of alcohol that was consumed in public places. Future research should provide answers to the differences in these drinking patterns.

Adult children of alcoholics (COAs) Adult children of alcoholics have an increased risk for ALCOHOLISM in their own adulthood. In one study reported in *Psychology of Addictive Behaviors* in 2005, researchers David B. Flora and Laurie Chassin studied whether alcoholism in parents related to the subsequent drug abuse in young adults. They also studied whether marriage was a mitigating factor decreasing the abuse of drugs.

The researchers found that adult children of alcoholics were significantly *less* likely to be married than non-COAs; however, for male COAs, marriage was linked to a *decrease* in drug use in their mid- to late twenties.

TABLE IV: PERCENTAGE DISTRIBUTION OF USUAL DRINKING LOCATION BY BEVERAGE TYPE AMONG YOUNG ADULT CURRENT DRINKERS AGES 21–24, ACCORDING TO SEX, RACE/ETHNICITY, AND COLLEGE ENROLLMENT STATUS, BY PERCENTAGE 2001–2002

Beverage	Sex/Race/Ethnicity, College Enrollment Status	In Own Home	In Homes of Friends or Relatives	In Public Places
Coolers	Total	37.8	33.0	29.2
	Men	37.6	37.6	24.8
	Women	38.0	29.7	32.3
	White	35.6	35.0	29.4
	Black	43.2	28.4	28.4
	American Indian/Alaska Native	66.1	19.4	14.5
	Asian/Native Hawaiian/Other Pacific Islander	39.0	25.8	35.2
	Hispanic	39.6	31.8	28.6
	College, full-time	29.5	37.2	33.3
	College, part-time	40.6	29.1	30.3
	Noncollege	42.6	31.1	26.3
Beer	Total	37.0	25.7	37.4
	Men	41.2	29.9	28.9
	Women	30.2	19.0	50.7
	White	33.1	23.8	43.0
	Black	41.5	34.0	24.5
	American Indian/Alaska Native	25.9	27.0	47.1
	Asian/Native Hawaiian/Other Pacific Islander	29.3	31.5	29.2
	Hispanic	51.4	26.8	21.8
	College, full-time	27.3	24.5	48.3
	College, part-time	34.6	24.5	40.9
	Noncollege	42.8	26.5	30.7
Wine	Total	42.8	26.5	30.7
	Men	34.9	34.1	31.1
	Women	42.2	28.7	29.2
	White	40.9	30.0	29.1
	Black	31.8	23.8	44.4
	American Indian/Alaska Native	75.2	7.5	17.3
	Asian/Native Hawaiian/Other Pacific Islander	26.0	56.9	26.3
	Hispanic	35.4	36.6	28.0
	College, full-time	39.8	30.8	29.4
	College, part-time	37.2	34.7	28.0
	Noncollege	38.8	30.2	31.0
Liquor	Total	20.5	22.5	57.1
	Men	22.7	29.4	47.9
	Women	18.3	15.6	66.0
	White	20.0	19.3	60.8
	Black	29.5	34.5	45.0
	American Indian/Alaska Native	9.9	11.6	78.4
	Asian/Native Hawaiian/Other Pacific Islander	17.7	31.4	50.9
	Hispanic	27.0	29.7	43.3
	College, full-time	14.6	21.9	63.4
	College, part-time	20.7	20.3	59.0
	Noncollege	24.5	23.3	52.2

Source: Adapted from Chen, Chiung M., Mary C. Dufour, M.D., and Hsiao-ye Yi. "Alcohol Consumption among Young Adults Ages 18–24 in the United States: Results from the 2001–2002 NESARC Survey." *Alcohol Research & Health* 28, no. 4 (2004/2005), p. 278.

Emergency Treatment

Young adults are more likely than those in any other age group in the United States to seek emergency room attention for their alcohol-related problems. This is in part because many of them are uninsured and/or they do not have personal physicians, but it is also because they are more likely than individuals of other ages to engage in drinking and driving. (See EMERGENCY TREATMENT.)

See also ADOLESCENTS.

Chen, Chiung M., Mary C. Dufour, M.D., and Hsiao-ye Yi. "Alcohol Consumption among Young Adults Ages 18–24 in the United States: Results from the 2001–2002 NESARC Survey." *Alcohol Research & Health* 28, no. 4 (2004/2005): 269–280.

Flora, David B., and Laurie Chassin. "Changes in Drug Use during Adulthood: The Effects of Parent Alcoholism and Transition into Marriage." *Psychology of Addictive Behaviors* 19, no. 19 (2005): 352–362.

Kashdan, Todd B., Charlene J. Vetter, and R. Lorraine Collins. "Substance Use in Young Adults: Associations with Personality and Gender." *Addictive Behaviors* 30, no. 2 (February 2005): 259–269.

Johnston, Lloyd D., et al., *Monitoring the Future: National Survey Results on Drug Use, 1975–2004.* Vol. 2, *College Students and Adults Ages 19–45.* Bethesda, Md.: National Institute on Drug Abuse, National Institutes of Health, 2005.

Substance Abuse and Mental Health Services Administration. *Overview of Findings for the 2004 National Survey on Drug Use and Health.* Rockville, Md.: Department of Health and Human Services, September 2005.

zero tolerance laws   State laws that allow for little or no leeway with regard to the abuse of alcohol and/or drugs; for example, zero tolerance state laws with regard to driving stipulate that either any or a very small amount of alcohol (well below the level of legal intoxication for the state, which is often a blood alcohol level of 0.8) detected in a blood alcohol test or breath test is a violation of the zero tolerance law.

State laws vary, but in general, the blood alcohol levels above which a person below age 21 is deemed to have committed a criminal act range from 0.0 to 0.02. These state laws were passed as a result of an amendment to the National Minimum Drinking Age of 1995, a federal law. The federal government required all the states to pass a zero tolerance law related to minors' drinking and driving or to risk losing federal funds. Since then, all 50 states and the District of Columbia have passed such laws.

There are many reasons to curtail drinking among young drivers; for example, young adult drivers who drink or use drugs are at high risk for accidents and fatalities. Some studies show that drivers who are below the age of 21 years have about double the rate of alcohol-involved crashes of older individuals. In addition, according to the 2003 Youth Risk Behavior Survey, 18 percent of youths reported that they never or rarely wore seat belts and 30 percent said they rode with a drinking driver in the past month. In addition, nearly half (45 percent) said they drank alcohol in the past month, while 22 percent used marijuana in the past month.

According to a study reported in *Injury Prevention* in 2002, drivers ages 18–20 years old are more likely to drive when they are impaired than all other age groups. Younger male drivers are also more likely to speed and to take chances when they drive. All of these acts further impair the already inexperienced young driver's ability to avoid car crashes.

The penalties for violating the zero tolerance driving laws vary from state to state and range from fines to community service to the loss of the driver's license.

Pros and Cons of Zero Tolerance

In general, most people support zero tolerance drinking laws. Some studies have shown that such laws have already decreased drinking among young adults. For example, in an article reported in the *Journal of Health Economics* in 2004, on the basis of data from the Behavior Risk Factor Surveillance System, the researcher Christopher Carpenter concludes, "results indicate that the laws reduced heavy episodic drinking (five or more drinks at one sitting) among underage males by 13%."

Carpenter adds that "further examination reveals that the reductions in heavy episodic drinking were accompanied by similarly sized increases in the likelihood of being a light drinker, as well as a decrease in overall number of drinks consumed by young males." (The results were mixed for young females.)

Carpenter hypothesizes, "One answer is that ZT [zero tolerance] laws work by inducing moderation by those individual who—despite drinking heavily in the pre–zero tolerance regime—were still under their state's legal adult threshold in the absence of a ZT law." Thus, in the past, a young man could probably have five or more drinks over a period of several hours but still be within a state's blood alcohol level of 0.08, even when he was a minor. However, with the zero tolerance law, many young men realize that the same level of drinking would cause them to exceed the allowable limit and incur severe penalties, such as losing their driver's licenses.

Concludes Carpenter:

My results are consistent with previous research suggesting that the main route through which alcohol control policies relate to drunk driving behavior is via sharp reductions in heavy drinking for the targeted groups. Overall, then, these findings advance our understanding of the way in which drunk driving policies "work," providing evidence as to their economic efficiency and highlighting an effective public health mechanism for curbing heavy alcohol use among adult young males.

In another study, by Voas and colleagues reporting in 2003 in *Accident Analysis and Prevention,* the researchers looked at fatality rates among drivers younger than age 21 from 1982 to 1987. They concluded that a significant reduction of fatalities resulted from both raising the drinking age to 21 nationwide and passing zero tolerance laws. The researchers state that "reinforcing this action by making it illegal for underage drivers to have any alcohol in their system appears to have been effective in reducing the proportion of fatal crashes involving drinking drivers."

However, those who *oppose* zero tolerance laws often argue that such laws demonize young people and unfairly and unreasonably stigmatize and punish their behavior. Critics also argue that zero tolerance laws are rigid and unreasonable, not allowing for individual circumstances to be considered. In addition, some critics say that zero tolerance policies are taken much too far; for example, with regard to zero tolerance for drugs in schools, as discussed later, some schools may expel students simply for taking an aspirin to school, applying the same punishment as if the student had taken in HEROIN or COCAINE.

School and Work Zero Tolerance Policies

There are other forms of zero tolerance policies. Some workplaces as well as many public and private schools also have zero tolerance policies, usually with regard to drug abuse but also for alcohol abuse. If employees or students violate these policies, the penalties may be severe. For example, companies may fire employees who drink or use drugs during working hours.

Schools may have a policy to expel students who are discovered to be using alcohol or drugs on the school grounds (and they may also contact law enforcement officials for further punitive action).

In most cases, zero tolerance policies are actively promoted within the workplace or school, and these sites often require a written signature from the individual that he or she understands the policies.

See also ABUSE, ALCOHOL; ADOLESCENTS; ALCOHOLISM; YOUNG ADULTS.

Carpenter, Christopher. "How Do Zero Tolerance Drunk Driving Laws Work?" *Journal of Health Economics* 23, no. 1 (2004): 61–83.

Centers for Disease Control and Prevention. "Youth Risk Behavior Surveillance—United States, 2003." *Morbidity and Mortality Weekly Report* 3, no. 2 (May 21, 2004).

Shults, R. A., et al. "Association between State Level Drinking and Driving Countermeasures and Self Reported Alcohol Impaired Driving." *Injury Prevention* 8 (2002): 106–110.

Voas, R. B., A. S. Tippetts, and J. C. Fell. "Assessing the Effectiveness of Minimum Legal Drinking Age and Zero Tolerance Laws in the United States." *Accident Analysis and Prevention* 35, no. 4 (July 2003): 579–587.

APPENDIXES

APPENDIX I
STATE AND TERRITORIAL SUBSTANCE ABUSE OFFICES IN THE UNITED STATES

This listing is of state government contacts with information on substance abuse treatment and issues in each state as well as in U.S. territories. When available, electronic mail addresses are provided.

Alabama

Mr. J. Kent Hunt
Associate Commissioner for Substance Abuse
Alabama Department of Mental Health and
　　Mental Retardation
RSA Union Building
100 North Union Street
P.O. Box 301410
Montgomery, AL 36130
(334) 242-3953
khunt@mh.state.al.us

Alaska

Ms. Melissa Witler Stone
Director
Division of Behavioral Health
Alaska Department of Health and Social Services
3601 C Street, Suite 934
Anchorage, AK 99503
(907) 269-3410
melissa.stone@alaska.gov

Arizona

Ms. Christy Dye
Program Manager
Bureau of Substance Abuse Treatment and
　　Preventive Services
Division of Behavioral Health Services
Arizona Department of Health Services
150 North 18th Avenue
Suite 220
Phoenix, AZ 85007
(602) 364-4558
dye@hs.state.az.us

Arkansas

Mr. Joe M. Hill
Director
Arkansas Department of Human Services
Division of Behavioral Health Services
Alcohol and Drug Abuse Prevention
4313 West Markham
Third Floor Administration
Little Rock, AR 72205
(501) 686-9871
joe.hill@mail.state.ar.us

California

Ms. Kathryn Jett
Director
Department of Alcohol and Drug Programs
1700 K Street
Fifth Floor
Executive Office
Sacramento, CA 95814
(916) 445-1943
kjett@adp.state.ca.us

Colorado

Ms. Janet Wood
Director

Alcohol and Drug Abuse Division
Colorado Department of Human Services
4055 South Lowell Boulevard
Building K-8
Denver, CO 80236
(303) 866-7480
Janet.wood@state.co.us

Connecticut

Dr. Thomas Kirk
Commissioner
Department of Mental Health and Addiction
    Services
P.O. Box 341431
Hartford, CT 06134
(860) 418-6969
thomas.kirk@po.state.ct.us

Delaware

Ms. Renata Henry
Director
Delaware Health and Social Services
Division of Alcoholism, Drug Abuse and Mental
    Health
Administration Building, DHHS Campus
1901 North DuPont Highway
Room 192
New Castle, DE 19720
(303) 255-9426
rehenry@state.de.us

District of Columbia

Mr. Robert Johnson
Administrator
Senior Deputy Director for Substance Abuse
    Services
Department of Operations Addiction Prevention
    and Recovery Administration
825 North Capitol Street NE
Suite 3125
Washington, D.C. 20002
(202) 442-9155
Robert.Johnson1@dc.gov

Florida

Mr. Ken DeCerchio
Director
Substance Abuse Program Office
Department of Children and Families
1317 Winewood Boulevard
Building 6
Third Floor
Tallahassee, FL 32399
(850) 921-2495
ken_decerchio@cdf.state.fl.us

Georgia

Mr. Bruce Hoopes
Chief
Substance Abuse Program
Division of Mental Health, Developmental
    Disabilities and Addictive Diseases
Georgia Department of Human Resources
2 Peachtree Street NW
Fourth Floor
Atlanta, GA 30303
(404) 657-2135
blhoopes@dhr.state.ga.us

Hawaii

Ms. Elaine Wilson
Chief
Alcohol and Drug Abuse Division
Hawaii Department of Health
Kakuhihewa Building
601 Kamokila Boulevard
Room 360
Kapolei, HI 96707
(808) 692-7507
ejwilson@mail.health.state.hi.us

Idaho

Mr. Pharis Stanger
Substance Abuse Project Manager
Bureau of Mental Health and Substance Abuse
Division of Family and Community Services
Idaho Department of Health and Welfare

450 West State Street
Fifth Floor
Boise, ID 83720
(208) 334-4944
stangerp@idhw.state.id.us

Illinois

Ms. Theodora Binion-Taylor
Associate Director
Illinois Department of Children and Family
    Services
Office of Alcoholism and Substance Abuse
James R. Thompson Center
100 West Randolph Street
Suite 5-600
Chicago, IL 60601
(312) 814-2300
DHSASA4@dhs.state.il.us

Indiana

Mr. John Viernes
Director
Division of Mental Health
Indiana Family and Social Services
    Administration
Indiana Government Building
402 West Washington Street
Room W353
Indianapolis, IN 46204
(317) 232-7844
jviernes@fssa.state.in.us

Iowa

Ms. Janet Zwick
Director
Division of Health Promotion, Prevention and
    Addictive Behaviors
Iowa Department of Public Health
Lucas State Office Building
321 East 12th Street
Fourth Floor
Des Moines, IA 50319
(515) 281-4417
jzwick@idph.state.ia.us

Kansas

Ms. Donna Doolin
Acting Director
Kansas Department of Social and Rehabilitation
    Services
Division of Health Care Policy, Addiction and
    Prevention Services
Docking State Office Building
915 Southwest Harrison Street
10th Floor, North
Topeka, KS 66612
(785) 296-7272
dxmd@srskansas.org

Kentucky

Ms. Karyn Hascal
Director
Division of Substance Abuse
Kansas Department for Mental Health and Mental
    Retardation Services
1000 Fair Oaks Lane
Frankfort, KY 40621
(502) 564-2880
karyn.hascal@mail.state.ky.us

Louisiana

Mr. Michael Duffy
Assistant Secretary
Office for Addictive Disorders
Louisiana Department of Health and Hospitals
1201 Capitol Access Road
Fourth Floor
P.O. Box 2790, BIN # 18
Baton Rouge, LA 70821
(225) 342-6717
mduffy@dhh.stae.la.us

Maine

Ms. Kimberly Johnson
Director
Maine Office of Substance Abuse
Augusta Mental Health Complex
Marquardt Building
159 State House Station
Third Floor

Augusta, ME 04333
(207) 287-2595
kimberly.johnson@state.me.us

Maryland

Dr. Peter Luongo
Director
Alcohol and Drug Abuse Administration
Maryland Department of Health and Mental Hygiene
55 Wade Avenue
Catonsville, MD 21228
(410) 402-8600
pluongo@dhmh.state.md.us

Massachusetts

Mr. Michael Botticelli
Associate Commissioner
Bureau of Substance Abuse Services
Massachusetts Department of Public Health
250 Washington Street
Third Floor
Boston, MA 02108
(617) 624-5111
Michael.Botticelli@state.ma.us

Michigan

Ms. Doris Gellert
Director
Bureau of Substance Abuse and Addiction Services
Michigan Department of Community Health
Lewis Cass Building
320 South Walnut Street
Fifth Floor
Lansing, MI 48909
(517) 373-2412
gellert:Michigan.gov

Minnesota

Mr. Donald R. Eubanks
Director
Chemical Health Division
Minnesota Department of Human Services
444 Lafayette Road North
St. Paul, MN 55155

(651) 582-1856
don.eubanks@state.mn.us

Mississippi

Mr. Herbert L. Loving
Director
Division of Alcohol and Drug Abuse
Mississippi Department of Mental Health
1101 Robert E. Lee Building
239 North Lamar Street
Jackson, MS 39201
(601) 359-6220
hloving@msdmh.org

Missouri

Mr. Michael Couty
Director
Division of Alcohol and Drug Abuse
Missouri Department of Mental Health
1706 East Elm Street
Jefferson City, MO 65102
(573) 751-4942
mzcoutm@mail.dmh.stae.mo.us

Montana

Ms. Joan Cassidy
Bureau Chief
Chemical Dependency Bureau
Addictive and Mental Disorders Division
555 Fuller Avenue
P.O. Box 202905
Helena, MT 59620
(406) 444-7924
jcassidy@state.mt.us

Nebraska

Mr. Ron Sorensen
Director
Division of Mental Health, Substance Abuse and
    Addictions Services
Nebraska Department of Health and Human
    Services Systems
Folsom Street & West Prospector Place
Building 14, West Campus

P.O. Box 98925
Lincoln, NE 68509
(402) 479-5583
ron.sorensen@hhss.state.ne.us

Nevada

Ms. Maria Canfield
Chief
Bureau of Alcohol and Drug Abuse, Health Division
Department of Human Resources
505 East King Street
Room 500
Carson City, NV 89701
(775) 684-4190
mcanfield@nvhd.state.nv.us

New Hampshire

Mr. Joseph Harding
Director
Community and Public Health Services
Office of Alcohol and Drug Policy
Main Building
105 Pleasant Street
Third Floor North
Concord, NH 03301
(603) 271-6105
jharding@dhhs.state.nh.us

New Jersey

Ms. Carolann Kane-Cavaiola
Assistant Commissioner
New Jersey Department of Health and Senior
   Services
Division of Addiction Services
120 South Stockton Street
Third Floor
P.O. Box 362
Trenton, NJ 08625
(609) 292-5760
carolann.kane-cavaiola@doh.state.nj.us

New Mexico

Mr. Richard Tavares
Acting Director

Behavioral Health Services Division
New Mexico Department of Health
Harold Runnels Building
1190 St. Francis Drive
Suite 3300 North
Santa Fe, NM 87502
(505) 827-2658

New York

Dr. William Gorman
Commissioner
New York State Office of Alcoholism and
   Substance Abuse Services
1450 Western Avenue
Albany, NY 12203
(518) 457-2061
BillGorman@oasas.state.ny.us

North Carolina

Ms. Flo Stein
Chief Community Policy Management
Division of Mental Health, Development
   Disabilities and Substance Abuse Services
North Carolina Department of Health and Human
   Services
3007 Mail Service Center
Raleigh, NC 27699
(919) 733-4670
flo.stein@ncmail.net

North Dakota

Mr. Don Wright
Unit Manager
Substance Abuse Services
Division of Mental Health and Substance Abuse
   Services
North Dakota Department of Human Services
Professional Building
600 South Second Street
Suite 1E
Bismarck, ND 58504
(701) 328-8922
sowrid@state.nd.us

Ohio

Mr. Gary Q. Tester
Director
Ohio Department of Alcohol and Drug Addiction
    Services
Two Nationwide Plaza
280 North High Street
12th Floor
Columbus, OH 43215
(614) 466-3445
tester@ada.state.oh.us

Oklahoma

Mr. Ben Brown
Deputy Commissioner
Substance Abuse Services
Oklahoma Department of Mental Health and
    Substance Abuse Services
1200 NE 13th Street
P.O. Box 53277
Oklahoma City, OK 73152
(405) 522-3877
bbrown@odmhsas.org

Oregon

Mr. Bob Nikkel
Administrator
Department of Human Services
Health Services Building
Office of Mental Health and Addiction Services
2575 Bittern Street NE
P.O. Box 14250
Salem, OR 97309
(503) 945-9700
Robert.E.Nikkel@state.or.us

Pennsylvania

Mr. Gene Boyle
Director
Bureau of Drug and Alcohol Programs
Pennsylvania Department of Health
02 Klein Plaza
Suite B
Harrisburg, PA 17104

(717) 783-8200
eboyle@state.pa.us

Rhode Island

Ms. Kim Harris
Executive Director
Behavioral Health Care Services
Department of Mental Health, Retardation and
    Hospitals
14 Harrington Road-Barry Hall
Cranston, RI 02920
(401) 462-2339
kharris@mhrh.state.ri.us

South Carolina

Mr. W. Lee Catoe
Director
South Carolina Department of Alcohol and Other
    Drug Abuse Services
101 Business Park Boulevard
Columbia, SC 29203
(803) 896-5551
LeeCatoe@daodas.state.sc.us

South Dakota

Mr. Gilbert Sudbeck
Director
Division of Alcohol and Drug Abuse
South Dakota Department of Human Services
East Highway 34, Hillsview Plaza
c/o 500 East Capitol
Pierre, SD 57501
(605) 773-3123
gib.sudbeck@state.sd.us

Tennessee

Dr. Stephanie W. Perry
Assistant Commissioner
Bureau of Alcohol and Drug Abuse Services
Tennessee Department of Health
Cordell Hull Building
425 Fifth Avenue North
Third Floor
Nashville, TN 37247

(615) 741-1921
Stephanie.perry@state.tn.us

Texas

Dr. Dave Wanser
Deputy Commissioner
Teas Department of State Health Services
1100 West 49th Street
M-751
Austin, TX 78756
(512) 458-7376
dave.wanser@dshs.state.tx.us

Utah

Mr. Randall Bachman
Director
Division of Substance Abuse and Mental Health
Utah Department of Human Services
120 North 200 West
Room 201
Salt Lake City, UT 84103
(801) 538-3939
rbachman@utah.gov

Vermont

Ms. Barbara Cimaglio
Deputy Commissioner and Director, Alcohol and
    Drug Abuse Programs
Vermont Department of Health
108 Cherry Street
Burlington, VT 05402
(802) 651-1553
bcimagl@vdh.state.vt.us

Virginia

Mr. Kenneth Batten
Director
Substance Abuse Specialty Services
Virginia Department of Mental Health, Mental
    Retardation and Substance Abuse
1220 Bank Street
Eighth Floor
Richmond, VA 23218
(804) 786-3906
kbatten@dmhmrsas.state.va.us

Washington

Mr. Kenneth D. Stark
Director
Division of Alcohol and Substance Abuse
Washington Department of Social and Health
    Services
P.O. Box 45330
Olympia, WA 98504
(360) 438-8200
StarkKD@dshs.wa.gov

West Virginia

Mr. Steve Mason
Director
Division of Alcohol and Drug Abuse
Office of Behavioral Health Services
West Virginia Department of Health and Human
    Services
1900 Kanawha Boulevard, Capitol Complex
Building 6
Room 738
Charleston, WV 25305
(304) 558-2276
stevemason@wvdhhr.org

Wisconsin

Mr. John Easterday
Director
Associate Administrator for Mental Health and
    Substance Abuse Services
Department of Health and Family Services
1 West Wilson Street
P.O. Box 7851
Madison, WI 53708
(608) 267-9391
easterjt@dhfs.state.wi.us

Wyoming

Ms. Alfrieda Gonzalez
Administrator
Department of Health Substance Abuse Division
2424 Pioneer Avenue
Suite 306
Cheyenne, WY 82002

(307) 777-6494
agonzalez@state.wy.us

American Samoa

L'aulualo Faafetai Talia
Director
Department of Human and Social Services
997534 Utulei Street
P.O. Box 9997534
Pago Pago, American Samoa 96799
(684) 633-2696
pmageo@hotmail.com

Guam

Mr. Peter Roberto
Director
Department of Mental Health and Substance
    Abuse
Government of Guam
790 Governor Carlos G. Camacho Road
Tamuning, Guam 96911
(671) 647-5445
mtlozada@mail.gov.gu

Marshall Islands

Ms. Saeko Shoniber
Ministry of Finance Office
Republic of the Marshall Islands
P.O. Box D
Majuro, MH 96960
011-692-625-8311
clrounds@hotmail.com

Micronesia

Mr. Nens S. Nena
Secretary
Department of Health, Education and Social
    Affairs
Federated States of Micronesia
P.O. Box PS 70
Palikir, Pohnpei Micronesia 96941
(691) 320-2619
jeffb@mail.fm

Northern Mariana Islands

Dr. James Hofschneider
Secretary of Health
Department of Public Health
Commonwealth of the Northern Mariana Islands
P.O. Box 500409 CK
Saipa, Northern Mariana Islands 96950
(670) 234-8950, extension 2001
health7@saipan.com

Palau

Ms. Sandra S. Pierantozzi
Minister of Health
Ministry of Human Services
Palau National Hospital
Republic of Palau
P.O. Box 6027
Koro, Republic of Palau 96940
(680) 488-2813
bhd@palaunet.com

Puerto Rico

Dr. Jose Galarza
Administrator
Puerto Rico Mental Health and Anti-Addiction
    Services Administration
Avenida Barbosa #414
GPO Box 70184
San Juan, Puerto Rico 0928
(787) 274-3795
JRullan@ salud.gov.pr

Virgin Islands

Dr. Brent Woodard
Acting Director
Mental Health, Alcoholism & Drug Dependency
Virgin Islands Department of Health
Barbel Plaza South
Second Floor
St. Thomas, Virgin Islands 00801
(340) 77304888

APPENDIX II
STATE MENTAL HEALTH AGENCIES

Alabama

Department of Mental Health and Mental Retardation
RSA Union Building
100 North Union Street
Montgomery, AL 36130-3417
(334) 242-3454
(800) 367-0955 (toll-free)
http://www.mh.state.al.us

Alaska

Division of Mental Health and Developmental Disabilities
Department of Health and Social Services
P.O. Box 110620
Juneau, AK 99811-0620
(907) 465-3370
(800) 465-4828 (toll-free)
(907) 465-2225 (TDD)
http://www.hss.state.ak.us/dbh/

Arizona

Department of Health Services
Division of Behavioral Health Services
150 North 18th Avenue
#200
Phoenix, AZ 85007
(602) 364-4558
http://www.hs.state.az.us/bhs/index.htm

Arkansas

Division of Mental Health Services
Department of Human Services
4313 West Markham Street
Little Rock, AR 72205-4096
(501) 686-9164
(501) 686-9176 (TDD)
http://www.state.ar.us/dhs/dmhs/

California

Department of Mental Health
Health and Welfare Agency
1600 Ninth Street
Room 151
Sacramento, CA 95814
(916) 654-3565
(800) 896-4042 (toll-free)
(800) 896-2512 (TDD)
http://www.dmh.cahwnet.gov

Colorado

Colorado Mental Health Services
3824 West Princeton Circle
Denver, CO 80236
(303) 866-7400
http://www.cdhs.state.co.us/ohr/mhs/

Connecticut

Department of Mental Health and Addictions Services
410 Capitol Avenue
Hartford, CT 06106
(860) 418-6700
(800) 446-7348 (toll-free)
(888) 621-3551 (TDD)
http://www.dmhas.state.ct.us

Delaware

Division of Substance Abuse and Mental Health
Department of Health and Social Services
Main Building
1901 N. DuPont Highway
New Castle, DE 19720
(302) 255-9427
http://www.state.de.us/dhss/dsamh/dmhhome.htm

District of Columbia

Department of Mental Health Services
77 P Street, NE
4th Floor
Washington, D.C. 20002
(202) 673-7440
(888) 793-4357 (toll-free)
http://dmh.dc.gov/dmh/site/default.asp

Florida

Department of Children and Families
Building 1
1317 Winewood Boulevard
Room 202
Tallahassee, FL 32399-0700
(850) 487-1111
http://www.state.fl.us/cf_web/

Georgia

Division of Mental Health, Mental Retardation and Substance Abuse
Department of Human Resources
2 Peachtree Street NW
Suite 22-224
Atlanta, GA 30303
(404) 657-2168
www.state.ga.us/departments/dhr/mhmrsa/
    index.html

Hawaii

Behavioral Health Services Administration
Department of Health
P.O. Box 3378

Honolulu, HI 96801
(808) 586-4419
http://www.state.hi.us/doh/about/behavior.html

Idaho

Department of Health and Welfare
450 West State Street
Boise, ID 83720-0036
(208) 334-5500
http://www2.state.id.us/dhw/index.htm

Illinois

Office of Mental Health
Department of Human Services
Centrum Building
319 East Madison Street
Third Floor
Springfield, IL 62701
(217) 785-6023
http://www.dhs.state.il.us

Indiana

Division of Mental Health
Department of Family and Social Services
    Administration
402 West Washington Street
Room W-353
Indianapolis, IN 46204-2739
(317) 232-7844

Iowa

Division of Mental Health and Developmental Disabilities
Hoover State Office Building
1305 East Walnut Street
Des Moines, IA 50319-0114
(515) 281-3573

Kansas

Department of Social and Rehabilitation Services
Docking State Office Building
915 SW Harrison Street

Topeka, KS 66612
(785) 296-3959
http://www.srskansas.org

Kentucky

Department for Mental Health and Mental Retardation Services

Cabinet for Human Resources
100 Fair Oaks Lane
Frankfort, KY 40621-0001
(502) 564-4527
http://mhmr.chs.ky.gov/Default.asp

Office of Mental Health

P.O. Box 4049, Bin #12
Baton Rouge, LA 70821-4049
(225) 342-2540
http://www.dhh.state.la.us/OMH/index.htm

Maine

Adult Mental Health Services

Department of Behavioral and Developmental
    Services
40 State House Station
Augusta, ME 04333
(207) 287-4200
(888) 568-1112 (toll-free)
http://www.state.me.us/dmhmrsa

Maryland

Department of Health and Mental Hygiene

201 West Preston Street
Baltimore, MD 21201
(410) 767-6860
(877) 463-3464 (toll-free)
(800) 735-2258 (TDD)
http://www.dhmh.state.md.us

Massachusetts

Department of Mental Health

25 Staniford Street
Boston, MA 02114
(617) 626-8000
(617) 727-9842 (TDD)
http://www.state.ma.us/dmh/_MainLine/
    MissionStatement.HTM

Michigan

Department of Community Health

Lewis-Cass Building
320 South Walnut Street
Sixth Floor
Lansing, MI 48913
(517) 373-3500
(517) 373-3573 (TDD)
http://www.michigan.gov/mdch

Minnesota

Department of Human Services

Mental Health Program Division
Human Services Building
444 Lafayette Road
Saint Paul, MN 55155-3828
(651) 297-3510
http://www.dhs.state.mn.us/Contcare/mentalhealth/
    default.htm

Mississippi

Department of Mental Health

Robert E. Lee Building
239 North Lamar Street
Suite 1101
Jackson, MS 39201
(601) 359-1288
(601) 359-6230 (TDD)
http://www.dmh.state.ms.us

Missouri

Department of Mental Health

P.O. Box 687
Jefferson City, MO 65102
(800) 364-9687 (toll-free)
(573) 526-1201 (TDD)
http://www.dmh.missouri.gov

Montana

Addictive and Mental Disorders Division

Department of Public Health and Human Services
555 Fuller
Helena, MT 59620
(406) 444-4928
http://www.dphhs.state.mt.us

Nebraska

Office of Mental Health, Substance Abuse and Addictions Services
P.O. Box 98925
Lincoln, NE 68509
(402) 479-5166
http://www.hhs.state.ne.us/beh/mhsa.htm

Nevada

Mental Health & Developmental Services Division
Department of Human Resources
Kinkead Building
505 East King Street
Room 602
Carson City, NV 89701
(775) 684-5943
http://www.mhds.state.nv.us

New Hampshire

Division of Behavioral Health
Department of Health and Human Services
State Office Park South
105 Pleasant Street
Concord, NH 03301
(603) 271-8140
(800) 852-3345 (toll-free)
(800) 735-2964 (TDD)
http://www.dhhs.state.nh.us

New Jersey

Division of Mental Health Services
50 East State Street
Capitol Center, Post Office 727
Trenton, NJ 08625-0727
(609) 777-0702
http://www.state.nj.us/humanservices/dmhs

New Mexico

Behavioral Health Services Division
Harold Runnels Building
1190 Saint Francis Drive
Room North 3300
Santa Fe, NM 87505-6110

(505) 827-2601
(800) 362-2013 (toll-free)
http://www.nmcares.org

New York

Office of Mental Health
44 Holland Avenue
Albany, NY 12229
(518) 474-4403
(800) 597-8481 (toll-free)
http://www.omh.state.ny.us

North Carolina

Division of Mental Health, Developmental Disabilities, and Substance Abuse Services
Department of Health & Human Resources
3001 Mail Service Center
Raleigh, NC 27699-3001
(919) 733-7011
(919) 733-1221 (fax)
http://www.dhhs.state.nc.us/mhddsas

North Dakota

Division of Mental Health & Substance Abuse Services
600 South Second Street
Suite 1D
Bismarck, ND 58504-5729
(701) 328-8940
(800) 755-2719 (toll-free)

Ohio

Department of Mental Health
30 East Broad Street
Eighth Floor
Columbus, OH 43215
(614) 466-2337
http://www.mh.state.oh.us

Oklahoma

Department of Mental Health and Substance Abuse Services
P.O. Box 53277, Capitol Station
Oklahoma City, OK 73152

(405) 522-3908
(800) 522-9054 (toll-free)
(800) 522-7233 (Domestic Violence Safeline)
http://www.odmhsas.org

Oregon

Oregon Department of Human Services
Mental Health and Addiction Services
500 Summer Street NE
E86
Salem, OR 97301
(503) 945-5763
(503) 947-5330 (TDD)
http://www.dhs.state.or.us/mentalhealth/

Pennsylvania

**Office of Mental Health and Substance Abuse
  Services**
P.O. Box 2675
Harrisburg, PA 17105-2675
(717) 787-6443
(877) 356-5355 (toll-free)
http://www.dpw.state.pa.us/omhsas/dpwmh.asp

Rhode Island

**Department of Mental Health, Mental
  Retardation and Hospitals**
14 Harrington Road
Cranston, RI 02920
(401) 462-3201
http://www.mhrh.state.ri.us

South Carolina

Department of Mental Health
2414 Bull Street
P.O. Box 485
Columbia, SC 29202
(803) 898-8581
http://www.state.sc.us/dmh

South Dakota

Division of Mental Health
Department of Human Services
Hillsview Plaza

East Highway 34
c/o 500 East Capitol
Pierre, SD 57501-5070
(605) 773-5991
(800) 265-9684 (toll-free)
http://www.state.sd.us/dhs/dmh

Tennessee

**Department of Mental Health and
  Developmental Disabilities**
Cordell Hull Building
425 Fifth Avenue North
Third Floor
Nashville, TN 37243
(615) 532-6500
http://www.state.tn.us/mental/

Texas

**Texas Department of Mental Health and
  Mental Retardation**
Central Office
909 West Forty Fifth Street
Austin, TX 78751
(512) 454-3761
(800) 252-8154 (toll-free)
http://www.mhmr.state.tx.us

Utah

Division of Mental Health
Department of Human Services
120 North 200 West
Fourth Floor, Suite 415
Salt Lake City, UT 84103
(801) 538-4270
http://www.hsmh.state.ut.us

Vermont

**Department of Developmental and Mental
  Health Services**
Weeks Building
103 South Main Street
Waterbury, VT 05671-1601
(802) 241-2610
http://www.state.vt.us/dmh

Virginia

**Department of Mental Health, Mental
  Retardation and Substance Abuse Services**
P.O. Box 1797
Richmond, VA 23218
(804) 786-3921
(804) 371-8977 (TDD)
(800) 451-554 (toll-free)
http://www.dmhmrsas.state.va.us/

Washington

Mental Health Division
Department of Social and Health Services
P.O. Box 45320
Olympia, WA 98504-5320
(360) 902-0790
(800) 446-0259 (toll-free)
http://www.wa.gov/dshs/

West Virginia

**Bureau for Behavioral Health and Health
  Facilities**
Department of Health and Human Resources
350 Capitol Street
Room 350
Charleston, WV 25301-3702
(304) 558-0627
http://www.wvdhhr.org/

Wisconsin

Bureau of Community Mental Health
Department of Health and Family Services
1 West Wilson Street
Room 433
P.O. Box 7851
Madison, WI 53702-7851
(608) 267-7792
http://www.dhfs.state.wi.us/mentalhealth

Wyoming

Mental Health Division
Department of Health
6101 Yellowstone Road
Room 259-B
Cheyenne, WY 82002
(307) 777-7094
http://mhd.state.wy.us/

APPENDIX III
STATE CONTROLLED SUBSTANCES SCHEDULING AUTHORITIES

This appendix provides state contacts for authorities involved in scheduled drugs, such as narcotics.

Alabama

Department of Public Health
P.O. Box 30317
Montgomery, AL 36130
(334) 206-5300

Alaska

Division of Occupational Licensing
P.O. Box 110806
Juneau, AK 99811
(907) 465-2589

Arizona

Board of Pharmacy
4425 West Olive Avenue
Suite 140
Glendale, AZ 85302

Arkansas

**Division of Pharmacy Services and Drug
    Control**
Arkansas Department of Public Health
4815 West Markham Street
Slot 25
Little Rock, AR 72205
(501) 661-2325

California

Board of Pharmacy
400 R Street
Suite 4070
Sacramento, CA 95814

Colorado

Board of Pharmacy
1560 Broadway
Suite 1301
Denver, CO 80202
(303) 894-7753

Connecticut

Drug Control Division
Department of Consumer Protection
165 Capitol Avenue
Hartford, CT 06106
(860) 713-6079

Delaware

Board of Pharmacy
P.O. Box 637
Dover, DE 19901
(302) 739-4978

District of Columbia

**Bureau of Food, Drugs & Radiological
    Protection**
Department of Health
51 N Street NE

Sixth Floor
Washington, DC 20002
(202) 535-2188

Florida

Assistant Attorney General
Administrative Law Section
The Capitol
Room LL-04
Tallahassee, FL 32399
(850) 414-3300

Georgia

Georgia Drugs & Narcotics Agency
40 Pryor Street SW
Suite 2000
Atlanta, GA 30303
(404) 656-5100

Hawaii

Department of Public Safety
Bureau of Narcotic Enforcement
3375 Koapaka Street
Suite D100
Honolulu, HI 96819
(808) 837-8470

Idaho

Board of Pharmacy
3380 Americana Terrace
Suite 320
Boise, ID 83706
(208) 334-2356

Illinois

Illinois Prescription Monitoring Program
Department of Human Services
401 North Fourth Street
Room 133
Springfield, IL 62701
(217) 524-9074

Indiana

Board of Pharmacy
Health Professions Bureau
402 West Washington Street
Room 041
Indianapolis, IN 46204
(317) 234-2067

Iowa

Controlled Drug Division
Board of Pharmacy Examiners
400 Southwest Eighth Street
Suite E
Des Moines, IA 50319
(515) 281-5944

Kansas

Kansas State Board of Pharmacy
900 Jackson Avenue
Room 560
Topeka, KS 66612
(785) 296-4056

Kentucky

Department for Public Health
Drug Enforcement Branch
275 East Main Street HS2GW-B
Frankfort, KY 40621
(502) 564-7985

Louisiana

Louisiana Board of Pharmacy
Corporate Boulevard
Suite 8E
Baton Rouge, LA 70808
(225) 925-6496

Maine

Board of Commissioners & Pharmacy
State House Station Number 35
Augusta, ME 04333
(207) 582-8723

Maryland

Maryland Board of Pharmacy
4201 Patterson Avenue
Baltimore, MD 21215
(410) 764-4794

Massachusetts

Drug Control Program
Department of Public Health, Division of Food and
    Drugs
305 South Street
Jamaica Plains, MA 02130
(617) 983-6700

Michigan

Bureau of Health Services
Health Regulatory Division
6546 Mercantile Way
Suite 2
P.O. Box 30454
Lansing, MI 48909
(517) 335-1769

Minnesota

Board of Pharmacy
2829 University Avenue SE
Suite 530
Minneapolis, MN 55414
(612) 617-2201

Mississippi

**Pharmacy Department, Division of Public
    Health**
P.O. Box 1700
Jackson, MS 39205
(601) 713-3471

Missouri

Bureau of Narcotics & Dangerous Drugs
Department of Health and Senior Services
P.O. Box 570
Jefferson City, MO 65102
(573) 751-6321

Montana

Board of Pharmacy
P.O. Box 200513
Helena, MT 59620
(406) 841-2355

Nebraska

**Professional and Occupational Licensing
    Division**
Department of Health
P.O. Box 94986
Lincoln, NE 68509
(402) 471-2118

Nevada

Board of Pharmacy
555 Double Eagle Court
Suite 1100
Reno, NV 89502
(775) 850-1440

New Hampshire

New Hampshire Board of Pharmacy
57 Regional Drive
Concord, NH 03301
(603) 271-2350

New Jersey

Drug Control
Department of Law and Public Safety
P.O. Box 45045
Newark, NJ 07101
(973) 504-6561

New York

Bureau of Controlled Substances
New York State Department of Health
433 River Street
Fifth Floor
Troy, NY 12180
(518) 402-0707

North Carolina

Controlled Substances Regulatory Branch
Alcohol & Drug Abuse Services
3824 Barrett Drive
Suite 308
Raleigh, NC 27609
(919) 420-7932

North Dakota

North Dakota Board of Pharmacy
P.O. Box 1354
Bismarck, ND 58502
(701) 328-9535

Ohio

Board of Pharmacy
77 South High Street
Room 1702
Columbus, OH 43215
(614) 466-4143

Oklahoma

Bureau of Narcotics and Dangerous Drugs
4545 North Lincoln Boulevard
Suite 11
Oklahoma City, OK 73105
(405) 521-2885

Oregon

Board of Pharmacy
State Office Building
800 Northeast Oregon
Suite 9
Portland, OR 97232
(503) 731-4032

Pennsylvania

**Bureau of Narcotic Investigations and Drug
    Control**
106 Lowther Street
Lemoyne, PA 17043
(717) 783-2600

Rhode Island

Compliance and Regulatory Section
Division of Drug Control
205 Cannon Office Building
3 Capitol Hill
Suite 205
Providence, RI 02908
(401) 222-2837

South Carolina

Bureau of Drug Control
Department of Health and Environmental Control
2600 Bull Street
Columbia, SC 29201
(803) 896-0636

South Dakota

Department of Health
Licensure and Certification
615 East Fourth Street
Pierre, SD 57501
(605) 773-3356

Tennessee

Tennessee Board of Pharmacy
Davy Crockett Tower
500 James Robinson Parkway
Second Floor
Nashville, TN 37243
(615) 741-2718

Texas

Texas State Department of Health
1100 West 49th Street
Austin, TX 78756
(512) 719-0237

Utah

Division of Professional Licensing
P.O. Box 146741
Salt Lake City, UT 84114
(801) 530-6721

Vermont

Vermont Department of Health
108 Cherry Street
P.O. Box 70
Burlington, VT 05042
(802) 863-7281

Virginia

Board of Pharmacy
6603 West Broad Street
Fifth Floor
Richmond, VA 23230-1712
(804) 662-9911

Washington

Board of Pharmacy
P.O. Box 47863
Olympia, WA 98504
(360) 236-4825

West Virginia

West Virginia Board of Pharmacy
232 Capitol Street
Charleston, WV 25301
(304) 558-0558

Wisconsin

Department of Regulation and Licensing
Controlled Substances Board
P.O. Box 8935
Madison, WI 53708
(608) 266-8098

Wyoming

State Board of Pharmacy
1720 South Poplar Street
Suite 4
Casper, WY 82601
(307) 234-0294

APPENDIX IV
STATE HEALTH DEPARTMENTS

Alabama

Alabama Department of Public Health
The RSA Tower
201 Monroe Street
Montgomery, AL 36104
(334) 206-5300
http://www.adph.org

Alaska

Office of the Commissioner
Health and Social Services
350 Main Street
Room 404
P.O. Box 110601
Juneau, AK 99811
(907) 465-3030
http://health.hss.state.ak.us/commissioner

Arizona

Arizona Department of Health Services
150 North 18th Avenue
Phoenix, AZ 85007
(602) 542-1000
http://www.azdhs.gov

Arkansas

Department of Health
4815 West Markham
Little Rock, AR 72203
(501) 661-2000
http://www.healthyarkansas.com/health.html

California

California Department of Health
714 P Street

Room 1253
Sacramento, CA 95899
(916) 440-7400
http://www.dhs.ca.gov

Colorado

Colorado Department of Public Health and Environment
4300 Cherry Creek Drive South
Denver, CO 80246
(303) 692-2000
http://www.cdphe.state.co.us/ic/infohom.html

Connecticut

Connecticut Department of Public Health
410 Capitol Avenue
P.O. Box 340308
Hartford, CT 06134
(860) 509-8000
http://www.dph.state.ct.us/

Delaware

Delaware Health and Social Services
1901 North DuPont Highway
New Castle, DE 19720
(302) 255-9040
http://www.state.de.us/dhss

District of Columbia

Department of Health
825 North Capitol Street, NE
Washington, DC 20002
(202) 671-5000
http://doh.dc/gov/doh/site/default.asp

Florida

Department of Health
4052 Bald Cypress Way
Tallahassee, FL 32399-3291
(850) 245-4147
http://esetappsdoh.doh.state.fl.us

Georgia

Georgia Department of Community Health
2 Peachtree Street
40th Floor
Atlanta, GA 30303
(404) 656-4507
http://dch.georgia.gov

Hawaii

Hawaii State Department of Health
1250 Punchbowl Street
Honolulu, HI 96813
(808) 586-4400
http://www.hawaii.gov/health

Idaho

Idaho Department of Health and Welfare
450 West State Street
Boise, ID 83720
(208) 334-5500
http://www.healthandwelfare.idaho.gov

Illinois

Illinois Department of Public Health
535 West Jefferson Street
Springfield, IL 62761
(217) 782-4977
http://www.idph.state.il.us

Indiana

Indiana State Department of Health
2 North Meridian Street
Indianapolis, IN 46204
(317) 233-1325
http://www.in.gov/isdh

Iowa

Iowa Department of Public Health
321 East 12th Street
Des Moines, IA 50319
(515) 281-7689
http://www.idph.state.is.us/

Kansas

Kansas Department of Health and Environment
Curtis State Office Building
1000 SW Jackson
Topeka, KS 66612
(785) 296-1500
http://www.kdheks.gov

Kentucky

Cabinet for Health and Family Services
Office of the Secretary
275 East Main Street
Frankfort, KY 40621
(800) 372-2973
http://chfs.ky.gov

Louisiana

Louisiana Department of Health & Hospitals
628 North 4th Street
P.O. Box 629
Baton Rouge, LA 70821
(225) 342-5568
http://www.dhh.louisiana.gov

Maine

Maine Center for Disease Control and Prevention
286 Water Street
State House Station 11
Augusta, ME 04333
(207) 287-8016
http://www.maine.gov/dhhs/boh

Maryland

Maryland Department of Health & Mental Hygiene
201 West Preston Street
Baltimore, MD 21201
(410) 767-8500
http://www.dhmh.state.md.us/

Massachusetts

Massachusetts Department of Public Health
250 Washington Street
Boston, MA 02108
(617) 624-6000
http://www.mass.gov/dph/dphhome.htm

Michigan

Michigan Department of Community Health
Capitol View Building
201 Townsend Street
Lansing, MI 48913
(517) 373-3740
http://www.michigan.gov/mdch

Minnesota

Minnesota Department of Health
P.O. Box 64975
St. Paul, MN 55164
(651) 201-5000
http://www.health.state.mn.us

Mississippi

Mississippi Department of Health
570 East Woodrow Wilson Drive
Jackson, MS 39216
(601) 576-7400
http://www.msdh.state.ms.us

Missouri

Missouri Department of Health & Senior Services
P.O. Box 570
Jefferson City, MO 65102

(573) 751-6400
http://www.dhss.mo.gov

Montana

Montana Department of Public Health and Human Services
1400 Broadway
Helena, MT 59620
(406) 444-1861
http://www.dphhs.mt.gov/

Nebraska

Nebraska Department of Health and Human Services
P.O. Box 95944
Lincoln, NE 68509
(402) 471-2306
http://www.hhs.state.ne.us

Nevada

Nevada Department of Health and Human Services
505 East King Street
Room 600
Carson City, NV 89710
(775) 684-4000
http://www.hr.state.nv.us/

New Hampshire

New Hampshire Department of Health and Human Services
State Office Park South
129 Pleasant Street
Concord, NH 03301
(603) 271-4688
http://www.dhhs.state.nh.us

New Jersey

Department of Health and Senior Services
P.O. Box 360
Trenton, NJ 08625
(609) 292-7837
http://www.state.nj.us/health/

New Mexico

New Mexico Department of Health
1190 South St. Francis Drive
Santa Fe, NM 87502
(505) 827-2613
http://www.health.state.nm.us

New York

New York State Department of Health
Corning Tower
Empire State Plaza
Albany, NY 12237
http://www.health.state.ny.us

North Carolina

**North Carolina Department of Health and
    Human Services**
2001 Mail Service Center
Raleigh, NC 27699
(919) 733-4534
http://www.dhhs.state.nc.us

North Dakota

North Dakota Department of Health
600 East Boulevard Avenue
Bismarck, ND 58505
(701) 328-2372
http://www.ndhan.gov

Ohio

Ohio Department of Health
246 North High Street
Columbus, OH 43126
(614) 644-8562
http://www.odh.ohio.gov

Oklahoma

Oklahoma Health Care Authority
4545 North Lincoln Boulevard
Suite 124
Oklahoma City, OK 73105
(405) 522-7300
http://www.ohca.state.ok.us

Oregon

Oregon Public Health Division
800 NE Oregon Street
Portland, OR 97232
(503) 731-4000
http://oregon.gov/DHS/ph

Pennsylvania

Pennsylvania Department of Health
Health and Welfare Building
7th and Forster Streets
Harrisburg, PA 17120
(717) 787-6436
http://www.health.state.pa.us/

Rhode Island

Rhode Island Department of Health
3 Capitol Hill
Providence, RI 02908
(401) 222-2231
http://www.health.state.ri.us

South Carolina

**South Carolina Department of Health and
    Human Services**
P.O. Box 8206
Columbia, SC 29202
(803) 898-2500
http://www.dhhs.state.sc.us

South Dakota

South Dakota Department of Health
600 East Capitol Avenue
Pierre, SD 57501
(605) 773-3361
http://www.state.sd.us/doh

Tennessee

Tennessee Department of Health
Cordell Hull Building
Third Floor
Nashville, TN 37247

(615) 741-3111
http://state.tn.us/health

Texas

Texas Department of State Health Services
1100 West 49th Street
Austin, TX 78756
(512) 458-7111
http://www.dshs.state.tx.us

Utah

Utah Department of Health
288 North 1460 West
Salt Lake City, UT 84114
(801) 538-6101
http://www.health.utah.gov

Vermont

Vermont Department of Health
108 Cherry Street
Burlington, VT 05402
(802) 863-7200
http://healthvermont.gov

Virginia

Virginia Department of Health
P.O. Box 2448
Richmond, VA 23218
(804) 864-7001
http://www.vdh.state.va.us

Washington

**Washington Department of Social and Health
    Services**
P.O. Box 45010
Olympia, WA 98504
(360) 902-7800
http://www1.dshs.wa.gov

West Virginia

Office of Community Health Systems
350 Capitol Street
Room 515
Charleston, WV 25301
(304) 558-3210
http://www.wvochs.org

Wisconsin

Department of Health and Family Services
1 West Wilson Street
Madison, WI 53702
(608) 266-1865
http://www.shfs.state.wi.us

Wyoming

Wyoming Department of Health
117 Hathaway Building
2300 Capitol Avenue
Cheyenne, WY 82002
(307) 777-7656
http://wdh.state.wy.us

APPENDIX V
IMPORTANT NATIONAL ORGANIZATIONS

Adult Children of Alcoholics World Service Organization
P.O. Box 3216
Torrance, CA 90510
(310) 534-1815
http://www.adultchildren.org

Al-Anon
1600 Corporate Landing Parkway
Virginia Beach, VA 23454
(757) 563-1600
http://www.al-anon.org

Alateen
1600 Corporate Landing Parkway
Virginia Beach, VA 23454
(888) 425-2666 (toll-free)
http://www.ai-anon.alateen.org

Alcoholics Anonymous World Services, Inc.
Grand Central Station
P.O. Box 459
New York, NY 10163
(212) 870-3400
http://www.alcoholics-anonymous.org

A Matter of Degree
Office of Alcohol and Other Drug Abuse
American Medical Association
515 North State Street
Chicago, IL 60610
(312) 464-5687

American Academy of Addiction Psychiatry
1010 Vermont Avenue NW
Suite 710
Washington, DC 20005
(202) 393-4484
http://www.aaap.org

American Academy of Pain Medicine
4700 West Lake Avenue
Glenview, IL 60025
(847) 375-4731
http://www.painmed.org

American Association for the Treatment of Opioid Dependence
217 Broadway
Suite 304
New York, NY 10007
(212) 566-5555
http://www.aatod.org

American Association of Suicidology
5221 Wisconsin Avenue NW
Washington, DC 20015
(202) 237-2280
http://www.suicidology.org

American Chronic Pain Association
P.O. Box 850
Rocklin, CA 95677
(916) 632-0922
http://www.theacpa.org

American Council for Drug Education
164 West 74th Street
New York, NY 10023
(800) 488-3784 (toll-free)
http://www.acde.org

American Council on Alcoholism
1000 East Indian School Road
Phoenix, AZ 85014
(703) 248-9005
http://www.aca-usa.org

American Foundation for Suicide Prevention
120 Wall Street

22nd Floor
New York, NY 10005
(888) 333-2377 (toll-free)
http://www.asfsp.org

American Hospital Association (AHA)
One North Franklin
Chicago, IL 60606
(312) 422-3000
http://www.aha.org

American Medical Association
515 North State Street
Chicago, IL 60610
(312) 464-5000
http://www.ama-assn.org

American Nurses Association
600 Maryland Avenue SW
Suite 100 West
Washington, DC 20024
(202) 554-4444
http://www.nursingworld.org

American Pharmaceutical Association
2215 Constitution Avenue NW
Washington, DC 20037
(202) 628-4410
http://www.aphanet.org

American Psychiatric Association
1400 K Street NW
Washington, DC 20005
(202) 682-6000
http://www.psych.org

American Psychological Association
750 First Street NE
Washington, DC 20002
(202) 336-5500
http://www.apa.org/

American Society of Addiction Medicine
4601 North Park Avenue Arcade
Suite 101
Chevy Chase, MD 20815
(301) 656-3920
http://www.asam.org

Anxiety Disorders Association of America
8730 Georgia Avenue
Suite 600

Silver Spring, MD 20910
(240) 485-1001
http://www.adaa.org

Association of State and Territorial Health Officials
1275 K Street NW
Suite 800
Washington, DC 20005
(202) 371-9090
http://www.astho.org

Attention Deficit Disorder Association
P.O. Box 543
Pottstown, PA 19464
(484) 945-2101
http://www.add.org

Center for Substance Abuse Prevention (CSAP)
Substance Abuse and Mental Health Services
  Administration
1 Choke Cherry Road
Rockville, MD 20857
(240) 276-2000
http://prevention.samhsa.gov/

Center for Substance Abuse Treatment (CSAT)
Substance Abuse and Mental Health Services
  Administration
1 Choke Cherry Road
Room 2-1075
Rockville, MD 20857
(240) 276-2700

Centers for Disease Control and Prevention (CDC)
1600 Clifton Road NE
Atlanta, GA, 30333
(404) 639-3311
http://www.cdc.gov

Centers for Medicare and Medicaid Services
7500 Security Boulevard
Baltimore, MD 21244
(410) 786-3000

Chemically Dependent Anonymous
General Service Office
P.O. Box 423
Severna Park, MD 21146

(888) 232-4673 (toll-free)
http://www.cdaweb.org

Children and Adults with Attention Deficit Disorders (CHADD)
8181 Professional Place
Suite 150
Landover, MD 20785
(800) 233-4050
http://www.chadd.org

Child Welfare Information Gateway
Children's Bureau/ACYF
1250 Maryland Avenue SW, Eighth Floor
Washington, DC 20024
(703) 385-7565
http://www.childwelfare.gov

Child Welfare League of America
Headquarters
440 First Street NW
Third Floor
Washington, DC 20001
(202) 638-2952
http://www.cwla.org

Children of Alcoholics Foundation
164 West 74th Street
New York, NY 10023
(212) 595-55810, extension 7760
http://www.coaf.org

Cocaine Anonymous World Services Organization
P.O. Box 2000
Los Angeles, CA 90049
(310) 559-5833
http://www.ca.org

College on Problems of Drug Dependence
3420 North Broad Street
Philadelphia, PA 19140
(215) 707-1904
http://www.cpdd.vcu.edu/pages

Depression and Bipolar Support Alliance
730 N. Franklin
Suite 501
Chicago, IL 60610
(800) 826-3632 (toll-free)
http://dbsalliance.org

Depression and Related Affective Disorders Association
8201 Greensboro Drive
Suite 300
McLean, VA 22102
(703) 610-9026
http://www.drada.org

Dual Recovery Anonymous
World Services Central Office
P.O. Box 8107
Prairie Village, KS 66208
(877) 883-2332 (toll-free)

Emergency Nurses Association
915 Lee Street
Des Plaines, IL 60016
(800) 900-9659 (toll-free)
http://www.ena.org

Food and Drug Administration (FDA)
5600 Fishers Lane
Rockville, MD 20857
(888) 463-6332 (toll-free)
http://www.fda.org

Governors Highway Safety Association
750 First Street NE
Suite 720
Washington, DC 20002
(202) 789-0942
http://www.naghsr.org

Group for the Advancement of Psychiatry
P.O. Box 570218
Dallas, TX 75357
(972) 613-3044
http://www.groupadpsych.org

Hepatitis B Coalition/Immunization Action Coalition
1573 Selby Avenue
Suite 234
St. Paul, MN 55104
(651) 647-9009
http://www.immunize.org

Hepatitis B Foundation
700 East Butler Avenue
Doylestown, PA 18901
(215) 489-4900
http://www.hepb.org

Hepatitis Foundation International
504 Blick Drive
Silver Spring, MD 20904
(301) 622-4200
(800) 891-0707 (toll-free)
http://www.hepfi.org

**The Higher Education Center for Alcohol and
    Other Drug Prevention**
Education Development Center, Inc.
55 Chapel Street
Newton, MA 02458
(800) 676-1730 (toll-free)
http://www.higheredcenter.org

**International Foundation for Research &
    Education on Depression (iFRED)**
7040 Bembe Beach Road
Suite 100
Annapolis, MD 21403
(410) 268-0044
http://www.ifred.org

LifeRing Service Center
1440 Broadway
Suite 312
Oakland, CA 94612
(510) 763-0779
http://www.lifering.org

Marijuana Anonymous World Services
P.O. Box 2912
Van Nuys, CA 91404
(800) 766-6779 (toll-free)
http://www.marijuana-anonymous.org

Men for Sobriety
P.O. Box 618
Quakertown, PA 18951
(215) 536-8026

Mood and Anxiety Disorder Programs (MAP)
National Institute of Mental Health
9000 Rockville Pike
Bethesda, MD 20892
(866) 627-6464
http://intramural.nimh.nih.gov/mood

Mothers Against Drunk Driving (MADD)
511 East John Carpenter Freeway
Suite 700
Irving, TX 75062

(800) 438-6233
http://www.madd.org

Nar-Anon Family Group Headquarters, Inc.
22527 Crenshaw Boulevard
#200
Torrance, CA 90505
(310) 534-8188
http://www.nar-anon.org

Narcotics Anonymous World Services, Inc.
P.O. Box 9999
Van Nuys, CA 91409-9099
(818) 773-9999
http://www.na.og

**National Association for Children of
    Alcoholics**
11426 Rockville Pike
Suite 100
Rockville, MD 20852
(888) 554-2627 (toll-free)
http://www.nacoa.net

**National Association for Native American
    Children of Alcoholics**
P.O. Box 2708
Seattle, WA 98111
(206) 903-6574

**National Association of Drug Court
    Professionals**
4900 Seminary Road
Suite 320
Alexandria, VA 22311
(703) 575-9400
http://www.nadcp.org

**National Association of State Controlled
    Substances Authorities**
72 Brook Street
Quincy, MA 02170
(617) 472-0520
http://www.nascsa.org

**National Center on Addiction and Substance
    Abuse at Columbia University**
633 Third Avenue
New York, NY 10017
(212) 841-5200
http://www.casacolumbia.org

National Center on Substance Abuse and Child Welfare
4940 Irvine Boulevard
Suite 202
Irvine, CA 92620
(714) 505-3525
http://www.ncsacw.samhsa.gov

National Clearinghouse for Alcohol and Drug Information (NCADI)
11426-28 Rockville Pike
Rockville, MD 20852
(800) 729-6686 (toll-free)
http://www.health.org

National Council on Alcoholism and Drug Dependence (NCADD)
22 Cortlandt Street
Suite 801
New York, NY 10007
(212) 269-7797
http://www.ncadd.org

National Council on Child Abuse and Family Violence
1025 Connecticut Avenue NW
Suite 1000
Washington, DC 20036
(202) 429-6695
http://www.nccafv.org

National Drug Court Institute
4900 Seminary Road
Suite 320
Alexandria, VA 22311
(703) 575-9400
http://www.ndci.org

National Drug Intelligence Center
319 Washington Street
Fifth Floor
Johnstown, PA 15901
(814) 532-4690
http://www.usdoj.gov/ndic

National Empowerment Center
599 Canal Street
Lawrence, MA 01840
(800) 769-3728 (toll-free)
http://www.power2u.org

National Highway Traffic Safety Administration (NHTSA)
400 Seventh Street SW
Washington, DC 20590
(888) 327-4236 (toll-free)
http://www.nhtsa.dot.gov

National Institute of Mental Health
NIMH Public Inquiries
6001 Executive Boulevard
Room 8184, MSC 9663
Bethesda, MD 20892
(301) 443-4513
www.nimh.nih.gov

National Institute on Alcohol Abuse and Alcoholism
5635 Fishers Lane
MSC 9304
Bethesda, MD 20892
(301) 443-0595
http://www.niaaa.nih.gov

National Institute on Drug Abuse
National Institutes of Health
6001 Executive Boulevard
Room 5213
Bethesda, MD 20892
(301) 443-1124
http://www.nida.nih.gov

National Mental Health Association
1021 Prince Street
Alexandria, VA 22314
(703) 684-7722
www.nmha.org

National Mental Health Consumers' Self-Help Clearinghouse
1211 Chestnut Street
Suite 1207
Philadelphia, PA 19107
(215) 751-1810
(800) 553-4539 (toll-free)

National Organization on Fetal Alcohol Syndrome (NOFAS)
900 17th Street NW
Suite 910
Washington, DC 20006
(202) 785-4585
www.nofas.org

National Self-Help Clearinghouse
365 Fifth Avenue
Suite 3300
New York, NY 10016
(212) 817-1822
www.selfhelpweb.org

National Sheriffs' Association
1450 Duke Street
Alexandria, VA 22314
(703) 836-7827
http://www.sheriffs.org

National Women's Health Network
514 10th Street NW
Suite 400
Washington, DC 20004
(202) 347-1140
http://www.womenshealthnetwork.org

Office of Safe and Drug-Free Schools
U.S. Department of Education
400 Maryland Avenue SW
Washington, DC 20202
(202) 260-3954
http://www.ed.gov/about/offices/list/osdfs/index.
   html

Partnership for a Drug-Free America
405 Lexington Avenue
Suite 1601
New York, NY 10174
http://www.drugfree.org

Psychologists Helping Psychologists
3484 South Utah Street
Arlington, VA 22206
(703) 243-4470

Recovery, Inc.
802 North Dearborn Street
Chicago, IL 60610
(312) 337-5661
http://www.recovery-inc.org

Robert Wood Johnson Foundation
College Road East and Route 1
P.O. Box 2316

Princeton, NJ 08543
(888) 631-9989 (toll-free)
http://www.rwif.org

**SAMHSA Fetal Alcohol Spectrum Disorders
   Center for Excellence (FASD Center)**
2101 Gaither Road
Suite 600
Rockville, MD 20850
http://fascenter.samhsa.gov

SMART Recovery
7537 Mentor Avenue
Suite 306
Mentor, OH 44060
(866) 951-5357 (toll-free)

Social Security Administration (SSA)
Office of Public Inquiries
6401 Security Boulevard
Baltimore, MD 21235
(800) 772-1213 (toll-free)
http://www.ssa.gov

**Substance Abuse and Mental Health Services
   Administration (SAMSHA)**
Department of Health and Human Services
1 Choke Cherry Road
Rockville, MD 20857
(240) 276-2000
http://www.samhsa.gov

**U.S. Department of Health and Human
   Services**
Administration for Children and Families
200 Independence Avenue SW
Washington, DC 20201
(202) 619-0257
http://www.acf.hhs.gov/

Women for Sobriety
P.O. Box 618
Quakertown, PA 18951
(215) 536-8026
http://www.womenforsobriety.org

APPENDIX VI
ADMISSIONS TO SUBSTANCE ABUSE TREATMENT CENTERS, BY PRIMARY SUBSTANCE OF ABUSE, 1998–2003

Primary Substance	1998	1999	2000	2001	2002	2003
Alcohol	828,252	824,641	824,888	795,663	818,003	767,998
Alcohol only	462,692	461,532	459,541	436,142	450,263	426,720
Alcohol w/secondary drug	365,560	363,109	365,347	359,521	367,740	341,278
Opiates	267,010	280,145	302,673	316,864	334,983	323,886
Heroin	247,069	257,508	273,952	278,693	289,056	272,815
Other opiates/synthetics	19,941	22,637	28,721	38,171	45,927	51,071
Nonprescription methadone	1,576	1,606	1,863	2,033	2,550	2,614
Other opiates/synthetics	18,365	21,031	26,858	36,138	43,377	48,457
Cocaine	254,365	242,143	240,756	231,219	245,332	249,556
Smoked cocaine	186,973	176,507	175,904	168,814	178,820	180,851
Nonsmoked cocaine	67,392	65,636	64,852	62,405	66,512	68,705
Marijuana/hashish	220,173	232,105	252,728	267,121	289,299	284,532
Stimulants	71,356	73,568	84,614	101,081	127,276	136,964
Methamphetamine	56,517	58,801	67,467	82,005	105,754	116,604
Other amphetamines	14,010	13,890	15,893	17,637	20,172	19,133
Other stimulants	829	877	1,254	1,439	1,350	1,227
Other drugs	21,718	26,702	31,296	33,330	30,620	29,169
Tranquilizers	5,369	5,913	6,679	7,496	8,337	7,993
Benzodiazepines	4,524	5,048	5,799	6,514	7,345	7,227
Other tranquilizers	845	865	880	982	992	766
Sedatives/hypnotics	3,459	3,459	3,640	3,975	4,478	4,134
Barbiturates	1,232	1,148	1,241	1,289	1,552	1,265
Other sedatives/hypnotics	2,227	2,311	2,399	2,686	2,926	2,869
Hallucinogens	2,378	2,789	3,178	3,200	2,805	2,190
PCP	1,846	2,321	2,813	3,135	3,911	4,086
Inhalants	1,603	1,423	1,334	1,271	1,219	1,170
Over-the-counter	486	1,091	775	636	647	695
Other	6,577	9,706	12,877	13,617	9,223	8,901

Source: Adapted from Office of Applied Studies. *Treatment Episode Data Set (TEDS) Highlights—2003: National Admissions to Substance Abuse Treatment Services.* Rockville, Md.: Substance Abuse and Mental Health Services Administration, Drug and Alcohol Services Information System Series: S-27, June 2005, p. 6.

APPENDIX VII
ADMISSIONS BY PRIMARY SUBSTANCE OF ABUSE, PERCENTAGE, 1998–2003

Primary Substance	1998	1999	2000	2001	2002	2003
Total	100.0	100.0	100.0	100.0	100.0	100.0
Alcohol	27.0	26.7	25.8	24.3	23.6	23.2
Alcohol only	27.0	26.7	25.8	24.3	23.6	23.2
Alcohol w/secondary drug	21.3	21.0	20.5	20.0	19.3	18.5
Opiates	15.6	16.2	17.0	17.7	17.5	17.6
Heroin	15.6	16.2	17.0	17.7	17.5	17.6
Other opiates/synthetics	14.4	14.9	15.4	15.5	15.1	14.8
Nonprescription methadone	1.2	1.3	1.6	2.1	2.4	2.8
Other opiates/synthetics	0.1	0.1	0.1	0.1	0.1	0.1
Cocaine	14.9	14.0	13.5	12.9	12.8	13.6
Smoked cocaine	10.9	10.2	9.9	9.4	9.4	9.8
Nonsmoked cocaine	3.9	3.8	3.6	3.5	3.5	3.7
Marijuana/hashish	12.9	13.4	14.2	14.9	15.1	15.5
Stimulants	4.2	4.3	4.7	5.6	6.7	7.4
Methamphetamine	3.3	3.4	3.8	4.6	5.5	6.3
Other amphetamines	0.8	0.8	0.9	1.0	1.1	1.0
Other stimulants	—	0.1	0.1	0.1	0.1	0.1
Other drugs	1.3	1.5	1.8	1.9	1.6	1.6
Tranquilizers	0.3	0.3	0.4	0.4	0.4	0.4
Benzodiazepines	0.3	0.3	0.3	0.4	0.4	0.4
Other tranquilizers	—	0.1	—	0.1	0.1	—
Sedatives/hypnotics	0.2	0.2	0.2	0.2	0.2	0.2
Barbiturates	0.1	0.1	0.1	0.1	0.1	0.1
Other sedatives/hypnotics	0.1	0.1	0.1	0.1	0.1	0.1
Hallucinogens	0.1	0.2	0.2	0.2	0.1	0.1
PCP	0.1	0.1	0.2	0.2	0.2	0.2
Inhalants	0.1	0.1	0.1	0.1	0.1	0.1
Over-the-counter	—	0.1	—	—	—	—
Other	0.4	0.6	0.7	0.8	0.5	0.5

Source: Adapted from Office of Applied Studies. *Treatment Episode Data Set (TEDS) Highlights—2003: National Admissions to Substance Abuse Treatment Services.* Rockville, Md.: Substance Abuse and Mental Health Services Administration, Drug and Alcohol Services Information System Series: S-27, June 2005, p. 7.

APPENDIX VIII
TYPES OF ILLICIT DRUG USE IN LIFETIME AND PAST YEAR AMONG PERSONS AGES 12 AND OLDER: NUMBERS IN THOUSANDS, 2002–2004

	Lifetime			Past Year		
Drug	2002	2003	2004	2002	2003	2004
ILLICIT DRUG[1]	108,255	110,205	110,057	35,132	34,993	34,807
Marijuana and Hashish	94,946	96,611	110,057	35,132	34,993	34,807
Cocaine	33,910	34,891	34,153	25,755	25,231	25,451
Crack cocaine	8,402	7,949	7,840	1,554	1,406	1,304
Heroin	3,668	3,744	3,145	404	314	398
Hallucinogens	34,314	34,363	34,333	4,749	3,936	3,878
LSD	24,516	24,424	23,398	999	558	592
PCP	7,418	7,107	6,762	235	219	210
Ecstasy	10,150	10,904	11,130	3,167	2,119	1,915
Inhalants	22,870	22,995	22,798	2,084	2,075	2,255
Nonmedical Use of Psychotherapeutics	46,558	47,882	48,013	14,680	14,986	14,643
Pain relievers	29,611	31,207	31,768	10,992	11,671	11,256
OxyContin	1,924	2,832	3,072	—	—	1,213
Tranquilizers	19,267	20,220	19,852	4,849	5,051	5,068
Stimulants	21,072	20,798	19,982	3,181	2,751	2,918
Methamphetamine	12,383	12,303	11,726	1,541	1,315	1,440
ILLICIT DRUG OTHER THAN MARIJUANA	70,300	71,128	70,657	20,423	20,305	19,658

[1] Illicit drugs include marijuana/hashish, cocaine (including crack cocaine), heroin, hallucinogens, inhalants, or prescription-type psychotherapeutics used nonmedically. Illicit drugs other than marijuana include cocaine (including crack cocaine), heroin, hallucinogens, inhalants, or prescription-type psychotherapeutics used nonmedically.

[2] Nonmedical use of prescription-type pain relievers, tranquilizers, stimulants, or sedatives; does not include over-the-counter drugs.

Source: Substance Abuse and Mental Health Services Administration. *Overview of Findings from the 2004 National Survey on Drug Use and Health.* Rockville, Md.: Department of Health and Human Services, September 2005, p. 46.

APPENDIX IX

TYPES OF ILLICIT DRUG USE IN LIFETIME AND PAST YEAR AMONG PERSONS AGES 12 AND OLDER: NUMBERS IN PERCENTAGES, 2002–2004

Drug	Lifetime			Past Year		
	2002	2003	2004	2002	2003	2004
ILLICIT DRUG[1]	46.0	46.4	45.8	14.9	14.7	14.5
Marijuana and hashish	40.4	40.6	40.2	11.0	10.6	10.6
Cocaine	14.4	14.7	14.2	2.5	2.5	2.4
Crack cocaine	3.6	3.3	3.3	0.7	0.6	0.5
Heroin	1.6	1.6	1.3	0.2	0.1	0.2
Hallucinogens	14.6	14.5	14.3	2.0	1.7	1.6
LSD	10.4	10.3	9.7	0.4	0.2	0.2
PCP	3.2	3.0	2.8	0.1	0.1	0.1
Ecstasy	4.3	4.6	4.6	1.3	0.9	0.8
Inhalants	9.7	9.7	9.5	0.9	0.9	0.9
Nonmedical use of psychotherapeutics	19.8	20.1	20.0	6.2	6.3	6.1
Pain relievers	19.8	20.1	20.0	6.2	6.3	6.1
OxyContin	0.8	1.2	1.3	—	—	—
Tranquilizers	8.2	8.5	8.3	2.1	2.1	2.1
Stimulants	9.0	8.8	8.3	1.4	1.2	1.2
Methamphetamine	5.3	5.2	4.9	0.7	0.6	0.6
ILLICIT DRUG OTHER THAN MARIJUANA	29.9	29.9	29.4	8.7	8.5	8.2

[1] Illicit drugs include marijuana/hashish, cocaine (including crack cocaine), heroin, hallucinogens, inhalants, or prescription-type psychotherapeutics used nonmedically. Illicit drugs other than marijuana include cocaine (including crack cocaine), heroin, hallucinogens, inhalants, or prescription-type psychotherapeutics used nonmedically.
[2] Nonmedical use of prescription-type pain relievers, tranquilizers, stimulants, or sedatives; does not include over-the-counter drugs.
Source: Substance Abuse and Mental Health Services Administration. *Overview of Findings from the 2004 National Survey on Drug Use and Health.* Rockville, Md.: Department of Health and Human Services, September 2005, p. 47.

APPENDIX X

TYPES OF ILLICIT DRUG USE, PAST YEAR AND PAST MONTH, AGES 12 AND OLDER: PERCENTAGES, 2002–2004, UNITED STATES

Drug	Past Year			Past Month		
	2002	2003	2004	2002	2003	2004
ILLICIT DRUG[1]	14.9	14.7	14.5	8.4	8.2	7.9
Marijuana and hashish	11.0	10.6	10.6	6.2	6.2	6.1
Cocaine	2.5	2.5	2.4	0.9	1.0	0.8
Crack	0.7	0.6	0.5	0.2	0.3	0.2
Heroin	0.2	0.1	0.2	0.1	0.1	0.1
Hallucinogens	2.0	1.7	1.6	0.5	0.4	0.4
LSD	0.4	0.2	0.2	0.0	0.0	0.0
PCP	0.1	0.1	0.1	0.0	0.0	0.0
Ecstasy (MDMA)	1.3	0.9	0.8	0.3	0.2	0.3
Inhalants	0.9	0.9	0.9	0.3	0.2	0.3
Medical use of psychotherapeutics[2]	6.2	6.3	6.1	2.6	2.7	2.5
Pain relievers	4.7	4.9	4.7	1.9	2.0	1.8
OxyContin	—	—	0.5	—	—	0.1
Tranquilizers	2.1	2.1	2.1	0.8	0.8	0.7
Stimulants	1.4	1.2	1.2	0.5	0.5	0.5
Methamphetamine	0.7	0.6	0.6	0.3	0.3	0.2
Sedatives	0.4	0.3	0.3	0.2	0.1	0.1
ILLICIT DRUG OTHER THAN MARIJUANA[1]	8.7	8.5	8.2	3.7	3.7	3.4

[1] Illicit drugs include marijuana/hashish, cocaine (including crack), heroin, hallucinogens, inhalants, or prescription-type psychotherapeutics used nonmedically. Illicit drugs other than marijuana include cocaine (including crack), heroin, hallucinogens, inhalants, or prescription-type psychotherapeutics used nonmedically.
[2] Nonmedical use of prescription-type pain relievers, tranquilizers, stimulants, or sedatives; does not include over-the-counter drugs.
Source: Substance Abuse and Mental Health Services Administration. *Overview of Findings from the 2004 National Survey on Drug Use and Health.* Rockville, Md.: Department of Health and Human Services, September 2005, p. 233.

APPENDIX XI

TYPES OF ILLICIT DRUG USE, PAST YEAR AND PAST MONTH, PERSONS AGES 18 TO 25 AND OLDER: PERCENTAGES, 2002–2004, UNITED STATES

Drug	Past Year			Past Month		
	2002	2003	2004	2002	2003	2004
ILLICIT DRUG[1]	35.5	34.6	33.9	20.2	20.3	19.4
Marijuana and hashish	29.8	28.5	27.8	17.3	17.0	16.1
Cocaine	6.7	6.6	6.6	2.0	2.2	2.1
Crack	0.9	0.9	0.8	0.2	0.2	0.3
Heroin	0.4	0.3	0.4	0.1	0.1	0.1
Hallucinogens	8.4	6.7	6.0	1.9	1.7	1.5
LSD	1.8	1.1	1.0	0.1	0.2	0.3
PCP	0.3	0.4	0.3	0.0	0.1	0.1
Ecstasy	5.8	3.7	3.1	1.1	0.7	0.7
Inhalants	2.2	2.1	2.1	0.5	0.4	0.4
Nonmedical use of psychotherapeutics	14.2	14.5	14.8	5.4	6.0	6.1
Pain relievers	11.4	12.0	11.9	4.1	4.7	4.7
OxyContin	—	—	1.7	—	—	0.4
Tranquilizers	4.9	5.3	5.2	1.6	1.7	1.8
Stimulants	3.7	3.5	3.7	1.2	1.3	1.4
Methamphetamine	1.7	1.6	1.6	0.5	0.6	0.6
Sedatives	0.5	0.5	0.5	0.2	0.2	0.2
ILLICIT DRUG OTHER THAN MARIJUANA[1]	20.2	19.7	19.3	7.9	8.4	8.1

[1] Illicit drugs include marijuana/hashish, cocaine (including crack cocaine), heroin, hallucinogens, inhalants, or prescription-type psychotherapeutics used nonmedically. Illicit drugs other than marijuana include cocaine (including crack cocaine), heroin, hallucinogens, inhalants, or prescription-type psychotherapeutics used nonmedically.
[2] Nonmedical use of prescription-type pain relievers, tranquilizers, stimulants, or sedatives; does not include over-the-counter drugs.
Source: Substance Abuse and Mental Health Services Administration. *Overview of Findings from the 2004 National Survey on Drug Use and Health.* Rockville, Md.: Department of Health and Human Services, September 2005, p. 49.

APPENDIX XII

USE OF SELECTED SUBSTANCES IN THE PAST MONTH BY PERSONS 12 YEARS OF AGE AND OLDER, ACCORDING TO AGE, SEX, RACE, AND HISPANIC ORIGIN: UNITED STATES, 2002–2003, BY PERCENTAGE OF POPULATION

Age, Sex, Race and Hispanic Origin	Any Illicit Drug		Marijuana		Nonmedical Use of Any Psychotherapeutic Drug	
	2002	2003	2002	2003	2002	2003
12 years and older	8.3	8.2	6.2	6.2	2.6	2.7
Age						
12–13 years	4.2	3.8	1.4	1.0	1.7	1.8
14–15 years	11.2	10.9	7.6	7.3	4.0	4.1
16–17 years	19.8	19.2	15.7	15.6	6.2	6.1
18–25 years	20.2	20.3	17.3	17.0	5.4	6.0
26–34 years	10.5	10.7	7.7	8.4	3.6	3.4
35 years and older	4.6	4.4	3.1	3.0	1.6	1.5
Sex						
Male	10.3	10.0	8.1	8.1	2.7	2.7
Female	6.4	6.5	4.4	4.4	2.6	2.6
Age and sex						
12–17 years	11.6	11.2	8.2	7.9	4.0	4.0
Male	12.3	11.4	9.1	8.6	3.6	3.7
Female	10.9	11.1	7.2	7.2	4.3	4.2
Hispanic origin and race						
Not Hispanic or Latino:						
White only	8.5	8.3	6.5	6.4	2.8	2.8
Black or African American only	9.7	8.7	7.4	6.7	2.0	1.8
American Indian and Alaska Native only	10.1	12.1	6.7	10.3	3.2	4.8
Native Hawaiian and Other Pacific Islander only	7.9	11.1	4.4	7.3	3.8	3.2
Asian only	3.5	3.8	1.8	1.9	0.7	1.7
Two or more races	11.4	12.0	9.0	9.3	3.5	2.4
Hispanic or Latino	7.2	8.0	4.3	4.9	2.9	3.0

Source: Health, United States, 2005 with Chartbook on Trends in the Health of Americans. Hyattsville, Md.: Centers for Disease Control and Prevention, 2005, p. 259.

APPENDIX XIII
FEDERAL TRAFFICKING PENALTIES FOR SCHEDULED DRUGS

Federal penalties for the selling of drugs (trafficking) are severe. The greater the quantity of drug that is sold, the harsher the penalty in terms of prison time and fines. In addition, the penalty is more severe with each progressive offense. If another person is seriously injured or killed, often the penalty is further increased.

This table shows the first- and second-offense penalties for trafficking in different types of drugs.

The left-hand Quantity column shows the penalties for lower quantities of drugs, while the Quantity column farther to the right shows the penalties for selling greater amounts of drugs. In some cases, any amount of drug that is sold is subject to penalties.

Note: trafficking penalties for selling marijuana are provided in the text entry on marijuana.

Drug and Schedule	Quantity	First Offense	Second Offense	Quantity	First Offense	Second Offense
Methamphetamine Schedule II	5–49 g pure or 50–499 g mixture	Not less than 5 years and not more than 40 years. If death or serious injury, not less than 20 or more than life. Fine of not more than $2 million if an individual, $5 million if other than an individual.	Not less than 10 years and not more than life. If death or serious injury, not less than life or more than life. Fine of not more than $4 million if an individual, $10 million if other than an individual.	50 g or more pure or 500 g or more mixture	Not less than 10 years and not more than life. If death or serious injury, not less than 20 years or more than life. Fine of not more than $4 million if an individual, $10 million if other than an individual.	Not less than 20 years and not more than life. If death or serious injury, not less than life. Fine of not more than $8 million if an individual, $20 million if other than an individual.
Heroin Schedule I	100–999 g mixture			1 kg or more mixture		
Cocaine Schedule II	500–4,999 g mixture			5 kg or more mixture		
Cocaine Base Schedule II	5–49 g mixture			50 g or more mixture		
PCP Schedule II	10–99 g pure or 100–999 g			100 g or more pure or 1 kg or more mixture		
LSD Schedule I	1–9 g mixture			10 g or more mixture		
Fentanyl Schedule II	40–399 g mixture			400 g or more mixture		
Fentanyl Analogue Schedule I	10–99 g mixture			100 g or more mixture		

Drug and Schedule	Quantity	First Offense	Second Offense	Quantity	First Offense	Second Offense
Others Schedules I & II (Includes 1 g or more flunitrazepam and gamma-hydroxybu-tyric [GHB] acid)	Any	Not more than 20 years. If death or serious injury, not less than 20 years not more than life. Fine of $1 million if an individual, $5 million if other than an individual	Not more than 30 years. If death or serious injury, life. Fine of $2 million if an individual, $10 million if other than an individual.			

Drug and Schedule	Quantity	First Offense		Second Offense		
Others Schedule III (Includes 30 mg–999 mg flunitrazepam)	Any	Not more than 5 years. Fine not more than $250,000 if an individual, $1 million if other than an individual.		Not more than 10 years. Fine not more than $500,000 if an individual, $2 million if other than an individual.		
Others* Schedules IV (Includes less than 30 mg flunitrazepam)	Any	Not more than 3 years. Fine not more than $250,000 if an individual, $1 million if other than an individual		Not more than 6 years. Fine not more than $500,000 if an individual, $2 million if other than an individual.		
All Schedules V	Any	Not more than 1 year. Fine not more than $100,000 if an individual, $250,000 if other than an individual		Not more than 2 years. Fine not more than $200,000 if an individual, $500,000 if other than an individual.		

* Although flunitrazepam is a Schedule IV controlled substance, quantities of 30 mg or more m of flunitrazepam are subject to greater statutory maximal penalties than the penalties referenced for Schedule IV controlled substances. See 21 U.S. C. §841(b)(1)(C) and (D).
Source: Adapted from: Joseph, Donald E., ed., Drug Enforcement Administration. *Drugs of Abuse.* Washington, D.C.: U.S. Department of Justice, 2005, p. 10.

APPENDIX XIV
TABLE OF SCHEDULED DRUGS

These are drugs that are under the control of the Drug Enforcement Administration (DEA) on the basis of the Controlled Substances Act. Some of these drugs are illegal (all Schedule I drugs) and some are legally prescribed medications, although they are monitored by the DEA. There are five drug schedules, from Schedule I, the most dangerous, to Schedule V, which has the least risk of these potentially addictive medications. The Food and Drug Administration (FDA) also has jurisdiction over legally prescribed medications.

Controlled Substances by Controlled Substances Act (CSA) Schedule

Substance	CSA Schedule	Narcotic (Y = yes, N = no)	Other Names
Schedule I Drugs			
1-(1-Phenylcyclohexyl)pyrrolidine	I	N	PCPy, PHP, rolicyclidine
1-(2-Phenylethyl)-4-phenyl-4-acetoxypiperidine	I	Y	PEPAP, synthetic heroin
1-[1-(2-Thienyl)cyclohexyl]piperidine	I	N	TCP, tenocyclidine
1-[1-(2-Thienyl)cyclohexyl]pyrrolidine	I	N	TCPy
1-Methyl-4-phenyl-4-propionoxypiperidine	I	Y	MPPP, synthetic heroin
2,5-Dimethoxy-4-propylthiophenethylamine	I	N	2C-T-7
2,5, Dimethoxy-4-ethylamphetamine	I	N	DOET
2,5-Dimethoxyamphetamine	I	N	DMA, 2.5-DMA
3,4,5-Trimethoxyamphetamine	I	N	TMA
3,4-Methylenedioxyamphetamine	I	N	MDA, Love Drug
3,4-Methylenedioxymethamphetamine	I	N	MDMA, Ecstasy, XTC
3,4-Methylenedioxy-N-ethylamphetamine	I	N	N-ethyl MDA, MDE, MDEA
3-Methfentanyl	I	Y	China White, fentanyl
3-Methylthio-fentanyl	I	Y	Chin White, fentanyl
4-Bromo-2,5-dimethoxyamphetamine	I	N	DOB, 4-bromo-DMA
4-Bromo-2,5-dimethoxyphenethylamine	I	N	2C-B, Nexus, has been sold as Ecstasy, i.e., MDMA
4-Methoxyamphetamine	I	N	PMA
4-Methyl-2,5-dimethoxyampheatmine	I	N	DOM, STP
4-Methylaminorex	I	N	U4Euh, McN-422
5-Methoxy-3,4-methylenedioxyamphetamine	I	N	MMDA
5-Methoxy-N,N-diisopropyltrytamine	I	N	5-MeO-DIPT
Acetorphine	I	Y	
Acetyl-alpha-methylfentanyl	I	Y	

Substance	CSA Schedule	Narcotic (Y = yes, N = no)	Other Names
Acetyldihydrocodeine	I	Y	Acetylcodone
Acetylmethadol	I	Y	Methadylacetate
Allylprodine	I	Y	
Alphacetylmethadol except levo-alphacetylmetahdol	I	Y	
Alpha-ethyltryptamine	I	N	ET, Trip
Alphameprodine	I	Y	
Alphamethadol	I	Y	
Alpha-methylfentanyl	I	Y	China White, fentanyl
Alpha-methylthiofentanyl	I	Y	China White, fentanyl
Alpha-methyltryptamine	I	N	AMT
Aminorex	I	N	Has been sold as methamphetamine
Benzethidine	I	Y	
Benzylmorphine	I	Y	
Betacetylmethadol	I	Y	
Beta-hydroxy-3-methylfentanyl	I	Y	China White, fentanyl
Beta-hydroxyfentanyl	I	Y	China White, fentanyl
Betameprodine	I	Y	
Betamethadol	I	Y	
Betaprodine	I	Y	
Bufotenine	I	N	Mappine, N, N-dimethylserotonin
Cathinone	I	N	Constituent of "khat" plant
Clonitazene	I	Y	
Codeine methylbromide	I	Y	
Codeine-N-oxide	I	Y	
Cyprenorphine	I	Y	
Desomorphine	I	Y	
Dextromoramide	I	Y	Palfium, Jetrium, Narcolo
Diampromide	I	Y	
Diethylthiambutene	I	Y	
Diethyltrytamine	I	N	NDET
Difenoxin	I	Y	Lyspafen
Dihydromorphine	I	Y	
Dimenoxadol	I	Y	
Dimepheptanol	I	Y	
Dimethylthiambutene	I	Y	
Dimethyltryptamine	I	N	DMT
Dioxaphetyl butyrate	I	Y	
Dipipanone	I	Y	Dipipan, phenylpiperone HCl, Diconal, Wellconal
Drotebanol	I	Y	Metebanyl, oxymethebanol
Ethylmethylthiambutene	I	Y	
Etonitazene	I	Y	
Etorphine (except HCl)	I	Y	
Etoxeridine	I	Y	
Fenethylline	I	N	Captagon, amfetyline, ethyltheophylline amphetamine

(table continues)

Substance	CSA Schedule	Narcotic (Y = yes, N = no)	Other Names
Furethidine	I	Y	
Gamma-Hydroxybutyric Acid	I	N	GHB, gamma-hydroxybutyrate, sodium oxybate
Heroin	I	Y	Diacetylmorphine, diamorphine
Hydromorphinol	I	Y	
Hydroxypethidine	I	Y	
Ibogaine	I	N	Constituent of *Tabernanthe iboga* plant
Ketobemidone	I	Y	Cliradon
Levomoramide	I	Y	
Levophenacylmorphan	I	Y	
Lysergic acid diethyamide	I	N	LSD, lysergide
Marihuana	I	N	Cannabis, marijuana
Mecloqualone	I	N	Nubarene
Mescaline	I	N	Constituent of "peyote" cacti
Methaqualone	I	N	Quaalude, Parest, Somnafac, Optimil, Mandrax
Methcathinone	I	N	N-Methylcathinone, "cat"
Methyldesorphine	I	Y	
Methyldihydromorphine	I	Y	
Morpheridine	I	Y	
Morphine methylbromide	I	Y	
Morphine methylsulfonate	I	Y	
Morphine-N-oxide	I	Y	
Myrophine	I	Y	
N, N-Dimethylamphetamine	I	Y	
N-Benzylpiperazine	I	N	BZP,1-benzylpiperazine
N-Ethyl-1-phenylcyclohexylamine	I	N	PCE
N-Ethyl-3-piperdyl benzilate	I	N	JB323
N-Ethylamphetamine	I	N	NEA
N-Hydroxy-3,4-methylenedioxyamphaetamine	I	N	N-hydroxy MDA
Nicocodeine	I	Y	
Nicomorphine	I	N	Vilan
N-Methyl-3-piperidyl benzilate	I	Y	JB336
Noracymetadol	I	Y	
Norlevorphanol	I	Y	
Normethadone	I	Y	Phenyldimazone
Normorphine	I	Y	
Norpipanone	I	Y	
Para, Fluorofentanyl	I	Y	China White, fentanyl
Parahexyl	I	N	Synhexyl
Peyote	I	N	Cactus that contains mescaline
Phenadoxone	I	Y	
Phenampromide	I	Y	
Phenormorphan	I	Y	
Phenoperidine	I	Y	Operidine, Lealgin

Substance	CSA Schedule	Narcotic (Y = yes, N = no)	Other Names
Pholcodine	I	Y	Copholco, Adaphol, codisol, Lantuss, Pholcolin
Piritramide	I	Y	Piridolan
Proheptazine	I	Y	
Properidine	I	Y	
Propiram	I	Y	Algeel
Psilocybin	I	N	Constituent of "magic mushrooms"
Psilocyn	I	N	Psilocin, constituent of "magic mushrooms"
Racemoramide	I	Y	
Tetrahydrocannabinols	I	N	THC, Delta-8 THC, Delta-9 THC, dronabinol and others
Thebacon	I	Y	Acetylhydrocodone, Acedicon, Thebacetyl
Thiofentanyl	I	Y	China White, fentanyl
Tilidine	I	Y	Tilidate, Valoron, Kitadol, Lak, Tilsa
Trimeperidine	I	Y	Promedolum

Schedule II Drugs

Substance	CSA Schedule	Narcotic (Y = yes, N = no)	Other Names
1-Phenylcyclohexylamine	II	N	PCP precursor
1-Piperidinocyclohexanecarbonitrile	II	N	PCC, PCP precursor
Alfentanil	II	Y	Alfenta
Alphaprodine	II	Y	Nisentil
Amorbarbital	II	N	Amytal, Tuinal
Amphetamine	II	N	Dexedrine, Adderall, Obetrol
Anileridine	II	Y	Leritine
Benzoylecgonine	II	Y	Cocaine metabolite
Bezitramide	II	Y	Burgodin
Carfentanil	II	Y	Wildnil
Coca leaves	II	Y	
Cocaine crack	II	Y	Methyl benzoylecgonine,
Codeine	II	Y	Morphine methyl ester, methyl morphine
Dextropropoxyphine, bulk (nondosage forms)	II	Y	Propoxyphene
Dihydrocodeine	II	Y	Didrate, Parzone
Dihydroetorphine	II	Y	DHE
Diphenoxylate	II	Y	
Diprenorphine	II	Y	M50-50
Ecgonine	II	Y	Cocaine precursor, in coca leaves
Ethylmorphine	II	Y	Dionin
Etorphine HCl	II	Y	M99
Fentanyl	II	Y	Duragesic, Oralet, Actiq, Sublimaze, Innovar

(table continues)

Substance	CSA Schedule	Narcotic (Y = yes, N = no)	Other Names
Glutethimide	II	N	Doriden, Dorimide
Hydrocodone[1]	II	Y	dihydrocodeinone
Hydromorphone	II	Y	Dilaudid, dihydromorphenone
Isomethadone	II	Y	Isoamidone
Levo-alphacetylmethadol	II	Y	LAAM, long-acting methadone, levomethadyl acetate
Levomethorphan	II	Y	
Levorphanol	II	Y	Levo-Dromoran
Meperidine	II	Y	Demerol, Mepergan, pethidine
Meperidine intermediate-A	II	Y	Meperidine precursor
Meperidine intermediate-B	II	Y	Meperidine precursor normeperdine
Meperidine intermediate-C	II	Y	Meperidine precursor
Metazocine	II	Y	
Methadone	II	Y	Dolphine, Methadose, Amidone
Methadone intermediate	II	Y	Methadone precursor
Methamphetamine	II	N	Desoxyn, D-desoxyephedrine, ICE, Crank, Speed
Methylphenidate	II	N	Concerta, Ritalin, Methylin
Metopon	II	Y	
Moramide-intermediate	II	Y	
Morphine	II	Y	Ms-Contin, Roxanol, Oramoprh, RMS, MSIR
Nabilone	II	N	Cesamet
Opium extracts	II	Y	
Opium fluid extract	II	Y	
Opium poppy	II	Y	*Papaver somniferum*
Opium tincture	II	Y	Laudanum
Opium, granulated	II	Y	Granulated opium
Opium, powdered	II	Y	Powdered opium
Opium, raw	II	Y	Raw opium, gum opium
Oxycodone	II	Y	OxyContin, Percocet, Endocet, Roxicodone, Roxicet
Oxymorphone	II	Y	Numorphan
Pentobarbital	II	N	Nembutal
Phenazocine	II	Y	Narphen, Prinadol
Phencyclidine	II	N	PCP, Sernylan
Phenmetrazine	II	N	Preludin
Phenylacetone	II	N	P2P, phenyl-2-propanone, benzyl methyl ketone
Piminodine	II	Y	
Poppy Straw	II	Y	Opium poppy capsules, poppy heads
Poppy Straw concentrate	II	Y	Concentrate of Poppy Straw, CPS
Racemethorphan	II	Y	
Racemorphan	II	Y	Dromoran

Substance	CSA Schedule	Narcotic (Y = yes, N = no)	Other Names
Remifentanil	II	Y	Ultiva
Secobarbital	II	N	Seconal, Tuinal
Thebaine	II	Y	Precursor of many narcotics

Schedule III Drugs

Substance	CSA Schedule	Narcotic (Y = yes, N = no)	Other Names
13Beta-ethyl-17beta-hydroxgon-4-en-3-one	III	N	
17Alpha-methyl-3alpha,17beta-dihydroxy-5alpha-androstane	III	N	
17Alpha-methyl-3beta-dihydroxy-5alpha-androstane	III	N	
17Alpha-methyl-3beta,17beta-dihydroxyandrost-4-ene	III	N	
17Alpha-methyl-4-hydroxynandrolone (17alpha-methyl-4-hydroxy-17beta0hydroxyestr-4-en3-one	III	N	
17Alpha-methyl-delta1-dinydrotestoserone (17beta-hydroxy-17almpha0methyl-5alpha-androst-1-en-3-one)	III	N	
19-Nor-4-androstenediol (3beta, 17 beta-dihydroxyestr-r-ene;3 alpha, 17beta-dihydorxyestr-4-ene)	III	N	
19-Nor-4androstenedione (estr-4-en,3,17 dione)	III	N	
19-Nor-5-androstenediol (3beta,17beta-dihydroxyestri-e-ene, 3alpha,17beta-dihydroxyestr-5-ene)	III	N	
19-Nor5-androstenedione (estr-5-en,3,17 dione)	III	N	
1-Androstenediol (3beta,17bet-dihydrixt-5alpha-androst-1-ene;3alpha,17beta-dihyrroxy-5alpha-androst-1-ene	III	N	
1-Androstenedione (5alpha-androst-1-en-3,17-dione)	III	N	
3Alpha,17beta-dihydroxy-5alpha-androstane	III	N	
3Beta,17bet-dihyroxy-5alpha-androstane	III	N	
4-Androstenediol (3beta,17beta-dihydroxy-androstate-4-ene)	III	N	
4-Androstenedione (androst-4-en-3,17-dione)	III	N	
4-Dihydrotestoserone (17beta-hydroxyandrostan-3-one)	III	N	
4-Hydroxy-19-nortestosterone (4,17beta-dihydroxyestr-4-ene-3-one)	III	N	
4-Hydroxytestoserone (4,17beta-dihydroxyandrost-4-en-3-one)	III	N	
5-Androstenediol (3beta-dihydroxyandrost-4-en-3-one	III	N	
5-Androstenedione (androst-5-en-3,17-dione)	III	N	
Amobarbital & noncontrolled active form	III	N	
Amobarbital suposity dosage form	III	N	
Anabolic steroids	III	N	"Bodybuilding" drugs
Androstanedione (5alpha-androstan-3,17-dione)	III	N	
Aprobarbital	III	N	Alurate
Barbituric acid derivative	III	N	Barbiturates not specifically listed
Benzphetamine	III	N	Didrex, Inapetyl

(table continues)

Substance	CSA Schedule	Narcotic (Y = yes, N = no)	Other Names
Bolasterone (7alpha,17alpha-dimethyl-17beta-hydroxyandrost-4-en-3-one)	III	N	
Boldenenone (17beta-hydrosyandrost-1,4-diene-3-one)	III	N	Equipose, Parenbol, Vebonel, dehydrostestosterone
Buprenorphine	III	N	Buprenex, Temgesic, Subutex, Suboxone
Butalbital	III	N	Fiornal, Butalbital with aspirin
Butobarbital (butethal)	III	N	Soneryl (UK)
Calusterone (7beta,17alpha-dimethyl-17beta-hydroxyandrost-4-en-3-one)	III	N	Methosarb
Chlorhexadol	III	N	Mechloral, Mecoral, medo-dorm, Chloralodol
Chlorphentermine	III	N	Pre-Sate, Lucogen, Apsedon, Desopimon
Clortermine	III	N	Voranil
Clostebol (4-chloro-17beta0hydroxyandrost-4-en3-)	III	N	Alfra, Trofodermin, Clostene, 4-chlorotestosterone
Codeine & isoquinoline alkaloid 90 mg	III	Y	Codeine with papaverine or noscapine
Codeine combination product 90 mg	III	Y	Empirin, Fiornal, Tynol, ASA or APAP with codeine
Dehydrochlormethyltestosterone (4-chloro-17beta-hydroxy-17alpha-methylandrost-1,4-dien-3-one)	III	N	Oral-Turinabol
Delta-1-dihydrotestosterone (17beta-hydorxy-alpha-androst-1-en-3-one)	III	N	1-Testosterone
Dihydrocodeine combination product 90 mg/du	III	Y	Synalgos-DC, Compal
Dronabinol in sesame oil in soft gelatin capsule	III	N	Marinol, synthetic THC in sesame oil/soft gelatin
Drostanolone (17beta-hydroxy-2alpha-methyl-5alpha-androstan-3-one)	III	N	Drolban, Masterid, Permastril
Ethylestrenol (17alpha-ethyl-17beta-hydroxyestr-4	III	N	Maxibolin, Orabolin, Durabo-lin-O, Duraboral
Ethylmorphine combination product 15 mg/du	III	Y	
Fluoxymesterone (9fluoro-17alpha-methyl-11beta,17beta-dihydroxyandrost-1,4-dien-3-one)	III	N	Anadroid-F, Halotestin, Ora-Testryl
Formebolone (2-formyl-17alpha-methyl-11alpha,17beta-dihydroxyandrost-1,4-dine-3-one	III	N	Esiciene, Hubernol
Furazabol (17alpha-methyl-17beta-hydroxyandrostanol[2,3-c]-fruazan	III	N	Zyrem
Gamma-hydroxybutyric acid preparations	III	N	Zyrem
Hydrocone & isoquinoline alkaloid <15 mg	III	Y	Dihydrocoeineinone + papaverine or noscapine
Hydrocodone combination product <15 mg	III	Y	Lorcet, Lortab, Vicodin, Vicoprofen, Tussionex, Norco
Ketamine	III	N	Ketaset, Ketalar, Special K, K
Lysergic acid	III	N	LSD precursor
Lysergic acid amide	III	N	LSD precursor

Substance	CSA Schedule	Narcotic (Y = yes, N = no)	Other Names
Mestanolone (17alpha-methyl-17beta-hydroxy-5alpha-androstan-3-one)	III	N	Assimil, Ermalone, Methybok, Tantarone
Mesteralone (1alpha-methyl-17beta-hydroxy-5alpha-androstan-3-one)	III	N	Androviron, Proviron, Testiwop
Methandienone (17alpha-methyl-17beta-hydroxyandrost-1,4-diene-3-one)	III	N	Dianabol, Metabolina, Nerobol, Perbolin
Methandriol (17alpha-methyl-3beta,17beta-dihydroxyandrost-5-ene)	III	N	Sinesex, Stenediol, Troformone
Methenolone (1-methyl-17beta-hydroxy-5alpha-androst-1-en-3-one)	III	N	Primobolan, Primobolan Depot, Primobolan S
Methydienolone (17alpha-methyl-17beta-hydroxyestr-4,9 (10)-dien-3-one)	III	N	
Methyltestosterone (17alpha-methyl-17beta-hydroxyandrost-4-en-3-one)	III	N	Android, Oreton, Testred, Virilon
Methyltrienolone (17alpha-methyl-17beta-hydroxyestr-4,9,11-trien-3-one)	III	N	Metribolone
Methyprylon	III	N	Noludar
Mibolerone (7alpha, 17alpha-dimethyl-17beta-hydroxyestr-4-en-3-one)	III	N	Cheque, Matenon
Morphine combination product/50 mg/100 mL or g	III	Y	
Nalorphine	III	Y	Nalline
Nandrolone (17beta-hydroxyestr-4-en-3-one)	III	N	Deca-Durabolin, Durabolin, Durabolin-50
Norbolethone (13beta017alpha-diethyl-17beta-hydroxgon-4-en-3-one)	III	N	Genabol
Norclostebol (4-chloro-17beta-hydroxyestr-4-en-3-one	III	N	Anabol-4, 19, Lentabol
Norethandrolone (17alpha-ethyl-17beta-hydroxyestr-4-en-3-one)	III	N	Nilevar, Pronabol, Solevar
Opium combination product 25 mg	III	Y	Paregoric, other combination products
Oxandrolone (17alpha-methyl-17beta-hydroxy-2-oxa-5alpha-androstan-3-one)	III	N	Anavar, Lonavar, Oxandrin, Provitar Vasorome
Oxymesterone (17alpha-methyl-2-hydroxymethyele-17beta-hydroxy-5alpha-androsan-3-one)	III	N	Anamidol, Bainimax, Oranabol, Oranabol 10
Oxymethalone (17alpha-methyl-2-hydroxymethyene-17beta-hydroxy-5alpha-androstan-3-one)	III	N	Anadrol-50, Adroyd, Anapolon, Anasteron, Pardroyd
Pentobarbital and noncontrolled active ingredient	III	N	FP-3
Pentobarbital suppository dosage form	III	N	WANS
Phendimetrazine	III	N	Plegine, Prelu-2, Bontril, Melfiat, Statobex
Secobarbital and noncontrolled active ingredient	III	N	

(table continues)

Substance	CSA Schedule	Narcotic (Y = yes, N = no)	Other Names
Secobarbital suppository dosage form	III	N	
Stanzolol (17alpha-methyl-17beta-hydroxy-5alpha-androst-1-eno[3,2-c]-pyrazole)	III	N	Winstrol, Winstrol-V
Stenbolone (17beta-hydroxy-2-methyl-5alpha-androst-1-en-3-one)	III	N	
Stimulant compounds previously excepted	III	N	Mediatric
Sulfondiethylmethane	III	N	
Sulfonethylmethane	III	N	
Talbutal	III	N	Lotusate
Testolactone (13-hydroxy-3-oxo-13,17-secoandrosta-1,4-dien-17-oic acid lactone)	III	N	Teolit, Teslac
Testosterone (17beta-hydroxyanrost-4-en-3-one)	III	N	Android-T, Androlan, Depotest, Delatestryl
Tetrahydrogestrinone (13beta, 17alpha-diethyl-17beta-hydroxygon-4,9,11-trien-3-one)	III	N	THG
Thiamytal	III	N	Surital
Thiopental	III	N	Pentothal
Tiletamine and zolazepam combination product	III	N	Telazol
Trenbolone (17beta-hydroxyestr-4,9,11-trien-3-one)	III	N	Finaplix-S, Finajet, parabolan
Vinbarbital	III	N	Delvinal, vinbarbitone

Schedule IV Drugs

Substance	CSA Schedule	Narcotic (Y = yes, N = no)	Other Names
Alprazolam	IV	N	Xanax
Barbital	IV	N	Veronal, Plexonal, barbitone
Bromazepam	IV	N	Lexotan, Lexatin, Lexotanil
Butorphanol Torbutrol	IV	N	Stadol, Stadol NS, Torbugesic
Camazepam	IV	N	Albego, Lipidon, Paxor
Cathine	IV	N	Constituent of "khat" plant
Chloral betaine	IV	N	Beta Chlor
Chloral hydrate	IV	N	Noctec
Chlordizepoxide SK-Lygen	IV	N	Librium, Libritabs, Limbritrol,
Clobazam	IV	N	Urbadan, Urbany
Clonazepam	IV	N	Klonopin
Clorazepate	IV	N	Tranxene
Clotiazepam	IV	N	Trecalmo, Rize, Clozan, Vertran
Clozazolam	IV	N	Akton, Lubaliz, Olcadil, Sepazon
Delorazepam	IV	N	
Dexfenfluramine	IV	N	Redux
Dextropropoxyphene dosage forms	IV	N	Darvon, propoxyphene, Darvocet, Propacet
Diazepam	IV	N	Valium, Diastat
Dichloralphenazone	IV	N	Midrin, dichloralantipyrine
Diethylpropion	IV	N	Tenuate, Tepanil
Difenoxin	IV	Y	Motofen

Substance	CSA Schedule	Narcotic (Y = yes, N = no)	Other Names
Estrazolam	IV	N	ProSom, Domnamid, Eurodin, Nuctalon
Ethinamate	IV	N	Valmid, Valamin
Ethchlorvynol	IV	N	Placidyl
Ethyl loflazepate	IV	N	
Fencamfamiin	IV	N	Reactivan
Fenfluramin	IV	N	Pondimin, Ponderal
Fenproporex	IV	N	Gacilin, Solvolip
Fludiazepam	IV	N	
Flunitrazepman	IV	N	Rohypnol, Narcozep, Darkene, Roipnol
Flurazepam	IV	N	Dalmane
Halezepam	IV	N	Paxipam
Haloxazolam	IV	N	
Ketazolam	IV	N	
Loprazolam	IV	N	Anxon, Loftran, Solatran, Contamex
Lorazepam	IV	N	Ativan
Lormetazepam	IV	N	Noctamid
Mazindol	IV	N	Sanorex, Mazanor
Mebutamate	IV	N	Capla
Medazepan	IV	N	Nobrium
Mefenorex	IV	N	Anorexic, Amexate, Doracil, Pondinil
Meprobamate	IV	N	Milltown, Equanil, Micrainin, Equagesic, Meprospan
Methohexital	IV	N	Brevital
Methylphenobarbital (mephobarbital)	IV	N	Mebaral, mephobarbital
Midazolam	IV	N	Versed
Modafinil	IV	N	Provigil
Nimetazepam	IV	N	Erimin
Nitrazepam	IV	N	Mogadon
Nordizepam	IV	N	Nordazepam, Demadar, Madar
Oxazepam	IV	N	Serax, Serenid-D
Oxazolam	IV	N	Serenal, Convertal
Paraldehyde	IV	N	Paral
Pemoline	IV	N	Cylert
Pentazocine	IV	N	Talwin, Talwin N X, Talacen, Talwin Compound
Petrichloral	IV	N	Pentaerythritol chloral, Periclor
Phenobarbital	IV	N	Luminal, Donnatal, Bellergal-S
Phentermine	IV	N	Ionamin, Fastin, Adipex-P, Obe-Nix, Zantryl
Pinazepam	IV	N	Domar
Pipradrol	IV	N	Detaril, Stimolag Fortis
Prazepam	IV	N	Centrax

(table continues)

Substance	CSA Schedule	Narcotic (Y = yes, N = no)	Other Names
Quazepam	IV	N	Doral
Sibutramine	IV	N	Meridia
SPA	IV	N	1-Dimethylamino-1,2-diphe-nylethane, Lefetamine
Temazepam	IV	N	Restoril
Tetrazepam	IV	N	Myolastan, Musaril
Triazolam	IV	N	Halcion
Zaleplon	IV	N	Sonata
Zolpidem	IV	N	Ambien, Ivadal, Stillnoct, Stillnox
Zopiclone	IV	N	Lunesta
Schedule V Drugs			
Codeine preparations: 200 mg/100 mL or 100 g	V	Y	Cosanyl, RobitussinA-C, Cheracol, Cerose, Pediacof
Difenoxin preparations: 0.5 mg/25 ug AtSOR/du	V	Y	Motofen
Dihydorcodeine preparations: 10 mg/100 mL or 100 g	V	Y	Cophene-S, various others
Diphenoxylate preparations: 2.5 mg/25 ur AtSO4	V	Y	Lomotil, Logen
Ethylmorphine preparations: 100 mg/100 mL or 100 g	V	Y	
Opium preparations: 100 mg/100 mg or 100 g	V	Y	Parepectolin, Kapectolin PG, Kaolin Pectin P.G.
Pyrovalerone	V	N	Centroton, Thymergix

[1] Some forms of hydrocodone are Schedule III drugs.

Source: Adapted from Office of Diversion Control, Drug Enforcement Administration. *Lists of: Scheduling Actions, Controlled Substances, Regulated Chemicals.* Washington, D.C.: U. S. Department of Justice, April 2005. Available online. URL: http://www.deadiversion.usdoj.gov/schedules/orangebook2007.pdf. Downloaded on August 21, 2007.

APPENDIX XV
MEDICATIONS USED TO TREAT ALCOHOL DEPENDENCE

	Disulfiram (Antabuse)	Naltrexone (ReVia)	Acamprosate (Campral)
Action	Inhibits intermediate metabolism of alcohol, causing a buildup of acetaldehyde and a reaction of flushing, sweating, nausea, and tachycardia if a patient drinks alcohol	Blocks opioid receptors, resulting in reduced craving and reduced reward in response to drinking	Affects glutamate and g-aminobutyrate GABA neurotransmitter systems, but alcohol-related action unclear
Contraindications	Concomitant use of alcohol or alcohol-containing preparations or metronidazole; coronary artery disease; severe myocardial disease	Currently using opioids or in acute opioid withdrawal; anticipated need for opioid analgesics, acute hepatitis or liver failure	Severe renal impairment
Precautions	High impulsivity; likely to drink while using it; psychoses (current or history); diabetes mellitus; epilepsy; hepatic dysfunction; hypothyroidism; renal impairment; rubber contact dermatitis	Other hepatic disease; renal impairment; history of suicide attempts. If opioid analgesia is required, larger doses may be required, and respiratory depression may be deeper and more prolonged	Moderate renal impairment; depression or suicidality
Serious adverse reactions	Hepatitis; optic neuritis; peripheral neuropathy; psychotic reactions. Pregnancy Category C Pregnancy Category C is a labeling designation used by the Food and Drug Administration (FDA). It is used when animal reproduction studies of animals using a drug have shown an adverse effect on the fetus but there are no adequate and well-controlled studies of the use of this drug in humans. In addition, the benefits from the use of the drug in pregnant women may be acceptable despite its potential risks. The drug is only given to pregnant women if clearly needed.	Will precipitate severe withdrawal if patient is dependent on opioids; hepatoxicity (uncommon at usual doses). Pregnancy Category C.	Anxiety; depression. Rare events include suicide attempt, acute kidney failure, heart failure, mesenteric arterial occlusion, cardiomyopathy, deep thrombophlebitis, and shock. Pregnancy Category C

(table continues)

	Disulfiram (Antabuse)	Naltrexone (ReVia)	Acamprosate (Campral)
Common side effects	Metallic after-taste; dermatitis	Nausea, abdominal pain, constipation; dizziness; headache; anxiety; fatigue	Diarrhea; flatulence, nausea; abdominal pain; headache; back pain; infection, flu syndrome; chills; somnolence; decreased libido; amnesia; confusion
Examples of drug interactions	Amitryptiline; anticoagulants, such as warfarin; diazepam; isoniazid; metronidazole; phenytoin; theophylline; any nonprescription drug containing alcohol	Opioid analgesics (blocks action); yohimbine (use with naltrexone increases negative drug effects)	No clinically relevant interactions known
Usual adult dosage	*Oral dose*: 250 mg daily (range 125 mg to 500 mg) *Before prescribing*: (1) warn that patient should not take disulfiram for at least 12 hours after drinking and that a disulfiram-alcohol reaction can occur up to 2 weeks after the last dose; (2) warn about alcohol in the diet (e.g., sauces and vinegars) and in medications and toiletries *Follow-up*: monitor liver function test results periodically	*Oral dose*: 50 mg daily *Before prescribing*: evaluate for possible current opioid use; consider a urine toxicology screen for opioids, including synthetic opioids. Obtain liver function test *Follow-up*: monitor liver function test results periodically	*Oral dose*: 666 mg (two 333-mg tablets) three times daily, or, for moderate renal impairment, reduce to 333 mg (one tablet) three times daily *Before prescribing*: establish abstinence

Source: Adapted from National Institute on Alcohol Abuse and Alcoholism. *Helping Patients Who Drink Too Much: A Clinician's Guide.* Rockville, Md.: National Institutes of Health, 2005, p. 20.

APPENDIX XVI
STATE LAWS ON CHILD ABUSE IN RELATION TO DRUG ABUSE

There are federal laws on abuse and neglect, but each state also has its own laws to define what constitutes abuse and neglect. Some states include circumstances that are related to substance abuse affecting children of all ages or substance abuse that affects newborn children. (Note that the states do not limit their definition of abuse and neglect to substance abuse only.)

Alabama

Not addressed in statutes reviewed.

Alaska

Not addressed in statutes reviewed.

Arizona

The terms *endangered* and *abuse* include but are not limited to circumstances in which a child or vulnerable adult is permitted to enter or remain in any structure or vehicle in which volatile, toxic, or flammable chemicals are found or equipment is possessed by any person for the purpose of manufacturing a dangerous drug in violation of state law.

A health care professional, who, after a routine newborn physical assessment of a newborn infant's health status, or notification of positive results of toxicology screens of a newborn infant, reasonably believes that the newborn infant may be affected by the presence of alcohol or a drug listed in state law shall immediately report this information, or cause a report to be made, to child protective services in the Department of Economic Security. For the purpose of this subsection, *newborn infant* means a newborn infant who is less than 30 days of age.

Arkansas

This issue is not addressed in the statutes reviewed.

California

A positive toxicology screen result at the time of the delivery of an infant is not in and of itself a sufficient basis for reporting child abuse or neglect. However, any indication of maternal substance abuse shall lead to an assessment of the needs of the mother and child pursuant to law.

If other factors are present that indicate risk to a child, then a report shall be made. However, a report based on risk to a child that relates solely to the inability of the parent to provide the child with regular care because of the parent's substance abuse shall be made only to county welfare departments and not to a law enforcement agency.

Colorado

Abuse or *child abuse* or *neglect* means an act or omission that threatens the health or welfare of a child:

- any case in which, in the presence of a child, on the premises where a child is found, or where a child resides, a controlled substance is manufactured

Connecticut

This issue is not addressed in the statutes reviewed.

Delaware

This issue is not addressed in the statutes reviewed.

District of Columbia

Any licensed health professional or a law enforcement officer, except an undercover officer whose identity or investigation might be jeopardized, shall report immediately, in writing, to the Child Protective Services Division of the Department of Human Services, that the law enforcement officer or health professional has reasonable cause to believe that a child is abused as a result of inadequate care, control, or subsistence in the home environment due to drug-related activity.

Neglected child means a child

- who is born addicted to or dependent on a controlled substance or has a significant presence of a controlled substance in his or her system at birth
- in whose body there is a controlled substance as a direct and foreseeable consequence of the acts or omissions of the child's parent
- who is regularly exposed to illegal drug-related activity in the home

Florida

Harm to a child's health or welfare can occur when the parent, legal custodian, or caregiver responsible for the child's welfare

- inflicts, or allows to be inflicted upon the child physical, mental, or emotional injury. In determining whether harm has occurred, the following factors must be considered in evaluating any physical, mental, or emotional injury to the child:
  - the age of the child; any prior history of injuries to the child; the location of the injury on the body of the child; the multiplicity of the injury, and the type of trauma inflicted
  - such injury includes, but is not limited to, purposely giving a child poison, alcohol, drugs, or other substances that substantially affect the child's behavior, motor coordination, or judgment or that result in sickness or internal injury. For the purpose of this subparagraph, the term *drugs* means prescription drugs not prescribed for the child or not administered as prescribed, and controlled substances
- exposes the child to a controlled substance or alcohol. Exposure to a controlled substance or alcohol is established by
  - use by the mother of a controlled substance or alcohol during pregnancy when the child, at birth, is demonstrably adversely affected by such usage or
  - continued chronic and severe use of a controlled substance or alcohol by a parent when the child is demonstrably adversely affected by such usage

Georgia

Any person who intentionally causes or permits a child to be present where any person is manufacturing methamphetamine or possessing a chemical substance with the intent to manufacture methamphetamine shall be guilty of a felony and, upon conviction thereof, shall be punished by imprisonment for not less than two nor more than 15 years.

Any person who violates (1) of this subsection wherein a child receives serious injury as a result of such violation shall be guilty of a felony and, upon conviction therof, shall be punished by imprisonment for not less than five nor more than 20 years.

Hawaii

Child abuse or neglect means the acts or omissions of any person who, or legal entity that, is in any manner or degree related to the child, is residing with the child, or is otherwise responsible for the child's care, that have caused the physical or psychological health or welfare of the child, who is under the age of 18, to be harmed, or to be subject to any reasonably foreseeable, substantial risk of being harmed. The acts or omissions are indicated for the purposes of reports by circumstances that includes but are not limited to *when the child is provided with dangerous, harmful, or detrimental drugs, provided that this paragraph shall not apply to the child pursuant to the direction or prescription of a practitioner

Idaho

Except as authorized in this chapter, it is unlawful for any person to manufacture or deliver, or possess with the intent to manufacture or deliver, a controlled substance as defined in Schedules I, II, III and IV in this chapter, upon the same premises where a child under the age of 18 years is present.

As used in this section, *premises* means any

- motor vehicle or vessel
- dwelling or rental unit, including, but not limited to, apartment, townhouse, condominium, mobile home, manufactured home, motel room, or hotel room
- dwelling house, and any other outbuildings

Illinois

The term *abused child* means a child whose parent or immediate family member, or any person responsible for the child's welfare, or any individual residing in the same home as the child, or a paramour of the child's parent

- causes to be sold, transferred, distributed, or given to such child under 18 years of age a controlled substance, as defined by law, except for controlled substances that are prescribed in accordance with the Illinois Controlled Substances Act and dispensed to the child in accordance in a manner that substantially complies with the prescription

Neglected child means any child who is not receiving the proper or necessary nourishment or medically indicated treatment including food or care not provided solely on the basis of the present or anticipated mental or physical impairment as determined by a physician acting alone or in consultation with other physicians or otherwise is not receiving the proper or necessary support or medical or other remedial care recognized under state law as necessary for a child's well-being, or other care necessary for his or her well-being, including adequate food, clothing and shelter; or who is abandoned by his or her parents or other person responsible for the child's welfare without a proper plan of care; or who is a newborn infant whose blood, urine, or meconium contains any amount of a controlled substance as defined inn the Illinois Controlled Substances Act or a metabolite thereof.

All persons required to report may refer to the Department of Human Services any pregnant person in this "state who is addicted as defined in the Alcoholism and Other Drug Abuse and Dependency Act."

The department of Human Services shall notify the local Infant Mortality Reduction Network service provided for Department-funded prenatal care provided in the area in which the person resides. The service provided shall prepare a case management plan and assist the pregnant woman in obtaining counseling and treatment from a local substance use service provider licensed by the Department of Human Services or a licensed hospital that provides substance abuse treatment services. The local Infant Mortality Reduction Network service provider and Department-funded prenatal care provider shall monitor the pregnant woman through the service program.

Those who are neglected include any newborn infant whose blood, urine, or meconium contains any amount of a controlled substance or a metabolite of a controlled substance, with the exception of controlled substances or metabolites of such substances, the presence of which in the newborn infant is the result of medical treatment administered to the mother or the newborn infant.

Indiana

A child is a *child in need of services,* if before the child becomes 18 years of age

- the child's physical or mental health is seriously endangered due to injury by the act or omission of the child's parent, guardian, or custodian, and
- the child needs care, treatment, or rehabilitation that the child is not receiving and is unlikely to

be provided or accepted without the coercive intervention of the court

Evidence that the illegal manufacture of a drug or controlled substance is occurring on property where a child resides creates a rebuttable presumption that the child's physical or mental health is seriously endangered.

A child is a *child in need of services* if before the child becomes 18 years of age

- the child is born with fetal alcohol syndrome, or any amount, including a trace amount, of a controlled substance or a legend drug in the child's body
- the child has an injury; has abnormal physical or psychological development; or is at substantial risk of a life-threatening condition that arises or is substantially aggravated because the child's mother used alcohol, a controlled substance, or a legend drug during pregnancy; and
- the child needs care, treatment, or rehabilitation that the child is not receiving or is unlikely to be provided or accepted without the coercive intervention of the court

Iowa

A *medically relevant test* means a test that produces results of exposure to cocaine, heroin, amphetamines, methamphetamines, or other illegal drugs, or combinations or derivatives of the illegal drugs, including a drug urine screen test.

Child abuse or *abuse* means

- an illegal drug is present in a child's body as a direct and foreseeable consequence of the acts or omissions of the person responsible for the care of the child
- the person responsible for the care of a child has, in the presence of the child, manufactured a dangerous substance, possesses a product containing ephedrine, its salts, optical isomers, salts of optical isomers, or pseudoephedrine, its salts, optical isomers, or salts of optical isomers, with the intent to use the product as a precursor or an intermediary to a dangerous substance

If a health practitioner discovers in a child physical or behavioral symptoms of exposure to cocaine, heroin, amphetamine, methamphetamine, or other illegal drugs, or combinations or derivatives thereof, that were not prescribed by a health practitioner; or if the health practitioner has determined through examination of the natural mother of the child that the child was exposed in utero, the health practitioner may perform or cause to be performed a medically relevant test.

The practitioner shall report any positive results of such a test on the child to the Department of Human Services. The Department shall begin an investigation pursuant to law upon receipt of such a report.

A positive test result obtained prior to the birth of a child shall not be used for the criminal prosecution of a parent for acts and omissions resulting in intrauterine exposure of the child to an illegal drug.

Kansas

This issue is not addressed in the statutes reviewed.

Kentucky

Abused or neglected child means a child whose health or welfare is harmed or threatened with harm when his parent, guardian, or other person exercising custodial control or supervision of the child engages in a pattern of conduct that renders the parent incapable of caring for the immediate and ongoing needs of the child including, but not limited to, parental incapacity due to alcohol and other drug abuse.

Any physician or person legally permitted to engage in attendance upon a pregnant woman may administer to each newborn infant born under that person's care a toxicology test to determine whether there is evidence of prenatal exposure to alcohol, a controlled substance, or a substance identified on the list provided by the Cabinet for Health Services, if the attending person has reason to believe, on the basis of a medical assessment of the mother or the infant, that the mother used any such substance for a nonmedical purpose during the pregnancy.

The circumstances surrounding any positive toxicology finding shall be evaluated by the attending person to determine whether abuse or neglect of an infant, as defined under state law, has occurred and where investigation by the Cabinet for Health Services is necessary.

Louisiana

This issue is not addressed in the statutes reviewed.

Maine

This issue is not addressed in the statutes reviewed.

Maryland

Within one year after a child's birth, there is a presumption that a child is not receiving proper care an attention from the mother for proposes of state law of this subtitle if

- the child was born exposed to cocaine, heroin, or a derivative of cocaine or heroin as evidenced by any appropriate tests of the mother or child; or
- upon admission to a hospital for delivery of the child, the mother tested positive for cocaine, heroin, or a derivative of cocaine or heroin as evidenced by any appropriate toxicology test; and
- drug treatment is made available to the mother and the mother refuses the recommended level of drug treatment, or does not successfully complete the recommended level of drug treatment.

Promptly after receiving a report from a hospital or health practitioner of suspected neglect related to drug abuse and conducting an appropriate investigation, the local department may

- file a petition alleging that the child is in need of assistance under state law; and
- offer the mother admission into a drug treatment program

The local department may initiate a judicial proceeding to terminate a mother's parental rights, if the local department offers the mother admission into a drug treatment program under this subsection within 90 days after the birth of the child and the mother

- does not accept admission to the program or its equivalent within 45 days after the offer is made
- does not accept the recommended level of drug treatment within 45 days after the offer is made; or
- fails to participate fully in the program or its equivalent

Petition for study custody: A Child in Need of Assistance petition shall be filed on behalf of a child who is born drug exposed, if

- the mother refused the recommended level of drug treatment or does not successfully complete the recommended level of drug treatment
- the mother is unable to provide adequate care for the child; and
- the father is unable to provide adequate care for the child.

Massachusetts

Injured, abused or neglected child includes a child under the age of 18 years who is determined to be physically dependent upon an addictive drug at birth.

Any mandated reporter who, in his professional capacity, shall have reasonable cause to believe that a child is suffering physical or emotional injury resulting from abuse . . . or who is determined to be physically dependent upon an addictive drug at birth, shall immediately report such condition to the Department by oral communication and by making a written report within 48 hours after such oral communication.

Michigan

A person who is required to report suspected child abuse or neglect, and who knows, or from the child's symptoms has reasonable cause to suspect, that a newborn infant has any amount of alcohol, a controlled substance, or a metabolite of a controlled substance in his or her body shall report to the Department in the same manner as required of other reports.

A report is not required under this section if the person knows that the alcohol, controlled substance, or metabolite, or the child's symptoms are the result of medical treatment administered to the newborn infant or his or her mother.

Minnesota

A physician shall administer a toxicology test to a pregnant woman under the physician's care or to a woman under the physician's care within eight hours after delivery to determine whether there is evidence that she has ingested a controlled substance, if the woman has obstetrical complications that are a medical indication of possible use of a controlled substance for a nonmedical purpose. If the test results are positive, the physician shall report the results. A negative test result does not eliminate the obligation to report if other evidence gives the physician reason to believe the patient has used a controlled substance for a nonmedical purpose.

A physician shall administer to each newborn infant born under the physician's care a toxicology test to determine whether there is evidence of prenatal exposure to a controlled substance if the physician has reason to believe, on the basis of a medical assessment of the mother or the infant, that the mother used a controlled substance for a nonmedical purpose during the pregnancy. If the test results are positive, the physician shall report the results as neglect. A negative test result does not eliminate the obligation to report if other medical evidence of prenatal exposure to a controlled substance is present.

Physicians shall report to the Department of Health the results of tests performed. A report shall be made on the Certificate of Live Birth Medical Supplement or the Report of Fetal Death Medical Supplement filed on or after February 1, 1991.

Any physician or other medical personnel administering a toxicology test to determine the presence of a controlled substance in a pregnant woman, in a woman within eight hours after delivery, or in a child at birth or during the first month of life is immune from civil or criminal liability arising from administration of the test, if the physician ordering the test believes in good faith that the test is required under this law and the test is administered in accordance with an established protocol and reasonable medical practice.

A positive test result reported under this law must be obtained from a confirmatory test performed by a drug testing laboratory that meets the requirements of the law and must be performed according to the requirements for performance of confirmatory test imposed by the licensing, accreditation, or certification program listed in the law in which the laboratory participates.

Neglect includes

- prenatal exposure to a controlled substance, used by the mother for a nonmedical purpose, as evidenced by withdrawal symptoms in the child at birth, results of a toxicology test performed on the mother at delivery or the child at birth, or medical effects or developmental delays during the child's first year of life that medically indicated prenatal exposure to a controlled substance
- chronic and severe use of alcohol or a controlled substance by a parent or person responsible for the care of the child that adversely affects the child's basic needs and safety

Physical abuse includes purposely giving a child poison, alcohol, or dangerous, harmful, or controlled substances that were not prescribed for the child by a practitioner, in order to control or punish the child; or other substances that substantially affect the child's behavior, motor coordination, or judgment or that result in sickness or internal injury, or subject the child to medical procedures that would be unnecessary if the child were not exposed to the substances.

A mandatory reporter shall immediately report to the local welfare agency if the person knows or has reason to believe that a woman is pregnant and has used a controlled substance for a nonmedical purpose during pregnancy.

Any person may make a voluntary report if the person knows or has reason to believe that a woman is pregnant and has used a controlled substance for a nonmedical purpose during the pregnancy. An oral report shall be made immediately by telephone or otherwise.

An oral report made by a person required to report shall be followed within 72 hours, exclusive of weekends and holidays, by a report in writing to the local welfare agency. Any report shall be of sufficient content to identify the pregnant woman, the nature and extent of the abuse, if known, and the name and address of the reporter.

If the report alleges a pregnant woman's use of a controlled substance for a nonmedical purpose, the local welfare agency shall immediately conduct an appropriate assessment and offer services indicated under the circumstances. Services offered may include, but are not limited to, a referral for chemical dependency assessment, a referral for chemical dependency treatment of recommended, and a referral for prenatal care. The local welfare agency also may take any appropriate action, including seeking an emergency admission pursuant to the law. The local welfare agency shall seek an emergency admission if the pregnant woman refuses recommended voluntary services or fails recommended treatment.

A person making a voluntary or mandated report under this law or assisting in an assessment is immune from any civil or criminal liability that otherwise might result from the person's actions, if the person is acting in good faith. This does not provide immunity to any person for failure to make a required report or for omitting neglect, physical abuse, or sexual abuse of a child.

Mississippi

This issue is not addressed in the statutes reviewed.

Missouri

Notwithstanding the physician-patient privilege, any physician or health care provider may refer to the Department of Health families in which children may have been exposed to a controlled substance as defined by law or alcohol as evidenced by

- medical documentation of signs and symptoms consistent with controlled substances or alcohol exposure in the child at birth; or

- results of a confirmed toxicology test for controlled substances performed at birth on the mother or the child; and

- a written assessment made or approved by a physician, health care provider, or the Division of Family Services that documents the child as being at risk of abuse or neglect

Nothing in the section shall preclude a physician or other mandated reporter from reporting abuse or neglect of a child as required pursuant to the provisions of the reporting laws.

Any physician or health care provider complying with this law, in good faith, shall have immunity from any civil liability that might otherwise result by reasons of such actions.

Montana

Child abuse or neglect includes exposing a child to the criminal distribution of dangerous drugs, as prohibited by state law; the criminal production or manufacture of dangerous drugs, as prohibited by state law; or the production of an unlawful clandestine laboratory, as prohibited by state law.

Nebraska

This issue is not addressed in the statutes reviewed.

Nevada

This issue is not addressed in the statutes reviewed.

New Hampshire

This issue is not addressed in the statutes reviewed.

New Jersey

This issue is not addressed in the statutes reviewed.

New Mexico

Evidence that demonstrates that a child has been negligently allowed to enter or remain in a motor vehicle, building, or another premise that contains chemicals, materials, or equipment used or intended for use in the manufacture of a controlled substance shall be deemed prima facie evidence of abuse of a child.

New York

Neglected child means a child less than 18 years of age, whose physical, mental, or emotional condition has been impaired or is in imminent danger of becoming impaired as a result of the failure of his parent or other person legally responsible for his care to exercise a minimum degree of care by misusing a drug or drugs; or by using alcoholic beverages to the extent that he loses self-control of his actions; or by any other acts of a similarly serious nature requiring the act of the court; provided, however, that where the respondent is voluntarily and regularly participating in a rehabilitative program, evidence that the respondent has repeatedly misused a drug or drugs or alcoholic beverages to the extent that he loses self-control of his actions shall not establish that the child is a neglected child in the absence of evidence establishing that the child's physical, mental, or emotional condition has been impaired or is in imminent danger becoming impaired.

North Carolina

This issue is not addressed in the statutes reviewed.

North Dakota

Deprived child means a child who

- was subject to prenatal exposure to chronic and severe use of alcohol or any controlled substance in a manner not lawfully prescribed by a practitioner
- is present in an environment subjecting the child to exposure to a controlled substance or drug paraphernalia

Ohio

No person shall . . . allow the child to be on the same parcel of real property and within 100 feet of, or, in the case of more than one housing unit on the same parcel of real property, in the same housing unit and within 100 feet of, an act in violation of state law [prohibiting the cultivation of marijuana or the manufacture of a controlled substance] or [prohibiting the possession of any of the chemicals used in the manufacture of a controlled substance] when the person knows that the act is occurring, whether or not any person is prosecuted or convicted of the violation that is the basis for the violation of this section.

Oklahoma

Every physician or surgeon, including doctors of medicine, osteopathic physicians, residents, and interns, or any other health care professional attending the birth of a child who appears to be a child born in a condition of dependence on a controlled dangerous substance, shall promptly report the matter to the county office of the Department of Human Services in the county in which such birth occurred.

Oregon

This issue is not addressed in the statutes reviewed.

Pennsylvania

This issue is not addressed in the statutes reviewed.

Rhode Island

Abused and/or neglect child means a child whose physical or mental health or welfare is harmed or threatened with harm when his or her parent or other person responsible for his or her welfare fails to provide the child with a minimum degree of care or proper supervision or guardianship because of his or her unwillingness or inability to do so by situations or conditions such as, but not limited to, social problems, mental incompetnecy, or the use of a drug, drugs, or alcohol to the extent that the parent or other person responsible for the child's welfare loses his or her ability or is unwilling to properly care for the child.

South Carolina

It is presumed that a newborn is an abused or neglected child as defined in state law and that the child cannot be protected from further harm without being removed from the custody of the mother upon proof that

- a blood or urine test of the child at birth or a blood or urine test of the mother at birth shows the presence of any amount of a controlled substance or a metabolite of a controlled substance unless the presence of the substance or the metabolite is the result of medical treatment administered to the mother of the infant or the infant; or
- the child has a medical diagnosis of fetal alcohol syndrome; and
- a blood or urine test of another child of the mother or a blood or urine test of the mother at the birth of another child showed the presence of any amount of a controlled substance or a metabolite of a controlled substance unless the presence of the substance or the metabolite was the result of medical treatment administered to the mother for the infant or the infant; or
- another child of the mother has the medical diagnosis of fetal alcohol syndrome

South Dakota

Abused or neglected child includes a child

- who was subject to parental exposure to abusive use of alcohol or any controlled drug or substance not lawfully prescribed by a practitioner as authorized by statute; or
- whose parent, guardian, or custodian knowingly exposes the child to an environment that is being used for the manufacturing of methamphetamines

Tennessee

Severe child abuse means

- knowingly allowing a child to be present within a structure where the act of creating methamphetamine is occurring

Texas

Abuse includes the following acts or omissions by a person:

- causing or permitting the child to be in a situation in which the child sustains a mental or emotional injury that results in an observable and material impairment in the child's growth, development, or psychological functioning
- the current use by a person of a controlled substance as defined by the Health and Safety Code, in a manner or to the extent that the use results in physical, mental, or emotional injury to a child or
- causing, expressing permitting, or encouraging a child to use a controlled substance

Born addicted to alcohol or a controlled substance means a child

- who is born to a mother who, during the pregnancy, used a controlled substance, as defined by the Health and Safety Code, other than a controlled substance legally obtained by prescription, or alcohol; and
- who, after birth as a result of the mother's use of the controlled substance or alcohol
  - experiences observable withdrawal from the alcohol or controlled substance
  - exhibits observable or harmful effects in the child's physical appearance of functioning; or
  - exhibits the demonstrable presence of alcohol or a controlled substance in the child's bodily fluids

Utah

When any person, including a licensee under the Medical Practice Act or the Nurse Practice Act, attends the birth of a child or care for a child, and determines that the child, at the time of birth, has fetal alcohol syndrome or fetal drug dependency, he shall report that determination to the Division of Child and Family Services as soon as possible.

Vermont

This issue is not addressed in the statutes reviewed.

Virginia

For purposes of the reporting law, *reason to suspect that a child is abused or neglected* shall include

- a finding made by an attending physician within seven days of a child's birth that the results of a blood or urine test conducted within 48 hours of the birth of the child indicate the presence of a controlled substance not prescribed for the mother by a physician
- a finding by an attending physician made within 48 hours of a child's birth that the child was born dependent on a controlled substance that was not prescribed by a physician for the mother and has demonstrated withdrawal symptoms
- a diagnosis by an attending physician made within seven days of a child's birth that the child was born dependent on a controlled substance that was not prescribed by a physician for the mother and has demonstrated withdrawal symptoms
- a diagnosis by an attending physician made within seven days of a child's birth that the child has an illness, disease, or condition that, to a reasonable degree of medical certainty, is attributable to in utero exposure to a controlled substance that was not prescribed by a physician for the mother or the child; or
- a diagnosis by an attending a physician made with seven days of a child's birth that the child has fetal alcohol syndrome attributable to in utero exposure to alcohol

When *reason to suspect* is based upon this subsection, such fact shall be included in the report along with the fact relied upon by the person making the report.

Abused or neglected child means any child less than 18 years of age

- whose parent or other person responsible for his care creates or inflicts, threatens to create or inflict, or allows to be created or inflicted upon such child a physical or mental injury by other than accidental means, or creates a substantial risk of death, disfigurement, or impairment of bodily or mental functions, including but not limited to, a child who is with his parent or other person responsible for his care either (i) during the manufacture or attempted manufacture of a Schedule I or II controlled substance, or (ii) during the unlawful sale of such substance by that child's parent or other person responsible for his care, where such manufacture, or attempted manufacture or unlawful sale would constitute a felony violation

Washington

When, as a result of a report of alleged child abuse or neglect, an investigation is made that includes an in-person contact with the person who is alleged to have committed the abuse or neglect, there shall be a determination of whether it is probable that the use of alcohol or controlled substances is a contributing factor to the alleged abuse or neglect.

In a criminal case where

- the defendant has been convicted of manufacture of a controlled substance under law relating to manufacture of methamphetamine; or possession of ephedrine or any of its salts or isomers or salts of isomers, pseudoephedrine or any of its salts or isomers or salts of isomers, pressurized ammonia gas, or pressurized ammonia gas solution with intent to manufacture methamphetamine, and
- there has been a special allegation prelade and proven beyond a reasonable doubt that the defendant committed the crime when a person under the age of 18 was present in or upon the premises of manufacture

The court shall make a finding of fact of the special legation, or if a jury trial is had, the jury shall, if it finds the defendant guilty, also find a special verdict as to the special allegation.

A law enforcement agent in the course of investigating an allegation related to manufacture of methamphetamine or an allegation related to possession of ephedrine or any of its salts or isomers or salts of isomers, epipherine or any of its salts or isomers or salts of isomers, pressurized ammonia gas, or pressurized ammonia gas solution with intent to manufacture methamphetamine, that discovers a child present at the site, shall contact the detente immediately.

West Virginia

This issue is not addressed in the statutes reviewed.

Wisconsin

Abuse other than when used in referring to abuse of alcohol beverages or other drugs, means any of the following:

• when used in referring to an unborn child, serious physical harm inflicted on the unborn child, and the risk of serious physical harm to the child when born, caused by the habitual lack of self-control of the expectant mother of the unborn child in the use of alcohol beverages, controlled substances, or controlled substance analogs, exhibited to a severe degree

Wyoming

No person shall knowingly sell, give, or otherwise furnish a child any drug prohibited by law without a physician's prescription.

A person violating this section is guilty of a misdemeanor punishable by imprisonment for not more than one year, a fine of not more than $1,000, or both. A person convicted of a second violation of this section is guilty of a felony punishable by imprisonment for not more than five years, a fine of not more than $5,000, or both.

Source: Adapted from information provided by the National Clearinghouse on Child Abuse and Neglect's *Parental Drug Use as Child Abuse,* 2004. Available online. URL: http://www.nccanch.acf.hhs.gov/general/legal/statutes/drugexposcd.cfm. Downloaded January 18, 2006.

BIBLIOGRAPHY

Abarbanel, Gail. "Learning from Victims," *National Institute of Justice Journal* (April 2000): 11–12.

Adlaf, E. M., P. Begin, and E. Swaka, eds. *Canadian Addiction Survey (CAS: A National Survey of Canadians' Use of Alcohol and Other Drugs: Prevalence of Use and Related Harms: Detailed Report).* Ottawa, Canada: Canadian Centre on Substance Abuse, 2005. Available online. URL: http://www.ccsa.ca/NR/reonlyres/6806130B-C314-4C96-95CC-075D14CD83DE/0/ccsa0040 282005.pdf. Downloaded June 27, 2006.

Adlaf, E. M., Andrée Demers, and Gouis Gliksman, eds. *Canadian Campus Survey 2004.* Toronto, Canada: Centre for Addiction and Mental Health, 2005. Available online. URL: http://www.camh.net/Research/Areas_of_research/Population_Life_Course_Studies/CCS_200 4_report.pdf. Downloaded June 27, 2006.

Administration on Children, Youth, and Families. *Child Maltreatment 2003.* Washington, D.C.: Children's Bureau, U.S. Department of Health and Human Services, 2005.

American Psychiatric Association. *Diagnostic and Statistical Manual of Mental Disorders.* 4th ed. Washington, D.C.: American Psychiatric Association, 2000.

Anda, Robert F., M.D., et al. "Adverse Childhood Experiences, Alcoholic Parents, and Later Risk of Alcoholism and Depression." *Psychiatric Services* 53, no. 8 (August 2002): 1,001–1,009.

Anton, Raymond F., M.D. "Combined Pharmacotherapies and Behavioral Interventions for Alcohol Dependence: The COMBINE Study: A Randomized Controlled Trial." *Journal of the American Medical Association* 295, no. 17 (May 2006): 2,003–2,017.

Arria, Amelia M., et al. "Methamphetamine and Other Substance Use during Pregnancy: Preliminary Estimates from the Infant Development, Environment, and Lifestyle (IDEAL) Study." *Maternal and Child Health* 10, no. 3 (May 2006): 1–10.

Arseneault, Louise. "Cannabis Use in Adolescence and Risk for Adult Psychosis: Longitudinal Prospective Study." *British Medical Journal* 325 (November 2002): 1,212–1,213.

Atluri, Sairam, M.D., et al. "Guidelines for the Use of Controlled Substances in the Management of Chronic Pain." *Pain Physician* 6 (2003): 233–257.

Bagnardi, Vincenzo, et al. "Alcohol Consumption and the Risk of Cancer: A Meta-Analysis." *Alcohol Research & Health* 25, no. 4 (2001): 263–270.

Bartels, Stephen J., M.D., et al. *Substance Abuse and Mental Health among Older Americans: The State of the Knowledge and Future Directions.* Rockville, Md.: Substance Abuse and Mental Health Services Administration, 2005. Available online. URL: http://www.samhsa.gov/aging/SA_MH_%20AMongOlderAdultsfinal102105.pdf. Downloaded January 5, 2006.

Bassuk, Ellen, M.D., John C. Buckner, Jennifer N. Perloff, and Shari S. Bassuk. "Prevalence of Mental Health and Substance Use Disorders among Homeless and Low-Income Housed Mothers." *American Journal of Psychiatry* 155 (1998): 1,561–1,564.

Belmaker, R. H., M.D. "Bipolar Disorder." *New England Journal of Medicine* 351, no. 5 (July 2004): 476–486.

Black, Donald W., M.D., et al. "Family History and Psychiatric Comorbidity in Persons with Compulsive Buying: Preliminary Findings." *American Journal of Psychiatry* 155, no. 7 (July 1998): 960–963.

Blanchard, Christopher M. *Afghanistan: Narcotics and U.S. Policy.* Washington, D.C.: Congressional Research Service, updated May 26, 2005. Available online. URL: http://www.usembassy.at/en/download/pdf/afgh_narcs.pdf. Downloaded January 19, 2006.

Bouchard, Jr., Thomas J., and Matt McGue. "Genetic and Environmental Influences on Human Psychological Differences." *Journal of Neurobiology* 54 (2003): 40–45.

Brady, Kathleen T., M.D., and Susan C. Sonne. "The Role of Stress in Alcohol Use, Alcoholism Treatment, and Relapse." *Alcohol Research & Health* 23, no. 4 (1999): 263–271.

Brady, Thomas M., and Olivia Silber Ashley, eds. *Women in Substance Abuse Treatment: Results from the Alcohol and Drug Services Study (ADSS).* Rockville, Md.: Substance Abuse and Mental Health Services Administration, 2005.

Brecht, Mary Lynn, et al. "Methamphetamine Use Behaviors and Gender Differences." *Addictive Behaviors* 29 (2004): 89–106.

Breshears, E. M., S. Yeah, and N. K. Young. *Understanding Substance Abuse and Facilitating Recovery: A Guide for Child Welfare Workers.* Rockville, Md.: U.S. Department of Health and Human Services, Substance Abuse and Mental Health Services Administration, 2004.

Brewer, Robert D., M.D., and Monica H. Swahn. "Binge Drinking and Violence." *Journal of the American Medical Association* 294, no. 5 (August 2005): 616–618.

Bureau for International Narcotics and Law Enforcement Affairs. "Canada, Mexico, and Central America." International Narcotics Control Strategy Report, Department of State, March 2006. Available online. URL: http://www.state.gov/p/inl/rls/nrcrpt/2006/vol1/html/62107.htm. Downloaded May 3, 2006.

Bureau of Justice Assistance. *2005 National Gang Threat Assessment.* Washington, D.C.: Department of Justice, 2005.

Campbell, Jacquelyn C. "Health Consequences of Intimate Partner Violence." *Lancet* 359 (April 2002): 1,331–1,336.

Carpenter, Christopher. "How Do Zero Tolerance Drunk Driving Laws Work?" *Journal of Health Economics* 23, no. 1 (2004): 61–83.

Centers for Disease Control and Prevention. "Alcohol Consumption among Women Who Are Pregnant or Who Might Become Pregnant—United States, 2002." *Morbidity and Mortality Weekly Review* 53, no. 50 (December 2004): 1,178–1,181.

———. "Atypical Reactions Associated with Heroin Use—Five States, January–April 2005." *Morbidity and Mortality Weekly Report* 54 (2005): 793–796.

———. "Cases of HIV/AIDS, by Area of Residence, Diagnosed in 2004—33 States with Confidential Name-Based HIV Infection Reporting." *HIV/AIDS Surveillance Report* 16 (2006).

———. "A Glance at the HIV/AIDS Epidemic." Available online. URL: http://www.cdc.gov/hiv/resources/factsheets/At-A-Glance.htm. Downloaded May 11, 2006.

———. "Youth Risk Behavior Surveillance—United States, 2003." *Morbidity and Mortality Weekly Report* 3, no. 2 (May 2004): 1–100.

Chen, Chiung M., Mary C. Dufour, M.D., and Hsiao-ye Yi. "Alcohol Consumption among Young Adults Ages 18–24 in the United States: Results from the 2001–2002 NESARC Survey." *Alcohol Research & Health* 28, no. 4 (2004/2005): 269–280.

Cicero, Theodore J., James A. Inciardi, and Alvaro Muñoz. "Trends in Abuse of OxyContin and Other Opioid Analgesics in the United States: 2002–2004." *Journal of Pain* 6, no. 10 (October 2005): 662–672.

Clark, Kathryn Anderson, et al. "Treatment Compliance among Prenatal Care Patients with Substance Abuse Problems." *American Journal of Drug and Alcohol Abuse* 27, no. 1 (2001): 121–136.

Clark, Robin E., Judith Freeman Clark, with Christine Adamec. *The Encyclopedia of Child Abuse.* New York: Facts On File, 2006.

Cnattingius, Sven, M.D., et al. "Caffeine Intake and the Risk of First-Trimester Spontaneous Abortion." *New England Journal of Medicine* 343, no. 25 (December 2000): 1,839–1,945.

Coleman, Eric. "Anorectics on Trial: A Half Century of Federal Regulation of Prescription Appetite Suppressants." *Annals of Internal Medicine* 143 (2005): 380–385.

Collins, Eric D., M.D., et al. "Anesthesia-Assisted vs Buprenorphine- or Clonidine-Assisted Heroin Detoxification and Naltrexone Induction: A Randomized Trial." *Journal of the American Medical Association* 294, no. 8 (August 2005): 903–913.

Compton III, Wilson M., M.D. "Prevalence of Marijuana Use Disorders in the United States 1991–1992 and 2001–2002." *Journal of the American Medical Association* 291, no. 17 (May 2004): 2,114–2,121.

Compton III, William M., M.D, et al. "The Role of Psychiatric Disorders in Predicting Drug Dependence Treatment Outcomes." *American Journal of Psychiatry* 160, no. 5 (May 2003): 890–895.

Condren, Rita M., John O'Connor, and Roy Browne. "Prevalence and Patterns of Substance Misuse in Schizophrenia." *Psychiatric Bulletin* 25 (2001): 17–20.

Copeland, Lorraine, et al. "Changing Patterns in Cause of Death in a Cohort of Injecting Drug Users, 1980–2001." *Archives of Internal Medicine* 165 (June 2004): 1,214–1,220.

Cramer, Robert J. "Internet Pharmacies: Hydrocodone, an Addictive Narcotic Pain Medication, Is Available without a Prescription through the Internet." Washington, D.C.: General Accounting Office, 2004. Available online. URL: http://www.gao.gov/new.items/do4892t.pdf. Downloaded February 22, 2006.

Crosse, Marcia. *Testimony before the Subcommittee on Health, Committee on Energy and Commerce, House of Representatives, Prescription Drugs: State Monitoring Programs May Help to Reduce Illegal Diversion.* Washington D.C.: General Accounting Office, 2004.

Department of Mental Health and Substance Abuse. *Global Status Report on Alcohol 2004.* Geneva, Switzerland: World Health Organization, 2004.

Dervaux, Alain, M.D., et al. "Is Substance Abuse in Schizophrenia Related to Impulsivity, Sensation Seeking, or Anhedonia?" *American Journal of Psychiatry* 158, no. 3 (March 2001): 492–494.

DeVoe, Jill F., et al. *Indicators of School Crime and Safety: 2005.* Washington, D.C.: U.S. Department of Education and U.S. Department of Justice, 2005.

Doctor, Ronald M., and Ada P. Kahn. *The Encyclopedia of Phobias, Fears, and Anxieties*. 2nd ed. New York: Facts On File, 2000.

D'Onofrio, Gail, M.D., and Linda C. Degutis. "Screening and Brief Intervention in the Emergency Department." *Alcohol Research & Health* 28, no. 2 (2004/2005): 63–72.

Dorsey, Tina L., Marianne W. Zawitz, and Priscilla Middleton. *Drugs and Crime Facts*. Washington, D.C.: U.S. Department of Justice, Office of Justice Programs, Bureau of Justice Statistics. Available online. URL: http://www.ojp.usdoj.gov/bjs/pub/pdf/dcf.pdf. Downloaded July 16, 2006.

Drake, Robert E., M.D., and Kim T. Mueser. "Co-Occurring Alcohol Use Disorder and Schizophrenia." *Alcohol Research & Health* 26, no. 2 (2002): 99–102.

Drug Enforcement Administration. *Steroid Abuse in Today's Society: A Guide to Understanding Steroids and Related Substances*. Washington, D.C.: U.S. Department of Justice, 2004.

Dube, Shanta R., et al. "Childhood Abuse, Neglect, and Household Dysfunction and the Risk of Illicit Drug Use: The Adverse Childhood Experiences Study." *Pediatrics* 111, no. 3 (March 2003): 564–572.

Edwards, Valerie, et al. "The Wide-Ranging Health Outcomes of Adverse Childhood Experiences." In *Child Victimization*. Kingston, N.J.: Civic Research Institute, 2005.

Emanuele, Mary Ann, M.D., Frederick Wezeman, and Nicholas V. Emanuele, M.D. "Alcohol's Effects on Female Reproductive Function." *Alcohol Research & Health* 26, no. 4 (2002): 274–281.

English, Brett A., et al. "Treatment of Chronic Post-traumatic Stress Disorder in Combat Veterans with Citalopram: An Open Trial." *Journal of Clinical Psychopharmacology* 26, no. 1 (February 2006): 84–88.

Evans, Charity, et al. "Use and Abuse of Methylphenidate in Attention-Deficit/Hyperactivity Disorder." *Canadian Pharmacists Journal* 137, no. 6 (July–August 2004): 30–35.

Evans, Christopher, J. "Secrets of the Opium Poppy Revealed." *Neuropharmacology* 47 (2004): 293–299.

Executive Office of the President. *Synthetic Drug Control Strategy: A Focus on Methamphetamine and Prescription Drug Abuse*. Washington, D.C.: Office of National Drug Control Policy, 2006.

Fals-Stewart, W., and J. Schafer. "The Treatment of Substance Abusers Diagnosed with Obsessive-Compulsive Disorder: An Outcome Study." *Journal of Substance Abuse Treatment* 9, no. 4 (Fall 1992): 365–370.

Farrell, M., et al. "Psychosis and Drug Dependence: Results for a National Survey of Prisoners." *British Journal of Psychiatry* 181, no. 5 (2002): 393–398.

Feeney, Gerald F. X., et al. "Combined Acamprosate and Naltrexone, with Cognitive Behavioural Therapy Is Superior to Either Medication Alone for Alcohol Abstinence: A Single Centre's Experience with Pharmacotherapy." *Alcohol and Alcoholism* 41, no. 3 (2006): 321–327.

Findling, Robert L., M.D., et al. "A Double-Blind Pilot Study of Resperidone in the Treatment of Conduct Disorder." *Journal of the American Academy of Child & Adolescent Psychiatry* 39, no. 4 (April 2000): 509–516.

Fitzgerald, Nora, and K. Jack Riley. "Drug Facilitated Rape: Looking for the Missing Pieces." *National Institute of Justice Journal*, April 2000, 8–15. Available online. URL: http://www.ncjrs.gov/pdffiles1/jr000243c.pdf. Downloaded March 16, 2006.

Flora, David B., and Laurie Chassin. "Changes in Drug Use during Adulthood: The Effects of Parent Alcoholism and Transition into Marriage." *Psychology of Addictive Behaviors* 19, no. 19 (2005): 352–362.

Fricchione, Gregory, M.D. "Generalized Anxiety Disorder." *New England Journal of Medicine* 351, no. 17 (August 2004): 675–682.

Friedman, Richard A., M.D. "The Changing Face of Teenage Drug Abuse—the Trend toward Prescription Drugs." *New England Journal of Medicine* 354, no. 14 (April 2006): 1,448–1,450.

Frisher, Martin, et al. "Prevalence of Comorbid Psychiatric Illness and Substance Misuse in Primary Care in England and Wales." *Journal of Epidemiology and Community Health* 58 (2004): 1,036–1,041.

Garbutt, James C., M.D., et al. "Efficacy and Tolerability of Long-Acting Injectable Naltrexone for Alcohol Dependence: A Randomized Controlled Trial." *Journal of the American Medical Association* 293, no. 13 (April 2005): 1,617–1,625.

Garfinkel, Doron, M.D., et al. "Facilitation of Benzodiazepine Discontinuation by Melatonin." *Archives of Internal Medicine* 159 (November 1999): 2,456–2,460.

General Accounting Office. *Anabolic Steroids Are Easily Purchased without a Prescription and Present Significant Challenges to Law Enforcement Officials*. Washington, D.C.: General Accounting Office, 2005.

———. "Internet Pharmacies: Some Pose Safety Risks for Consumers." Washington, D.C.: General Accounting Office, 2004. Available online. URL: http://www.gao.gov/new.items/do4820.pdf. Downloaded February 23, 2006.

General Accounting Office, Report to Congressional Requesters. *Prescription Drugs: OxyContin Abuse and Diversion and Efforts to Address the Problem*. Washington, D.C.: General Accounting Office, 2003.

General Accounting Office, Report to the Subcommittee on Oversight and Investigations, Committee on

Energy and Commerce, House of Representatives. *Prescription Drugs: State Monitoring Programs Provide Useful Tool to Reduce Diversion.* Washington, D.C.: General Accounting Office, 2002.

Gordon, Rachel J., M.D., and Franklin D. Lowy, M.D. "Bacterial Infections in Drug Users." *New England Journal of Medicine* 353, no. 18 (November 2005): 1,945–1,954.

Gossop, Michael, Victoria Manning, and Gayle Ridge. "Concurrent Use of Alcohol and Cocaine: Differences in Patterns of Use and Problems among Users of Crack Cocaine and Cocaine Powder." *Alcohol and Alcoholism* 41, no. 2 (2006): 121–125.

Grant, Bridget F., et al. "Prevalence, Correlates and Disability of Personality Disorders in the United States: Results from the National Epidemiologic Survey on Alcohol and Related Conditions." *Journal of Clinical Psychiatry* 65 (2004): 948–958.

Grant, Bridget F., et al. "The 12-Month Prevalence and Trends in DSM-IV Alcohol Abuse and Dependence: United States, 1991–1992 and 2001–2002." *Drug and Alcohol Dependence* 74, (2004): 223–234.

Green, Carla A. "Gender and Use of Substance Abuse Treatment Services." *Alcohol Research & Health* 29, no. 1 (2006): 55–62.

Grilo, Carlos M., Rajita Sinha, and Stephanie S. O'Malley. "Eating Disorders and Alcohol Use Disorders." *Alcohol Research & Health* 26, no. 2 (2002): 51–160.

Grisso, Jeane Ann, M.D., et al. "Violent Injuries among Women in an Urban Area." *New England Journal of Medicine* 341, no. 25 (December 1999): 1,899–1,905.

Gwinnell, Esther, M.D., and Christine Adamec. *The Encyclopedia of Addictions and Addictive Behaviors.* New York: Facts On File, 2006.

Hall, Ryan C. W., M.D., Richard C. W. Hall, M.D., and Marcia J. Chapman. "Psychiatric Complications of Anabolic Steroid Abuse." *Psychosomatics* 46, no. 4 (July–August 2005): 285–290.

Hampton, Tracy. "Interplay of Genes and Environment Found in Adolescents' Alcohol Abuse." *Journal of the American Medical Association* 295, no. 15 (April 2006): 1,760, 1,762.

———. "Researchers Address Use of Performance-Enhancing Drugs in Nonelite Athletes." *Journal of the American Medical Association* 295, no. 6 (February 2006): 607–608.

Harocops, Alex, and Mike Hough. *Drug Dealing in Open-Air Markets.* Washington, D.C.: Office of Community Oriented Policing Services, U.S. Department of Justice, 2005.

Hénquet, Cecile, et al. "Prospective Cohort Study of Cannabis Use, Predisposition for Psychosis, and Psychotic Symptoms in Young People." *British Medical Journal* 330 (2005): 11–15.

Hingson, Ralph, and Michael Winter. "Epidemiology and Consequences of Drinking and Driving." *Alcohol Research & Health* 27, no. 1 (2003): 63–70.

Howe, David. *Child Abuse and Neglect: Attachment, Development and Intervention.* New York: Palgrave Macmillan, 2005.

Hubbard, William K. "Statement of William K. Hubbard, Associate Commissioner for Policy and Planning, before the Committee on Government Reform, U.S. House of Representatives Hearing on Internet Drug Sales. March 18, 2004." Available online. URL: http://www.fda.gov/ola/2004/internetdrugs0318.html. Downloaded January 15, 2006.

Huddleston III, C. West, Karen Freeman-Wilson, and Daniel Boone. *Painting the Current Picture: A National Report Card on Drug Courts and Other Problem Solving Court Programs in the United States.* Alexandria, Va.: National Drug Court Institute, 2004.

International Narcotics and Law Enforcement Affairs. "Canada, Mexico and Central America." *International Narcotics Control Strategy Report.* March 2006. Available online. URL: http://www.state.gov/p/inl/rls/nrcrpt/2006/vol1/html/62107.htm. Downloaded May 3, 2006.

Johnson, Dick. *Meth: The Home-Cooked Menace.* Center City, Minn.: Hazelden, 2005.

Johnston, Lloyd D., et al. *Monitoring the Future: National Survey Results on Drug Use, 1975–2004.* Vol. 2, *College Students and Adults Ages 19–45.* Bethesda, Md.: National Institute on Drug Abuse, National Institutes of Health, 2005.

Johnston, Lloyd D., et al. *Monitoring the Future: National Results on Adolescent Drug Use. Overview of Key Findings 2004.* Bethesda, Md.: National Institute of Drug Abuse, 2005.

Joseph, Donald E., et al., eds. *Drugs of Abuse.* Washington, D.C.: U.S. Department of Justice, 2005.

Kadison, Richard, M.D. "Getting an Edge—Use of Stimulants and Antidepressants in College." *New England Journal of Medicine* 353, no. 11 (September 2005): 1,089–1,091.

Kalso, E. "Oxycodone." *Journal of Pain Symptom Management* 29, no. 5 (May 2005): S47–S56.

Kampman, Kyle M., M.D. "New Medications for the Treatment of Cocaine Dependence." *Psychiatry* 2, no. 12 (December 2005): 44–48.

Karberg, Jennifer C., and Doris J. James. *Substance Dependence, Abuse, and Treatment of Jail Inmates, 2002.* Washington, D.C.: U.S. Department of Justice, 2005.

Karch, Steven B., M.D. "Cocaine: History, Use, Abuse." *Journal of the Royal Society of Medicine* 92 (August 1999): 393–397.

Kashdan, T. B., John D. Elhai, and B. Christopher Frueh. "Anhedonia and Emotional Numbing in Combat Veterans with PTSD." *Behaviour Research and Therapy* 44 (2006): 457–467.

Kashdan, T. B., C. J. Vetter, and R. L. Collins. "Substance Use in Young Adults: Associations with Personality and Gender." *Addictive Behaviors* 30, no. 2 (February 2005): 259–269.

Katz, Debra A., M.D., and Lon R. Hays, M.D. "Adolescent OxyContin." *Journal of the American Academy of Child & Adolescent Psychiatry* 43, no. 2 (February 2004): 231–234.

Kendall-Tackett, Kathleen, and Sarah M. Giacomoni, eds. *Child Victimization.* Kingston, N.J.: Civic Research Institute, 2005.

Kessler, Ronald C., et al. "The Prevalence and Correlates of Adult ADHD in the United States: Results from the National Comorbidity Survey Replication." *American Journal of Psychiatry* 163, no. 4 (April 2006): 716–723.

Kessler, Ronald C., et al. "Prevalence and Treatment of Mental Disorders, 1990 to 2003." *New England Journal of Medicine* 352, no. 24 (June 2005): 2,515–2,523.

Khouzam, Hani Raoul, M.D. "Obsessive-Compulsive Disorder: What to Do If You Recognize Baffling Behavior." *Postgraduate Medicine* 106, no. 7 (December 1999). Available online. URL: http://www.postgradmed. com/issues/1999/12_99/khouzam.htm. Downloaded March 12, 2006.

Kosten, Thomas R., M.D., and Patrick G. O'Connor, M.D. "Management of Drug and Alcohol Withdrawal." *New England Journal of Medicine* 348, no. 18 (May 2003): 1,786–1,795.

Kraman, Pilar. *Prescription Drug Diversion.* Lexington, Ky.: Council of State Governments, 2004.

Krantz, Mori J., M.D., and Philip S. Mehler, M.D. "Treating Opioid Dependence: Growing Implications for Primary Care." *Archives of Internal Medicine* 164 (February 2004): 277–288.

Krystal, John H., M.D., et al. "Naltrexone in the Treatment of Alcohol Dependence." *New England Journal of Medicine* 345, no. 24 (December 2001): 1,734–1,739.

Kupfner, David. "The Increasing Medical Burden in Bipolar Disorder." *Journal of the American Medical Association* 293, no. 20 (May 2005): 2,528–2,530.

Kyle, Angelo D., and Bill Hansell. *The Meth Epidemic in America: Two Surveys of U.S. Counties: The Criminal Effect of Meth on Communities: The Impact of Meth on Children.* Washington, D.C.: National Association of Counties, 2005.

Kyriacou, Demetrios, M.D., et al. "Risk Factors for Injury to Women from Domestic Violence." *New England Journal of Medicine* 341, no. 25 (December 1999): 1,892–1,898.

Lakins, Nekisha, et al. *Apparent per Capita Alcohol Consumption, National State and Regional Trends, 1977–2003, Surveillance Report # 73.* Bethesda, Md.: National Institute of Alcohol Abuse and Alcoholism, 2005.

Lamberg, Lynne. "Advances in Eating Disorders Offer Food for Thought." *Journal of the American Medical Association* 290, no. 11 (September 2003): 1,437–2,442.

———. "All Night Diners: Researchers Take a New Look at Night Eating Syndrome." *Journal of the American Medical Association* 290, no. 11 (September 2003): 1,442.

Lange, Richard A., M.D., and L. David Hillis, M.D. "Cardiovascular Complications of Cocaine Use." *New England Journal of Medicine* 345, no. 6 (August 2001): 351–358.

Lantz, Melinda S., M.D. "Prescription Drug and Alcohol Abuse in an Older Woman." *Clinical Geriatrics* 13, no. 1 (January 2005): 39–43.

Leitzmann, Michael F., M.D., et al. "A Prospective Study of Coffee Consumption and the Risk of Symptomatic Gallstone Disease in Men." *Journal of the American Medical Association* 281, no. 22 (June 1999): 2,106–2,112.

Levinthal, Charles F. *Drugs, Society, and Criminal Justice.* New York: Pearson Education, 2006.

Library of Congress. "Today in History: May 8 Coca Cola." Available online. URL: http://memory.loc.gov/ammem/ today/may08.html. Downloaded July 3, 2006.

Longo, Lance P., M.D., and Brian Johnson, M.D. "Addiction: Part I. Benzodiazepines—Side Effects, Abuse Risk and Alternatives." *American Family Physician* 61 (2000): 2,121–2,128. Available online. URL: http://www.aafp. org/afp/2000401/2121.html. Downloaded January 15, 2006.

Mann, J. John, M.D. "The Medical Management of Depression." *New England Journal of Medicine* 353, no. 17 (October 2005): 1,819–1,834.

Martis, Brian, M.D., et al. "Obsessive-Compulsive Disorder." In *Clinical Manual of Anxiety Disorders.* Washington, D.C.: American Psychiatric Press, 2004.

Marzuk, Peter M., M.D. "Fatal Injuries after Cocaine Use as Leading Cause of Death among Young Adults in New York City." *New England Journal of Medicine* 332 (1995): 1,753–1,757.

Matochik, John A., et al. "Altered Brain Tissue Composition in Heavy Marijuana Users." *Drug and Alcohol Dependence* 77 (2005): 23–30.

McCabe, S. E., C. J. Teter, and C. J. Boyd. "Illicit Use of Prescription Pain Medication among College Students." *Drug and Alcohol Dependence* 77 (2005): 37–47.

———. "The Use, Misuse and Diversion of Prescription Stimulants among Middle and High School Students." *Substance Use and Misuse* 39, no. 7 (2004): 1,095–1,116.

McClanahan, Susan F., Gary M. McClelland, Karen M. Abram, and Linda A. Teplin. "Pathways into Prostitution among Female Jail Detainees and Their Implications for Mental Health Services." *Psychiatric Services* 50, no. 12 (December 1999): 1,606–1,613.

McGinn, Cynthia G., M.D. "Close Calls with Club Drugs." *New England Journal of Medicine* 352, no. 26 (June 2005): 2,671–2,672.

Miller, Normal S., and Andrea Greenfield. "Patient Characteristics and Risk Factors for Development of Dependence on Hydrocodone and Oxycodone." *American Journal of Therapeutics* 11, no. 1 (January/February 2004): 26–32.

Minocha, Anil, M.D., and Christine Adamec. *The Encyclopedia of the Digestive System and Digestive Disorders.* New York: Facts On File, 2004.

Mokdad, Ali H., et al. "Actual Causes of Death in the United States, 2000." *Journal of the American Medical Association* 291, no. 10 (March 2004): 1,238–1,245.

Mueller, Mark R., et al. "Unintentional Prescription Drug Overdose Deaths in New Mexico, 1994–2003." *American Journal of Preventive Medicine* 30, no. 5 (2006): 423–429.

Murphy, James G., Meghan E. Mc-Devitt Murphy, and Nancy P. Barnett. "Drink and Be Merry? Gender, Life Satisfaction, and Alcohol Consumption among College Students." *Psychology of Addictive Behaviors* 19, no. 2 (2005): 184–191.

National Center for Health Statistics. *Health United States, 2005 with Chartbook on Trends in the Health of Americans.* Hyattsville, Md.: National Center for Health Statistics, 2005.

National Center for Statistics and Analysis. *Alcohol-Related Fatalities in 2004.* Washington, D.C.: National Highway Safety Transportation Administration, 2005.

National Center on Addiction and Substance Abuse at Columbia University. *Food for Thought: Substance Abuse and Eating Disorders.* New York: National Center on Addiction and Substance Abuse at Columbia University, 2003.

———. *Under the Counter: The Diversion and Abuse of Controlled Prescription Drugs in the U.S.* New York: National Center on Addiction and Substance Abuse at Columbia University, 2005.

National Clearinghouse on Child Abuse and Neglect information. *Definitions of Child Abuse and Neglect: Summary of State Laws.* Available online URL: http://www.nccanch.acf.hhs.gov/general/legal/statutes/define.cfm. Downloaded December 10, 2005.

National Drug Intelligence Center. "Drug-Facilitated Sexual Assault Fast Facts: Questions and Answers." Johnston, Pa.: National Drug Intelligence Center, 2004. Available online. URL: http://www.usdoj.gov/ndic/pubs/8/8872/8872p.pdf. Downloaded March 16, 2006.

National Highway Traffic Safety Administration. *Drugs and Human Performance Fact Sheets.* Washington, D.C.: U.S. Department of Transportation, 2004.

National Institute of Justice, Office of Justice Programs. *2000 Arrestee Drug Abuse Monitoring: Annual Report.* Washington, D.C.: U.S. Department of Justice, 2003.

National Institute of Mental Health. "The Numbers Count: Mental Disorders in America." National Institutes of Health. Available online. URL: http://www.nimh.nih.gov/publicat/numbers.cfm#readNow. Downloaded April 22, 2006.

National Institute on Alcohol Abuse and Alcoholism. "Alcohol Use and Alcohol Use Disorders in the United States: Main Findings from the 2001–2002 National Epidemiologic Survey on Alcohol and Related Conditions (NESARC)." *U.S. Alcohol Epidemiologic Data Reference Manual* 8, no. 1 (January 2006), pp. 1–247.

———. "Changing the Culture of Campus Drinking." *Alcohol Alert* 58 (October 2002).

———. *Helping Patients Who Drink Too Much: A Clinician's Guide.* Rockville, Md.: National Institutes of Health, 2005.

National Institute on Alcohol Abuse and Alcoholism, National Advisory Council on Alcohol Abuse and Alcoholism Task Force on College Drinking. *High-Risk Drinking in College: What We Know and What We Need to Learn: Final Report of the Panel on Contexts and Consequences.* Rockville, Md.: National Institutes of Health, 2002.

National Institute on Drug Abuse. "Childhood Sexual Abuse Increases Risk for Drug Dependence in Adult Women." Available online. URL: http://www.nida.nih.gov/NIDA_Notes/NNVol17N1/childhood.html. Downloaded December 29, 2005.

National Institute on Drug Abuse. *Drug Use among Racial/Ethnic Minorities.* Bethesda, Md.: National Institutes of Health, 2003.

———. *Epidemiologic Trends in Drug Abuse: Advance Report and Highlights/Executive Summary: Abuse of Stimulants and Other Drug: Proceedings of the Community Epidemiology Work Group.* Bethesda, Md.: Division of Epidemiology Services and Prevention Research, 2005.

———. *Epidemiologic Trends in Drug Abuse.* Vol. 1, *Proceeding of the Community Epidemiology Work Group: Highlights and Executive Summary.* Bethesda, Md.: National Institutes of Health, 2005.

———. "HIV/AIDS, Research Report Series." Available online. URL: http://www.drugabuse.gov/PDF/Rrhiv.pdf. Downloaded April 7, 2006.

———. *Inhalant Abuse.* Bethesda, Md.: National Institutes of Health, 2005.

———. *MDMA (Ecstasy) Abuse.* Available online. URL: http://wwwdrugabuse.gov/PDF/RR mdma.pdf. Downloaded April 6, 2006.

———. *Principles of Drug Abuse Treatment for Criminal Justice Populations: A Research-Based Guide.* Rockville, Md.: National Institutes of Health, U.S. Department of Health and Human Services, 2006. Available online. URL: http://www.drugabuse.gov/PODAT_CJ/PODAT_CJ.pdf. Downloaded August 6, 2006.

———. *Principles of Drug Addiction Treatment: A Research-Based Guide.* Bethesda, Md.: National Institutes of Health, 1999.

National Survey on Drug Use and Health. "Methamphetamine Use, Abuse, and Dependence: 2002, 2003, and 2004." *The NSDUH Report.* Available online. URL: http://www.oas.samhsa.gov/2k5/meth/meth.htm. Downloaded March 11, 2006.

———. "Substance Use during Pregnancy: 2002 and 2003." *The NSDUH Report.* Office of Applied Studies, Substance Abuse and Mental Health Services Administration, 2005.

National Task Force on Fetal Alcohol Syndrome and Fetal Alcohol Effect. *Fetal Alcohol Syndrome: Guidelines for Referral and Diagnosis.* Atlanta: Centers for Disease Control and Prevention, 2004.

Negrusz, Adam, Matthew Juhascik, and R. E. Gaensslen. "Estimate of the Incidence of Drug-Facilitated Sexual Assault in the United States." Washington, D.C.: U.S. Department of Justice, 2005. Available online. URL: http://www.ncjrs.gov/pdffiles1/nij/grants/21200.pdf. Downloaded June 19, 2006.

Ness, Roberta B., M.D., et al. "Cocaine and Tobacco Use and the Risk of Spontaneous Abortion." *New England Journal of Medicine* 340, no. 5 (February 1999): 333–339.

Newlin, David B., et al. "Environmental Transmission of DSM-IV Substance Use Disorders in Adoptive and Step Families." *Alcoholism* 24, no. 12 (December 2000): 1,785–1,794.

Nnadi, Charles U., et al. "Neuropsychiatric Effects of Cocaine Use Disorders." *Journal of the National Medical Association* 97, no. 11 (November 2005): 1,504–1,515.

Noakes, Timothy D., M.D. "Tainted Glory—Doping and Athletic Performance." *New England Journal of Medicine* 351, no. 9 (August 2004): 847–849.

Nock, Matthew K., et al. "Prevalence, Subtypes, and Correlates of DSM-IV Conduct Disorder in the National Comorbidity Survey Replication." *Psychological Medicine* 36 (2006): 688–710.

Nordahl, Thomas E., M.D. "Methamphetamine Users in Sustained Abstinence: A Proton Magnetic Resonance Spectroscopy Study." *Archives of General Psychiatry* 62 (April 2005): 444–452.

Nordstrom Bailey, Beth, et al. "Prenatal Exposure to Binge Drinking and Cognitive and Behavioral Outcomes at Age 7 Years." *American Journal of Obstetrics and Gynecology* 191 (2004): 1,037–1,043.

Nunes, Edward V., M.D., and Frances R. Levin, M.D. "Treatment of Depression in Patients with Alcohol or Other Drug Dependence." *Journal of the American Medical Association* 291, no. 15 (April 2004): 1,887–1,896.

O'Brien, Charles P., M.D. "Anticraving Medications for Relapse Prevention: A Possible New Class of Psychoactive Medications." *American Journal of Psychiatry* 162 (2005): 1,423–1,431.

O'Connor, Patrick G., M.D. "Methods of Detoxification and Their Role in Treating Patients with Opioid Dependence." *Journal of the American Medical Association* 294, no. 8 (August 2005): 961–963.

Office of Applied Studies. "Age at First Use of Marijuana and Past Year Serious Mental Illness." *The NSDUH Report.* Rockville, Md.: Office of Applied Studies, 2005.

———. *DAWN Series D-26.* Rockville, Md.: Department of Health and Human Services, 2004.

———. "Emergency Department Visits Involving Underage Drinking." *The DAWN Report* 1 (2006): 3.

———. "Facilities Offering Special Programs of Groups for Clients with Co-Occurring Disorders: 2004." *The DASIS Report* 2 (2006).

———. "Injection Drug Use Update: 2002 and 2003." *The NSDUH Report.* Rockville, Md.: Substance Abuse and Mental Health Services Administration, 2005.

———. "Marijuana Use and Delinquent Behaviors among Youths." *The NSDUH Report.* Rockville, Md.: Substance Abuse and Mental Health Services Administration, 2004.

———. "Methamphetamine Use, Abuse, and Dependence: 2002, 2003, and 2004." *The NSDUH Report.* Rockville, Md.: National Survey on Drug Use and Health, 2005.

———. *National Survey of Substance Abuse Treatment Services (N-SSATS): 2004: Data on Substance Abuse Treatment Facilities.* Rockville, Md.: Substance Abuse and Mental Health Services Administration, 2005.

———. *Overview of Findings from the 2004 National Survey on Drug Use and Health.* Rockville, Md.: Department of Health and Human Services, 2005.

———. *Treatment Episode Data Set (TEDS): 1993–2004. National Admissions to Substance Abuse Treatment Services.* Rockville, Md.: Substance Abuse and Mental Health Services Administration, 2005.

———. *Treatment Episode Data Set (TEDS) Highlights—2003: National Admissions to Substance Abuse Treatment Services.*

Rockville, Md.: Substance Abuse and Mental Health Services Administration, 2005.

———. "Trends in Methamphetamine/Amphetamine Admissions to Treatment: 1993–2003." *The DASIS Report* 9 (2006), pp. 1–4.

———. "Youth Violence and Illicit Drug Use." *The NSDUH Report* (2006). Available online. URL: http://www. drugabusestatistics.samhsa.gov/2k6/youthViolence/youthViolence.pdf. Downloaded February 7, 2006.

Office of Diversion Control, Drug Enforcement Administration. *Lists of: Scheduling Actions, Controlled Substances, Regulated Chemicals.* Washington, D.C.: U. S. Department of Justice, 2007. Available online. URL: http://www.deadiversion.usdoj.gov/schedules/orangebook 2005.pdf. Downloaded August 21, 2007.

Office of National Drug Control Policy. *Girls and Drugs: A New Analysis: Recent Trends, Risk Factors and Consequences.* Washington, D.C.: Executive Office of the President, 2006.

———. *Marijuana Myths and Facts: The Truth behind 10 Popular Misperceptions.* Available online. URL: http://www. whitehousedrugpolicy.gov/publications/marijuana_ myths_facts/marijuana_myths_fats.pdf. Downloaded January 16, 2006.

———. *Predicting Heavy Drug Use.* Washington, D.C.: Executive Office of the President, 2004.

Okie, Susan, M.D. "Medical Marijuana and the Supreme Court." *New England Journal of Medicine* 353, no. 7 (August 2005): 648–651.

Oldfield, V., and C. M. Perry. "Oxycodone/Ibuprofen Combination Tablet: A Review of Its Use in the Management of Acute Pain." *Drugs* 65, no. 16 (2005): 2,337–2,354.

O'Malley, Stephanie S., et al. "Initial and Maintenance Naltrexone Treatment for Alcohol Dependence Using Primary Care vs. Specialty Care." *Archives of Internal Medicine* 163 (July 2003): 1,695–1,704.

Ompad, Danielle, et al. "Childhood Sexual Abuse and Age at Initiation of Injection Drug Use." *American Journal of Public Health* 95 (2005): 703–709.

Oscar-Berman, Marlene, and Ksenija Marinkovic. "Alcoholism and the Brain: An Overview." *Alcohol Research & Health* 27, no. 3 (2003): 125–133.

Osmond, Dennis H. "Epidemiology of HIV/AIDS in the United States." March 2003. Available online. URL: http://hivinsite.ucsf.edu/InSite?page=kb–01–03.Downloaded May 11, 2006.

Pecora, Peter J., et al. *Improving Family Foster Care: Findings from the Northwest Foster Care Alumni Study.* Seattle: Casey Family Services, 2005.

Petrakis, Ismene L., M.D., et al. "Comorbidity of Alcoholism and Psychiatric Disorders." *Alcohol Research & Health* 26, no. 2 (2002): 81–89.

Pi-Sunyer, F. Xavier, M.D., et al. "Effect of Rimonabant, a Cannabinoid-1 Receptor Blocker, on Weight and Cardiometabolic Risk Factors in Overweight or Obese Patients." *Journal of the American Medical Association* 295, no. 7 (February 2006): 761–775.

Potter, Jennifer Sharpe, et al. "Substance Use Histories in Patients Seeking Treatment for Controlled-Release Oxycodone Dependence." *Drug and Alcohol Dependence* 76 (2004): 213–215.

Poulin, Christiane. "Medical and Nonmedical Stimulant Use among Adolescents: From Sanctioned to Unsanctioned Use." *Canadian Medical Association Journal* 165, no. 8 (2001): 1,039–1,044.

Quigley, Robert M., and Kenneth E. Leonard. "Alcohol Use and Violence among Young Adults." *Alcohol Research & Health* 28, no. 4 (2004/2005): 191–194.

Raskind, Muray A., M.D. "Reduction of Nightmares and Other PTSD Symptoms in Combat Veterans by Prazosin: A Placebo-Controlled Study." *American Journal of Psychiatry* 160, no. 2 (February 2003): 371–373.

Rehm, Jürgen, et al. "Alcohol-Related Morbidity and Mortality." *Alcohol Research & Health* 27, no. 1 (2002): 39–51.

Rey, Joseph M., and Christopher C. Tennant. "Cannabis and Mental Health." *British Medical Journal* 325 (November 2002): 1,183–1,184.

Richard, Jack, M.D., and Marcus M. Reidenberg, M.D. "The Risk of Disciplinary Action by State Medical Boards against Physicians Prescribing Opioids." *Journal of Pain and Symptom Management* 29, no. 2 (February 2005): 206–212.

Rosack, Jim. "Methylphenidate Skin Patch Approved for ADHD." *Psychiatric News* 41, no. 1 (January 2006): 1, 37.

Ross, G. Webster, M.D. "Association of Coffee and Caffeine Intake with the Risk of Parkinson's Disease." *Journal of the American Medical Association* 283, no. 20 (March 2000): 2,674–2,679.

Rouse, Beatrice A., ed. *Substance Abuse and Mental Health Services Administration (SAMHSA) Statistics Source Book, 1998.* Rockville, Md.: Office of Applied Studies, 1998.

Sattar, S. Pirzada, M.D., and Subhash Bhatia, M.D. "Benzodiazepines for Substance Abusers: Yes or No?" *Current Psychiatry Online* 2, no. 5 (May 2003). Available online. URL: http://www.currentpsychiatry.com/2003_05/0503_benzodiazepines.asp. Downloaded July 15, 2006.

Schneider, Jennifer P., M.D. "Chronic Pain Management in Older Adults." *Geriatrics* 60, no. 5 (May 2005): 26–31.

Shanti, Chrtina M., M.D., and Charles E. Lucas, M.D. "Cocaine and the Critical Care Challenge." *Critical Care Medicine* 31, no. 6 (2003): 1,851–1,859.

Shiskin, Philip, and David Crawford. "In Afghanistan, Heroin Trade Soars Despite U.S. Aid." *Wall Street Journal,* 14 January 2006, A1, A8.

Shivani, Ramesh, M.D., R. Jeffrey Goldsmith, M.D., and Robert M. Anthenelli, M.D. "Alcoholism and Psychiatric Disorders: Diagnostic Challenges." *Alcohol, Research & Health* 26, no. 2 (2002): 90–98.

Shults, R. A., et al. "Association between State Level Drinking and Driving Countermeasures and Self Reported Alcohol Impaired Driving." *Injury Prevention* 8 (2002): 106–110.

Snead III, O. Carter, M.D., and K. Michael Gibson. "γHydroxybutyric Acid." *New England Journal of Medicine* 353, no. 26 (June 2005): 2,727–2,732.

Snyder, Howard N., and Melissa Sickmund. *Juvenile Offenders and Victims: 2006 National Report.* Washington D.C.: National Center for Juvenile Justice, 2006.

Sokol, Robert J., M.D., Virginia Delaney-Black, M.D., and Beth Nordstrom. "Fetal Alcohol Spectrum Disorder." *Journal of the American Medical* Association 290, no. 22 (December 2003): 2,996–2,999.

Solowij, Nadia, et al. "Cognitive Functioning of Long-Term Heavy Cannabis Users Seeking Treatment." *Journal of the American Medical Association* 287, no. 9 (March 2002): 1,123–1,131.

Sonne, Susan C., and Kathleen T. Brady, M.D. "Bipolar Disorder and Alcoholism." National Institute on Alcohol Abuse and Alcoholism. Available online. URL: http://www.niaaa.nih.gov/publicatons/arh26-2/103–108.htm. Downloaded March 25, 2006.

Stahl, Stephen M. *Essential Psychopharmacology: The Prescriber's Guide.* Cambridge: Cambridge University Press, 2005.

Stein, Gideon Y., M.D., et al. "Phencyclidine-Induced Multi-Organ Failure." *Israel Medical Association Journal* 7 (August 2005): 535–537.

Stein, Murray B., M.D., Neal A. Kline, M.D., and Jeffrey L. Matloff. "Adjunctive Olanzapine for SSRI-Resistant Combat-Related PTSD: A Double-Blind, Placebo-Controlled Study." *American Journal of Psychiatry* 159, no. 10 (October 2002): 1,777–1,779.

Streissguth, Ann P., et al. "Risk Factors for Adverse Life Outcomes in Fetal Alcohol Syndrome and Fetal Alcohol Effects." *Journal of Developmental and Behavioral Pediatrics* 25, no. 4 (2004): 228–238.

Substance Abuse and Mental Health Services Administration. *Overview of Findings for the 2004 National Survey on Drug Use and Health.* Rockville, Md.: Maryland Department of Health and Human Services, 2005.

Sullivan, Michael, and John Wodarski. "Rating College Students' Substance Abuse: A Systematic Literature Review." *Brief Treatment and Crisis Intervention* 4 (2004): 71–91.

Swofford, Cheryl D. "Double Jeopardy: Schizophrenia and Substance Use." *American Journal of Drug and Alcohol Abuse* (August 2000).

Tapert, Susan F., Lisa Caldwell, and Christina Burke. "Alcohol and the Adolescent Brain: Human Studies." *Alcohol Research & Health* 28, no. 4 (2004/2005): 205–212.

Tjaden, Patricia, and Nancy Thoennes. *Full Report of the Prevalence, Incidence, and Consequences of Violence against Women: Findings from the National Violence against Women Survey.* Washington, D.C.: Office of Justice Programs, U.S. Department of Justice, 2000.

Trivedi, Madhukar H., M.D, et al. "Medication Augmentation after the Failure of SSRIs for Depression." *New England Journal of Medicine* 354, no. 12 (March 2006): 1,243–1,252.

Tuomilehto, Jaako, M.D. "Coffee Consumption and Risk of Type 2 Diabetes Mellitus among Middle-Aged Finnish Men and Women." *Journal of the American Medical Association* 291, no. 10 (March 2004): 1,213–1,219.

United Nations Office on Drugs and Crime. *The Opium Situation in Afghanistan as of 29 August 2005.* Available online. URL: http://www.unodc.org/pdf/afghanistan_2005/opium-afghanistan_2005–08–26.pdf. Downloaded January 19, 2006.

———. *2004 World Drug Report.* Vol. 1, *Analysis.* New York: United Nations, 2004.

United States Customs and Border Protection. "Buying Prescription Medicine from Internet Foreign Pharmacies." February 22, 2006. Available online. URL: http://www.cbp.gov/xp/cgov/newsroom/highlights/foreign_medication.xml. Downloaded February 23, 2006.

Van Gaal, Luc F., et al. "Effects of the Cannabinoid-1 Receptor Blocker Rimonabant on Weight Reduction and Cardiovascular Risk Factors in Overweight Patients: 1-Year Experience from the RIO-Europe Study." *The Lancet* 365 (April 2005): 1,389–1,397.

Vastag, Brian "What's the Connection? No Easy Answers for People with Eating Disorders and Drug Abuse." *Journal of the American Medical Association* 285, no. 8 (February 2001): 1,006–1,007.

Voas, R. B., A. S. Tippetts, and J. C. Fell. "Assessing the Effectiveness of Minimum Legal Drinking Age and Zero Tolerance Laws in the United States." *Accident Analysis and Prevention* 35, no. 4 (July 2003): 579–587.

Vocci, Frank, Jane Acri, and Ahmed Elkasef. "Medication Development for Addictive Disorders: The State of the Science." *American Journal of Psychiatry* 162, no. 8 (August 2005): 1,432–1,440.

Vocci, Frank, and Ahmed Elkasef. "Pharmacotherapy and Other Treatments for Cocaine Abuse and Dependence." *Current Opinion in Psychiatry* 18, no. 3 (May 2005): 265–270.

von Syndow, Kirsten, et al. "Use, Abuse and Dependence of Ecstasy and Related Drugs in Adolescents and Young Adults—a Transient Phenomenon? Results from a Longitudinal Community Study." *Drug and Alcohol Dependence* 66 (2002): 147–159.

Weatherall, Miles. "Drug Treatment and the Rise of Pharmacology." In the *Cambridge Illustrated History of Medicine,* edited by Ray Porter, 246–278. Cambridge: Cambridge University Press, 2001.

Weathermon, Ron, and David W. Crabb, M.D. "Alcohol and Medication Interactions." *Alcohol Research & Health* 23, no. 1 (1999): 40–54.

Weitzman, Elissa R. "Poor Mental Health, Depression, and Associations with Alcohol Consumption, Harm, and Abuse in a National Sample of Young Adults in College." *Journal of Nervous and Mental Disease* 192, no. 4 (April 2004): 269–277.

Wells, Kathryn M. "Substance Abuse and Child Maltreatment." In *Understanding the Medical Diagnosis of Child Maltreatment: A Guide for Nonmedical Professionals.* New York: Oxford University Press, 2006.

Welsh, Christopher, M.D., and Adela Valadez-Meltzer, M.D. "Buprenorphine: A (Relatively) New Treatment for Opioid Dependence." *Psychiatry* 2, no. 12 (December 2005): 29–39.

White, Alan G., et al. "Direct Costs of Opioid Abuse in an Insured Population in the United States." *Journal of Managed Care Pharmacy* 11, no. 6 (July/August 2005): 469–479.

Whitten, Lori. "Topiramate Shows Promise in Cocaine Addiction." *NIDA Notes* 19, no. 6 (May 2005): 1, 6.

Wilens, Timothy E., M.D. "Attention-Deficit/Hyperactivity Disorder and the Substance Use Disorders: The Nature of the Relationship, Subtypes at Risk, and Treatment Issues." *Psychiatric Clinics of North America* 27 (2004): 283–301.

Wilens, Timothy E., et al. "Characteristics of Adolescents and Young Adults with ADHD Who Divert or Misuse Their Prescribed Medications." *Journal of the American Academy of Child & Adolescent Psychiatry* 45, no. 4 (2006): 408–414.

Wilens, Timothy E., M.D., et al. "Does Stimulant Therapy of Attention-Deficit/Hyperactivity Disorder Beget Later Substance Abuse? A Meta-Analytic Review of the Literature." *Pediatrics* 111, no. 1 (2003): 179–185.

Winger, Gail, James H. Woods, and Frederick G. Hofmann. *A Handbook on Drug and Alcohol Abuse: The Biomedical Aspects.* New York: Oxford University Press, 2004.

Wolf, B. C., et al. "One Hundred Seventy Two Deaths Involving the Use of Oxycodone in Palm Beach County." *Journal of Forensic Science* 50, no. 1 (January 2005): 192–195.

Wyatt, Stephen A. "Medical Education in Substance Abuse: From Student to Practicing Osteopathic Physician." *Journal of the American Osteopathic Academy* 105, no. 6 (June 2005): S18–S25.

Yager, Joel, M.D., and Arnold E. Andersen, M.D. "Anorexia Nervosa." *New England Journal of Medicine* 353, no. 14 (October 2005): 1,481–1,488.

Yang, Yi-Chang, et al. "The Protective Effect of Habitual Tea Consumption." *Archives of Internal Medicine* 164 (July 2004): 1,534–1,540.

Yehuda, Rachel. "Post-Traumatic Stress Disorder." *New England Journal of Medicine* 346, no. 2 (January 2002): 108–114.

Zacny, James, et al. "College on Problems of Drug Dependence Taskforce on Prescription Opioid Non-Medical Use and Abuse: Position Statement." *Drug and Alcohol Dependence* 69 (2003): 215–232.

Zickler, Patricia. "Modafinil Improves Behavioral Therapy Results in Cocaine Addiction." *NIDA Notes* 20, no. 5 (2005): 1, 11.

INDEX

Boldface page numbers denote main entries. *t* denotes a table.